T0337373

THE WASHINGTON MANUAL®

Infectious Diseases

Subspecialty Consult

THIRD EDITION

THE WASHINGTON MANUAL®

Infectious Diseases

Subspecialty Consult

THIRD EDITION

Editors

Nigar Kirmani, MD

Professor of Medicine
Division of Infectious Diseases
Department of Internal Medicine
Washington University School of Medicine
St. Louis, Missouri

Michael J. Durkin, MD

Assistant Professor of Medicine
Division of Infectious Diseases
Department of Internal Medicine
Washington University School of Medicine
St. Louis, Missouri

Stephen Y. Liang, MD

Assistant Professor of Medicine
Divisions of Infectious Diseases and
    Emergency Medicine
Department of Internal Medicine
Washington University School of Medicine
St. Louis, Missouri

Series Editors

Thomas M. Ciesielski, MD

Assistant Professor of Medicine
Associate Program Director
Division of Medical Education,
    Department of Medicine
Washington University School of
    Medicine
St. Louis, Missouri

Thomas M. De Fer, MD, FACP

Executive Editor
Professor of Medicine
Associate Dean for Medical Student
    Education
Division of Medical Education,
    Department of Medicine
Washington University School of
    Medicine
St. Louis, Missouri

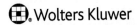. Wolters Kluwer

Philadelphia • Baltimore • New York • London
Buenos Aires • Hong Kong • Sydney • Tokyo

Acquisitions Editor: Rebecca Gaertner
Product Development Editor: Liz Schaeffer
Editorial Coordinators: Tim Rinehart, Katie Sharp
Production Project Managers: Linda Van Pelt, Sadie Buckallew
Design Coordinator: Holly McLaughlin
Manufacturing Coordinator: Beth Welsh
Prepress Vendor: TNQ Technologies

Third edition

Copyright © 2020 by Department of Medicine, Washington University School of Medicine.
Copyright © 2013 by Department of Medicine, Washington University School of Medicine.
Copyright © 2006 by Department of Medicine, Washington University School of Medicine.

All rights reserved. This book is protected by copyright. No part of this book may be reproduced or transmitted in any form or by any means, including as photocopies or scanned-in or other electronic copies, or utilized by any information storage and retrieval system without written permission from the copyright owner, except for brief quotations embodied in critical articles and reviews. Materials appearing in this book prepared by individuals as part of their official duties as U.S. government employees are not covered by the above-mentioned copyright. To request permission, please contact Wolters Kluwer at Two Commerce Square, 2001 Market Street, Philadelphia, PA 19103, via email at permissions@lww.com, or via our website at shop.lww.com (products and services).

9 8 7 6 5 4

Printed in The United States of America

Library of Congress Cataloging-in-Publication Data

Names: Kirmani, Nigar, editor. | Durkin, Michael J. (Michael Joseph), 1981- editor. | Liang, Stephen Y., editor. | Washington University (Saint Louis, Mo.). School of Medicine, sponsoring body.
Title: The Washington manual infectious diseases subspecialty consult / editors, Nigar Kirmani, Michael J. Durkin, Stephen Y. Liang.
Other titles: Infectious diseases subspecialty consult | Washington manual subspecialty consult series.
Description: Third edition. | Philadelphia : Wolters Kluwer, [2020] | Series: Washington manual subspecialty consult series | Includes bibliographical references and index.
Identifiers: LCCN 2019011923 | ISBN 9781975113421
Subjects: | MESH: Communicable Diseases | Diagnosis, Differential | Patient Care Planning | Handbook
Classification: LCC RC111 | NLM WC 39 | DDC 616.9–dc23
LC record available at https://lccn.loc.gov/2019011923

This work is provided "as is," and the publisher disclaims any and all warranties, express or implied, including any warranties as to accuracy, comprehensiveness, or currency of the content of this work.

This work is no substitute for individual patient assessment based upon healthcare professionals' examination of each patient and consideration of, among other things, age, weight, gender, current or prior medical conditions, medication history, laboratory data and other factors unique to the patient. The publisher does not provide medical advice or guidance and this work is merely a reference tool. Healthcare professionals, and not the publisher, are solely responsible for the use of this work including all medical judgments and for any resulting diagnosis and treatments.

Given continuous, rapid advances in medical science and health information, independent professional verification of medical diagnoses, indications, appropriate pharmaceutical selections and dosages, and treatment options should be made and healthcare professionals should consult a variety of sources. When prescribing medication, healthcare professionals are advised to consult the product information sheet (the manufacturer's package insert) accompanying each drug to verify, among other things, conditions of use, warnings and side effects and identify any changes in dosage schedule or contraindications, particularly if the medication to be administered is new, infrequently used or has a narrow therapeutic range. To the maximum extent permitted under applicable law, no responsibility is assumed by the publisher for any injury and/or damage to persons or property, as a matter of products liability, negligence law or otherwise, or from any reference to or use by any person of this work.

shop.lww.com

Dedication

For our families, without whose patience, encouragement, and many sacrifices this work would not be possible.

—Nigar Kirmani, Michael J. Durkin, Stephen Y. Liang

In memoriam

We are eternally grateful to Gerald Medoff, MD, the former chief of the Infectious Diseases Division at Washington University School of Medicine, who passed away shortly before publication of this book. He was an extraordinary clinician, scientist, and teacher who trained generations of Infectious Disease fellows to push the boundaries of current knowledge. He taught us all to take care of patients with compassion and respect.

Contributing Authors

Abdullah Aljorayid, MD
Clinical Fellow
Division of Infectious Diseases
Department of Internal Medicine
Washington University School of Medicine
St. Louis, Missouri

Merilda Blanco, MD
Assistant Professor of Medicine
Division of Infectious Diseases
Department of Internal Medicine
Washington University School of Medicine
St. Louis, Missouri

Philip Budge, MD
Assistant Professor of Medicine
Division of Infectious Diseases
Department of Internal Medicine
Washington University School of Medicine
St. Louis, Missouri

Juan J. Calix, MD
Clinical Fellow
Division of Infectious Diseases
Department of Internal Medicine
Washington University School of Medicine
St. Louis, Missouri

Abigail L. Carlson, MD
Instructor in Medicine
Division of Infectious Diseases
Department of Internal Medicine
Washington University School of Medicine
St. Louis, Missouri

Maren Cowley, MD
Pharmacy Resident, Infectious Diseases
Barnes-Jewish Hospital
St. Louis, Missouri

Michael J. Durkin, MD
Assistant Professor of Medicine
Division of Infectious Diseases
Department of Internal Medicine
Washington University School of Medicine
St. Louis, Missouri

Gerome Escota, MD
Assistant Professor of Medicine
Division of Infectious Diseases
Department of Internal Medicine
Washington University School of Medicine
St. Louis, Missouri

Ige George, MD
Assistant Professor of Medicine
Division of Infectious Diseases
Department of Internal Medicine
Washington University School of Medicine
St. Louis, Missouri

Yasir Hamad, MD
Assistant Professor of Medicine
Division of Infectious Diseases
Department of Internal Medicine
Washington University School of Medicine
St. Louis, Missouri

Jeffrey P. Henderson, MD
Associate Professor of Medicine
Division of Infectious Diseases
Department of Internal Medicine
Washington University School of Medicine
St. Louis, Missouri

Matifadza Hlatshwayo, MD
Clinical Fellow
Division of Infectious Diseases
Department of Internal Medicine
Washington University School of Medicine
St. Louis, Missouri

Kevin Hsueh, MD
Assistant Professor of Medicine
Division of Infectious Diseases
Department of Internal Medicine
Washington University School of Medicine
St. Louis, Missouri

Nigar Kirmani, MD
Professor of Medicine
Division of Infectious Diseases
Department of Internal Medicine
Washington University School of Medicine
St. Louis, Missouri

Robyn S. Klein, MD
Professor of Medicine
Division of Infectious Diseases
Department of Internal Medicine
Washington University School of Medicine
St. Louis, Missouri

F. Matthew Kuhlmann, MD
Assistant Professor of Medicine
Division of Infectious Diseases
Department of Internal Medicine
Washington University School of Medicine
St. Louis, Missouri

Jennie H. Kwon, MD
Assistant Professor of Medicine
Division of Infectious Diseases
Department of Internal Medicine
Washington University School of Medicine
St. Louis, Missouri

Michael A. Lane, MD
Assistant Professor of Medicine
Division of Infectious Diseases
Department of Internal Medicine
Washington University School of Medicine
St. Louis, Missouri

Steven J. Lawrence, MD
Associate Professor of Medicine
Division of Infectious Diseases
Department of Internal Medicine
Washington University School of Medicine
St. Louis, Missouri

Stephen Y. Liang, MD
Assistant Professor of Medicine
Division of Infectious Diseases
Divisions of Infectious Diseases and
    Emergency Medicine
Washington University School of Medicine
St. Louis, Missouri

Darrell McBride, MD
Clinical Fellow
Division of Infectious Diseases
Department of Internal Medicine
Washington University School of Medicine
St. Louis, Missouri

Carlos Mejia-Chew, MD
Clinical Fellow
Division of Infectious Diseases
Department of Internal Medicine
Washington University School of Medicine
St. Louis, Missouri

Caline S. Mattar, MD
Assistant Professor of Medicine
Division of Infectious Diseases
Department of Internal Medicine
Washington University School of Medicine
St. Louis, Missouri

Lemuel B. Non, MD
Assistant Professor of Medicine
Division of Infectious Diseases
Department of Internal Medicine
Washington University School of Medicine
St. Louis, Missouri

Jane O'Halloran, MD
Clinical Fellow
Division of Infectious Diseases
Department of Internal Medicine
Washington University School of Medicine
St. Louis, Missouri

Anupam Pande, MD
Assistant Professor of Medicine
Division of Infectious Diseases
Department of Internal Medicine
Washington University School of Medicine
St. Louis, Missouri

Shadi Parsaei, DO
Clinician, Infectious Diseases
Norton Hospital
Louisville, Kentucky

Rachel Presti, MD
Assistant Professor of Medicine
Division of Infectious Diseases
Department of Internal Medicine
Washington University School of Medicine
St. Louis, Missouri

Krunal Raval, MD
Clinical Fellow
Division of Infectious Diseases
Washington University School of Medicine
St. Louis, Missouri

Hilary Reno, MD
Assistant Professor of Medicine
Division of Infectious Diseases
Department of Internal Medicine
Washington University School of Medicine
St. Louis, Missouri

David J. Ritchie, PharMD
Clinical Pharmacist, Infectious Diseases
Barnes-Jewish Hospital
Professor of Pharmacy Practice
St. Louis College of Pharmacy
St. Louis, Missouri

Mohammad J. Saeed, MD
Instructor in Medicine
Division of Infectious Diseases
Department of Internal Medicine
Washington University

Andrej Spec, MD
Assistant Professor of Medicine
Division of Infectious Diseases
Department of Internal Medicine
Washington University School of Medicine
St. Louis, Missouri

Michael Tang, MD
Instructor in Medicine
Division of Hospital Medicine
Washington University School of Medicine
St. Louis, Missouri

Derek Yee, MD
Instructor in Medicine
Division of Hospital Diseases
Department of Internal Medicine
Washington University School of Medicine
St. Louis, Missouri

Chairman's Note

It is a pleasure to present the new edition of *The Washington Manual® Infectious Diseases Subspecialty Consult*. This pocket-size book remains a primary reference for medical students, interns, residents, and other practitioners who need ready access to practical clinical information to diagnose and treat patients with a wide variety of infectious diseases. Infectious diseases continue to be major causes of morbidity and mortality around the world. New and emerging pathogens and increasing antimicrobial drug resistance have created major challenges in many healthcare settings. Medical knowledge surrounding microbial pathogenesis, host pathogen interactions, and mechanisms of drug resistance has grown dramatically. There have also been significant advances in rapid molecular diagnostics for infectious diseases as well as new therapeutic and preventive strategies. The astounding rate of scientific discoveries in the area of infectious diseases creates a challenge for physicians to keep up with the biomedical discoveries and novel therapeutics that can positively impact patient outcomes. This manual addresses this challenge by concisely and practically providing current scientific information for clinicians to aid them in the diagnosis, investigation, and treatment of infectious diseases.

I want to personally thank the authors, who include the residents, fellows, and attendings at Washington University School of Medicine and Barnes-Jewish Hospital. Their commitment to patient care and education is unsurpassed, and their efforts and skill in compiling this manual are evident in the quality of the final product. In particular, I would like to acknowledge our editors, Drs. Nigar Kirmani, Michael J. Durkin, and Stephen Y. Liang, and the series editors, Drs. Tom De Fer and Thomas Ciesielski, who have worked tirelessly to produce another outstanding edition of this manual. I would also like to thank Dr. Melvin Blanchard, Chief of the Division of Medical Education in the Department of Medicine at Washington University School of Medicine, for his advice and guidance. I believe this subspecialty manual will meet its desired goal of providing practical knowledge that can be directly applied at the bedside and in outpatient settings to improve patient care.

Victoria J. Fraser, MD
Adolphus Busch Professor
Chair of the Department of Medicine
Washington University School of Medicine

Preface

We are delighted to introduce the third edition of *The Washington Manual®
Infectious Diseases Subspecialty Consult*. The chapters have been contributed primarily by faculty and fellows from the Infectious Diseases Division in the Department of Internal Medicine at the Washington University School of Medicine in St. Louis. In this edition, we have added chapters on antimicrobial stewardship, arboviruses, and hemorrhagic fevers, and we updated content in all other chapters.

Infectious disease is an exciting field in constant evolution. Even since the release of the last edition of this manual, there have been new diseases, new diagnostic methods, and new treatment challenges with the development of multiple-drug–resistant organisms. There continues to be a need for specialists in this field. Infectious disease specialists treat patients of all ages, deal with all organ systems, and collaborate with nearly all other medical specialties and subspecialties. In infectious disease, no case is exactly the same, so there is no "cookbook" approach to these problems. This makes each case intriguing, and even the most mundane cases have appeal. It is our hope that this manual stimulates interest in infectious disease among its readers and inspires them to pursue a career in this specialty.

This manual complements the *Washington Manual of Medical Therapeutics* by providing more in-depth coverage of infectious diseases. We have focused on providing easy-to-follow guidance for the diagnosis and treatment of infectious diseases likely to be seen by trainees and practicing physicians. Diseases are organized primarily by organ system to facilitate generating a useful differential diagnosis based on a patient's presentation. By providing practical guidance for common problems, the manual serves not as a comprehensive textbook, but rather as a go-to reference that can be kept handy on the wards.

It should be noted that the dosing information in the text assumes normal renal function unless otherwise indicated. Dosing information for impaired renal function is available in a chapter dedicated to antimicrobial agents.

We would like to offer special thanks to Katie Sharp for her extensive assistance in keeping the project organized and moving forward. This book wouldn't have been possible without her. We would also like to thank Dr. Tom De Fer in the Department of Medicine for his editorial guidance, and Dr. Thomas Ciesielski for reviewing each and every chapter. Finally, we would like to recognize Dr. William G. Powderly, the J. William Campbell Professor in the Department of Medicine and Co-Chief of the Infectious Diseases Division, and Dr. Victoria Fraser, the Adolphus Busch Professor and Chair of the Department of Medicine, for their leadership, mentorship, and unwavering support.

N.K.
M.J.D.
S.Y.L.

Contents

Approach to the Infectious Disease Consultation

Stephen Y. Liang, Michael J. Durkin, and Nigar Kirmani

1

THE VALUE OF THE INFECTIOUS DISEASE CONSULTATION

Infectious disease consultation is associated with high quality care. The value of an infectious disease consultation has been borne out in studies demonstrating reduced mortality for a number of conditions including *Staphylococcus aureus* bacteremia,[1] solid organ transplant infections,[2] infections due to multidrug-resistant pathogens,[3] cryptococcal infections,[4] and candidemia.[5] It is likely that these benefits stem from improved adherence to evidence-based clinical practice guidelines.[4,5] Infectious disease physicians are also more likely to prescribe the most appropriate antibiotics and decrease overall antibiotic utilization in hospitals.[6] By following the approaches described in this chapter, we believe that you can provide outstanding and high-quality patient care while effectively communicating with your colleagues.

GENERAL PRINCIPLES

- The greatest challenge of the infectious disease consultation is the breadth of the subspecialty. Disease manifestations can involve multiple organ systems, expanding across a broad range of medical and surgical disciplines. Infectious disease consultation requires thorough evaluation, organized thought processes, and an ability to appropriately consider rare but significant diagnoses.
- **Infectious disease consultations can be divided into four general categories:**
  - **Diagnostic dilemmas** are by far the most challenging consultation; these are consults in which a diagnosis remains elusive (e.g., fever of unknown origin). A thorough history detailing potential exposures and systematic physical examination is critical.
  - **Therapeutic management** involves treatment of a specific infection as it relates to the overall care of the patient, such as an infected prosthetic joint.
  - **Antibiotic management** ensures appropriate selection, dosing, and duration of antibiotics for a given infection.
  - **Occupational health and infection prevention** address the health of employees, patients, and visitors within health care facilities.
- **Ten commandments for effective consultation.** Introduced in 1983 and modified in 2007, these rules provide a framework for effective patient care and communication with requesting physicians.[7,8] Understanding the specific expectations of the requesting physician allows one to address the underlying concerns prompting an infectious disease consultation. Always remember that a physician requests a service from the consultant much like a consumer buys products from a vendor.
  - **Determine your customer.** Are you providing **management** for a surgeon or **guidance** for an internist? What specific question(s) need to be answered?
  - **Establish urgency.** How quickly should the patient be seen? Several infectious diseases (e.g., necrotizing fasciitis, cerebral malaria) require emergent consultation to initiate proper therapy.
  - **Look for yourself.** Although one does not need to repeat every excruciating detail in written consultation, each important detail should be reconfirmed.

- ○ **Be as brief as appropriate.** Write concise assessments that adequately explain your rationale.
- ○ **Be specific and humble.** Write clear plans. Provide help in executing the plans when requested. Such help may include writing orders or obtaining additional information from other hospitals or health departments.
- ○ **Provide contingency plans.** Determine likely problems and provide guidance for their remediation. Provide around-the-clock contact information to assist in addressing such problems when they arise.
- ○ **Determine the appropriate level of management.** How much should you intervene regarding writing orders and dictating patient care? This should be agreed on with the requesting physician during initial discussions.
- ○ **Teach with tact and pragmatism.** Provide educational materials or discussions appropriate to the given situation.
- ○ **Talk is essential.** Always call the requesting physician with your recommendations.
- ○ **Follow up daily.** Daily written/electronic notes should be provided until problems are no longer active as determined by yourself and the requesting physician. Provide appropriate long-term follow-up care.
- **The "curbside" consultation.** Requesting physicians frequently seek opinions based on limited conversations. Such "curbside consultations" are considered a courtesy and promote collegiality. When providing curbside consultation, one should always speak in general terms and avoid providing absolute recommendations. Frequently, important historical details are unintentionally omitted, limiting the ability to provide accurate advice. Generalized guidelines for providing curbside consultation are as follows:
  - ○ **Appropriate for curbside consultation**
    - Dose or duration of antibiotics for simple infections
    - Choice of antibiotics for simple infections
  - ○ **Inappropriate for curbside consultation**
    - Complex patient problems
    - Uncertainty regarding the question being asked by the requesting physician
    - Infections due to highly resistant organisms, rare organisms, or bloodstream infections
- **Addressing patient concerns.** Many patients may feel that additional questioning by a consultant is redundant or insulting. Frequently, a thorough review of the medical record followed by empathetic consultations strengthens rapport with the patient. The following suggestions can aid in alleviating patient fear:
  - ○ Advise patients that you are visiting them on the request of their primary physician and that you will work closely with that physician to provide the best possible care.
  - ○ Consider telling the patient that you have reviewed his/her history and have additional specific questions that you would like to ask before providing an opinion on his/her care.
  - ○ Ask the patient to confirm your brief understanding of his/her history and to supplement information with important details. After the initial conversation, specific or open-ended questions regarding the history of the patient's illness can be asked.
  - ○ Do not provide information that directly contradicts the clinical care of the primary provider. Reasons for following a specific care plan may not be readily apparent at the time of the patient encounter and should be clarified with the requesting physician before instituting changes.

STRUCTURE OF CONSULT NOTES

- Consult notes should be written in a fashion similar to that of an admission history and physical, supplemented with details unique to the epidemiology and clinical presentation of infectious diseases.

- **History of present illness (HPI).** Provide a thorough review of the patient's current illness (i.e., onset, severity, duration, location, etc.) and hospital course. Specific details of positive findings or pertinent negative findings from the review of systems, past medical/surgical history, family history, and social history should be included.
- **Review of systems.** Be thorough and comprehensive in characterizing the presence or absence of signs and symptoms of disease. Patients may neglect significant details of the history in their initial encounters that may shed additional light on potential diagnoses.
- **Past medical and surgical history**
  ○ Provide pertinent details in the HPI and supplement additional information in the body of the consultation note.
  ○ Identify and characterize immunosuppression due to illness or medication.
  ○ Create a timeline of relevant surgeries and summarize operative findings related to infection.
  ○ Document relevant vaccinations that can modify a patient's risk for infection.
- **Medications**
  ○ Detail all antibiotics the patient has received over the past several months, including doses, durations, and any drug levels obtained.
  ○ Note all immunosuppressive medications.
  ○ Pay attention to drugs that frequently interact with antimicrobials, particularly warfarin.
- **Allergies.** List the medication and describe the type of reaction (e.g., rash, gastrointestinal intolerance, anaphylaxis), paying particular attention to antibiotics.
- **Social history**
  ○ Many behaviors can place patients at risk for specific infections. A detailed exposure history is one of the hallmarks of an infectious disease consultation (Table 1-1).
  ○ **Animal exposures.** Has the patient had contact with domestic or wild animals associated with specific zoonoses?
  ○ **Occupational exposures.** What types of jobs has the patient worked, and have any of these involved exposures to potentially infectious or toxic agents?
  ○ **Travel history.** Has the patient ever traveled to an area known to harbor specific infections, even within their native country? Any travel history over a patient's lifetime should be considered potentially important.
  ○ **Hobbies.** What recreational activities does the patient enjoy engaging in and do these involve environmental exposures?
  ○ **Sexual exposures.** Number and gender of sex partners, nature of contact, use of barrier protection, and history of prior sexually transmitted infections are all important factors in assessing risk for specific infections.
  ○ **Illicit drug use.** What substances has the patient used and by what route?
  ○ **Housing.** In what geographical region does the patient reside? Does the patient live in a stable home or is he/she homeless? Does the patient live in an urban or rural environment? Has the patient ever been incarcerated in the past?
- **Physical examination.** A detailed examination can provide additional clues to the cause of a patient's illness or complications from a patient's medical interventions. Thorough dermatological, oral, ocular, and lymph node examinations are especially important. Rashes are highly indicative of specific infections or toxicities from antibiotics. Detailed descriptions of infected lesions remain essential.
- **Laboratory data and imaging**
  ○ Heed trends in laboratory data. Look for neutropenia and lymphopenia. In patients receiving long-term antibiotics, new abnormal liver or kidney function testing may be indicative of drug toxicity.
  ○ Note specific details of microbiological culture data, both positive and negative, including body site, date and time of collection, and any microorganism isolated along with its antibiotic susceptibility profile.

TABLE 1-1	IMPORTANT QUESTIONS RELATED TO SOCIAL HISTORY AND THEIR ASSOCIATION WITH SPECIFIC INFECTIONS

Animal Exposure

Do you have a pet?	Birds	*Chlamydophila psittaci* (psittacosis)
	Cats	*Bartonella henselae* (cat-scratch disease)
		Coxiella burnetii (Q fever)
		Pasteurella multocida
		Toxocara cati
		Toxoplasma gondii (toxoplasmosis)
	Dogs	*Capnocytophaga canimorsus*
		Pasteurella multocida
		Toxocara canis
	Reptiles	*Salmonella* spp. (salmonellosis)
	Fish	*Mycobacterium marinum* (fish tank granuloma)
Have you been bitten by an animal?	Bats, domestic dogs, and wild carnivorous animals	Rabies
	Monkeys	Herpes B virus
Do you hunt?	Skinning rabbits	*Francisella tularensis* (tularemia)
	Eating undercooked wild boar	*Trichinella spiralis* (trichinosis)
	Tick exposure	*Rickettsia rickettsii* (Rocky mountain spotted fever)
		Francisella tularensis (tularemia)
		Anaplasma phagocytophilum (anaplasmosis)
		Babesia microti (babesiosis)
		Borrelia burgdorferi (Lyme disease)
		Ehrlichia chaffeensis (ehrlichiosis)

Occupational exposures

What is your occupation?	Farmers, veterinarians, and slaughterhouse workers	*Brucella melitensis*
		Coxiella burnetii
	Construction workers	*Blastomyces dermatitidis* (blastomycosis, moist soil)
		Histoplasma capsulatum (histoplasmosis, contaminated soil)
		Leptospira spp. (leptospirosis, exposure to rat urine)
	Fishing industry	*Erysipelothrix rhusiopathiae* (erysipeloid)

TABLE 1-1	IMPORTANT QUESTIONS RELATED TO SOCIAL HISTORY AND THEIR ASSOCIATION WITH SPECIFIC INFECTIONS (CONTINUED)

Travel history

What areas of the United States have you visited?	Southwestern United States	*Coccidioides immitis* (coccidioidomycosis)
	Ohio and Mississippi River Valleys	*Blastomyces dermatitidis* (blastomycosis)
		Histoplasma capsulatum (histoplasmosis)
	Southeastern and South Central United States	*Ehrlichia* spp. (ehrlichiosis)
	Northeast and upper Midwest	*Borrelia burgdorferi* (Lyme disease)
		Babesia microti (babesiosis)
Have you traveled internationally?	Africa, Asia, parts of Central and South America	*Plasmodium* spp. (malaria)
		Dengue virus (dengue fever)
		Salmonella typhi (typhoid fever)
	Brazil	Yellow fever virus
	Latin America	*Trypanosoma cruzi* (Chagas disease)
		Zika virus
		Paracoccidioides brasiliensis (paracoccidioidomycosis)
	Northern Australia/ Southeast Asia	*Burkholderia pseudomallei* (melioidosis)
Type of travel	Cruise ship	Norovirus

Hobbies

What are your hobbies?	Gardening	*Aspergillus* spp. (mulching)
		Sporothrix schenckii (sporotrichosis, rose thorns)
	Spelunking	*Histoplasma capsulatum* (histoplasmosis)
	Water sports	*Naegleria fowleri* (naegleriasis, warm water)
		Leptospira spp. (leptospirosis)

Sexual exposures

Are you sexually active?	Painful penile ulcer	*Haemophilus ducreyi* (chancroid)
		Herpes simples virus

(Continued)

TABLE 1-1	IMPORTANT QUESTIONS RELATED TO SOCIAL HISTORY AND THEIR ASSOCIATION WITH SPECIFIC INFECTIONS (CONTINUED)		
	Painless penile ulcer	*Treponema pallidum* (syphilis)
		Klebsiella granulomatis (granuloma inguinale, also known as donovanosis)
		Chlamydia trachomatis L1, L3, L3 serovars (lymphogranuloma venereum)
	Vaginal/urethral discharge	*Chlamydia trachomatis*
		Neisseria gonorrhoeae
	Blood-borne viruses	HIV
		Hepatitis B virus
		Hepatitis C virus
Illicit drug use		
Have you ever injected drugs?	Blood-borne viruses	HIV
		Hepatitis B virus
		Hepatitis C virus
	Black tar heroin	*Clostridium botulinum* (botulism)
		Clostridium tetani (tetanus)
Housing		
Where do you live?	Rural area	*Coxiella burnetii* (Q fever, direct animal contact)
What is your water supply?	Well water	Hepatitis A virus
		Giardia lamblia (giardiasis)
		Campylobacter jejuni
		Escherichia coli
		Shigella spp. (shigellosis, dysentery)
		Salmonella spp. (salmonellosis)
		Cryptosporidium spp. (cryptosporidiosis)

Courtesy of Jane O'Halloran. Washington University School of Medicine, St. Louis, MO.

○ Individualized discussion and review of microbiologic or pathologic specimens with a clinical microbiologist or pathologist wherever appropriate can provide invaluable insight into the disease process. Likewise, review of imaging with a radiologist can often help refine and narrow the radiographic differential diagnosis.
○ When available, historical laboratory data (e.g., past microbiologic cultures, organism-specific serologies) can provide an important context for understanding the patient's present condition.

- **Assessment and plan**
  - Briefly summarize the case.
  - Outline your recommendations in an easy-to-read format and describe the rationale for your recommendations.
  - Include next steps and contingency plans.
  - Communicate your assessment directly to the requesting physician.

REFERENCES

1. Honda H, Krauss MJ, Jones JC, et al. The value of infectious diseases consultation in *Staphylococcus aureus* bacteremia. *Am J Med*. 2010;123:631-637.
2. Hamandi B, Husain S, Humar A, Papadimitropoulos EA. Impact of infectious disease consultation on the clinical and economic outcomes of solid organ transplant recipients admitted for infectious complications. *Clin Infect Dis*. 2014;59:1074-1082.
3. Burnham JP, Olsen MA, Stwalley D, et al. Infectious diseases consultation reduces 30-day and 1-year all-cause mortality for multidrug-resistant organism infections. *Open Forum Infect Dis*. 2018;5(3):ofy026.
4. Spec A, Olsen MA, Raval K, Powderly WG. Impact of infectious diseases consultation on mortality of cryptococcal infection in patients without HIV. *Clin Infect Dis*. 2017;64:558-564.
5. Mejia C, Kronen R, Lin C, et al. Impact of infectious diseases consultation on mortality in patients with candidemia. *Open Forum Infect Dis*. 2017;4(suppl_1):S52.
6. Pulcini C, Botelho-Nevers E, Dyar OJ, Harbarth S. The impact of infectious disease specialists on antibiotic prescribing in hospitals. *Clin Microbiol Infect*. 2014;20:963-972.
7. Goldman L, Lee T, Rudd P. Ten commandments for effective consultations. *Arch Intern Med*. 1983;143:1753-1755.
8. Salerno SM, Hurst FP, Halvorson S, Mercado DL. Principles of effective consultation: an update for the 21st-century consultant. *Arch Intern Med*. 2007;167:271-275.

The Acute Febrile Patient and Sepsis

Yasir Hamad and Stephen Y. Liang

2

Approach to the Acute Febrile Patient

GENERAL PRINCIPLES

Definition

- Fever has classically been defined as a body temperature of ≥38°C (100.4°F). Recent evidence suggests that the upper limit of normal oral temperature may be 37.2°C (98.9°F) in the early morning and 37.7°C (99.9°F) overall in healthy adults, though significant variability exists between individuals.[1]
- Febrile response in the elderly patient is frequently blunted, leading some to define fever in this population as a persistent oral temperature ≥37.2°C (98.9°F), rectal temperature ≥37.5°C (99.5°F), or a rise in temperature of ≥1.3°C (2.3°F) above baseline.[2]
- Oral temperatures are generally 0.4°C (0.7°F) lower than rectal temperatures. Axillary and tympanic temperatures may be unreliable.

Etiology

- Infectious causes of fever lasting less than 2 weeks are legion and may range from self-limited viral to serious bacterial infections. Differential diagnosis hinges heavily on the history and physical examination. Fevers of unknown origin lasting more than 3 weeks are discussed in Chapter 3.
- Noninfectious causes of fever may include neoplastic, rheumatologic, endocrine, thromboembolic, and medication-related disorders.
- While hyperpyrexia (>41.5°C or 106.7°F) may be encountered with severe infection, it is more common with central nervous system hemorrhage.
- **Hyperthermia** is a distinct entity apart from fever and may result from environmental factors, endocrine disorders (hyperthyroidism), and certain medications (e.g., anesthetics, neuroleptic agents, recreational drugs).

Pathophysiology

- Thermoregulation is mediated by the hypothalamus.
- Exogenous pyrogens (e.g., microbes, toxins) induce host macrophages and other phagocytic cells, triggering the release of endogenous cytokines (e.g., interleukin [IL]-1, IL-6, tumor necrosis factor [TNF]-α, interferons).
- These endogenous pyrogens modulate an inflammatory acute phase response and promote prostaglandin E2 (PGE2) synthesis. It is thought that PGE2 acts on the hypothalamus, precipitating a rise in body temperature.

DIAGNOSIS

Clinical Presentation

History
- **Clarify the patient's definition of "fever,"** whether it is subjective, tactile, or measured, and if so, by what route. Characterize the magnitude, duration, and consistency of the fever.

- **Establish a time line of all symptoms** in relation to the start of the fever. While the cause may be obvious in many cases, a thorough review of systems may uncover additional symptomatology characteristic of specific infections (e.g., myalgias, rashes, lymphadenopathy). Look for temporal relationships between fever and medical interventions (e.g., surgeries, catheters, mechanical ventilation, antibiotics, prolonged hospitalizations).
- **Ascertain the immune status of the patient.** Neoplasm, chemotherapy, immunosuppressive therapy (to prevent transplant rejection or treat rheumatologic disorders), corticosteroid use, HIV infection, and primary immunodeficiency disease (e.g., humoral immune or severe combined immunodeficiencies) all influence the spectrum of infections possible.
- Obtain a complete past medical history, surgical history (including all prosthetics, foreign materials, and implantable devices), and medication list (prescription, over-the-counter, alternative). Use of antipyretics should be noted. When available, a vaccination record should be reviewed, particularly in asplenic and immunocompromised patients.
- A social history should identify environmental, occupational, recreational, sexual, dietary, animal, and travel exposures as well as sick contacts.
- Family members can frequently provide additional insight into the patient's illness and exposure history.

Physical Examination

A thorough and methodical approach to the physical examination helps ensure that subtle findings are not missed (see Table 2-1).

Febrile Syndromes

- When used in conjunction with the history and physical, common febrile syndromes help guide the differential diagnosis by suggesting organ-specific disease processes.
- Fever and headache is concerning for meningitis, whereas fever with focal neurologic deficits or seizure may suggest encephalitis, cerebral abscess, subdural empyema, or epidural abscess.
- Fever and chest pain mandate a search for pneumonia, but may also be seen with pericarditis, esophagitis, and mediastinitis.
- Depending on the location and history, fever and abdominal pain may raise the suspicion of cholecystitis, appendicitis, intra-abdominal abscess, peritonitis, diverticulitis, colitis, or a host of other pathologies.
- Other febrile syndromes (e.g., rash [see Table 2-2], lymphadenopathy [see Table 2-3], jaundice, and splenomegaly) may be indicative of an underlying systemic infection (see Table 2-4).

Diagnostic Testing

Laboratories

- **Initial testing**
  - Laboratory evaluation of fever should be driven by the nature and severity of the patient's symptoms. In the inpatient setting, the following tests are a reasonable starting point to screen for abnormalities:
    - Complete blood count with differential (leukocytosis, neutrophilia, bandemia, neutropenia, anemia, thrombocytopenia)
    - Metabolic panel (hyponatremia, acidosis, impaired renal function)
    - Liver tests (transaminitis, cholestasis)
    - Coagulation studies (disseminated intravascular coagulation)
    - Urinalysis (urinary tract infection, active urinary sediment)
  - HIV screening is strongly recommended, particularly in high-prevalence areas.

TABLE 2-1	PHYSICAL EXAMINATION FINDINGS AND CLINICAL SYNDROMES TO CONSIDER IN THE PATIENT WITH FEVER
Location	**Findings and Associations**
Eyes	Retinitis and other lesions (e.g., Roth spots), uveitis, hypopyon, conjunctival suffusion/hemorrhage, conjunctivitis, visual field deficits
Ears	Otitis media/externa, mastoiditis
Face, nose, throat	Sinus tenderness, pharyngitis (erythema, exudate), mucosal lesions, thrush, periodontitis, peritonsillar abscess, muffled voice (epiglottitis)
Neck	Neck stiffness (meningitis, retropharyngeal abscess), tenderness along the sternocleidomastoid muscle (internal jugular septic thrombophlebitis), thyromegaly
Heart	Murmurs (endocarditis), rubs, distant sounds
Lungs	Crackles, rhonchi, wheezes, dullness to percussion
Abdomen	Focal tenderness, peritoneal signs, hepatomegaly, splenomegaly, ascites
Genitourinary/rectum	Male: urethritis, prostatitis, orchitis, epididymitis Female: cervicitis, adnexal mass/tenderness, foreign body (e.g., tampon) Rectum: perirectal fluctuance (abscess), ulcers, Fournier gangrene
Back	Pressure sores, decubitus ulcers, costovertebral angle tenderness
Extremities	Stigmata of endocarditis (Osler nodes, Janeway lesions, splinter hemorrhages), clubbing, palmar/plantar rashes, track marks
Neuro	Altered mental status, focal neurologic deficits, ataxia
Skin	Cellulitis, cutaneous abscess, sinus tracts, crepitus, necrotizing soft tissue infection, rash (petechiae, purpura, macules, papules, vesicles, ulcers, eschars)
Musculoskeletal	Effusion, septic arthritis, spinous process tenderness
Lymph	Any lymphadenopathy, lymph node fluctuance or drainage
Devices	Pacemaker/defibrillator, tunneled intravenous catheter, implantable port, orthopedic hardware

- **Cultures should be obtained before antimicrobials whenever possible.** However, collection of cultures should not delay antimicrobial administration in an unstable patient.
- Blood cultures (preferably a minimum of 2–3 sets) should be obtained from a febrile patient within the first 24 hours of presentation when endocarditis, bacteremia, or catheter-associated bloodstream infection is suspected. Each culture should consist of 20 to 30 mL of blood drawn from a single site at a single time point. In the case

| TABLE 2-2 | DIFFERENTIAL DIAGNOSIS OF INFECTIONS CAUSING FEVER AND RASH |

Rash	Potential Causes	
Petechiae/ purpura	Meningococcemia Gonococcemia Subacute bacterial endocarditis Enterovirus EBV Rubella	RMSF Relapsing fever Rat bite fever Hepatitis B (acute) Viral hemorrhagic fevers
Macules/ papules	Lyme disease Meningococcemia Gonococcemia Mycoplasma Adenovirus Enterovirus EBV HHV-6 Coxsackievirus	Typhoid fever (rose spots) Syphilis (secondary) RMSF and other *Rickettsia* Typhus (epidemic, murine, and scrub) Parvovirus B19 Hepatitis B Rubeola Rubella HIV Dengue
Nodules	Ecthyma gangrenosum (*Pseudomonas* sepsis) Disseminated atypical mycobacterial infection	Disseminated fungal infection (candidiasis, histoplasmosis, blastomycosis, coccidioidomycosis, cryptococcosis, sporotrichosis)
Erythema nodosum	*Streptococcus* spp. *Yersinia* spp. *Mycoplasma pneumoniae* *Chlamydia* spp.	Mycobacteria Histoplasmosis Coccidioidomycosis
Vesicles	Enterovirus Echovirus HSV	VZV Coxsackievirus (hand-foot-mouth) Poxviruses
Pustules	*Pseudomonas aeruginosa* *Staphylococcus* spp.	Gonococcemia
Bullae	*Streptococcus* spp. (group A) *Staphylococcus* spp.	*Pseudomonas aeruginosa* *Vibrio vulnificus*
Ulcers	Anthrax Chancroid Glanders Granuloma inguinale Leprosy Lymphogranuloma venereum All invasive fungal infections HSV	Melioidosis Mycobacteria Plague Syphilis Tularemia Dracunculiasis Amebiasis Leishmania

TABLE 2-2	DIFFERENTIAL DIAGNOSIS OF INFECTIONS CAUSING FEVER AND RASH (CONTINUED)	
Rash	**Potential Causes**	
Eschars	*Rickettsia* spp. Anthrax Poxvirus Leishmaniasis	Tularemia Plague Disseminated aspergillosis Blastomycosis Mucormycosis
Lesions involving the palms and soles	Meningococcemia Subacute bacterial endocarditis Syphilis (secondary) Enterovirus	RMSF and other *Rickettsia* spp. Ehrlichiosis Rat bite fever VZV
Oral lesions	HSV VZV	Enterovirus Syphilis (secondary) Histoplasmosis (ulcer)

CMV, cytomegalovirus; EBV, Epstein–Barr virus; HSV, herpes simplex virus; HHV, human herpes virus; RMSF, Rocky Mountain spotted fever; VZV, varicella zoster virus.

of catheter-associated bloodstream infection, at least one culture should be obtained through the infected catheter. Specialized blood culture media may be required to effectively isolate fungi, mycobacteria, viruses, and rare organisms (e.g., *Brucella* spp.).
- Urine cultures should be obtained if a urinary tract infection is suspected.
- Sputum and bronchoalveolar lavage cultures may be obtained to guide antibiotic therapy of pneumonia, particularly in intensive care unit (ICU) and severely immunocompromised patients where fungal and mycobacterial infections are also suspected.
- Stool cultures, parasite examination, and tests for *Clostridium difficile* infection should be considered in a febrile patient with diarrhea.
- If osteomyelitis is suspected, an erythrocyte sedimentation rate and C-reactive protein may be helpful if highly elevated.
- **Subsequent testing**
  - In cases where meningitis or encephalitis is suspected, lumbar puncture should be performed before the initiation of antibiotics if possible. Cerebrospinal fluid should be sent for cell count, glucose, protein, Gram stain, culture, and other specialized tests based on clinical suspicion.
  - As a general rule, all fluid collections suspected of being infected (e.g., pleural fluid, ascites, abscess) should be sampled and sent for cell count, culture, and other appropriate analytic studies.
  - Superinfected chronic wounds (e.g., decubitus or diabetic foot ulcers) should be debrided first and then cultured from the base of the wound. Superficial cultures are contaminated with skin flora that may or may not be responsible for the infection.
  - Intravascular catheters strongly suspected as sources of infection should be removed after blood cultures are obtained through the lumen and the catheter tip should be sent for culture.

TABLE 2-3	DIFFERENTIAL DIAGNOSIS OF INFECTIONS CAUSING FEVER AND LYMPHADENOPATHY

Distribution	Potential Causes	
Generalized	Cat-scratch disease	Brucellosis
	Syphilis (secondary)	Mycobacteria
	Typhoid fever	Leptospirosis
	CMV	Rubella
	EBV	Rubeola
	HIV	Dengue
	Histoplasmosis	Toxoplasmosis
	Blastomycosis	Visceral leishmaniasis
	Coccidioidomycosis	
Cervical	Streptococci (group A)	Mycobacteria
	Diphtheria	EBV
	Numerous other viruses	
Regional	Streptococci	Mycobacteria
	Staphylococci	Tularemia
	Cat scratch disease	Plague
	Syphilis (secondary, epitrochlear)	Typhus
		Sporotrichosis
	HSV	Filariasis
	Toxoplasmosis	
	Trypanosomiasis	
Inguinal	Syphilis (primary)	Lymphogranuloma venereum
	Chancroid	
	HSV	Granuloma inguinale

CMV, cytomegalovirus; EBV, Epstein–Barr virus; HSV, herpes simplex virus.

○ Throat and nasopharyngeal sampling may help identify viral and streptococcal upper respiratory tract infections. Testing for influenza, particularly in immunocompromised and elderly patients, should be considered if the season is appropriate or an epidemic is underway.

○ Disease-specific serologies and other specialized laboratory tests (e.g., polymerase chain reaction [PCR]) may be indicated in the appropriate clinical context.

Imaging
• Chest radiography should be obtained if pulmonary complaints exist.
• Computed tomography (CT), magnetic resonance imaging, ultrasound, and nuclear studies may be indicated based on presenting symptoms and clinical suspicion. Consultation with a radiologist regarding the best modality for visualizing pathology (e.g., abscess, osteomyelitis, cerebral disease) can be helpful in avoiding excessive imaging.
• Echocardiography should be pursued if endocarditis is suspected based on the presence of a new heart murmur and other clinical criteria.

Diagnostic Procedures
• Tissue biopsy for pathology, culture, and other specialized testing may be needed to establish diagnoses of osteomyelitis, disorders associated with lymphadenopathy

TABLE 2-4	DIFFERENTIAL DIAGNOSIS OF INFECTIOUS CAUSES OF SELECTED FEBRILE SYNDROMES	
Syndrome	**Potential Causes**	
Fever and jaundice	Sepsis	Q fever
	Cholangitis	Leptospirosis
	Hepatic abscesses	Viral hepatitis
	CMV	Rift Valley fever
	EBV	Viral hemorrhagic fevers
	HIV	Fascioliasis
	Malaria	
	Hepatic flukes	
Fever and splenomegaly	Endocarditis	Brucellosis
	Typhoid fever	Rickettsiosis
	Miliary tuberculosis	CMV
	EBV	Echinococcosis
	Malaria	Trypanosomiasis
	Visceral leishmaniasis	
	Schistosomiasis	
Fever without localizing symptoms	Tuberculosis	Brucellosis
	Endocarditis	Q fever
	Mycotic aneurysm	Rat bite fever
	Intra-abdominal abscess	Leptospirosis
	Osteomyelitis	Rickettsiosis
	Typhoid fever	Ehrlichiosis
	Cat scratch disease	Whipple disease
	CMV	HIV
	Coccidioidomycosis	Toxoplasmosis
	Histoplasmosis	Malaria

CMV, cytomegalovirus; EBV, Epstein–Barr virus.

(e.g., cat-scratch disease, toxoplasmosis), and disseminated infections (e.g., tuberculosis, atypical mycobacteria, histoplasmosis).
- When possible, appropriate cultures should be obtained during any surgical intervention to treat an infectious complication (e.g., endocarditis, pacemaker lead infection, graft, or hardware infection).

TREATMENT

Antimicrobial Therapy

- In the outpatient setting, most fevers in healthy adults are associated with transient, self-limited viral infections and are frequently overtreated with antimicrobials.
- An emphasis should be placed on establishing an infectious etiology for the fever to guide appropriate antimicrobial coverage.
- Situations warranting empiric antimicrobial therapy before a definitive diagnosis can be made that include the following:
  - Acute clinical deterioration (e.g., respiratory distress, altered mental status, hemodynamic instability, sepsis)

   ○ Immunocompromised state (e.g., HIV, neoplasm, transplant, immunosuppressive therapy)
   ○ Elderly patients (in whom atypical and muted presentations of serious infection are common)
- Choice of empiric antimicrobial therapy should be based on the type of infection suspected (e.g., pneumonia, meningitis, cellulitis), common microorganisms implicated, concern for multidrug resistance among those organisms, and local antimicrobial susceptibility patterns.

Antipyretic Therapy

- Antipyretics can be given for symptom relief but they do not alter outcomes. In patients with cardiovascular or pulmonary disease, antipyretics may reduce some of the metabolic demands of fever.
- Acetaminophen and nonsteroidal anti-inflammatory drugs including ibuprofen and aspirin inhibit the synthesis of inflammatory prostaglandins through the cyclooxygenase pathway and trigger other antipyretic pathways, reducing hypothalamus-mediated fever.
- Corticosteroids also have antipyretic properties but generally are not indicated for fever control alone.
- External cooling methods including cooling blankets, fans, and water sponging effect heat loss through conduction, convection, and evaporation, respectively. Rebound hyperthermia may result if antipyretic medications are not used and shivering is not controlled.

SPECIAL CONSIDERATIONS

Fever in the Intensive Care Unit

- New, unexplained fevers complicate a significant number of ICU admissions and prolonged hospitalizations.[3,4] The causes can be wide ranging, underscoring the complexity of these patients (see Table 2-5).
- In reviewing the medical history of the ICU patient, a strong emphasis should be placed on understanding not only the patient's initial clinical presentation and primary diagnosis but also the sequence of medical interventions (e.g., new medications, procedures, surgeries, health care–associated devices, respiratory support) that have taken place since admission.
- Nursing observations regarding patient hemodynamics, oxygen requirements, tracheal secretions, catheter sites, skin breakdown, wounds, diarrhea, and other clinically relevant conditions can lend valuable insight into the patient's hospital course.
- **Health care–associated infections** are responsible for a sizable portion of these fevers.
   ○ **Intravascular catheter–associated bloodstream infection.**[5] Infection rates differ by type (uncuffed > tunneled > peripheral), location (femoral vein > internal jugular vein > subclavian vein), duration, frequency of manipulation, and method of placement (use of sterile precautions).
      ■ At least one blood culture should be obtained through the infected catheter and one culture from a peripheral site by venipuncture.
      ■ The intravascular catheter in question should be promptly removed and the catheter tip sent for culture if sepsis, embolic disease, or tunnel infection is suspected.
      ■ Peripheral intravenous catheters should be changed every 72 hours regardless of fever.
   ○ **Ventilator-associated pneumonia.** Infection occurring more than 48 hours after endotracheal intubation and mechanical ventilation.
      ■ Chest radiography or CT with evolving infiltrates coupled with clinical cues (increased purulent tracheal secretions and/or oxygen requirement) help secure the diagnosis.

TABLE 2-5	DIFFERENTIAL DIAGNOSIS OF A NEW FEVER IN THE INTENSIVE CARE UNIT	
Infectious	Intravascular catheter–related infection: Tunnel infection Bloodstream infection Suppurative phlebitis Pneumonia: Hospital acquired Ventilator associated	Urinary tract infection *Clostridium difficile* infection Surgical site infection Cellulitis/abscess Sinusitis Otitis media Parotitis Transfusion-related infection Retained foreign body (e.g., tampon)
Noninfectious	Drug fever: Antimicrobials Anticonvulsants Antihistamines Antihypertensives Antiarrhythmics Neuroleptic malignant syndrome Antipsychotics (haloperidol) Serotonin syndrome Selective serotonin reuptake inhibitors Malignant hyperthermia Succinylcholine Halothane Withdrawal syndromes: Alcohol Opiates Barbiturates Benzodiazepines	Acalculous cholecystitis Pancreatitis Adrenal insufficiency Hyperthyroidism (thyroid storm) Cerebrovascular accident Intracranial hemorrhage Acute myocardial infarction Mesenteric ischemia/infarction Thromboembolic diseases (deep vein thrombosis/pulmonary embolus) Transfusion reactions Tumor lysis syndrome Gout

- Bronchoscopy to obtain accurate lower respiratory tract cultures and Gram stains should be considered.
- Blood cultures and diagnostic thoracentesis of associated pleural effusions may also be helpful in identifying a causative organism.
  - **Urinary tract infection.**[6] Risk factors include having an indwelling urethral catheter, suprapubic catheter, ureteral stent, or nephrostomy.
    - Urinalysis and urine culture should be obtained from the sampling port of the catheter and never the drainage bag.
    - Infected catheters should be removed promptly if possible.
  - ***C. difficile* infection.**[7] Spectrum of disease may range from diarrhea to ileus and toxic megacolon. Leukemoid reactions with extremely high white blood cell counts are occasionally seen.
    - Send a stool specimen for *C. difficile* toxin by enzyme immunoassay or PCR and for fecal leukocytes.
    - Consider empiric therapy with oral vancomycin if illness is severe.

- **Sinusitis.** Nasotracheal/nasogastric intubations, nasal packing, and maxillofacial trauma may prevent drainage of the facial sinuses (especially maxillary) leading to bacterial overgrowth.
  - CT of the facial sinuses should be performed. Sinus puncture and aspiration under sterile conditions is diagnostic.
  - Empiric antibiotic therapy and removal of the nasotracheal or nasogastric tube are indicated in most cases.
- **Surgical site infection.** See discussion on postoperative fever.
- **Wound infection.** Prolonged or chronic debilitation increases the risk of pressure sores and decubitus ulcers, which are prone to infection.
  - Examine the back, sacrum, and other dependent areas thoroughly for wounds.
  - Document the number, size, and depth of any wounds and any signs of superinfection or necrosis.
- **Transfusion-related infection.** However rare, bacterial infection may be transmitted through blood product transfusion. Cytomegalovirus (CMV) transmitted by donor leukocytes present in the blood product can precipitate a mononucleosis-like syndrome in healthy adults or disseminated disease in the immunocompromised (particularly if the recipient is CMV seronegative).
  - Identify the timing of all blood product transfusions in relation to onset of fever. If a bacterial infection is suspected, obtain a recipient blood culture from a site opposite that of the transfusion and culture the donor blood product.
  - Administer leukocyte-reduced blood components to immunocompromised patients to prevent CMV disease.
- **Noninfectious causes** of a new, unexplained fever in the ICU include the following:
  - **Drug fever.** Antimicrobials (e.g., sulfonamides, penicillins, cephalosporins, vancomycin, nitrofurantoin), anticonvulsants (e.g., phenytoin, carbamazepine, barbiturates), H1- and H2-blocking antihistamines, antihypertensives (e.g., hydralazine, methyldopa), and antiarrhythmics (e.g., quinidine, procainamide) are common offenders. Relative bradycardia, rash, leukocytosis, and eosinophilia may or may not be present.
    - Establish a time line of start and stop dates for all suspect medications (particularly antimicrobials).
    - The time between discontinuation of the offending agent and resolution of fever can be variable and up to a week.
  - **Thromboembolic disease.** Deep vein thrombosis and pulmonary embolus occasionally present with isolated fever.
  - **Endocrine disease.** Adrenal insufficiency and thyroid storm may present with fever, tachycardia, and hypotension that can be easily mistaken for sepsis.
  - **Transfusion reactions**
    - **Febrile nonhemolytic transfusion reactions are common** (1 in 100 units) and occur when recipient antibodies react against antigens on donor leukocytes and platelets, triggering cytokine release anywhere from 30 minutes to several hours after a transfusion.
    - Acute hemolytic transfusion reactions result from ABO mismatch and occur when preformed recipient antibodies rapidly destroy donor erythrocytes leading to fever, flank pain, and hemoglobinuria. This is considered a medical emergency.
- Recent guidelines suggest that a body temperature of ≥38.3°C (100.9°F) or <36°C (96.8°F) is a reasonable threshold for initiating an evaluation for infection in the ICU patient. Remember that critically ill patients with serious infection may be normothermic or hypothermic in the context of extensive burns, open abdominal wounds, continuous renal replacement therapy, extracorporeal membrane oxygenation, or a host of medical illnesses (e.g., congestive heart failure, end-stage liver or renal disease, myxedema coma). Evaluation for infection should be guided ultimately by clinical suspicion.

- If infection is suspected, empiric antimicrobial therapy should be initiated immediately after appropriate cultures have been obtained. The risk of infection with multidrug-resistant pathogens should be taken into account along with local antimicrobial susceptibility patterns.

Postoperative Fever

- **Fever within the first 72 hours after surgery** is common and generally self-limited. Cytokine release from surgical trauma is thought to play a part.
  - **Wound infections are uncommon during the first three postoperative days.** When an early infection is evident, myonecrosis secondary to *Clostridium* species and group A streptococci must be considered and may require antibiotics and emergent surgical debridement. Toxic shock syndrome may accompany serious infection with group A streptococci or *Staphylococcus aureus.*
  - Noninfectious causes of fever may include thromboembolism, hematoma, transfusion reactions, and adrenal insufficiency. Malignant hyperthermia may manifest as muscle rigidity, tachycardia, and hyperthermia up to 10 hours after induction of general anesthesia.
- **Fever more than 72 hours after surgery** is significant and more likely to be associated with infection.
  - Wound infections, intra-abdominal infections, abscesses, infected hematomas, and the sequelae of anastomotic leaks are typically seen around the fourth or fifth day after surgery.
  - Health care–associated infections including pneumonia, urinary tract infection (in the setting of urinary catheterization), intravenous catheter–related infections (cellulitis, thrombophlebitis, bloodstream infection), and *C. difficile* infection related to antibiotic exposure are also more common.
  - Acalculous cholecystitis, pancreatitis, and thromboembolism are noninfectious etiologies that must also be considered.
- Postoperative fever may also result from surgical site inflammation, seroma, or hematoma without infection.
- Classic teaching maintains that the differential diagnosis of postoperative fever should focus on the **"5 Ws": wind** (pneumonia), **water** (urinary tract infection), **wound, walking** (thromboembolism), and **"wonder" drugs** (medication reaction). Opinions differ on whether atelectasis causes fever.
- History gathering should focus on understanding the preoperative presentation (including existing infection), surgical procedure (duration, complexity, blood products, perioperative prophylactic antibiotics, complications including intra-operative contamination; Table 2-6), and postoperative course (cough, diarrhea, pain, and changes in character or volume of surgical drain output or wound drainage). Hardware and foreign material inserted during the surgery should be documented. The possibility of drug fever should be examined through a chronology of all medications (e.g., antibiotics, anesthetics) received during and after surgery (see Table 2-6).
- Chest radiography, urinalysis, and urine culture are suggested for the evaluation of fever presenting more than 72 hours after surgery and for any febrile postoperative patient who has had a urinary catheter in place for ≥72 hours. Hemodynamic instability with concern for bacteremia or pending sepsis should prompt blood cultures.
- All surgical wounds should be examined daily for erythema, induration, and purulent discharge. Surgical and percutaneous drain reservoirs and their exit sites should likewise be inspected for evidence of infection.
- All infected surgical wounds should be cultured and in many cases opened to facilitate drainage.

TABLE 2-6	COMMON CAUSES OF POSTOPERATIVE FEVER ASSOCIATED WITH SPECIFIC TYPES OF SURGERY	
Neurosurgery	Meningitis Deep vein thrombosis Intracranial hemorrhage	Posterior fossa syndrome Hypothalamic dysfunction
Cardiothoracic surgery	Pneumonia Endocarditis	Mediastinitis Sternal wound infection
Abdominal surgery	Abscess Infected hematoma/seroma Anastomotic leak (e.g., bowel, biliary)	Peritonitis Pancreatitis Splenoportal thrombosis
Obstetrical or gynecologic surgery	Urinary tract infection Pelvic abscess Postpartum endometritis	Pelvic thrombophlebitis Toxic shock syndrome (vaginal packing)
Urologic surgery	Urinary tract infection	Deep infection (prostate, perinephric)
Orthopedic surgery	Prosthetic infection Infected hematoma	Deep vein thrombosis Fat embolism
Vascular surgery	Graft infection Postimplantation syndrome	Blue toe syndrome (atherothrombotic embolism)

- **Superficial wound cultures are seldom helpful in the absence of a clinically apparent infection.**
- If an abscess or deep infection is suspected, be aggressive about obtaining further imaging and surgical evaluation to determine whether operative or radiology-guided drainage is necessary. All fluid collections requiring drainage should be sent for culture.
- Be vigilant of intravenous catheter–associated infections, *C. difficile* infection, and noninfectious causes of fever already discussed with fever in the ICU patient.
- Empiric antimicrobial therapy is generally unnecessary for fever presenting within the first 72 hours of surgery, unless infection is clinically evident or uncovered on laboratory evaluation or imaging. Continuation of perioperative prophylactic antibiotics for early postoperative fever does not prevent infection and likely selects for resistant organisms.

Fever in the Immunocompromised Patient

- Immunocompromised patients are at heightened risk not only for community-acquired infections but also for an extensive range of opportunistic infections.
- Atypical and nonspecific clinical presentations abound. Muted inflammatory responses arising from neutropenia, corticosteroids, and other forms of immunosuppressive therapy may conceal serious infections.
- The medical history should assess the severity of the patient's immunocompromised state and risk factors for primary infection or reactivation of latent disease (see Table 2-7).
- The etiology of fever in the immunocompromised patient varies depending on the underlying disease and its subsequent therapy. Markers of immune status and approximately derived windows of susceptibility to infection help inform the differential diagnosis.

TABLE 2-7	KEY ASPECTS OF THE MEDICAL HISTORY IN EVALUATING THE IMMUNOCOMPROMISED PATIENT WITH FEVER
All immuno-compromised patients	• Any history of tuberculosis • Chronic infections (e.g., hepatitis B and C) • Disseminated infections (e.g., mycobacteria, endemic mycoses) • Opportunistic infections (e.g., *Pneumocystis jiroveci*, *Cryptococcus neoformans*, *Toxoplasma gondii*, *Mycobacterium avium complex*) • Chemoprophylaxis against opportunistic infections (dose, duration) • Baseline serologies (e.g., CMV, *T. gondii*) • Known colonization with multidrug-resistant organisms • Presence of long-term intravascular access (tunneled catheters vs. implantable ports) • Sick contacts • Environmental exposures
HIV infection	• CD4+ cell count and HIV viral load • Antiretroviral therapy (date started, adherence) • Recent unprotected sex • Presence of immune reconstitution inflammatory syndrome
Chemotherapy-related neutropenia	• Type and location of neoplasm (solid organ vs. hematologic) • Chemotherapy (dose, duration, number of days since last cycle) • Other therapies (e.g., surgery, radiation) and any associated complications • Relapse versus remission of disease
Solid organ transplantation	• Date and type of organ transplant • Immediate and delayed surgical complications associated with transplant • Immunosuppressive regimens (dose, duration, serum levels) • Presence of graft rejection • Donor and recipient CMV serology
Hematopoietic stem cell transplantation	• Date and type of transplant (allogeneic vs. autologous) • Immunosuppressive regimen (dose, duration) • Presence of GVHD • Donor CMV serology (if allogeneic transplant)

CMV, cytomegalovirus; GVHD, graft versus host disease.

• In addition to the opportunistic infections discussed below, it is important to keep in mind that immunocompromised patients are also at risk for common community-acquired infections (e.g., bacterial pneumonia, influenza) as well as health care–associated infections (e.g., intravascular catheter–associated bloodstream infection, *C. difficile* infection), given their frequent contact with the hospital environment and exposure to antimicrobials either as chemoprophylaxis or to treat active infection.

○ **HIV**
- The CD4+ lymphocyte cell count is a reasonably accurate gauge of susceptibility to opportunistic infections in the HIV patient (see Table 2-8).
- Patients recently started on antiretroviral therapy may present with immune reconstitution inflammatory syndrome, an inflammatory immune response against pathogens that may have previously been clinically silent (e.g., mycobacteria, *Pneumocystis jiroveci*, endemic fungi, CMV).
- Noninfectious causes of fever particular to HIV include neoplasm (non–Hodgkin lymphoma and occasionally visceral Kaposi sarcoma), drug fever (e.g., trimethoprim–sulfamethoxazole, dapsone), hypersensitivity reaction (abacavir, nevirapine, efavirenz), and Castleman disease (angiofollicular lymph node hyperplasia).
○ **Chemotherapy-related neutropenia**
- **Neutropenic fever.**[8] Absolute neutrophil count of <500 cells/μL or <1000 cells/μL with an anticipated decline below 500 cells/μL over the next 48 hours coupled with the presence of a single temperature of ≥38.3°C (100.9°F) or a persistent temperature of ≥38.0°C (100.4°F) for more than an hour.

TABLE 2-8	DIFFERENTIAL DIAGNOSIS OF INFECTIOUS CAUSES OF FEVER IN A PATIENT WITH HIV
Meningitis/ encephalitis/ other CNS disorders	Any CD4+: *Streptococcus pneumoniae, Neisseria meningitidis, Listeria monocytogenes,* HSV CD4+ <100: *Cryptococcus neoformans, Toxoplasma gondii* (encephalitis, cerebral abscess) CD4+ <50: CMV and VZV (encephalitis), EBV-associated lymphoma,[a] JC polyomavirus (progressive multifocal leukoencephalopathy)[a]
Pneumonia	Any CD4+: *S. pneumoniae, Haemophilus influenzae, Mycoplasma pneumoniae, Legionella pneumophila, Staphylococcus aureus, Mycobacterium tuberculosis* CD4+ <200: *Pneumocystis jiroveci,* endemic fungi CD4+ <100: *C. neoformans, T. gondii* CD4+ <50: *Mycobacterium avium complex, Aspergillus* spp., CMV, VZV
Esophagitis	CD4 <200: *Candida albicans,* CMV, HSV
Diarrhea	Any CD4+: *Salmonella, Shigella, Campylobacter, Escherichia coli, L. monocytogenes, Clostridium difficile;* rotavirus, norovirus, *Giardia lamblia*[a] CD4+ <100: CMV (colitis), *Cryptosporidium,*[a] Microsporidia,[a] Cyclospora,[a] Isospora[a]
Rash	Any CD4+: *Staphylococcus and Streptococcus* spp. (cellulitis, abscess); VZV (herpes zoster)
Disseminated infection	CD4+ <100 (generally): *Mycobacterium avium complex, Mycobacterium tuberculosis, Histoplasma capsulatum, Coccidioides immitis, Bartonella henselae, Penicillium marneffei, Cryptococcus neoformans*

[a]For completeness, several important opportunistic infections not typically associated with fever are included as well.

CNS, central nervous system; CMV, cytomegalovirus; EBV, Epstein–Barr virus; HSV, herpes simplex virus; VZV, varicella zoster virus.

- Mucosal barriers compromised by chemotherapy may allow translocation of intestinal flora into the bloodstream, leading to bacteremia (*Enterococcus*, gram-negative bacteria) and candidemia. Hepatosplenic candidiasis, seen mostly in patients with acute leukemia, may present with fever, abdominal pain, and elevated alkaline phosphatase. Mucositis predisposes to bacteremia with oral flora (*Streptococcus viridans*, anaerobes). Cutaneous breakdown can lead to cellulitis, abscess, and bacteremia with gram-positive and gram-negative organisms alike.
- Neutropenic enterocolitis (typhlitis) manifesting as a necrotizing cecal infection can extend to the terminal ileum and ascending colon, leading to bowel perforation.
- Invasive mold infections (*Aspergillus*, *Fusarium*, *Zygomycetes*) presenting as pneumonia, sinusitis, central nervous system infection, or skin infections are also encountered.

○ **Solid organ transplantation**
  - Infections occurring shortly after organ transplant are largely related to surgical complications (e.g., anastomotic leaks, wound dehiscence, infected fluid collections) and prolonged hospitalization.
  - As immunosuppressive therapy to prevent acute rejection takes effect, opportunistic infections (e.g., mycobacteria, *Aspergillus*, *P. jiroveci*, herpesviruses) become more common by 1 month after transplant. CMV donor–recipient mismatch leading to primary CMV infection carries the highest risk of invasive disease (pneumonitis, hepatitis, colitis).
  - As the risk of acute graft rejection declines over time, the need for immunosuppression stabilizes and decreases. At 6 months posttransplant, community-acquired infections are more likely than opportunistic ones. Patients still on significant doses of immunosuppressive therapy remain prone to the latter.

○ **Hematopoietic stem cell transplantation**
  - The preengraftment phase comprises the first 3 weeks after conditioning chemotherapy and allogeneic stem cell transplant. Bone marrow suppression is profound and patients are at high risk for all of the infections associated with chemotherapy-related neutropenia.
  - Bone marrow recovery marks the beginning of the **immediate postengraftment phase** typically lasting from 3 weeks to 3 months after allogeneic stem cell transplant. Invasive fungal and viral infections (e.g., CMV) as well as other opportunistic infections (e.g., *P. jiroveci*) are possible depending on antimicrobial prophylaxis strategies. Acute graft versus host disease (GVHD) may necessitate additional immunosuppressive therapy.
  - Six months after transplant, the recipient enters the **late postengraftment phase.** If a recipient has not developed GVHD by this point, immune function may be largely restored within 1 to 2 years. However, recipients with chronic GVHD on immunosuppression remain prone to a wide array of opportunistic infections.

- A more comprehensive discussion of infections seen in each of these immunocompromised states and their management shall be undertaken in later chapters.
- Empiric broad-spectrum antimicrobial therapy is almost universally indicated in the initial management of fever in the immunocompromised patient pending a thorough investigation for infection.

Fever in the Returned Traveler

- Fever is a common complaint among returned travelers seeking medical care.[9]
- The differential diagnosis of fever in the returned traveler can be broad and elusive. Geographic-specific infections not routinely encountered in daily practice may present alongside globally distributed infections (e.g., influenza) and illnesses not necessarily specific to travel (e.g., pneumonia).
- A thorough travel history should include the following:
  ○ Departure and return dates
  ○ Itinerary (e.g., all geographic locations visited, length of stay at each site, urban vs. rural setting, nature of the accommodations, modes of transportation)

- ○ Purpose of travel (tourism, work, visiting family or friends)
- ○ Activities (e.g., freshwater swimming, caving, hunting, agriculture, missionary work, health care)
- ○ Sick contacts (including fellow travelers)
- ○ Sexual contacts
- ○ Animal contacts (e.g., domestic animals, rodents, exotic wildlife, insects, ticks)
- ○ Type of food consumed (e.g., undercooked food, unpasteurized dairy products)
- ○ Source of water
- ○ Childhood and pretravel immunizations
- ○ Chemoprophylaxis (start and start dates, adherence)
- Knowledge of geographic-specific infections and their usual incubation periods (Table 2-9) can help in narrowing the list of suspect pathogens. Published by the Centers for Disease Control and Prevention (www.cdc.gov), the Yellow Book can be an invaluable travel medicine asset. Likewise, ProMED-mail (www.promedmail.org), a global electronic reporting system sponsored by the International Society for Infectious Diseases, can provide timely information about outbreaks of emerging infectious diseases around the world (see Table 2-9).[10]
- **Malaria is the most common cause of fever in the returned traveler** and should always be considered highest on the differential if travel has occurred in an endemic area. Serial thick and thin blood smears should be obtained to evaluate for parasitemia.
- **Enteric fever** (*Salmonella typhi* or *Salmonella paratyphi*) acquired through fecal–oral spread may present as fever, abdominal discomfort, and constipation. Diarrhea may or may not be present early in the infection. **Dengue fever, rickettsioses**, and **leptospirosis** are also commonly encountered in tropical regions. Poor sanitation, inadequate hand hygiene, and food or waterborne exposures increase the risk of acquiring **viral hepatitis** and **infectious diarrheas** (bacterial, viral, or parasitic). Emerging infections involving Chikungunya and Zika virus should also be considered based on location of travel.
- Upper respiratory tract infections, bacterial pneumonia, urinary tract infections, and viral syndromes (including mononucleosis secondary to CMV or Epstein–Barr virus) that may occur irrespective of geography traveled are likewise common.

TABLE 2-9	INCUBATION PERIODS OF SELECTED CAUSES OF FEVER IN THE RETURNED TRAVELER		
Incubation Period	**<10 d**	**10–21 d**	**>21 d**
Bacterial Infections	Bacterial enteritis Bacterial pneumonia Meningococcemia Typhoid and paratyphoid Rickettsiosis (RMSF, African tick bite fever, Mediterranean spotted fever, scrub typhus, Q fever) Relapsing fever Leptospirosis	Typhoid and paratyphoid Rickettsiosis (flea-borne, louse-borne, and scrub typhus, Q fever) Brucella Leptospirosis	Tuberculosis Rickettsiosis (Q fever) Syphilis (secondary) Brucella Bartonellosis (chronic)

TABLE 2-9	INCUBATION PERIODS OF SELECTED CAUSES OF FEVER IN THE RETURNED TRAVELER (CONTINUED)		
Incubation Period	**<10 d**	**10–21 d**	**>21 d**
Viral/ Fungal Infections	Respiratory viruses (e.g., Chikungunya, influenza, SARS) Arboviruses (dengue, Japanese encephalitis, yellow fever) Viral hemorrhagic fevers	Acute HIV CMV Flaviviruses Viral hemorrhagic fevers Rabies Measles Histoplasmosis Coccidioidomycosis	Acute HIV CMV EBV Viral hepatitis Rabies
Parasitic Infections	Malaria Amebic dysentery Fascioliasis African trypanosomiasis (acute)	Malaria Babesiosis Giardia Toxoplasmosis Amebic dysentery African trypanosomiasis (acute)	Malaria (especially *Plasmodium vivax* or in the context of ineffective chemoprophylaxis) Babesiosis Amebic liver disease Schistosomiasis Leishmaniasis Filariasis African trypanosomiasis (chronic)

Adapted from Freedman DO. Infections in returning travelers. In: Mandell GL, Bennett JE, Dolin R, eds. *Mandell, Douglas, and Bennett's Principles and Practice of Infectious Diseases.* 7th ed. Philadelphia, PA: Elsevier; 2009:4019-4028.

CMV, cytomegalovirus; EBV, Epstein–Barr virus; RMSF, Rocky Mountain spotted fever; SARS, severe acute respiratory syndrome.

- Noninfectious causes of fever related to travel may include medications (e.g., chemoprophylaxis or antibiotic therapy prescribed during travel) and thromboembolism related to prolonged venous stasis during transit.
- Empiric antimicrobial therapy may be necessary in the clinically deteriorating patient with suspected malaria, rickettsiosis, leptospirosis, or other infection before a definitive diagnosis can be made.

Sepsis

GENERAL PRINCIPLES

Definitions

- Sepsis is a life-threatening organ dysfunction caused by dysregulated host response to infection.
- Clinically, sepsis is defined as infection in combination with organ dysfunction. The latter is identified by an acute change in Sequential Organ Failure Assessment (SOFA) score of ≥2 points[11] (see Table 2-10).

TABLE 2-10 SEQUENTIAL ORGAN FAILURE ASSESSMENT (SOFA) SCORE

System	0	1	Score 2	3	4
Respiration PaO₂/FIO₂ (mm Hg)	$\geq$400	<400	<300	<200	<100
Coagulation Platelets (× 1000/µL)	$\geq$150	<150	<100	<50	<20
Liver Bilirubin (mg/dL)	<1.2	1.2–1.9	2.0–5.9	6.0–11.9	>12
Cardiovascular	MAP $\geq$70 mm Hg	MAP <70 mm Hg	Dopamine <5 µg/kg/min or dobutamine (any dose)	Dopamine 5.1–15 µg/kg/min or epinephrine $\leq$0.1 µg/kg/min or norepinephrine $\leq$0.1 µg/kg/min	Dopamine >15 µg/kg/min or epinephrine >0.1 µg/kg/min or norepinephrine >0.1 µg/kg/min
Central nervous system Glasgow Coma Scale	15	13–14	10–12	6–9	<6
Renal Creatinine (mg/dL)	<1.2	1.2–1.9	2.0–3.4	3.5–4.9 or UOP <500 mL/d	>5 or UOP <200 mL/d

Adapted from Singer M, Deutschman CS, Seymour CW, et al. The third international consensus definitions for sepsis and septic shock (sepsis-3). *JAMA* 2016;315(8):801-810.

FIO₂, fraction of inspired oxygen; MAP, mean arterial pressure; PaO₂, partial pressure of oxygen.

- Septic shock is a subset of sepsis in which underlying circulatory and cellular/metabolic abnormalities are profound enough to substantially increase mortality. This is recognized clinically by:
  - Persistent hypotension requiring vasopressors *and*
  - Hyperlactatemia >2 mmol/L
- The quick SOFA (qSOFA) score is an abbreviated bedside tool that can help identify patients with sepsis likely to have a poor outcome outside the ICU. Patients with a qSOFA score ≥2 are at greater risk for death or prolonged ICU stay. Elements of the qSOFA score include:
  - Alteration in mental status
  - Systolic blood pressure ≤100 mm Hg
  - Respiratory rate ≥22/min

Pathophysiology

- The host response to infection is normally comprised of a localized inflammatory process mediated by phagocytic cells with little host tissue damage or physiologic derangement. Pattern recognition receptors on these immune cells, including toll-like receptors, selectively bind to damage-associated molecular patterns on invading pathogens, triggering a balance of proinflammatory and anti-inflammatory reactions, thereby eliminating the infection. In sepsis, this balance is unseated, leading to a predominantly proinflammatory, anti-inflammatory, or mixed picture.
- The systemic proinflammatory state of sepsis and septic shock is orchestrated by cytokine (e.g., IL-1, TNF-α) and noncytokine (e.g., nitric oxide) mediators, resulting in endothelial damage, microvascular dysfunction, impaired tissue oxygenation, and organ injury. The anti-inflammatory state is marked by immunosuppression and anergy.

Etiology

- Major causes of sepsis include respiratory, bloodstream, intra-abdominal, and urinary tract infections. Gram-positive and gram-negative bacteria comprise the majority of the causative organisms implicated in sepsis (Table 2-11).[12] Fungal sepsis (mainly with *Candida* spp.) has also become increasingly common, particularly among immunocompromised patients and patients receiving parenteral feeding (Table 2-11).[12]
- Fulminant sepsis can accompany bacteremia with *Neisseria meningitidis*, *S. aureus*, *Yersinia pestis*, *Bacillus anthracis*, and *Capnocytophaga canimorsus* among a handful of other organisms. Asplenic patients are at particular risk for fulminant sepsis with encapsulated organisms (*Streptococcus pneumoniae*, *Haemophilus influenzae*, and *N. meningitidis*).

DIAGNOSIS

- Blood cultures (minimum of 2–3 sets) should be obtained from separate sites preferably before antibiotics have been administered. In the case of catheter-associated bloodstream infection, at least one blood culture should be obtained through the infected catheter.
- Appropriate imaging to identify or confirm sites of infection should be sought as the patient's clinical and hemodynamic status permits.
- Additional diagnostic testing (e.g., lumbar puncture, abscess drainage) should be driven by the type of infection suspected.

TREATMENT

Antimicrobial Therapy

- Early empiric antimicrobial therapy reduces mortality and improves patient outcomes in sepsis.[13]

TABLE 2-11	BACTERIAL PATHOGENS FREQUENTLY ASSOCIATED WITH SEPSIS		
Meningitis	*Streptococcus pneumoniae* *Listeria monocytogenes*	*H. influenzae* *Neisseria meningitidis*	
Pneumonia	*S. pneumoniae* *Haemophilus influenzae* *Staphylococcus aureus*	*Klebsiella pneumoniae* *Pseudomonas aeruginosa*	
Biliary tract infection	*Enterococcus* spp. *Escherichia coli*	*K. pneumoniae*	
Intra-abdominal infection	*E. coli* *Bacteroides fragilis*	*Enterococcus* spp. (rare)	
Urinary tract infection	*E. coli* *Klebsiella* spp. *Enterobacter* spp.	*Proteus* spp. *P. aeruginosa* *Enterococcus* spp.	
Soft tissue and skin infection	*Staph. aureus* Group A streptococci	*Clostridium perfringens*	
Intravascular catheter infection	*Staph. aureus* *Enterococcus faecalis*	*P. aeruginosa*	

Adapted from Munford RS, Suffredini AF. Sepsis. In: Mandell GL, Bennett JE, Dolin R, eds. *Mandell, Douglas, and Bennett's Principles and Practice of Infectious Diseases.* 7th ed. Philadelphia, PA: Elsevier; 2009:987-1010.

- An empiric regimen should target anticipated pathogens and penetrate suspected sites of infection. As always, the risk of multidrug-resistant infection and local antimicrobial susceptibility patterns should be considered.
- Broad-spectrum empiric antimicrobial therapy should cover both gram-positive and gram-negative bacteria.
  - If **Pseudomonas is not suspected**, a combination of vancomycin with one of the following is generally acceptable:
    - Third- or fourth-generation cephalosporin (e.g., ceftriaxone, cefotaxime)
    - β-Lactam/β-lactamase inhibitor (e.g., ampicillin-sulbactam, piperacillin-tazobactam)
    - Carbapenem (e.g., meropenem, imipenem)
  - If **Pseudomonas is a concern,** a combination of vancomycin with one or two of the following is recommended:
    - Antipseudomonal cephalosporin (e.g., cefepime, ceftazidime)
      - Antipseudomonal β-lactam/β-lactamase inhibitor (e.g., piperacillin-tazobactam)
      - Antipseudomonal carbapenem (e.g., meropenem, imipenem)
      - Aminoglycoside (e.g., gentamicin, amikacin; although frequently added for synergy, this practice is not well supported by evidence)
      - Fluoroquinolone with antipseudomonal activity (e.g., ciprofloxacin)
    - Monobactam (e.g., aztreonam)
- For patients with documented colonization or previous infection with a multidrug-resistant organism or who have had prolonged or repeated hospitalizations or exposures to a health care setting, empiric therapy should include appropriate coverage:
  - Methicillin-resistant *S. aureus*: vancomycin
  - Vancomycin-resistant enterococcus: linezolid, daptomycin
  - Extended-spectrum β-lactamase producing gram-negative bacteria: carbapenem
  - Carbapenem-resistant Enterobacteriaceae: ceftazidime-avibactam

- In clinical situations where fungemia is strongly suspected, empiric coverage with an echinocandin or amphotericin B may be warranted until blood cultures have been finalized.
- **Once a pathogen has been isolated in culture and antibiotic susceptibilities determined, empiric antimicrobial therapy should be de-escalated and narrowed accordingly.**
- Duration of therapy should be individualized and guided by the patient's clinical improvement and type of infection (e.g., pneumonia, bloodstream infection).

Source Control

- In addition to antimicrobial therapy, physical interventions are frequently necessary to eradicate primary infectious foci and prevent spread.[13]
- **All abscesses and infected fluid collections** (e.g., empyema) **should be drained.** Complicated intra-abdominal infections (e.g., abscess, cholangitis, necrotizing pancreatitis, peritonitis secondary to organ perforation) may require laparotomy or percutaneous drainage. Necrotizing soft tissue infections mandate emergent surgical debridement.
- **Infected intravascular catheters, urinary catheters, and prosthetic devices should be removed promptly.**
- Endocarditis may necessitate valve replacement.

Other Therapies

- Supportive care of sepsis in the ICU focuses on aggressive volume resuscitation and hemodynamic stabilization to restore perfusion and limit organ dysfunction. Intravenous fluids, vasopressors, and red blood cell transfusions are administered to normalize physiologic parameters including mean arterial pressure, central venous pressure, central venous oxygenation saturation, and urine output.
- Mechanical ventilation may be necessary in the face of pending respiratory compromise in many cases.
- Glycemic control in critical illness contributes to improved outcomes and should aim for a target blood glucose level ≤ 180 mg/dL.

OUTCOME/PROGNOSIS

Even with appropriate and timely medical care, the overall mortality for sepsis remains as high as 40% in critically ill patients. The role of the infectious disease specialist in guiding appropriate antimicrobial therapy and advocating for source control in the patient with sepsis can be crucial in determining clinical outcomes.

REFERENCES

1. Mackowiak PA, Wasserman SS, Levine MM. A critical appraisal of 98.6°F, the upper limit of the normal body temperature, and other legacies of Carl Reinhold August Wunderlich. *JAMA.* 1992;268:1578-1580.
2. Norman DC. Fever in the elderly. *Clin Infect Dis.* 2000;31:148-151.
3. Dimopoulos G, Falagas ME. Approach to the febrile patient in the ICU. *Infect Dis Clin N Am.* 2009;23:471-484.
4. O'Grady NP, Barie PS, Bartlett JG, et al. Guidelines for evaluation of new fever in critically ill adult patients: 2008 update from the American college of critical care medicine and the infectious diseases society of America. *Crit Care Med.* 2008;36:1330-1349.
5. Mermel LA, Allon M, Bouza E, et al. Clinical practice guidelines for the diagnosis and management of intravascular catheter-related infection: 2009 update by the infectious diseases society of America. *Clin Infect Dis.* 2009;49:1-45.

6. Hooton TM, Bradley SF, Cardenas DD, et al. Diagnosis, prevention, and treatment of catheter-associated urinary tract infection in adults: 2009 international clinical practice guidelines from the Infectious Diseases Society of America. *Clin Infect Dis.* 2010;50:625-663.

7. Cohen SH, Gerding DN, Johnson S, et al. Clinical practice guidelines for Clostridium difficile infection in adults: 2010 update by the Society for Healthcare Epidemiology of American (SHEA) and the Infectious Diseases Society of America (IDSA). *Infect Control Hosp Epidemiol.* 2010;31:431-455.

8. Freifeld AG, Bow EJ, Sepkowitz KA, et al. Clinical practice guideline for the use of antimicrobial agents in neutropenic patients with cancer: 2010 update by the Infectious Diseases Society of America. *Clin Infect Dis.* 2011;52:e56-93.

9. Wilson ME, Weld LH, Boggild A, et al. Fever in returned travelers: results from the geosentinel surveillance network. *Clin Infect Dis.* 2007;44:1560-1568.

10. Freedman DO. Infections in returning travelers. In: Mandell GL, Bennett JE, Dolin R, eds. *Mandell, Douglas, and Bennett's Principles and Practice of Infectious Diseases.* 7th ed. Philadelphia, PA: Elsevier; 2009:4019-4028.

11. Singer M, Deutschman CS, Seymour CW, et al. The third international consensus definitions for sepsis and septic shock (sepsis-3). *JAMA.* 2016;315(8):801-810.

12. Munford RS, Suffredini AF. Sepsis. In: Mandell GL, Bennett JE, Dolin R, eds. *Mandell, Douglas, and Bennett's Principles and Practice of Infectious Diseases.* 7th ed. Philadelphia, PA: Elsevier; 2009:987-1010.

13. Rhodes A, Evans LE, Alhazzani W, et al. Surviving sepsis campaign: international guidelines for management of sepsis and septic shock: 2016. *Crit Care Med.* 2017;45(3):486-552.

Fever of Unknown Origin

Mohammad J. Saeed and Michael J. Durkin

3

GENERAL PRINCIPLES

Definition

Classic fever of unknown origin (FUO) is defined as an illness lasting >3 weeks with temperatures >38.3°C (101°F) on multiple occasions and no established etiology after 3 days of inpatient hospitalization or three outpatient visits, despite appropriate investigations.

Etiology

Infections account for 25% to 40% of all cases of FUO in the United States, followed by neoplasm (15%–30%), connective tissue disorders (10%–20%), and miscellaneous disorders (15%–20%). A definitive cause may not be found in up to 15% of cases. Over the years, advances in imaging and diagnostic microbiology have led to a decrease in infections and malignancies as a cause of FUO, while inflammatory diseases and unknown causes have increased.[1-4]

- The differential diagnosis of infectious causes of FUO can be extensive (see Table 3-1).[1]
- In many instances, FUO may constitute an atypical presentation of a common disease rather than a typical presentation of a rare disease.
- Causes of FUO vary significantly by geography. Infections acquired in endemic regions through travel or residence may present to care as FUO in nonendemic areas.

TABLE 3-1	CAUSES OF CLASSIC FEVER OF UNKNOWN ORIGIN	
Etiology	Common	Uncommon
Infectious diseases	*Bacteria*	*Bacteria*
	Abscess	Chronic sinusitis
	Subacute bacterial endocarditis	Brucellosis
	Culture-negative endocarditis	Q fever
		Rat bite fever
	Osteomyelitis	Leptospirosis
	Tuberculosis	Relapsing fever
	Typhoid fever	Ehrlichiosis
	Cat-scratch disease	Scrub and murine typhus
		Melioidosis
		Lymphogranuloma venereum
		Whipple disease

(Continued)

TABLE 3-1	CAUSES OF CLASSIC FEVER OF UNKNOWN ORIGIN (CONTINUED)	
Etiology	**Common**	**Uncommon**
	Virus	*Virus*
	Epstein–Barr virus	Parvovirus B19
	Cytomegalovirus	Chikungunya fever
	HIV	
		Fungus
		Coccidioidomycosis
		Histoplasmosis
		Parasite
		Malaria
		Babesiosis
		Toxoplasmosis
		Trichinosis
		Visceral leishmaniasis
Neoplastic disorders	Lymphoma	Atrial myxoma
	Leukemia	Central nervous system tumors
	Myelodysplastic syndrome	Multiple myeloma
	Renal cell carcinoma	Hemophagocytic lymphohistiocytosis
	Hepatocellular carcinoma	
	Liver metastases	Colon carcinoma
	Pancreatic carcinoma	
Rheumatic disorders	Temporal (giant cell) arteritis	Granulomatosis with polyangiitis (Wegener granulomatosis)
	Polymyalgia rheumatica	Takayasu arteritis
	Adult-onset Still disease	Behçet disease
	Polyarteritis nodosa	Cryoglobulinemic vasculitis
	Systemic lupus erythematosus	Kikuchi–Fujimoto disease
	Rheumatoid arthritis	Polyarticular gout/pseudogout
Miscellaneous disorders	Drug fever	Thromboembolic disease
	Hematoma	Periodic fever syndromes
	Alcoholic hepatitis	Sweet syndrome
	Inflammatory bowel disease	Schnitzler syndrome (with hives)
	Sarcoidosis	Hypothalamic dysfunction
	Subacute thyroiditis	Hyperthyroidism
		Pheochromocytoma
		Adrenal insufficiency
		Factitious fever

Adapted from Cunha BA. Fever of unknown origin: clinical overview of classic and current concepts. *Infect Dis Clin North Am.* 2007;21:867-915.

Bacterial Infections

- **Tuberculosis** remains an important cause of FUO. In particular, disseminated (miliary) and extrapulmonary tuberculosis (e.g., renal, mesenteric lymphadenitis) may present initially with vague and protean manifestations.
- **Subacute bacterial endocarditis** with *Streptococcus viridans* and **culture-negative endocarditis** with less virulent organisms (e.g., *Coxiella burnetii*, *Bartonella* spp., *Brucella*, HACEK [*Haemophilus parainfluenzae*, *Aggregatibacter* spp., *Cardiobacterium hominis*, *Eikenella corrodens*, *Kingella kingae*] group organisms) may manifest insidiously as FUO in the context of a new heart murmur with or without peripheral stigmata. Blood cultures can be negative if patients have received antibiotics.
- **Occult abscesses** in the abdomen or pelvis may arise in the context of recent surgery, infection (e.g., cholecystitis, cholangitis, appendicitis, diverticulitis, urinary tract infection), diabetes mellitus, or immunosuppression. Septic emboli from endocarditis commonly lead to splenic abscesses. Dental abscesses can also be a rare cause of FUO.
- **Occult osteomyelitis** may present as FUO accompanied by musculoskeletal complaints. Vertebral osteomyelitis should be suspected in elderly patients with a history of fever and recurrent urinary tract infections.
- **Typhoid fever** (*Salmonella typhi*), acquired through travel and ingestion of contaminated food or water, may present with persistent fever, abdominal pain, relative bradycardia, hepatosplenomegaly, rose spots, and leukopenia.
- **Cat-scratch disease** (*Bartonella henselae*) should be suspected in the patient with fever, lymphadenopathy, and recent history of a cat bite or scratch.
- **Q fever** (*C. burnetii*) may manifest as a flu-like illness after close contact with cattle, sheep, and goats or the consumption of contaminated dairy products.
- **Brucellosis** is marked by undulant fevers, sweating, and migratory arthralgias. It has been associated with the consumption of unpasteurized milk or goat cheese.

Viral Infections

- **Epstein-Barr virus** and **cytomegalovirus (CMV)** may present as fever, fatigue, lymphadenopathy, and transaminitis. Leukopenia and atypical lymphocytes seen on peripheral smear may aid in diagnosis.
- **HIV/AIDS** and associated opportunistic infections (e.g., mycobacteria, CMV) and neoplasms can manifest as FUO in the absence of antiretroviral therapy and adequate antibiotic prophylaxis.

Fungal Infections

- Endemic mycoses including **histoplasmosis** and **coccidioidomycosis** should be considered in patients reporting travel to or residence in geographic locations traditionally associated with these fungi.
- Disseminated histoplasmosis and tuberculosis bear many similarities.

Parasitic Infections

- **Toxoplasmosis** in immunocompetent patients may present with fever, lymphadenopathy, and myalgias in the setting of ingestion of raw or partially cooked meat or exposure to cat litter. A peripheral smear may reveal atypical lymphocytes.
- **Visceral leishmaniasis** (kala-azar) involving the liver, spleen, and bone marrow can manifest with FUO accompanied by weight loss, malaise, hepatosplenomegaly, anemia, and elevated liver function tests after travel to an endemic region.

Neoplasm

- **Lymphoma**, especially non-Hodgkin lymphoma, remains the most common neoplastic etiology of FUO. Fever, night sweats, weight loss, and lymphadenopathy warrant further evaluation with imaging and lymph node biopsy.

- **Leukemias** and **myelodysplastic syndromes** can be identified on peripheral smear but may ultimately require a bone marrow biopsy for diagnosis.
- **Renal cell carcinoma** may present with fever and hematuria. **Hepatocellular carcinoma** and **metastatic liver cancer** also frequently present as FUO.
- **Atrial myxoma** should be considered in the patient with fever, weight loss, a heart murmur, and negative blood cultures.

Connective Tissue Disorders
- In young and middle-aged adults, **adult-onset Still disease** ("juvenile rheumatoid arthritis") is marked by fever >39°C (102.2°F), arthritis, and an evanescent salmon-pink rash. Lymphadenopathy and splenomegaly coupled with leukocytosis and elevated erythrocyte sedimentation rate (ESR), C-reactive protein (CRP), ferritin (>1000 ng/mL), and liver enzymes may suggest the diagnosis.
- In a patient over age 50, **temporal arteritis** may present with a constellation of fever, headache, jaw claudication, and abrupt vision loss. Tenderness to palpation or diminished pulsation over the temporal artery coupled with an ESR >50 mm/h should prompt consideration of temporal artery biopsy.
- **Polymyalgia rheumatica** presents with bilateral aching and morning stiffness of the neck, torso, shoulders, and hip girdle with ESR >40 mm/h.

Miscellaneous Disorders
- **Drug fever** may arise from any number of medications. Antimicrobials (e.g., sulfonamides, penicillins, cephalosporins, vancomycin, nitrofurantoin), anticonvulsants (e.g., phenytoin, carbamazepine, barbiturates), H1 and H2 blocking antihistamines, antihypertensives (e.g., hydralazine, methyldopa), and antiarrhythmic drugs (e.g., quinidine, procainamide) are common causes. Rash and eosinophilia may or may not be present.
- **Factitious fever** is a psychiatric illness. Manipulation of thermometers may lead to spurious readings, while self-administration of nonsterile injections can cause intentional infections.
- **Periodic fever syndromes** (e.g., familial Mediterranean fever, tumor necrosis factor 1–associated periodic syndrome, hyperimmunoglobulinemia D syndrome) are autoinflammatory and hereditary in nature.
- **Sarcoidosis** manifesting with fever, night sweats, weight loss, fatigue, cough, and lymphadenopathy can be mistaken for other granulomatous diseases, notably tuberculosis and histoplasmosis.
- **Alcoholic hepatitis** may be characterized by low-grade fevers, jaundice, hepatosplenomegaly, and abnormal liver function tests with an aspartate aminotransferase: alanine aminotransferase ratio of 2:1.
- **Inflammatory bowel disease** frequently presents with fever, weight loss, abdominal pain, and diarrhea with or without gastrointestinal bleeding.
- Endocrine disorders including **hyperthyroidism**, **pheochromocytoma**, and **adrenal insufficiency** may occasionally surface as FUO.
- Unexplained fever may be the only presenting feature of a **deep vein thrombosis** or **pulmonary embolus**.

DIAGNOSIS

Clinical Presentation

A comprehensive history and physical examination focuses the diagnostic evaluation of FUO and spares the patient unnecessary tests and procedures.[5]

History
- Establish a time line of any and all symptoms.
- Characterize all prior infections, malignancies, and their subsequent medical management. All surgeries, postsurgical complications, foreign materials, and prosthetic devices should be identified.
- Review all current prescription and over-the-counter medications.
- Obtain a complete social history including environmental, occupational, recreational, sexual, dietary, animal, and travel exposures.
- A family history should identify inherited malignancies and inflammatory disorders, as well as any common symptomatology or prior infections between family members.

Physical Examination
- **Verify the presence of fever.** Comparison of temperatures taken from multiple sites (oral, rectal, voided urine) can aid in clarifying a factitious fever.
- Most fevers peak in the late or early afternoon. Abnormal fever patterns may be helpful in selected cases provided that antipyretic medications or body cooling devices have not altered their periodicity.
  - Morning fever spikes: typhoid fever, tuberculosis, polyarteritis nodosa.
  - Double quotidian fevers (two temperature spikes within 24 h): disseminated (miliary) tuberculosis, visceral leishmaniasis, or adult-onset Still disease.
  - Relative bradycardia: malaria, typhoid fever, drug fever, central nervous system disorder. Beware of confounding medications (e.g., β-blockers, calcium channel blockers).
- Inspect the eyes (including fundi). Palpate the sinuses and temporal arteries. Examine the oropharynx for ulcers, thrush, and evidence of dental infection. Look for thyromegaly.
- A new heart murmur may suggest bacterial endocarditis, marantic endocarditis (e.g., systemic lupus erythematosus), or atrial myxoma.
- Hepatomegaly, splenomegaly, and any abnormal abdominal masses should be noted. Genitourinary and rectal examination should be performed to look for ulcerative lesions and signs of perirectal abscess.
- Thoroughly examine the skin, joints, and all major lymph nodes.
- Repeat physical examination may be necessary to identify subtle and evolving findings as the FUO progresses with time.

Diagnostic Testing

Laboratories
- Basic laboratory evaluation should include a complete blood count with differential, liver function panel, urinalysis, and nonspecific inflammatory markers including an ESR, CRP, and ferritin level. Highly elevated ESR (>100 mm/h) can be suggestive of abscess, osteomyelitis, or endocarditis. Highly elevated ferritin levels favor noninfectious etiologies of FUO.[6]
- **At least three blood cultures should be obtained, while the patient is off antibiotics, preferably during febrile episodes and several hours apart.**
- All patients should be screened for HIV infection and syphilis.
- Purified protein derivative skin test or interferon gamma release assay is recommended. While a positive test may suggest infection, **a negative result cannot exclude it**.
- Additional laboratory tests may include antinuclear antibodies, rheumatoid factor, and serum protein electrophoresis if a rheumatologic diagnosis is being considered.
- Infection-specific serologies and other definitive diagnostic assays should be ordered based on the prevalence and degree of clinical suspicion for that disease in order to minimize the risk of false-positive results.

Imaging
- Obtain a screening chest radiogram if pulmonary complaints exist.
- Computed tomography (CT) of the chest, abdomen, and pelvis may be helpful in identifying occult abscesses, hematoma, or lymphadenopathy.
- Echocardiography should be reserved for patients with a heart murmur where endocarditis or other valvular abnormality is suspected.
- Nuclear medicine studies (e.g., gallium scintigraphy, indium white blood cell scanning, fluorodeoxyglucose positron emission tomography/CT) may be helpful in localizing occult infection, inflammation, or malignancy.

Diagnostic Procedures
- Tissue biopsy is frequently required to establish the etiology of FUO.
- All biopsied tissues should be sent for appropriate culture (e.g., bacterial, mycobacterial, fungal) and sensitivity in addition to pathology.
- **Liver biopsy** is useful in establishing the cause of granulomatous hepatitis, which may be seen in disseminated tuberculosis, histoplasmosis, or sarcoidosis.
- **Lymph node biopsy** is crucial in diagnosing lymphoma and can also aid with the identification of disseminated granulomatous infections, toxoplasmosis, and cat-scratch disease.
- **Bone marrow biopsy** may be necessary to confirm leukemia and myelodysplastic syndrome. It should be strongly considered with infections associated with bone marrow involvement (e.g., disseminated tuberculosis and histoplasmosis).
- **Exploratory laparotomy** is rarely indicated given modern imaging and guided biopsy techniques.

TREATMENT

Antimicrobial Therapy

- In the absence of clinical deterioration or a severely immunocompromised state (neutropenic fever, solid organ or hematopoietic stem cell transplant, advanced AIDS, asplenia), empiric antibiotics are **rarely** indicated in the initial management of fever without a clear source. In many cases, they may delay diagnosis and optimal antimicrobial therapy through partial treatment of infection (e.g., tuberculosis).
- Most infections associated with classic FUO are indolent and subacute. Emphasis should be placed on establishing a definitive diagnosis.
- Disseminated tuberculosis is one of the few exceptions where antimicrobial therapy is reasonable if the suspicion is high. Adequate cultures should be obtained **before** therapy to confirm diagnosis.
- Culture-negative endocarditis likewise warrants empiric therapy once adequate blood cultures have been obtained.

Other Interventions

- Withdrawal of offending medications frequently leads to resolution of a drug fever within 72 hours.
- Timely corticosteroid therapy and other immunosuppression are important in rheumatic disorders, particularly temporal arteritis.
- Chemotherapy, radiation, and surgery may be necessary depending on the type of neoplastic disorder identified.

PROGNOSIS

- Prognosis is dictated by timely diagnosis of life-threatening infections, malignancies, and other miscellaneous disorders.
- The longer the duration of FUO without progressive clinical deterioration, the less likely the FUO is infectious in nature.

- If no clear etiology of FUO has been found despite a thorough evaluation for infections, neoplasm, connective tissue disorders, and miscellaneous causes, patient mortality is generally low and prognosis is considered good. Spontaneous resolution of FUO is not uncommon. Long-term follow-up is indicated to monitor for recurrence of fever.

SPECIAL CONSIDERATIONS

In addition to the classic form, FUO has also been described in the context of several patient populations at heightened risk for infectious complications.

Health Care–Associated Fever of Unknown Origin

- Defined as fever >38.3°C (101°F) on several occasions in a hospitalized patient without an initial infection on admission and having no established cause after at least 3 days of investigation and 48 hours of culture incubation.
- Common etiologies include catheter-related infection, sinusitis, postoperative complications, *Clostridium difficile* infection, thromboembolic disease (deep vein thrombosis/pulmonary embolism), and drug fever (Table 3-2). Health care–associated and aspiration pneumonia must also be considered in the nonintubated patient.

Immunodeficiency (neutropenic) and Fever of Unknown Origin

- Defined as fever >38.3°C (101°F) on several occasions in a patient with an absolute neutrophil count <500 cells/μL (or anticipated decline below this level within the next 48 h) with no established cause after at least 3 days of investigation and 48 hours of culture incubation.
- Opportunistic infections, invasive fungal infections, health care–associated infections, and drug fever are most frequently implicated (Table 3-3).
- Repeated and prolonged hospitalization places immune-deficient patients at high risk of colonization and infection with multidrug-resistant organisms.
- Empiric antimicrobial therapy should be instituted promptly based on suspicion for serious bacterial or fungal infection.

TABLE 3-2	CAUSES OF HEALTH CARE–ASSOCIATED FEVER OF UNKNOWN ORIGIN
Risk Factor	**Complication**
Central venous catheter	Insertion site infection
	Catheter-related bloodstream infection
	Suppurative thrombophlebitis
	Endocarditis
Arterial catheter	Insertion site infection
	Catheter-related bloodstream infection
Nasogastric, nasoendotracheal, endotracheal tube	Sinusitis
Urinary catheter	Urinary tract infection
Mechanical ventilation	Ventilator-associated pneumonia
Surgery	Surgical site infection
Recent antibiotic exposure	*Clostridium difficile* infection

TABLE 3-3	CAUSES OF IMMUNE-DEFICIENT FEVER OF UNKNOWN ORIGIN
Bacteria	*Staphylococcus aureus*
	Coagulase-negative staphylococcus
	Streptococcus spp.
	Enterococcus spp.
	Pseudomonas aeruginosa
	Escherichia coli
	Enterobacteriaceae
	Klebsiella spp.
	Nocardia spp.
	Clostridium difficile
Virus	Human herpesviruses (HSV, CMV, EBV, VZV, HHV-6)
	Respiratory viruses (RSV, parainfluenza, influenza, adenovirus, rhinovirus, human metapneumovirus)
Fungi	*Candida* sp.
	Cryptococcus neoformans
	Aspergillus spp.
	Fusarium spp.
	Zygomycetes
	Histoplasma capsulatum
	Blastomyces dermatitidis
	Coccidioides immitis
	Pneumocystis jiroveci

CMV, cytomegalovirus; EBV, Epstein–Barr virus; HHV, human herpesvirus; HSV, herpes simplex virus; RSV, respiratory syncytial virus; VZV, varicella zoster virus.

HIV-Associated Fever of Unknown Origin

- Defined as fever >38.3°C (101°F) on several occasions in a patient with HIV infection, lasting more than 3 weeks with no established cause after 3 days of inpatient hospitalization and 48 hours of culture incubation.
- In patients with low CD4+ cell counts, opportunistic infections including infection with *Mycobacterium avium-intracellulare*, CMV, *Pneumocystis jiroveci*, *Cryptococcus neoformans*, and *Toxoplasma gondii* are frequently encountered, particularly in the absence of prophylactic antimicrobials. Tuberculosis, *Bartonella* infection, and endemic mycoses (histoplasmosis, coccidioidomycosis) remain important causes of FUO.
- Immune reconstitution inflammatory syndrome after the initiation of antiretroviral therapy can present as FUO with reactivation or worsening of preexisting opportunistic infections.
- Neoplastic disorders (lymphoma) and drug fever related to antiretroviral and prophylactic antimicrobial therapy are also common causes of FUO (Tables 3-3 and 3-4).

TABLE 3-4	CAUSES OF HIV-ASSOCIATED FEVER OF UNKNOWN ORIGIN
Infectious disorders	*Mycobacterium tuberculosis*
	Mycobacterium avium-intracellulare
	Bartonella spp.
	CMV
	Pneumocystis jiroveci
	Cryptococcus neoformans
	Aspergillus spp.
	Histoplasma capsulatum
	Coccidioides immitis
	Toxoplasma gondii
	Leishmania
	IRIS-associated opportunistic infection
Neoplastic disorders	Lymphoma (non-Hodgkin, central nervous system, B cell)
	Kaposi sarcoma
	Castleman disease
Rheumatic disorders	Systemic lupus erythematosus
Miscellaneous disorders	Drug fever

CMV, cytomegalovirus; IRIS, immune reconstitution inflammatory syndrome.

REFERENCES

1. Cunha BA. Fever of unknown origin: clinical overview of classic and current concepts. *Infect Dis Clin North Am.* 2007;21(4):867.
2. de Kleijn EM, Knoeckaert D, van der Meer JW. Fever of unknown origin (FUO). A prospective multicenter study of 167 patient, using fixed epidemiologic criteria. The Netherlands FUO Study Group. *Medicine (Baltimore).* 1997;76:392.
3. Zenone T. Fever of unknown origin in adults: evaluation of 144 cases in a non-university hospital. *Scan J Infect Dis.* 2006;38:632.
4. Horowitz HW. Fever of unknown origin or fever of too many origins? *N Engl J Med.* 2013;368:197.
5. Cunha BA, Lotholary O, Cunha CB. Fever of unknown origin: a clinical approach. *Am J Med.* 2015;128:1138e.
6. Bleeker-Rovers CP, Vos FJ, de Kleijn EM, et al. A prospective study on fever of unknown origin: the yield of a structured diagnostic protocol. *Medicine (Baltimore).* 2007;86:26.

Bacteremia and Infections of the Cardiovascular System

Merilda Blanco and Michael J. Durkin

4

Bacteremia and Fungemia

GENERAL PRINCIPLES

- Bacteremia is common in hospitalized patients, and the incidence is increasing. This is likely due to the increasing use of central venous catheters (CVCs) and implantable cardiac devices and the increased severity of illness in hospitalized patients.
- Fungemia is the presence of fungi in the blood. Many of the principles of bacteremia and fungemia are the same. For general principles, the term *bacteremia* will refer to both entities unless specified.

Definition

- Bacteremia is defined as the presence of bacteria in the bloodstream. Bacteremia is not an uncommon event even in healthy, asymptomatic people. Transient bacteremia can be provoked by eating, brushing teeth, or minor scrapes and cuts. These transient episodes of bacteremia are usually eliminated by the host immune system. Clinical disease occurs when bacteremia overcomes the host's immune defense.
- There are many potential causes of bacteremia. Primary bacteremia is due to an intravascular source of infection, such as the heart and a blood vessel. Primary bacteremia can also occur when normal barriers to the bloodstream are disrupted, as with a vascular catheter, or as a result of to trauma. Secondary bacteremia occurs when a bacterial infection of a noncardiovascular tissue is introduced into the vascular supply. Urinary tract infections, respiratory infections, infections of the gastrointestinal tract, and skin and soft tissue infections can all result in invasion of organisms into the bloodstream. Spontaneous secondary bacteremia may occur in immunosuppressed individuals owing to translocation of gut bacteria into the bloodstream.

Epidemiology

- Clinically significant bacteremia occurs most commonly in hospitalized patients. Because of more frequent use of home intravenous (IV) catheters for hemodialysis and administration of chemotherapy, antibiotics, or parenteral nutrition, as well as more frequent implantation of cardiovascular devices, bacteremia is also becoming a problem in the outpatient setting.
- Bacteremia should be considered in any patient with fever who has implanted vascular devices or implanted cardiac devices, in neutropenic patients, or in patients with evidence of bacterial infection at distant sites. It is critically important in these patient populations to obtain blood cultures before the institution of antibiotics to diagnose and identify the cause of bacteremia.

Etiology

- Many gram-negative, gram-positive, aerobic, or anaerobic bacteria can cause bacteremia. The source of infection can give clues to the possible organism involved. Clinical consideration should be given to the probable source of the infection.

- Urinary tract infections are most commonly caused by aerobic gram-negative bacteria, usually enterobacteriaceae. *Escherichia coli* accounts for >50% of bacteremias associated with infections of the urinary tract.
- Bacteremias with a respiratory source are commonly caused by *Streptococcus pneumoniae*, *Klebsiella pneumoniae*, and *Pseudomonas aeruginosa*.
- If skin or soft tissue infection is the source, the most common organisms include normal gram-positive skin flora such as *Streptococcus* and *Staphylococcus* spp.
- If an abdominal source is suspected, infection is likely from *E. coli* or other enterobacteriaceae, *Bacteroides* spp., other anaerobes, or mixed organisms.
- Neutropenic patients are particularly at risk for infection with gram-negative organisms such as *Pseudomonas aeruginosa*.
- Patients with prolonged hospitalization are at risk for bacteremia with resistant organisms such as *P. aeruginosa*, *Acinetobacter baumannii*, and methicillin-resistant *Staphylococcus aureus* (MRSA).
- Patients on antibiotics are also at risk for bacteremia caused by resistant organisms as well as fungi.
- Patients with *Staphylococcus aureus* bacteremia or bacteremia from highly resistant organisms have a much higher mortality.

DIAGNOSIS

- All patients presenting with fever, sepsis, altered sensorium, or shock should be suspected of potentially having bloodstream infections.
- If bloodstream infection is suspected, patients should be evaluated for the causative organism, the source of infection, and the severity of illness.
- Blood cultures should be obtained from two to three separate venipuncture sites, as well as from any indwelling vascular catheter, over 15 to 30 minutes. **Cultures should be obtained before starting antibiotics.**
- The source should also be determined. Common causes include CVCs (addressed in detail in a later section), the genitourinary tract, the respiratory tract, and the gastrointestinal tract. Additional workup, such as urinalysis, chest radiography, and abdominal imaging, should be determined based on clinical suspicion.
- Determining the causative organism as well as the source of bacteremia is of paramount importance, as this will determine the choice of treatment and the duration of therapy.

TREATMENT

- Empiric antimicrobial therapy should be based on the most likely causative organisms. Treatment should be initiated with parenteral antibiotics.
  - If the source of bacteremia is thought to be **skin or soft tissues**, the selected agent should be geared toward gram-positive organisms including streptococci and staphylococci. If there is a high local incidence of MRSA, vancomycin should be included in the initial empiric treatment. Otherwise, treatment may be initiated with nafcillin, oxacillin, clindamycin, or cephalosporins.
  - If the source is thought to be the urinary tract, treatment should be geared toward gram-negative organisms including *E. coli*. Empiric treatment could include a fluoroquinolone or a third-generation cephalosporin.
  - If the source is thought to be the **abdomen**, treatment should be effective against gram-negative and anaerobic organisms, specifically *E. coli* and *Bacteroides* spp. Empiric treatment could include a β-lactam combined with a β-lactamase inhibitor, a third- or fourth-generation cephalosporin combined with metronidazole, or a carbapenem.

- ○ In **neutropenic patients**, the initial antibiotic should be geared toward gram-negative organisms. The agent should have coverage against *P. aeruginosa*. Empiric treatment should be with an antipseudomonal cephalosporin, carbapenem, ciprofloxacin, or piperacillin/tazobactam. Neutropenic patients with hypotension, mucositis, evidence of a skin or catheter site infection, known MRSA colonization, or clinical deterioration should also be empirically covered with an agent effective against MRSA: vancomycin or daptomycin.
- ○ Patients who have been **hospitalized or are in a health care setting** should initially be treated with broad-spectrum antibiotics with coverage against resistant organisms such as *P. aeruginosa* and MRSA. Treatment options are similar to options for neutropenic patients.
- ○ **Critically ill patients** should be covered with broad-spectrum antibiotics until the causative organism is known. Consideration should also be given to antifungal coverage in critically ill patients.
- Definitive treatment should be tailored to the results of culture and sensitivity testing. In rare cases, route of antimicrobial therapy may be switched from parenteral to oral once the organism, susceptibilities, source, and extent of infection are known.
- Duration of treatment will be based on the source of infection and the severity of illness.
- **Fungemia** is the presence of fungi in the blood. The most common fungi found in the bloodstream are *Candida* spp. Empiric antifungal choice should depend on the severity of illness and the prevalence of non-albicans *Candida* spp. in the hospital population. Most *Candida albicans* are sensitive to fluconazole. *Candida glabrata* and *Candida krusei* are commonly resistant to fluconazole. Echinocandins are preferred for infections due to *C. glabrata* and *C. krusei*. *Candida parapsilosis* is less sensitive to the echinocandins, and fluconazole is the preferred agent.

Catheter-Related Bacteremia and Fungemia

GENERAL PRINCIPLES

- This section is devoted to the treatment of catheter-related bloodstream infections (CRBSIs). Many of the principles of diagnosis and treatment are the same as in the previous section. This section focuses on the differences from other sources of bacteremia.
- The use of CVCs is a necessary component of health care delivery in a hospitalized patient, and their use outside of hospitals is increasingly frequent.
- Complicated CRBSIs are catheter-related bacteremias with evidence of distant site seeding, for example, endocarditis, septic thrombophlebitis, osteomyelitis, and intracranial or distant abscesses.

Epidemiology

- The risk of developing a CRBSI is dependent on several factors, including the type of catheter used, the location of the catheter, the setting (i.e., inpatient or outpatient; intensive care unit [ICU] or general wards), the duration of catheter placement, frequency of catheter manipulation, and patient-dependent factors and comorbidities such as diabetes and obesity.
- Peripheral IV catheters are associated with low risk of bacteremia; however, inflammation or phlebitis is not uncommon when the catheter is left in place for a prolonged duration.
- **Temporary, nontunneled CVCs and pulmonary artery catheters have the highest risk of infection.** The risk of infection with CVCs is dependent on the site used. The subclavian vein is the preferred location with the lowest infection risk, followed by internal jugular vein. **Femoral venous catheters have the highest rates of infection and should be avoided whenever possible.** Catheters placed emergently are at higher risk for infection and should be replaced once a patient is stabilized.

- Tunneled CVCs have a lower risk of infection than nontunneled catheters. Peripherally inserted central venous catheters (PICCs) also have lower rates of infection than nontunneled CVCs.
- Totally implanted vascular access devices (ports) have the lowest overall risk of infection. Placement and removal of implanted venous catheters require a surgical procedure.
- Overall, nontunneled CVCs account for about 90% of all CRBSIs.

Etiology

- The most common organisms identified in CRBSIs are gram positive. Coagulase-negative staphylococci are the most common, followed by *Staphylococcus aureus*, gram-negatives, enterococci, and *Candida*. Among gram-negative organisms, the most common are enterobacteriaceae (*E. coli*, *Klebsiella* spp., and *Enterobacter* spp.) and *Pseudomonas aeruginosa*.
- CRBSI with *S. aureus* has the highest mortality with a rate of 8.2%.[1] Coagulase-negative staphylococcal CRBSI has the lowest associated mortality.
- Prolonged hospitalization, ICU admission, and prior antibiotic exposure increase the risk of more resistant organisms. Infection with *Candida* spp. should be considered in patients on broad-spectrum antibiotics and those receiving lipid-rich formulations, such as parenteral nutrition and propofol. Colonization of urinary catheters and endotracheal or tracheostomy tubes with *Candida* can predispose patients to fungemia.
- Bacteria usually enter the blood by migrating from the skin at the site of line insertion. Less commonly, the catheter may be hematogenously seeded by bacteria or fungi that entered the blood at a distant site.

Prevention

- **Most CRBSIs are preventable.** A multifaceted approach should be taken in attempts to prevent catheter infections.[2]
- Insertion of the catheter should be **performed** after proper hand hygiene, **with the use of maximal sterile barrier precautions**, including sterile gloves, cap, mask, gown, and full body drape. Skin cleansing should be performed using 2% chlorhexidine solution. The preferred site for insertion of a nontunneled CVC is the subclavian vein followed by the internal jugular vein.
- **The femoral vein should be used for CVC insertion only when there are no other options or in emergency situations. When a femoral CVC is placed, it should be removed as soon as alternative venous access can be established.**
- When the CVC is expected to be needed for a prolonged period of time, tunneled catheters, PICC, and totally implanted catheters should be used when feasible.
- CVCs should be **removed as soon as central venous access is no longer needed.** Routine catheter exchange and exchange of the catheter over a wire are not generally recommended.
- Systemic antimicrobial prophylaxis during insertion or use of a catheter for the purpose of preventing CRBSI is not recommended.

DIAGNOSIS

- The most common presentation of a CRBSI is a **new fever in a patient with an intravascular catheter.** Any patient with a new fever and an intravascular device should be evaluated by means of vital signs and physical examination.
- The catheter should be evaluated for obvious signs of infection such as erythema or purulent drainage, although these signs are not commonly present.
- The patient should also be evaluated for alternative sources of fever.
- The diagnosis of a CRBSI requires obtaining **a minimum of two cultures, with at least one via peripheral venipuncture.** The diagnosis is made if one or more cultures are positive with a pathogen associated with CRBSI in the absence of another source of bloodstream infection (i.e., pneumonia and urinary tract infection).

- If a common skin contaminant (diphtheroids, *Bacillus* spp., coagulase-negative *Staphylococcus*, and *Propionibacterium* spp.) is grown in culture, it should be confirmed by growth in two or more cultures drawn on separate occasions.
- Cultures should be **always** be drawn before the administration of antibiotics if possible.

TREATMENT

- **Empiric antibiotic coverage should target the most likely causative organisms.** The first-line agent for empiric treatment is **vancomycin**. In critically ill patients or patients with other comorbid conditions, the addition of gram-negative coverage or an antifungal agent should be considered.
- **Catheter removal is a key component** in the management of CRBSI. In general, all intravascular catheters should be removed if there is evidence of an insertion site infection (e.g., purulent drainage, erythema, induration, and pain at the site of insertion). Clinically unstable patients in whom CRBSI is suspected should have the catheter removed as soon as possible.
- Nontunneled, nonimplanted CVCs should be removed in almost all circumstances when CRBSI is suspected. If CRBSI is suspected, the patient should be evaluated for alternative sites for venous access. If central venous access is needed, the existing catheter should be removed once alternative access is achieved. If the patient does not need central venous access, the existing catheter should be removed and a peripheral catheter placed.
- If a patient has persistent fevers without a clear source, consideration should be given to CVC removal or exchange even in the absence of positive blood cultures or evidence of an insertion site infection.
- In rare cases, when a patient is stable and an uncomplicated CRBSI is due to coagulase-negative *Staphylococcus*, the physician may choose to retain the catheter if alternative access is problematic. If the catheter is retained, treatment should be with 10 to 14 days of effective parenteral antibiotics, accompanied by antibiotic lock therapy.[1]
- Infection of a long-term CVC (e.g., tunneled catheter or totally implanted catheter) presents a unique challenge when it comes to catheter removal. The choice to remove or retain the catheter is dependent on the causative organism, the indication for the long-term catheter, and the presence or absence of an alternative site for vascular access.
- In a patient with long-term CVC without exit site or tunnel infection, uncomplicated bacteremia with organisms other than *S. aureus* or *Candida* spp., and for whom alternative access is problematic, catheter salvage may be considered with use of systemic antibiotics plus antibiotic lock therapy for 2 weeks.[1]
- Antibiotic lock therapy is the instillation of a highly concentrated antibiotic solution into the lumen of a catheter to allow long dwelling times with the purpose of eliminating bacteria in biofilm. The lock will depend on the type of catheter, frequency of use, organism, and patient characteristics. Examples of solutions previously used for this purpose include vancomycin, cefazolin, ciprofloxacin, and gentamicin, either alone or in combination with heparin.[3]
- The following are details in the treatment of uncomplicated long-term CVC infection due to specific organisms:
  - *S. aureus.* Long-term CVC should be removed followed by 4 to 6 weeks of effective parenteral antibiotics. Shorter courses can **only** be considered if the patient is not diabetic or immunocompromised, the catheter is removed, and blood cultures are negative and if fevers have resolved at 72 hours, there is no evidence of endocarditis on transesophageal echocardiogram, and there is no evidence of suppurative thrombophlebitis or other metastatic infection. Because of the high morbidity and mortality, *S. aureus* bloodstream infections are best managed in consultation with an infectious disease specialist.[4]

- ○ **Gram-negative bacilli.** If possible, remove the long-term CVC and follow this with 7 to 14 days of effective parenteral antibiotics. If vascular access is difficult and infection is uncomplicated, it is reasonable to attempt to treat through the infection with 10 to 14 days of effective parenteral antibiotics, and antibiotic lock therapy should be considered in conjunction withdrugs. If there is persistent bacteremia or no clinical improvement, the catheter should be removed followed by 7 to 14 days of effective antibiotics.
- ○ *Candida* **spp.** Long-term CVC should be removed as soon as possible followed by 14 days of appropriate antifungal therapy in the absence of complicated infection.
- ○ *Enterococcus* **spp.** Long-term CVC may be retained if infection is uncomplicated. Treat with 10 to 14 days of effective parenteral antibiotics. Antibiotic lock therapy can be considered. If there is persistent bacteremia or no clinical improvement, the catheter should be removed followed by 7 to 14 days of effective antibiotics.
- ○ **Coagulase-negative** *Staphylococcus.* Long-term CVC may be retained if infection is uncomplicated. Treat with 10 to 14 days of effective parenteral antibiotics. Antibiotic lock therapy can be considered. If there is persistent bacteremia or no clinical improvement, the catheter should be removed followed by 7 to 14 days of effective antibiotics. The exception to this is infection with *Staphylococcus lugdunensis*, which should be treated more aggressively with catheter removal and further evaluation, as for *S. aureus.*
- ○ Figure 4-1 presents a summary of the management of CRBSIs.[1]

Native Valve Endocarditis

GENERAL PRINCIPLES

Definition

- Endocarditis is defined as inflammation of the endocardium (inner lining) of the heart and heart valves. Infections are the most common cause of endocarditis (i.e., infective endocarditis [IE]). Infection of the endocardium, most commonly the heart valves, is a serious and potentially life-threatening disease. Presentation may be acute or subacute. **Consultation with an infectious disease specialist is recommended in most cases of suspected or confirmed IE.**
- Acute IE has onset of symptoms within 3 to 10 days of presentation. The course of acute IE may be fulminant, and patients may rapidly become critically ill.
- Subacute IE is more indolent, and symptoms may be present for weeks or months. The frequent symptoms of subacute endocarditis are fever, fatigue, and weight loss, and patients may have evidence of embolic phenomena.
- This section reviews native valve endocarditis, but similar principles apply to prosthetic valve endocarditis (PVE). PVE is covered in a separate section.

Epidemiology

Risk factors for the development of IE include prior endocarditis, valve replacement, valvular damage (age-related sclerosis, mitral valve prolapse, history of rheumatic fever), and IV drug use (IVDU). Any condition that increases the risk of bacteremia will increase the risk of endocarditis.

Etiology

- **The organisms most commonly associated with native valve endocarditis are** *Staphylococcus aureus, Streptococcus* spp. (**classically** viridans group streptococci), and *Enterococcus* spp.

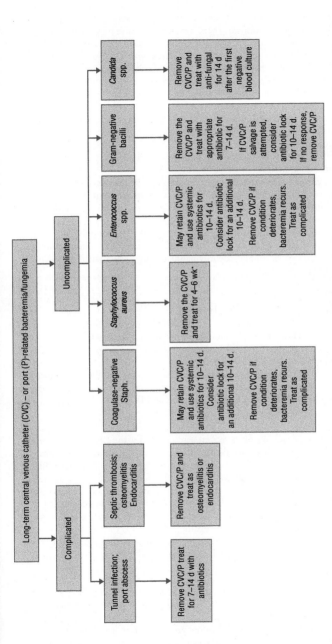

FIGURE 4-1 Management of central venous catheter–related bacteremia and fungemia. *A shorter course (≥14 d) may be considered if catheter is removed, infection is uncomplicated, bacteremia and fevers resolve within 72 hours, and the patient is nondiabetic, nonneutropenic, or nonimmunosuppressed, patient is without prosthetic intravascular device (e.g., graft and pacemaker), transesophageal echocardiogram is negative, and ultrasound is negative for septic thrombophlebitis. Adapted from Mermel LA, Allon M, Bouza E, et al. Clinical practice guidelines for the diagnosis and management of intravascular catheter-related infection: 2009 update by the Infectious Diseases Society of America. *Clin Infect Dis.* 2009;49:1-45.

- Less common causes of native valve endocarditis include gram-negative bacilli, HACEK organisms (*Haemophilus* spp., *Aggregatibacter actinomycetemcomitans, Cardiobacterium hominis, Eikenella corrodens,* and *Kingella kingae*), coagulase-negative staphylococci, fungi, *Bartonella* spp., *Tropheryma whipplii, Legionella* spp., *Chlamydia* spp., *Abiotrophia* spp. (previously nutritionally variant streptococci), and *Coxiella burnetii*. When no pathogen is identified but the diagnostic criteria are met, it is termed culture-negative endocarditis.
- Patient demographics may give a clue to the possible causative organism in IE.
  - Patients with poor dentition or following dental procedures are more commonly infected with viridans group streptococci.
  - Patients with indwelling venous catheters are at risk for staphylococcal endocarditis.
  - IVDU may lead to pseudomonal or fungal endocarditis, although *Staphylococcus* spp. are still more common.
  - Nosocomial infection may be due to any number of gram-negative organisms or staphylococci including MRSA.
- **Culture-negative endocarditis accounts** for approximately 5% of cases of endocarditis, when strict diagnostic criteria are followed. **The most common reason for negative cultures is antibiotic administration before blood cultures are drawn.** True culture-negative endocarditis presents a unique challenge and may prompt additional diagnostics such as serology or polymerase chain reaction (PCR) testing for organisms such as *Bartonella, Coxiella, Legionella,* and *T. whippelii*. Bacterial 16S ribosomal RNA gene sequencing has shown promise in identifying the etiologic agent when the valve is removed and subjected to testing.

Pathophysiology

- The classic lesion of endocarditis is valvular vegetation. Vegetations are made up of fibrin, platelets, microorganisms, and cells. The vegetation tends to form in areas of turbulent blood flow. This is most common when a valve is congenitally abnormal or damaged by some other factor. When microorganisms seed a damaged part of the endocardium, a vegetation forms, creating a protective barrier.
- The most commonly involved area is the ventricular surface of the mitral valve, followed by the aortic valve; however, any area of the endocardium may be involved. There is a classic relationship between tricuspid valve endocarditis and IVDU.

Prevention

- Antimicrobial prophylaxis against IE is recommended only for the patients at highest risk of acquiring the disease. These include patients with prosthetic heart valves, history of IE, unrepaired cyanotic congenital heart disease, or repaired congenital valvular disease with residual valvular dysfunction; during the first 6 months after a completely repaired congenital heart defect with prosthetic material without residual dysfunction; and with valvular dysfunction in a transplanted heart. It is no longer recommended to give antibiotic prophylaxis to patients with bicuspid aortic valve, mitral valve prolapse with regurgitation, or hypertrophic cardiomyopathy.[5]
- High-risk patients should receive antimicrobial prophylaxis against IE whenever they are undergoing a procedure that is likely to result in bacteremia with an organism with high potential for causing endocarditis.[5]
- High-risk procedures include dental work with invasive manipulation of the oral mucosa, gingival tissue, or periapical region of the teeth; procedures requiring incision or biopsy of the respiratory tract mucosa; and surgical procedures for management of skin, skin structure, or deep tissue infections.[5]
- Antibiotic prophylaxis is not recommended before procedures with lower associated risk of bacteremia such as gastrointestinal procedures (including colonoscopy with biopsy), genitourinary procedures, and vaginal or cesarean births.
- Please see Table 4-1 for information on prophylaxis.[5]

TABLE 4-1 INFECTIVE ENDOCARDITIS PROPHYLAXIS

I. **Endocarditis prophylaxis is recommended only for the following cardiac conditions:** prosthetic valves; previous endocarditis; unrepaired congenital heart disease, including palliative shunts or conduits; repaired congenital heart disease with prosthetic material during the first 6 mo after procedure or with residual defects at or adjacent to the site of the prosthetic device; and cardiac valvulopathy in transplant recipients.

II. Regimens for dental, oral, or respiratory tract procedures (including dental extractions, periodontal or endodontic procedures, professional teeth cleaning, bronchoscopy with biopsy, rigid bronchoscopy, surgery on respiratory mucosa, and tonsillectomy).

Clinical Scenario	Drug and Dosage
Standard prophylaxis	Amoxicillin 2 g PO 1 h before procedure
Unable to take PO	Ampicillin 2 g IM or IV or cefazolin or ceftriaxone 1–2 g IM or IV within 30 min before procedure
Penicillin-allergic patient	Clindamycin 600 mg PO, cephalexin 2 g PO, or clarithromycin or azithromycin 500 mg PO 1 h before procedure
Penicillin-allergic and unable to take PO	Clindamycin 600 mg IV or cefazolin or ceftriaxone 1 g IV within 30 min before procedure

III. Prophylaxis is recommended for procedures on infected skin, skin structures, or musculoskeletal tissue ONLY for patients with cardiac conditions outlined above. An antistaphylococcal penicillin or cephalosporin should be used.

Adapted from Wilson W, Taubert KA, Gewitz M, et al. Prevention of infective endocarditis: guidelines from the American Heart Association: a guideline from the American Heart Association Rheumatic Fever, Endocarditis, and Kawasaki Disease Committee, Council on Cardiovascular Disease in the Young, and the Council on Clinical Cardiology, Council on Cardiovascular Surgery and Anesthesia, and the Quality of Care and Outcomes Research Interdisciplinary Working Group. *Circulation.* 2007;116:1736-1754.

DIAGNOSIS

Clinical Presentation

History
- Patients with endocarditis may present with a wide spectrum of complaints.
- **The most common symptoms include fevers, weight loss, malaise, fatigue, night sweats, low-back pain, arthralgias, and evidence of embolic phenomenoa** (e.g., rash, hematuria, lung abscess, or stroke).
- Depending on the extent of the valve damage, patients may also present with symptoms of left- or right-sided heart failure, shortness of breath, syncope, or arrhythmias.

Physical Examination
- Physical examination may reveal fever, findings consistent with heart failure or valve regurgitation, new murmur, splenomegaly, and evidence of embolic phenomena.
- Central nervous system (CNS) embolism or ruptured mycotic aneurysm.
- Cutaneous findings may include petechiae, Osler nodes (painful subcutaneous nodules frequently on the pads of the fingers and toes), Janeway lesions (nonpainful hemorrhages found in the palms, soles, fingers, and toes), splinter hemorrhages (small linear hemorrhages underneath the fingernails or toenails), Roth spots (clear centered retinal hemorrhages), and subconjunctival hemorrhages.

Diagnostic Criteria

The most commonly used diagnostic criteria are the Duke criteria (Table 4-2).[6]

TABLE 4-2	DUKE CRITERIA FOR THE DIAGNOSIS OF ENDOCARDITIS

Definite endocarditis

Pathologic criteria:

Microorganisms demonstrated by culture of a vegetation, a vegetation that has embolized, or an intracardiac abscess specimen; or vegetation or intracardiac abscess showing active endocarditis by histological examination.

Clinical criteria:

Requires two major criteria; one major criterion and three minor criteria; or five minor criteria.

Possible endocarditis requires one major and one minor criterion; or three minor criteria.

No endocarditis: when the criteria above are not met and a firm alternative diagnosis explains findings suggestive of IE; resolution of syndrome with less than 4 d of antibiotic therapy; or no pathological evidence at surgery or autopsy with less than 4 d of antibiotics.

Major criteria

- Positive blood culture suggestive of IE:
  - Typical organism isolated from at least two separate blood cultures: viridans streptococci, *Staphylococcus aureus*, HACEK organisms, *Streptococcus bovis*, or *Enterococcus* spp. in the absence of an alternative primary site of infection OR
  - Persistently positive blood cultures: at least two cultures drawn 12 h apart or three cultures with first and last drawn at least 1 h apart OR
  - One culture (or phase 1 IgG > 1:800) for *Coxiella burnetii*
- Evidence of endocardial involvement: echocardiogram showing oscillating intracardiac mass without alternative explanation; abscess; new partial dehiscence of prosthetic valve; or new valvular regurgitation

---

Minor criteria

- Predisposition to IE: prior IE, IVDU, prosthetic heart valve, or cardiac lesion causing turbulent blood flow
- Documented fever ≥38°C (100.4°F)
- Vascular phenomenon: arterial embolism, pulmonary infarct, mycotic aneurysm, intracranial or conjunctival hemorrhage, or Janeway lesions
- Immunologic phenomena: Osler nodes, Roth spots, glomerulonephritis, or positive rheumatoid factor
- Microbiologic findings not meeting major criteria

Baddour LM, Wilson WR, Bayer AS, et al. Infective endocarditis in adults: diagnosis, antimicrobial therapy, and management of complications: a scientific statement for healthcare professionals from the American Heart Association. *Circulation.* 2015;132(15):1435-1486.

HACEK, *Haemophilus* spp. (*H. aphrophilus, H. parainfluenzae, H. paraphrophilus*), *Aggregatibacter actinomycetemcomitans, Cardiobacterium hominis, Eikenella corrodens,* and *Kingella kingae*; IE, infective endocarditis; IVDU, intravenous drug use.

TABLE 4-3	TREATMENT OF NATIVE VALVE ENDOCARDITIS CAUSED BY SPECIFIC ORGANISMS (CONTINUED)		
Organism	**Antibiotic Regimen**	**Duration**	**Notes**
Penicillin MIC >0.5 µg/mL	• Ampicillin or penicillin G **PLUS** gentamicin • Vancomycin	• 4–6 wk	Ceftriaxone combined with gentamicin may be a reasonable alternative for isolates susceptible to ceftriaxone
Enterococcus species (same as prosthetic valve endocarditis)			
Penicillin and gentamicin susceptible	• Ampicillin or penicillin G **PLUS** gentamicin • Ampicillin **PLUS** ceftriaxone	• 4–6 wk	
Penicillin-resistant	• Vancomycin **PLUS** gentamicin	• 6 wk	
Vancomycin- and ampicillin-resistant	• Linezolid or daptomycin	• ≥6 wk	• Consult infectious diseases specialist
Staphylococcus species			
Methicillin-sensitive _Staphylococcus aureus_ and coagulase-negative staphylococci	• Oxacillin/nafcillin • Cefazolin • Vancomycin if PCN allergic (daptomycin is a reasonable alternative to vancomycin)	• ≥6 wk	In cases of brain abscess, nafcillin should be used over cefazolin Gentamicin or Rifampin is nor recommended
Methicillin-resistant _Staphylococcus aureus_ and coagulase-negative staphylococci	• Vancomycin • Daptomycin is alternative	• ≥6 wk	
HACEK organisms and culture-negative IE	• Ceftriaxone or ampicillin or ciprofloxacin	• 4 wk	Ceftriaxone is the preferred option

Adapted from Baddour LM, Wilson WR, Bayer AS, et al. Infective endocarditis in adults: diagnosis, antimicrobial therapy, and management of complications: a scientific statement for healthcare professionals from the American Heart Association. _Circulation._ 2015;132(15):1435–1486.

Dosing: Ceftriaxone 2 g IV q24h; gentamicin 1 mg/kg IV q8h; vancomycin 15 mg/kg IV q12h for normal renal function; ampicillin–sulbactam 3 g IV q6h; ampicillin 2 g IV q4h; oxacillin/nafcillin 2 g IV q4h; rifampin 300 mg PO q8h; cefazolin 2 g IV q8h; daptomycin 6 mg/kg/d; linezolid 600 mg IV q12h; ciprofloxacin 400 mg IV q12h.

Baseline and weekly audiometry recommended for patients receiving aminoglycosides >7 d. Monitor aminoglycoside and vancomycin levels. Goal vancomycin trough levels are 15–20 µg/mL. IE, infective endocarditis; MIC, minimum inhibitory concentration; PCN, penicillin.

- Patients with recurrent emboli and persistent or enlarging vegetations despite appropriate antibiotics
- Patients with severe valvular regurgitation and mobile vegetations >10 mm, particularly when involving the anterior leaflet of the mitral valve, or if there are other relative surgical indications

COMPLICATIONS

- **Mycotic aneurysms** are abnormal aneurysmal dilations of arteries caused by IE.
  - They are caused by direct infection of the arterial wall, immune complex deposition in the blood vessel wall, or embolic occlusion of the vasa vasorum.
  - The incidence of mycotic aneurysms in IE is unknown.
  - Mycotic aneurysms are most commonly found in the cerebral circulation but may also exist in other vascular distributions.
  - Usually, these are clinically silent until they rupture. Ruptured CNS mycotic aneurysms have approximately 80% mortality.[6] Routine screening is not indicated; however, if CNS symptoms develop, the clinician should have a low threshold to evaluate with neurologic imaging and neurosurgical evaluation.
- Embolic events are common complications of endocarditis. Emboli most commonly travel to the cerebral, renal, splenic, pulmonary, coronary, and systemic circulation. This can result in abscess formation or ischemic damage to distant tissue.
- **Immunologic complications** are also common in IE. IE stimulates the cellular and humoral immune system, which may result in hypergammaglobulinemia, splenomegaly, and the deposition of immune complexes in distant organs such as the kidneys. Rheumatoid factor and antinuclear antibodies may develop and may play a role in the pathogenesis of IE.
- **Renal dysfunction** in IE is not uncommon. This may occur as a result of several different processes including abscess formation, infarction, and glomerulonephritis.

Prosthetic Valve Endocarditis

GENERAL PRINCIPLES

- Many of the principles are the same as in native valve endocarditis; however, the etiologic agents and the treatment are different.
- PVE frequently requires surgery to achieve a cure. Early surgical consultation with a cardiac surgeon is suggested in PVE.

Etiology

- PVE can be divided into early and late PVE based on the time from valve placement to the time of infection. There is no consensus regarding the cutoff between early- and late-onset PVE, but treatment recommendations use one year as a cutoff. The etiologic agents responsible are different between early and late PVE.
- **The vast majority of early-onset PVE is caused by *Staphylococcus aureus* and coagulase-negative staphylococci,** followed by gram-negative organisms and fungi.
- **Late-onset PVE is still predominantly caused by staphylococci; however, other organisms associated with native valve endocarditis begin to increase in frequency.**

Epidemiology

PVE accounts for up to a third of all cases of IE. IE is more common among patients with mechanical prosthetic valves rather than bioprosthetic valves. In the first year after implantation, the risk is between 1% and 3%. After the first year, the rate drops to about 0.5% per year. Contamination of the valve may occur at the time of implantation, or it may develop later by hematogenous seeding.

Pathophysiology

- Newly replaced valves are not yet endothelialized, which puts them at greater risk for the development of a sterile platelet fibrin thrombus. This thrombus provides a place for bacteria to adhere. This usually occurs at the interface between the cuff and the native tissue, and frequently perivalvular leaks will be present at diagnosis.
- Biofilm formation plays a large role in the pathogenesis of PVE. Biofilms are polysaccharide-enclosed matrices that protect the infecting organism from host defenses such as phagocytosis. Also, biofilms provide protection from antibiotic exposure. Many organisms in biofilms may lie dormant and many antibiotics require cell division to work effectively.

DIAGNOSIS

- Microbiologic diagnosis of PVE is the same as that for native valve IE. Physicians should have a high index of suspicion for PVE in a patient with fevers and a prosthetic valve. Extension into the myocardium is more common in PVE, and ECG abnormalities may be more common.
- Approximately 50% of patients with *Staphylococcus aureus* bacteremia and 40% of patients with coagulase-negative staphylococci bacteremia go on to develop endocarditis.[9]
- **TEE is required in all cases of suspected PVE.**
  - ○ TTE is inadequate to evaluate PVE owing to decreased sensitivity and specificity when prosthetic valve material is present.
  - ○ The initial TEE may be negative early in PVE or with a small abscess.
  - ○ If initial TEE is negative and suspicion remains high, a repeat TEE should be performed several days later.

TREATMENT

Medications

- The basic principles of medical management of PVE are similar to those of native valve IE. Treatment should be with **high-dose, parenteral, bactericidal antibiotics**.
- Empiric antibiotics should be started after blood cultures if the patient is acutely ill or clinically unstable. If the patient is clinically stable and there is a suspicion for subacute endocarditis, antibiotics need not be given until the culture results are known.
- Empiric antibiotic choice for either early or late PVE should initially include vancomycin 15 mg/kg IV q12h, **PLUS** rifampin 300 mg IV or PO q8h, **PLUS** gentamicin 1 mg/kg IV q8h.
- Culture-driven antibiotic therapy for PVE is detailed in Table 4-4.[6]
- For non-HACEK group gram-negative organisms, antipseudomonal penicillin or cephalosporin plus aminoglycoside is recommended. Infectious Disease consultation is also recommended. Fungal endocarditis should be initially treated with amphotericin B. Echinocandins have also been successfully used, but data are limited. The mortality of fungal endocarditis is high, and early surgical evaluation is suggested.
- Patients with mechanical valves on long-term oral anticoagulation should have warfarin and antiplatelet therapy held and IV heparin initiated on the diagnosis of IE, as surgery may be required. If the patient develops neurologic symptoms, heparin should be stopped until intracranial hemorrhage is ruled out.

TABLE 4-4	TREATMENT OF PROSTHETIC VALVE ENDOCARDITIS CAUSED BY SPECIFIC ORGANISMS		
Organism	Antibiotic Regimen	Duration	Notes
Viridians streptococci or *Streptococcus bovis*			
MIC <0.12 µg/mL	• Penicillin G or ceftriaxone with or without gentamicin • Vancomycin if PCN allergic	6 wk. If gentamicin added, use for 2 wk	Including gentamicin does not improve cure rates and should be used with caution
MIC ≥0.12 µg/mL	• Penicillin G or ceftriaxone **PLUS** gentamicin • Vancomycin if PCN allergic	6 wk	
Enterococcus species (same as native valve endocarditis)			
Penicillin-susceptible	• If gentamicin susceptible: ampicillin **PLUS** gentamicin or ampicillin **PLUS** ceftriaxone • If gentamicin resistant/streptomycin susceptible: ampicillin **PLUS** ceftriaxone or ampicillin **PLUS** streptomycin	4–6 wk	Substitute streptomycin 7.5 mg/kg q12h for high-level gentamicin resistance
Penicillin-resistant	• Vancomycin **PLUS** gentamicin	6 wk	
Vancomycin- and ampicillin-resistant	• Linezolid or daptomycin	>6 wk	Consult infectious diseases specialist
***Staphylococcus* species**			
Methicillin-sensitive *Staphylococcus aureus* and coagulase-negative staphylococci	Oxacillin/nafcillin **PLUS** rifampin **PLUS** gentamicin	≥6 wk with 2 wk of gentamicin	
Methicillin-resistant *S. aureus* and coagulase-negative staphylococci	Vancomycin **PLUS** rifampin **PLUS** gentamicin	≥6 wk with 2 wk of gentamicin	

TABLE 4-4	TREATMENT OF PROSTHETIC VALVE ENDOCARDITIS CAUSED BY SPECIFIC ORGANISMS (CONTINUED)		
Organism	**Antibiotic Regimen**	**Duration**	**Notes**
HACEK organisms and culture-negative IE	Ceftriaxone or ampicillin or ciprofloxacin	6 wk	

Adapted from Baddour LM, Wilson WR, Bayer AS, et al. Infective endocarditis in adults: diagnosis, antimicrobial therapy, and management of complications: a scientific statement for healthcare professionals from the American Heart Association. *Circulation.* 2015;132(15):1435-1486.

Dosing: Ceftriaxone 2 g IV q24h; gentamicin 2 g qd or 1 mg/kg q8h; vancomycin 1 g IV q24h; ampicillin–sulbactam 3 g IV q6h; ampicillin 2 g IV q4h; oxacillin 2 g IV q4h; rifampin 300 mg PO q8h; cefazolin 2 g IV q8h; daptomycin 6 mg/kg/d; linezolid 600 mg IV q12h; ciprofloxacin 400 mg IV q12h.

Baseline and weekly audiometry recommended for patients receiving aminoglycosides >7 d.

Monitor aminoglycoside and vancomycin levels. Goal vancomycin trough levels are near to 15 µg/mL.

IE, infective endocarditis; MIC, minimum inhibitory concentration; PCN, penicillin.

Surgical Management

- Cure with antibiotics alone is less likely than in native valve IE. A cardiac surgeon should be contacted early in patients with suspected or confirmed PVE.
- Indications for valve surgery in PVE include symptomatic congestive heart failure resulting from valve dehiscence, fistula or severe prosthetic valve dysfunction, bacteremia >5 to 7 days despite adequate effective antibiotics, vegetation >10 mm, PVE complicated by heart block, annular or aortic abscess, PVE with recurrent emboli, or PVE with fungus, *Pseudomonas*, *Staphylococcus aureus*, or most *Enterococcus* spp.
- Intracerebral hemorrhage is a contraindication to cardiac surgery, but cerebral embolism without evidence of hemorrhage is not.
- TEE is of the utmost importance to fully evaluate for dysfunction of the prosthetic valve.
- Postoperative antibiotics should be continued for a full course, starting from the time of surgery.

Infection of Implanted Cardiac Devices

GENERAL PRINCIPLES

- The devices most associated with infection are implanted electrophysiologic (EP) cardiac devices and mechanical circulatory support (MCS) devices.
- Implanted EP cardiac devices include permanent pacemakers (PPMs) and implanted cardioverter–defibrillators (ICD). These are being used at an increased rate in the United States with a corresponding increase in the rate of device-related infection.[10]
- MCS devices include left and right ventricular assist devices (LVAD and RVAD, respectively), biventricular devices (BiVADs), and total artificial hearts (TAH). LVADs are currently the most commonly implanted MCS devices. Despite changes in device size and functionality, infections remain a major complication and significant cause of morbidity and mortality in LVAD recipients.[11]
- Any implanted foreign material, such as cardiac stents, patches, and peripheral vascular grafts, may become infected; however, the rate of infection of these devices is much lower.

Epidemiology

- The overall rate of device infection has been previously reported to be between 0.13% and 19.9%. The higher rate was from the era of intra-abdominal implantation.[12] The current rate is closer to 1%. Risk factors for the development of EP cardiac device infections include fever within 24 hours of device implantation, lack of prophylactic antibiotic use, temporary pacing before permanent device placement, presence of a tunneled venous catheter, diabetes mellitus, renal failure, malignancy, operator inexperience, prior device infection, use of more than two leads, and anticoagulation.
- The reported rate of LVAD infection has been reported to be as high as 33%.[13] Risk factors for MCS device infection include older age, diabetes, renal failure, malnutrition, T-cell dysfunction associated to the device, hypogammaglobulinemia, obesity, delayed sternal closure, prolonged ICU, stay and prolonged duration of MCS.[11]

Etiology

- **Staphylococci account for the vast majority of PPM and ICD infections.** Coagulase-negative staphylococci account for 42%, of cases and *Staphylococcus aureus* accounts for 29%. The remaining cases are due to gram-negative bacilli (9%), other gram-positive cocci (4%), polymicrobial infection (7%), fungi (2%), and culture negative (7%).[14]
- *Staphylococcus aureus* **and** *Staphylococcus epidermidis* **account for greater than 50% of all MCS device–related infections.** Other common organisms include *Enterococcus* spp. (2%), *Pseudomonas aeruginosa* (22%–28%), *Klebsiella* (2%), and *Enterobacter* (2%). Since 2009, there has been a significant increase in resistant organisms such as vancomycin-resistant enterococci and multidrug-resistant gram negatives.[11]
- *Candida albicans* is the most common fungal organism to cause MCS infection followed by *Candida glabrata*. These MCS device–related infections are difficult to eradicate and carry an associated overall mortality rate of 15% to 25%.

Pathophysiology

- The pathogenesis of PPM and ICD infections is **contamination of the device with skin flora at the time of implantation or manipulation** (such as generator change).
- Alternatively, implanted cardiac devices may be secondarily infected by **seeding of the device during bacteremia from a distant source of infection** (i.e., vascular catheter infection, skin and soft tissue infections, urinary tract infections, pneumonia, or intra-abdominal infections) or ascending infection from the skin–device interface at the driveline site.
- **Biofilm formation** plays a large role in the pathogenesis of cardiac device infections.

Prevention

- The best way to prevent cardiovascular device–related infection is by practicing **meticulous aseptic technique with device implantation.** Skin preparation should be done with 2% chlorhexidine.
- **Antibiotic prophylaxis** with an appropriate antistaphylococcal agent should be given 30 to 60 minutes before surgery. MRSA coverage should be considered in patients with known MRSA colonization or in areas with high rates of MRSA.
- Antibiotic prophylaxis for patients with implanted cardiac devices before dental procedures or other medical procedures is not recommended by the guidelines of the American Heart Association. Although this is fully applicable to EP devices, in the case of MCS devices, the International Society for Heart and Lung Transplantation qualifies the use of secondary prophylaxis as a reasonable strategy with procedures at high risk for bacteremia, which may lead to seeding of the device and negative outcomes.[11]

DIAGNOSIS

Clinical Presentation

- The presentation can vary depending on the portion of the device that is infected and the organism causing the infection.
- With EP devices, the most common presentation is local infection at the site of the PPM or ICD implantation. Local infection may manifest itself as cellulitis overlying the pocket, abscess formation, surgical wound dehiscence, sinus tract formation, device migration, or erosion through the skin.
  - Patients may also present with occult bacteremia with no evidence of infection at the insertion site. Patients with an ICD or PPM and occult bacteremia should be evaluated for the presence of cardiac device infection, even in the absence of inflammation at the insertion site.
  - The final presentation is with symptoms of endocarditis. The symptoms of device-related endocarditis and other forms of endocarditis are very similar. Systemic septic embolism is rare, but pulmonary embolism is more common owing to the right-sided location of implanted cardiac devices.
  - A minimum of two blood cultures should be obtained before the initiation of antibiotics.
  - The implantation site can be evaluated for involvement by ultrasound, looking for fluid collection. Percutaneous aspiration of the generator pocket should not be performed as part of the diagnostic evaluation.
  - Indium-labeled leukocyte scan or gallium scanning may help differentiate an inflammatory fluid collection from a noninflammatory one.
  - Other laboratory findings are nonspecific and may include leukocytosis, anemia, or elevated inflammatory markers.
  - Generator-pocket tissue Gram stain and culture and lead-tip culture should be obtained when the device is explanted.
  - Patients with bacteremia or who have negative blood cultures but received antimicrobials before culture should undergo evaluation of endocarditis with transesophageal echocardiogram.
  - Patients with *Staphylococcus aureus* bacteremia, or persistent bacteremia with another organism, and no evidence of infection at the device insertion site (after a thorough evaluation) should also have a cardiac evaluation with TEE.
- Clinical manifestations of LVAD infection are often different than for other implanted cardiac devices.
  - The presentation will be dependent on the site involved. LVAD-specific infections are due to direct involvement of the device including driveline, pump, and/or cannulae and pocket. LVAD-related infections include the spaces contiguous to the LVAD such as mediastinum, bacteremia related to the device, and device-related endocarditis.
  - The most common presentations with LVAD infections are local symptoms and signs of inflammation at the driveline exit site and bacteremia related to device infection.
  - Less commonly patients may present with dysfunction of the LVAD, manifesting as worsening symptoms of heart failure. This is due to mechanical disruption of the lumen of the device from infection.
  - Diagnosis is made through physical examination of the percutaneous entry site of the driveline or cannula. Blood cultures as well as cultures of any drainage or aspirated fluid collection should be sent for microbiological confirmation.
  - If the device is revised or explanted, tissue and device surface cultures should be obtained.
  - Ultrasound or computed tomography (CT) imaging can be used to assess for drainable collections and inflammatory stranding of the driveline tunnel and pocket.

- ○ Indium-labeled leukocyte scans have been used to determine the extent of infection.
- ○ Echocardiogram may be required to evaluate for valvular infection in patients with bacteremia, although the data on its diagnostic utility in this setting are unclear and recommendations are derived from data on other device-related infections.

TREATMENT

- The basic management of implanted EP cardiac devices is presented in Figure 4-2.[10]
- **Device removal is required in all cases of suspected or confirmed PPM or ICD infection.**
  - ○ Trials of conservative management with antibiotics alone have an unacceptably high failure rate.
  - ○ The best strategy is a combination of complete removal of the implanted device AND the cardiac leads combined with parenteral antibiotics.
  - ○ Even if blood cultures are negative, the best strategy is removal of the entire device. In one study of 105 patients with implanted cardiac device infection, 79% had positive cultures of the intravascular portion of the leads, while only 5 patients had bacteremia.
- In some cases, removal of the device and the cardiac leads may either be impossible or it may carry too high a risk of complications. In these cases, as much of the device as possible should be removed. If the device cannot be removed at all, indefinite suppression with oral antibiotics should be considered, after a full treatment course of IV antibiotics.
- Patients with secondary bacteremia with no evidence of pocket inflammation and without evidence of cardiac lead or valve involvement on TEE can usually be managed with antibiotics alone without removal of the implanted device.
- **The antibiotic of choice should be tailored to the results of culture and sensitivity data.** Empiric antibiotics should be directed toward the most likely causative organisms. **Vancomycin is the drug of choice in most cases.**
- Compared with other implanted cardiac devices, **the removal of an LVAD is very complicated, expensive, and frequently unfeasible.**
  - ○ Local debridement of abscesses should be performed when possible.
  - ○ LVAD infections with bloodstream involvement should be treated initially with parenteral antibiotics. Successful suppression of symptomatic infection has been achieved with parenteral antibiotics followed by long-term suppression with oral antibiotics. Antibiotic suppression should be continued until the device is removed at the time of transplant or for the life of the patient when the LVAD is for destination therapy.
  - ○ Some patients with overwhelming LVAD infection eventually do require removal or exchange of the LVAD for successful treatment.
  - ○ LVAD infection is not a contraindication for heart transplantation.
- Please see Figure 4-2.[10]

Mediastinitis

GENERAL PRINCIPLES

Definition

- Mediastinitis refers to infection involving the structures of the mediastinum. There are acute and chronic forms.
- Primary infection involving the mediastinum is rare, and acute mediastinitis is usually due to the spread of infection from another space, due to trauma, or following a thoracic surgical procedure.
- Chronic or fibrosing mediastinitis is manifest by diffuse fibrosis of the tissues of the mediastinum.

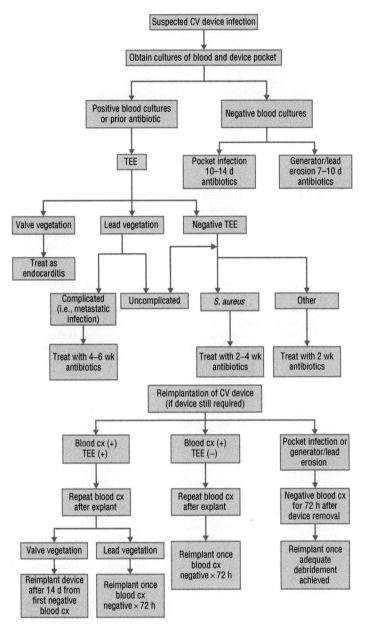

FIGURE 4-2 Management of implanted cardiovascular device infections. CV, cardiovascular; cx, culture; TEE, transesophageal echocardiogram. This algorithm applies to patients who have had complete device explantation. Duration of antibiotics should be from the time of device removal. Adapted from Baddour LM, Epstein AE, Erickson CC, et al. Update on cardiovascular implantable electronic device infections and their management: a scientific statement from the American Heart Association. *Circulation*. 2010;121(3):458-477.

Epidemiology

- The incidence of mediastinitis after surgery requiring median sternotomy is between 0.5% and 4.4%.[9]
- The incidence is higher in patients who undergo heart transplantation.
- Risk factors for the development of mediastinitis following cardiac surgery include obesity, diabetes mellitus, chronic obstructive pulmonary disease, renal failure, cigarette smoking, peripheral vascular disease, use of internal mammary artery for bypass, length of surgery, length of time on cardiopulmonary bypass, need for blood transfusion, length of preoperative hospitalization, and length of ICU stay.

Pathophysiology

- Before the advent of cardiothoracic surgery, the most common causes of mediastinitis were esophageal rupture and spread of infection from the oropharynx. Now **most cases of mediastinitis are caused by wound infection following cardiothoracic surgery.**
- Mediastinitis from **esophageal rupture is now most commonly iatrogenic** and may be due to esophageal endoscopic procedure, nasogastric tube placement, esophageal stenting, esophageal dilation, and endotracheal intubation. Other causes of esophageal rupture are spontaneous (also called Boerhaave syndrome), swallowed foreign bodies, penetrating trauma, blunt force trauma, excessive vomiting, and rupture secondary to neoplasm.
- Mediastinitis due to **spread from head and neck infections** occurs by spread along fascial planes into the mediastinum. Head and neck infections that may lead to mediastinitis include Ludwig angina (usually caused by infection of the second or third mandibular molar spreading to the submandibular space and then tracking along the parapharyngeal space or carotid sheath into the mediastinum), odontogenic infection, tonsillitis, pharyngitis, parotitis, epiglottitis, and Lemierre syndrome (septic thrombophlebitis of the jugular vein and superior vena cava).
- Rarely, mediastinitis may occur following infection of other structures in the chest or abdomen. Mediastinitis has occurred following pneumonia, empyema, infection of the bony structures of the thorax, pancreatitis, and subphrenic abscess.
- Fibrosing mediastinitis may occur as a response to infection. It is unclear how much of the pathophysiology is due to infection and how much is to an aberrant inflammatory response. It can also be caused by radiation therapy, sarcoidosis, and silicosis.

Etiology

- The bacteriology of mediastinitis depends on if it is postoperative or secondary to esophageal rupture or spread from head and neck infections.
- Postoperative mediastinitis is most commonly due to contamination of the surgical wound with the patient's endogenous flora. The causative organisms are most commonly gram-positive cocci. *Staphylococcus epidermidis*, followed by *Staphylococcus aureus*, **is the most common causative organism for postoperative mediastinitis**. Gram-negative organisms and fungal organisms are less likely causes.
- Mediastinitis due to esophageal perforation or spread from head and neck infections is frequently polymicrobial and may include anaerobes, gram-negative bacilli, and gram-positive oral flora. Common organisms include viridans group streptococci, *Peptostreptococcus* spp., *Bacteroides* spp., and *Fusobacterium* spp.
- **The most common underlying infections in chronic or fibrosing mediastinitis are** *Histoplasma capsulatum* **and tuberculosis**. It has also been described with *Nocardia asteroides*, *Actinomyces* spp., *Coccidioides immitis*, and *Blastomyces dermatitidis*.

DIAGNOSIS

Clinical Manifestations

- Postoperative patients may complain of out-of-proportion chest pain, which may be pleuritic in nature or may radiate to the neck, often accompanied by fevers. Patients may complain of dyspnea, dysphagia, or odynophagia. Instability of the sternotomy fusion is frequently present.
- Mediastinitis stemming from an infection in the head and neck will involve mouth, throat, or neck pain as the earliest manifestation, along with facial or neck swelling.
- Physical examination may reveal fever, tachycardia, crepitus, edema or erythema of the chest, and instability of the sternal fusion. Hamman sign is a crunching sound which is synchronous to the heart rhythm due to air in the mediastinum.
- **Lemierre syndrome** usually occurs following bacterial pharyngitis, although it has been described following otitis, mastoiditis, sinusitis, and dental infections.
  - Bacteria migrate along tissue planes to the carotid sheath.
  - The syndrome is characterized by antecedent infection followed by persistent fevers and septic pulmonary embolism.
  - This may be accompanied by neck swelling and induration. Fevers and bacteremia may persist despite adequate antibiotic therapy.
  - The diagnosis can be confirmed by CT scan of the neck or ultrasound demonstrating thrombosis of the jugular vein.
- Patients may also present with signs and symptoms of sepsis.
- Chest radiography may reveal widening of the mediastinum or air in the superior mediastinum. It is important to check a lateral film as some signs may not be apparent on frontal or posterior views. Chest radiography is less useful in poststernotomy mediastinitis as mediastinal air may be a normal postoperative finding.
- CT scan may be useful to determine the extent of infection or in cases where diagnosis is uncertain. CT scan is essential for the diagnosis of odontogenic or pharyngeal infections. Findings are usually fluid collections, with or without gas present, which track along soft tissue planes. The diagnosis of Lemierre syndrome can be confirmed by CT scan of the neck or ultrasound demonstrating thrombosis of the jugular vein.
- Esophageal rupture may be diagnosed with esophagography using water-soluble contrast material.
- Bacteremia is common in mediastinitis and frequently due to *Staphylococcus aureus* or gram-negative bacilli. Blood cultures should be obtained in all cases of suspected mediastinitis, preferably before antibiotics are administered.
- Symptoms of **chronic mediastinitis** can range from chronic cough, dyspnea, wheezing, and hemoptysis to pulmonary hypertension and cor pulmonale.
  - Many patients are asymptomatic.
  - Chronic mediastinitis is the most common, nonmalignant cause of **superior vena cava syndrome.**
  - The diagnosis of chronic mediastinitis is made by pathologic examination from tissue biopsy.

TREATMENT

Acute Mediastinitis

- **Combined medical and surgical treatment is essential in most cases of mediastinitis.** One exception is esophageal microperforation. If microperforation is diagnosed early, it can sometimes be managed by careful monitoring, nasopharyngeal suction, parenteral nutrition, and broad-spectrum antibiotics.

- Postoperative mediastinitis usually requires aggressive surgical debridement and drainage. Initial antibiotics should be broad spectrum and have activity against gram-positive and gram-negative organisms. Final antibiotic choice should be tailored to the organisms identified in cultures. Duration depends on the extent of infection. **Sternal osteomyelitis is common, and therefore, a prolonged treatment course is usually warranted.**
- Mediastinitis due to spread from head and neck infections should be treated with surgical debridement and drainage along with antibiotics. Frequently surgery is a combined effort with head and neck surgeons and cardiothoracic surgeons. The antibiotics chosen for mediastinitis from a suspected head and neck source should have activity against oral anaerobes and gram-negative organisms. Traditionally, penicillin G was the drug of choice but with emerging resistance of some oral anaerobes, combination therapy with β-lactam, β-lactamase inhibitors, carbapenems, or metronidazole or clindamycin combined with gram-negative coverage is usually chosen. Anaerobic coverage should be continued for the duration of therapy, even if no anaerobes are identified in culture, as they are frequently difficult to grow in culture.

Lemierre Syndrome

- Lemierre syndrome is septic thrombophlebitis of the internal jugular vein and/or the superior vena cava. Most commonly it occurs in young patients in the second or third decade of life. The most common causative organism is *Fusobacterium necrophorum*, although cases due to *Bacteroides* spp., *Peptostreptococcus* spp., *Staphylococcus aureus*, streptococci, and *Bacteroides fragilis* have been described.
- Empiric therapy should be directed toward oral anaerobes and should include a β-lactam/β-lactamase combination or a carbapenem. Vancomycin should be considered especially if the patient has a central venous catheter. Antibiotics should be tailored to the causative organism.
- Anticoagulation is controversial. Some authors suggest using anticoagulation only when there is evidence of thrombus extension.[15]
- Surgery may be warranted if an abscess is present, if empyema develops, or if the patient fails to improve despite adequate antibiotic therapy.

Chronic Mediastinitis

- There is no definitive or curative treatment for fibrosing mediastinitis.
- Antibiotics and antifungal agents and corticosteroids are usually not indicated, as there is typically no active infection.
- Airway stents can be placed by bronchoscopy and vascular stents percutaneously.
- Sometimes surgery may be required to remove scar tissue in severely symptomatic patients.

Acute Rheumatic Fever

GENERAL PRINCIPLES

- Acute rheumatic fever (ARF) is a nonsuppurative sequela of streptococcal pharyngitis. Most cases of ARF are self-limited; however, damage to the cardiac valves may persist and lead to long-term sequela such as progressive cardiac failure, valvular stenosis, and predisposition to endocarditis.
- Patients who recover from ARF are predisposed to future episodes of ARF following subsequent streptococcal infections.

Epidemiology

- The incidence of ARF in the United States and Western Europe has been in steady decline over the past 100 years. This is likely due to the increased antibiotic use for streptococcal pharyngitis and improved general hygiene standards.

- ARF remains a major cause of morbidity and mortality in the developing world. An estimated half-million people worldwide are affected each year. ARF is a disease associated with overcrowding and is more common in lower socioeconomic groups.
- ARF should be considered in people traveling to endemic regions.
- ARF commonly affects children between ages 5 and 15 years but can occur in adults as well. Recurrent episodes can occur in adults following an acute streptococcal infection.

Etiology

- ARF is a nonsuppurative sequela of Group A streptococcal pharyngitis. It is not known to occur following Group A streptococcal skin infections, implying that the abundant lymphoid tissue in the pharynx may play a role in the pathogenesis.
- The exact mechanism of ARF is not completely understood. It is known that some strains of Group A streptococci are more rheumatogenic than others. There are several theories regarding the pathogenesis of ARF. The first is that ARF is caused by the direct toxic effects of a streptococcal toxin. A second theory is that it is caused by a "serum sickness" leading to deposition of antigen–antibody complexes. The third, and the theory which garners the most attention, is that ARF occurs as an autoimmune response induced by **molecular mimicry of Group A streptococcal antigens**.

DIAGNOSIS

- Symptoms of ARF usually occur between 1 and 5 weeks following an episode of acute streptococcal pharyngitis.
- **Polyarthritis is the most common symptom** that occurs in about 75% of cases. Clinically evident carditis occurs in 40% to 50% of cases, whereas chorea, subcutaneous nodules, and erythema marginatum are less common, occurring less than 15% of the time.
- Most of the symptoms of ARF are self-limited and resolve without sequela. Carditis is the exception to this.
- Carditis can potentially lead to chronic heart failure, and it can rarely be fatal in the acute episode.
- The joint involvement ranges from arthralgias to true arthritis with swelling, erythema, and severe pain. Arthritis is frequently migratory. The most commonly affected joints are the knees, ankles, elbows, and wrists with the joints of the hands being less frequently involved. Typically it resolves within 4 weeks.
- Sydenham chorea is characterized by rapid involuntary movements associated with emotional lability.
- Subcutaneous nodules are firm, painless nodules that tend to occur overlying bony prominences.
- Erythema marginatum is a nonpainful, nonpruritic, erythematous eruption that commonly occurs on the trunk or proximal extremities. The erythema tends to migrate in patterns likened to smoke rings, progressing with the development of central clearing.
- ARF is a clinical diagnosis that is made by using the **Jones criteria**, which are divided into major and minor criteria. In 2015, the American Heart Association modified the cutoffs in some of the Jones criteria for diagnostic use in low- versus high-risk populations. Shown below are criteria in low-risk populations, with modifications for high-risk populations in parenthesis.[16,17]
  - The **major criteria** are as follows:
    - Carditis
    - Polyarthritis (mono- or polyarthritis, polyarthralgia)
    - Sydenham chorea
    - Subcutaneous nodules
    - Erythema marginatum

- ○ The **minor criteria** are as follows:
  - Polyarthralgias (monoarthralgia)
  - Fever >38.5°C (fever >38°C)
  - ESR ≥60 mm/h and/or CRP ≥3 mg/dl (ESR ≥30 mm/h and/or CRP ≥3 mg/dl)
  - Heart block (PR segment prolongation on electrocardiogram)
- ○ To make the diagnosis, there must be **evidence of a recent Group A streptococcal infection** (positive throat culture, positive rapid streptococcal antigen test, and elevated antistreptolysin O) in addition to either **two major criteria or one major criterion and two minor criteria.** For the diagnosis of recurrent ARF, three minor criteria plus evidence of preceding Group A streptococcal infection can also be used.

TREATMENT

- **Treatment of ARF is essentially supportive.** There are no therapies that prevent the progression to chronic disease. Mild to moderate disease, without carditis, is usually treated with analgesics alone. If carditis is present and there is no evidence of heart failure, **aspirin** is used. If there is evidence of heart failure, **corticosteroids** are used.
- Chorea may be treated with sedative medications or atypical antipsychotics.
- If ARF results in chronic heart failure, it is treated the same as heart failure from other causes.
- Recurrent episodes of ARF are common following an acute case. Prophylaxis against subsequent Group A streptococcal infections may be warranted in many situations (Table 4-5).[16]
- The duration of prophylaxis is variable based on the extent of the patient's acute illness and their risk of subsequent Group A streptococcal infections (Table 4-5).[16]

Myocarditis

GENERAL PRINCIPLES

- Myocarditis is inflammation of the myocardium. Inflammation may be infectious or noninfectious in etiology. The spectrum of illness ranges from asymptomatic cases to sudden death. Myocarditis is **a major cause of sudden death in patients under age 40 years.**
- The diagnosis of myocarditis should be considered in anyone presenting with new-onset heart failure, or new arrhythmias, especially in the setting of an acute febrile illness or viral upper respiratory syndrome. **Frequently patients may not remember an antecedent infection**, so the absence of prior acute illness does not rule out infectious myocarditis.
- Myocarditis has been identified histologically in 10% to 20% of cases of idiopathic dilated cardiomyopathy.[17]
- Numerous viral, bacterial, parasitic, and fungal agents are known to cause myocarditis. Table 4-6 lists potential etiologic agents.
- Although almost any infectious agent can cause myocarditis, viral agents are the most common in the United States and Western Europe. Many cases of idiopathic myocarditis are presumed to be viral in nature.
- **Members of the enterovirus family, specifically Coxsackie B virus, are the most commonly identified viral pathogens.**
- Bacteria may cause inflammation or infection of the myocardium via toxin production or by direct extension from endocarditis.
  - ○ *Corynebacterium diphtheriae.* Myocardial involvement is the most common cause of death in cases of diphtheria infection. Diphtheritic myocarditis is toxin mediated and not due to direct invasion by the organism.

TABLE 4-5	SECONDARY PREVENTION OF RHEUMATIC FEVER	
Agents	**Dosage**	**Route**
Benzathine penicillin G	600,000 U for children <27 kg, 1.2 million U for children >27 kg every 4 wk	Intramuscular
Penicillin V	250 mg twice daily	Oral
Sulfadiazine	0.5 g daily for children <27 kg, 1 g daily for children >27 kg	Oral
Macrolide or azalide	For individuals with penicillin/ sulfa allergy—dose variable	Oral
Indication	**Duration**	
Rheumatic fever with carditis and residual heart disease (persistent valvular disease)	10 y or until age 40 y, whichever is longer; sometimes lifetime prophylaxis	
Rheumatic fever with carditis but without residual heart disease (no valvular disease)	10 y or until age 21 y, whichever is longer	
Rheumatic fever without carditis	5 y or until age 21 y, whichever is longer	

Adapted from Gerber MA, Baltimore RS, Eaton CB, et al. Prevention of rheumatic fever and diagnosis and treatment of acute Streptococcal pharyngitis: a scientific statement from the American Heart Association Rheumatic Fever, Endocarditis, and Kawasaki Disease Committee of the Council on Cardiovascular Disease in the Young, the Interdisciplinary Council on Functional Genomics and Translational Biology, and the Interdisciplinary Council on Quality of Care and Outcomes Research: endorsed by the American Academy of Pediatrics. *Circulation*. 2009;119(11):1541-1551.

- ○ *Rickettsia* spp. Myocarditis is not uncommonly seen with rickettsial infections.
- ○ *Borrelia burgdorferi*. Up to 10% acute cases of Lyme disease can present with myocardial involvement, usually in the form of conduction abnormalities.[18] Most cases of Lyme myocarditis resolve entirely.
- In South America, the most common infectious agent causing myocarditis is *Trypanosoma cruzi*, the causative agent of **Chagas disease**.
  - ○ Chagas disease is one of the most common causes of dilated cardiomyopathy worldwide. Heart failure is the main feature of chronic Chagas disease.
  - ○ The agents of African trypanosomiasis, *Trypanosoma gambiense* and *Trypanosoma rhodesiense*, may also cause heart failure, although CNS involvement is most common.

DIAGNOSIS

- A high index of suspicion is required to make the diagnosis. Patient history may reveal symptoms of a recent viral infection involving the upper respiratory tract or the gastrointestinal tract. The presenting symptoms are indistinguishable from other more common causes of heart failure and can include dyspnea on exertion, orthopnea, cough, pink frothy sputum production, and peripheral edema; see Table 4-6.

TABLE 4-6 INFECTIOUS CAUSES OF MYOCARDITIS

Viruses

Coxsackie A and B	Influenza A and B	Lymphocytic choriomen-
Echoviruses	Respiratory syncytial	ingitis virus
Enteroviruses	virus	Lassa virus
Adenovirus	Rabies virus	Cytomegalovirus
Varicella zoster virus	Dengue virus	Epstein–Barr virus
Poliovirus	Chikungunya virus	Herpes simplex virus
Mumps virus	Yellow fever virus	Hepatitis B and C
Measles virus	Argentine hemorrhagic	Parvovirus B19
Rubella virus	fever (Junin virus)	Human immunodefi-
Variola virus	Bolivian hemorrhagic	ciency virus
Vaccinia virus	fever (Machupo virus)	

Bacteria

Corynebacterium diphtheriae	*Staphylococcus aureus*	*Chlamydophila pneumoniae*
Clostridium perfringens	*Listeria monocytogenes*	*Rickettsia rickettsii*
Neisseria meningitides	*Vibrio cholera*	*Rickettsia prowazekii*
Salmonella spp.	*Mycobacterium tuberculosis*	*Rickettsia tsutsugamushi*
Shigella spp.	*Legionella pneumophila*	*Coxiella burnetii*
Campylobacter jejuni	*Mycoplasma pneumoniae*	*Ehrlichia* spp.
Brucella	*Chlamydia psittaci*	*Borrelia burgdorferi*
Streptococcus pyogenes		*Tropheryma whippelii*

Fungi

Aspergillus spp.	*Blastomyces dermatitidis*	*Cryptococcus neoformans*
Candida spp.	*Coccidioides immitis*	*Histoplasma capsulatum*

Parasites

Trypanosoma cruzi	*Trypanosoma rhodesiense*	*Toxoplasma gondii*
Trypanosoma gambiense	*Trichinella spiralis*	*Toxocara canis*

- Infectious myocarditis should be strongly considered in younger patients and patients without prior history or risk factors for heart disease.
- Physical examination may reveal signs of heart failure. Peripheral edema, jugular venous distension, crackles on auscultation of the lungs, and the presence of a third heart sound may be physical examination clues.
- Electrocardiogram will usually give a clue to myocardial involvement. Abnormalities may include conduction abnormalities, supraventricular tachycardia, ventricular arrhythmias, ectopy, heart block, and ischemic changes.
- Abnormalities in laboratory tests may also be present including an elevation of cardiac enzymes. These enzymes usually peak early in infection and may return to normal after a few days. Leukocytosis may or may not be present.
- **Identification of the exact viral agent responsible is not routinely done.** Antibody titers to specific infective agents can be repeated to document a fourfold rise in the convalescent titer. Serum can be sent for PCR for viral agents, although with the exception of testing for treatable viruses such as influenza or human immunodeficiency virus (HIV); it is not clear that there is a clinical benefit to extensive testing.

- Echocardiography is an important component in the diagnosis of myocarditis. Although echocardiography will not reveal the cause of myocardial dysfunction, it may rule out other causes of heart failure such as hypertrophic cardiomyopathy and valvular disease. In general, the cardiac dysfunction caused by myocarditis is diffuse and involves both ventricles. Serial echocardiography may be important to monitor resolution or progression.
- Other imaging modalities have been used, such as cardiac magnetic resonance imaging (MRI) and indium 111–labeled antimyosin antibody scintigraphy, when the diagnosis is not established by echocardiography.
- Endomyocardial biopsy is the "gold standard" for diagnosis but is not routinely done. There are histopathologic criteria for the diagnosis of myocarditis, the Dallas criteria; however, the sensitivity and specificity of evaluating a single sample of myocardium has been questioned.[19]

TREATMENT

- **Supportive care is mainstay of treatment of myocarditis.**
- If the causative agent of infectious myocarditis is identified and if there is specific treatment available this should be initiated as soon as the diagnosis is made. Unfortunately, there are few antiviral agents available for the most common causes of infectious myocarditis.
- Treatment with diuretics, afterload reduction, and possible inotropic agents may be needed short term for heart failure management.
- Treatment with immunosuppression with glucocorticoids or cyclophosphamide has not been supported unless an autoimmune etiology is suspected. Other immunomodulatory agents such as Interferon α and β have been investigated, but data on their efficacy need to still be confirmed by large scale clinical trials.[20]
- Nonsteroidal anti-inflammatory drugs (NSAIDs) should generally be avoided, as they have been shown to worsen outcomes in animal models.
- Many patients with viral myocarditis recover completely with supportive care alone.
- Vaccination is a useful method for preventing infectious myocarditis caused by agents for which there are vaccines available.

Pericarditis

GENERAL PRINCIPLES

- Pericarditis, or inflammation of the pericardium, can be classified into several different types of clinical syndromes: acute, relapsing, tamponade, chronic, or constrictive.
- Most infectious etiologies have an acute presentation.
- Pericarditis, like myocarditis, may be infectious or noninfectious in etiology.
- **There is frequently overlap in the syndromes of pericarditis and myocarditis,** and likewise, there is overlap in many of the agents that can cause infectious pericarditis.
- **The etiology of pericarditis is most commonly idiopathic or due to viral infection.** Many idiopathic cases of pericarditis are likely due to viral infection that is undiagnosed. **The most common viral causes are enteroviruses,** as in myocarditis.
- There are no clinical distinctions between idiopathic and viral pericarditis.
- Pathogens associated with pericarditis are listed in Table 4-7.
- Bacterial causes of pericarditis, or purulent pericarditis, are usually due to extension from head and neck infections, mediastinitis, or postoperative infections. Anaerobic bacteria may cause pericarditis by direct extension from esophageal rupture or mediastinitis, or they may seed the pericardium via the bloodstream. *Neisseria meningitidis* can cause

TABLE 4-7 INFECTIOUS CAUSES OF PERICARDITIS

Viruses

Coxsackie A and B	Variola virus	Cytomegalovirus
Echoviruses	Vaccinia virus	Epstein–Barr virus
Adenovirus	Influenza A and B	Herpes simplex virus
Varicella zoster virus	Lymphocytic chorio-	Hepatitis B
Poliovirus	meningitis virus	Human immunodefi-
Mumps virus	Lassa virus	ciency virus

Bacteria

Streptococcus pneumoniae	*Pseudomonas*	*Nocardia asteroides*
Other *Streptococcus* spp.	*Campylobacter* spp.	*Actinomyces* spp.
Staphylococcus aureus	*Brucella melitensis*	Other anaerobic bacteria
Neisseria meningitidis	*Listeria*	*Legionella pneumophila*
Neisseria gonorrhea	*monocytogenes*	*Mycoplasma*
Haemophilus influenzae	*Mycobacterium*	*pneumoniae*
Salmonella spp.	*tuberculosis*	*Chlamydophila*
Yersinia enterocolitica	Nontuberculous	*pneumoniae*
Francisella tularensis	mycobacteria	*Coxiella burnetii*
		Borrelia burgdorferi

Fungi

Aspergillus spp.	*Blastomyces*	*Cryptococcus neofor-*
Candida spp.	*dermatitidis*	*mans, Histoplasma*
	Coccidioides immitis	*capsulatum*

Parasites

Entamoeba histolytica	*Toxocara canis*	*Paragonimus* spp.
Toxoplasma gondii	*Schistosoma* spp.	

pericarditis by direct bacterial invasion or through a reactive immune process. Primary pulmonary infection with *Mycobacterium tuberculosis* can progress to constrictive pericarditis in up to 1% of cases.[21]
- Fungal causes of pericarditis are rare and can develop from disseminated histoplasmosis, coccidioidomycosis, or even candidiasis. Pericarditis due to *Aspergillus* spp., *Candida* spp., or *Cryptococcus neoformans* is usually seen only in severely immunocompromised patients. The most common risk factor for fungal pericarditis is prior cardiothoracic surgery.
- Parasitic infection is a very rare cause of pericarditis.

DIAGNOSIS

- A high index of suspicion is required for the diagnosis of pericarditis.
- The presenting symptoms vary according to the causative agent of pericarditis.
  - Viral pericarditis is most commonly associated with chest pain. Pain is retrosternal and may be aggravated by breathing, swallowing, and lying flat. Pain relief by sitting up and leaning forward is classic. Frequently, patients will also present with fevers and upper respiratory symptoms. If a large pericardial effusion is present, patients may also have symptoms of heart failure.

- ○ Bacterial pericarditis is usually accompanied by severe systemic infection or local infection involving the head, neck, chest, mediastinum, and thorax.
- ○ Tuberculous pericarditis is frequently insidious in nature. Chest pain may or may not be a predominant feature. Constitutional symptoms are commonly seen, including fevers, cough, night sweats, and weight loss.
- ○ Pleural effusions are common in HIV-infected patients but are usually asymptomatic.
- Physical examination may reveal fevers and tachycardia. The classic finding on physical examination is the pericardial friction rub. The rub associated with pericarditis may be evanescent and difficult to perceive. If the pericardial effusion is large enough, there may be signs of cardiac tamponade, including jugular venous distension and pulsus paradoxus of more than 10 mm Hg.
- Chest radiography may be normal or if there is presence of an effusion greater than 250 mL, enlargement of the cardiac silhouette may be present.
- ECG is crucial in making the diagnosis of acute pericarditis. The classic ECG finding is diffuse ST segment elevations.
- Echocardiography is useful to determine the size of the effusion, to evaluate for tamponade, and to evaluate for underlying myocardial dysfunction or myocarditis.
- It is frequently difficult to identify the viral agent responsible for viral pericarditis. Virus can be potentially isolated by testing a specimen from a throat swab or from the stool. Acute and convalescent antibody titers can be evaluated for a fourfold increase.
- If the effusion is large enough to require drainage, the entire volume of fluid should be drained and sent for evaluation. Fluid should be evaluated for cytology and spun sediment should be ordered and stained for acid-fast bacilli. Viral isolation from the pericardial fluid is uncommon, even if viral etiology is highly suspected. Availability of virus-specific PCR could potentially increase the proportion of cases of pericarditis where the etiology is elucidated. Pericardiocentesis is rarely indicated in cases of presumed viral or idiopathic pericarditis and adds little to the diagnostic yield.
- Evaluation of the pericardial fluid by pericardiocentesis or pericardiotomy is not routinely indicated. If tamponade is present or if the pericardial fluid persists for longer than 3 weeks, evaluation of the fluid may be indicated. Pericardiotomy with biopsy is preferable to pericardiocentesis with regard to the potential diagnostic yield but pericardiotomy is not readily available in most situations.
- Cardiac tamponade is more common in noninfectious causes of pericardial effusions. Bacterial, tuberculous, and fungal pericardial effusions are more likely to cause hemodynamic complications and will likely require drainage.

TREATMENT

- Rest and symptomatic treatment with analgesics are the mainstays of treatment for **viral and idiopathic pericarditis.**
  - ○ **NSAIDs** are useful for the treatment of the chest pain associated with pericarditis. NSAIDs should be avoided if there is a significant component of myocarditis, as they can worsen outcomes in animal models.
  - ○ Steroids should be avoided as in myocarditis.
  - ○ **Colchicine** 0.6 mg twice daily has shown some benefit in acute pericarditis and may be useful to prevent recurrent episodes; however, prospective double-blind studies are lacking.[22] Colchicine should be monitored carefully.
  - ○ **Purulent pericarditis** should be diagnosed aggressively, as untreated purulent pericarditis is uniformly fatal.
  - ○ Pericardiocentesis should be performed, and empiric **antibiotics** should be given and appropriate antibiotics continued once the causative agent is identified.
  - ○ Cardiothoracic surgery should be notified for emergent drainage, as these effusions usually reaccumulate rapidly and must be surgically drained.

- **Tuberculous pericarditis** should be treated with **standard four-drug antituberculous treatment.**
  - Effusions should be drained if tamponade develops.
  - Steroids have previously been universally recommended in combination with antituberculous therapy; however, a recent clinical trial and additional systematic reviews did not find differences in mortality, constrictive pericarditis or tamponade when steroids were compared with placebo. Based on these, the 2016 guidelines for management of tuberculosis from the American Thoracic Society, Centers for Disease Control, and the Infectious Diseases Society of America no longer endorse the routine use of steroids in these patients. Selective use in patients with large pericardial effusions, high levels of inflammatory cells or markers in pericardial fluid, or early signs of constriction may be appropriate based on evidence suggesting lower risk of developing constrictive pericarditis.[23]

REFERENCES

1. Mermel LA, Allon M, Bouza E, et al. Clinical practice guidelines for the diagnosis and management of intravascular catheter-related infection: 2009 update by the Infectious Diseases Society of America. *Clin Infect Dis.* 2009;49(1):1-45.
2. O'Grady NP, Alexander M, Burns LA, et al. Guidelines for the prevention of intravascular catheter-related infections. *Clin Infect Dis.* 2011;52(9):e162-e193.
3. Yahav D, Rozen-Zvi B, Gafter-Gvili A, Leibovici L, Gafter U, Paul M. Antimicrobial lock solutions for the prevention of infections associated with intravascular catheters in patients undergoing hemodialysis: systematic review and meta-analysis of randomized, controlled trials. *Clin Infect Dis.* 2008;47(1):83-93.
4. Honda H, Krauss MJ, Jones JC, Olsen MA, Warren DK. The value of infectious diseases consultation in *Staphylococcus aureus* bacteremia. *Am J Med.* 2010;123(7):631-637.
5. Wilson W, Taubert KA, Gewitz M, et al. Prevention of infective endocarditis: guidelines from the American Heart Association: a guideline from the American Heart Association Rheumatic Fever, Endocarditis, and Kawasaki Disease Committee, Council on Cardiovascular Disease in the Young, and the Council on Clinical Cardiology, Council on Cardiovascular Surgery and Anesthesia, and the Quality of Care and Outcomes Research Interdisciplinary Working Group. *Circulation.* 2007;116(15):1736-1754.
6. Baddour LM, Wilson WR, Bayer AS, et al. Infective endocarditis in adults: diagnosis, antimicrobial therapy, and management of complications: a scientific statement for healthcare professionals from the American Heart Association. *Circulation.* 2015;132(15):1435-1486.
7. Bashore TM, Cabell C, Fowler V. Update on infective endocarditis. *Curr Probl Cardiol.* 2006;31(4):274-352.
8. McDonald JR. Acute infective endocarditis. *Infect Dis Clin North Am.* 2009;23(3):643-664.
9. Mandell GL, Bennett JE, Dolin R. *Mandell, Douglas and Bennett's Principles and Practices of Infectious Diseases.* 7th ed. Philadelphia, PA: Churchill Livingstone; 2009.
10. Baddour LM, Epstein AE, Erickson CC, et al. Update on cardiovascular implantable electronic device infections and their management: a scientific statement from the American Heart Association. *Circulation.* 2010;121(3):458-477.
11. Kusne S, Mooney M, Danziger-Isakov L, et al. An ISHLT consensus document for prevention and management strategies for mechanical circulatory support infection. *J Heart Lung Transplant.* 2017;36(10):1137-1153.
12. Baddour LM, Bettmann MA, Bolger AF, et al. Nonvalvular cardiovascular device-related infections. *Circulation.* 2003;108(16):2015-2031.
13. Kirklin JK, Cantor R, Mohacsi P, et al. First annual IMACS report: a global International Society for Heart and Lung Transplantation Registry for Mechanical Circulatory Support. *J Heart Lung Transplant.* 2016;35(4):407-412.
14. Sohail MR, Uslan DZ, Khan AH, et al. Management and outcome of permanent pacemaker and implantable cardioverter-defibrillator infections. *J Am Coll Cardiol.* 2007;49(18):1851-1859.
15. Armstrong AW, Spooner K, Sanders JW. Lemierre's syndrome. *Curr Infect Dis Rep.* 2000;2(2):168-173.

16. Gerber MA, Baltimore RS, Eaton CB, et al. Prevention of rheumatic fever and diagnosis and treatment of acute Streptococcal pharyngitis: a scientific statement from the American Heart Association Rheumatic Fever, Endocarditis, and Kawasaki Disease Committee of the Council on Cardiovascular Disease in the Young, the Interdisciplinary Council on Functional Genomics and Translational Biology, and the Interdisciplinary Council on Quality of Care and Outcomes Research: endorsed by the American Academy of Pediatrics. *Circulation.* 2009;119(11):1541-1551.

17. Knowlton KU. *Myocarditis and pericarditis. Mandell, Douglas, and Bennett's Principles and Practice of Infectious Diseases;* 2009.

18. Ciesielski CA, Markowitz LE, Horsley R, et al. Lyme disease surveillance in the United States, 1983–1986. *Rev Infect Dis.* 1989;11(Suppl 6):S1435-S1441.

19. Aretz HT, Billingham ME, Edwards WD, et al. Myocarditis. A histopathologic definition and classification. *Am J Cardiovasc Pathol.* 1987;1(1):3-14.

20. Magnani JW, Dec GW. Myocarditis: current trends in diagnosis and treatment. *Circulation.* 2006;113(6):876-890.

21. Larrieu AJ, Tyers GF, Williams EH, Derrick JR. Recent experience with tuberculous pericarditis. *Ann Thorac Surg.* 1980;29(5):464-468.

22. Lotrionte M, Biondi-Zoccai G, Imazio M, et al. International collaborative systematic review of controlled clinical trials on pharmacologic treatments for acute pericarditis and its recurrences. *Am Heart J.* 2010;160(4):662-670.

23. Nahid P, Dorman SE, Alipanah N, et al. Executive summary: official American Thoracic Society/Centers for Disease Control and Prevention/Infectious Diseases Society of America Clinical Practice Guidelines: Treatment of Drug-Susceptible Tuberculosis. *Clin Infect Dis.* 2016;63(7):853-867.

Respiratory Infections

Carlos Mejia-Chew and Michael A. Lane

5

Acute Pharyngitis

GENERAL PRINCIPLES

- Acute pharyngitis is one of the most common syndromes seen by primary care physicians.
- Pathogenesis may include inflammatory mediators, direct invasion of pharyngeal cells, and lymphoid hyperplasia.
- Viruses are the most common cause of pharyngitis.
- Group A streptococcal (GAS) pharyngitis is the most common bacterial cause of acute pharyngitis in both children (20%–30%) and adults (5%–15%).[1]
- In patients with HIV, *Candida albicans*, cytomegalovirus (CMV), and sexually transmitted infections such as *Neisseria gonorrhoeae* and herpes simplex virus should be considered.
- Table 5-1 presents pathogens that commonly cause respiratory infections, including pharyngitis.[1]

TABLE 5-1	ETIOLOGY OF RESPIRATORY INFECTIONS	
Microorganism	**Clinical Syndrome**	**Comments**
Virus		
Rhinovirus/coronavirus	Common cold Acute bronchitis	Most common cause.
Human metapneumovirus	Common cold Acute bronchitis	Can cause severe disease in infants, elderly, and immunocompromised persons.
Adenovirus	Pharyngoconjunctival fever Acute bronchitis Pneumonia	
Coxsackievirus	Herpangina	
Parainfluenza	Croup, pneumonia, bronchitis	
Influenza A and B	Influenza Acute bronchitis	Superinfection with *Staphylococcus aureus* is common.
Respiratory syncytial virus infection	Bronchiolitis in children Pneumonia	Likely to have sinus or ear involvement.

(Continued)

TABLE 5-1	ETIOLOGY OF RESPIRATORY INFECTIONS (CONTINUED)	
Microorganism	**Clinical Syndrome**	**Comments**
Viral		
Measles virus	Pneumonia Croup and bronchiolitis in children	Pneumonia is the most common cause of measles-associated death.
Rubella virus	Rubella	
Epstein–Barr virus	Mononucleosis/mononucleosis-like syndrome	Only serologies can distinguish them.
Cytomegalovirus		
Human immunodeficiency virus		Acute HIV infection can concomitantly have opportunistic infections.
Herpes simplex virus	Gingivostomatitis	Therapy within 72 h leads to faster healing.
Bacteria		
Group A β-hemolytic streptococci	Pharyngotonsillitis, scarlet fever	Group C and group G Streptococcus can also cause pharyngotonsillitis.
Arcanobacterium haemolyticum	Pharyngitis with scarlatiniform rash	
Corynebacterium diphtheriae	Diphtheria	
Bordetella pertussis	Acute bronchitis ("whooping cough")	
Fusobacterium necrophorum	Peritonsillar abscess, Lemierre syndrome	
Mixed anaerobes	Vincent angina	
Francisella tularensis	Tularemia: oropharyngeal or severe pneumonia	
Streptococcus pneumoniae	Pneumonia, sepsis	Most common cause of pneumonia
Haemophilus influenzae	Pneumonia, bronchitis	
Mycoplasma pneumoniae	Pneumonitis, bronchitis	
Chlamydia pneumoniae	Pneumonia, bronchitis	
Chlamydia psittaci	Psittacosis (Parrot fever)	Exposure to parrots or other birds.
Treponema pallidum	Syphilis	Dark field microscopy
Neisseria gonorrhoeae	Pharyngitis	

TABLE 5-1	ETIOLOGY OF RESPIRATORY INFECTIONS (CONTINUED)	

Microorganism	Clinical Syndrome	Comments
Coxiella burnetii	Q fever: from flu-like illness to pneumonia	A common cause of culture-negative endocarditis.
Mycobacterium tuberculosis	Pleural tuberculosis, pulmonary tuberculosis with or without cavitation, military tuberculosis	
Nontuberculosis mycobacterial infection	Lady Windermere syndrome, pneumonia, pulmonary cavitation	Most commonly due to MAC and M. kansasii
Nocardia spp	Pulmonary cavitations	
Fungi		
Aspergillus fumigatus	Aspergillosis	It is angioinvasive
Histoplasma capsulatum	Histoplasmosis	Hilar and mediastinal lymphadenopathy is common
Blastomyces dermatitis	Blastomycosis	Similar presentation as histoplasmosis, but bone and skin involvement is more common
Coccidioides immitis	*Coccidioidomycosis*	
Candida albicans	Thrush—pharyngitis/ esophagitis	
Mimics of Infection		
Kawasaki disease	Pharyngitis	Vasculitis typically having skin and renal disease (e.g., glomerulonephritis) involvement
Stevens–Johnson syndrome		
Behçet syndrome		
Cryptogenic organizing pneumonia (COP)	Pneumonia	COP commonly presents as recurrent pneumonia
ANCA-associated vasculitis		

ANCA, antineutrophil cytoplasmic antibodies; MAC, mycobacterium avium-intracellulare complex.

DIAGNOSIS

Clinical Presentation

- Patients typically have upper respiratory tract infection symptoms that begin with a prodrome of fever, malaise, and headache.
- Patients may have tonsillar exudates and anterior cervical lymphadenopathy.
- Patients should not have any signs of a lower respiratory tract infection such as productive cough or abnormal lung sounds.

TABLE 5-2	MODIFIED CENTOR CRITERIA (MCISAAC) TO DIAGNOSE GROUP A β-HEMOLYTIC STREPTOCOCCAL PHARYNGITIS	
Criteria	**Point**	
Tonsillar exudates	1	
Tender anterior cervical adenopathy	1	
History of fever (>38°C [100.4°F])	1	
Absence of cough	1	
Age 3–14	1	
Age 15–44	0	
Age ≥45	−1	
Score	**Action**	
0 criteria	No testing,[a] no antibiotics	
1 criterion	No testing, no antibiotics	
2 or 3 criteria	Perform testing, antibiotics if positive	
4–5 criteria	Empiric antibiotics	

Adapted from Mclsaac WJ, Goel V, To T, Low DE. The validity of a sore throat score in family practice. *CMAJ.* 2000;163:811-815.
[a]Throat culture or rapid antigen detection testing.

Diagnostic Criteria
- There are no diagnostic criteria for nonspecific pharyngitis.
- Clinical diagnosis of GAS pharyngitis can be aided by the **modified Centor Diagnostic Criteria** (Table 5-2).[2]

Diagnostic Testing
- Throat cultures are the gold standard for GAS pharyngitis; however, they can take 24 to 48 hours to grow.
- Rapid streptococcal antigen testing takes minutes and is often tested in the office while a patient is waiting. Newer assays have 90% to 99% sensitivity and 90% to 99% specificity.[1] Rapid tests should be performed in patients with 2 to 3 Centor criteria.
- Serologic tests, such as antistreptolysin O (ASO) and antideoxyribonuclease B, should only be performed in cases of suspected rheumatic fever and not routinely used for possible GAS pharyngitis.
- A broader differential diagnosis and additional testing should be considered for those patients with a Centor score of 3 or 4 with a negative rapid streptococcal test or in those that do not improve within 36 hours of antibiotic therapy.
- No further testing needs to be performed for patients with <2 Centor criteria.[3]

TREATMENT

- Most cases of pharyngitis do not require treatment (Centor criteria <2).
- However, all cases of GAS pharyngitis should be treated as indicated in Table 5-3,[1] for the following reasons:

○ Reduce risk of complications including rheumatic fever and peritonsillar abscess
○ Prevent transmission of GAS pharyngitis to other people
○ Reduce duration and severity of symptoms

COMPLICATIONS

- There are few complications for most causes of pharyngitis.
- However, GAS pharyngitis may lead to the following:
  ○ Acute rheumatic fever (see Table 5-4)
  ○ Peritonsillar abscess and retropharyngeal abscess
- Rheumatic heart disease is much more common in developing countries than in the United States. It may manifest years after initial symptoms of rheumatic fever.
- Throat cultures are negative in most patients with rheumatic fever, so ASO and other titers may be beneficial.
- Antibiotic treatment does not affect the risk of developing post-streptococcal glomerulonephritis.

TABLE 5-3	SUGGESTED ADULT REGIMENS FOR STREPTOCOCCAL PHARYNGITIS

Penicillin V 500 mg PO twice daily for 10 d

Amoxicillin 500 mg PO twice daily for 10 d

Cephalexin 500 mg PO twice daily for 10 d

Clindamycin 300 mg PO three times daily for 10 d

Azithromycin 500 mg PO once then 250 mg PO daily for 4 d[a]

[a]In some communities up to 15% of the group A streptococcal isolates can be resistant.

TABLE 5-4	JONES CRITERIA FOR RHEUMATIC FEVER	
History/examination	**Major criteria:**	**Minor criteria:**
	Migratory arthritis	Fever
	Sydenham chorea	Elevated acute phase reactants
	Erythema marginatum	
	Subcutaneous nodules	Prolonged PR interval
	Carditis	Arthralgias
Diagnosis	a. Serologic evidence of group A streptococcal infection **PLUS**	
	b. Two major criteria **or** one major **plus** two minor manifestations	

Acute Epiglottitis

GENERAL PRINCIPLES

- Acute epiglottitis is an inflammation of the epiglottis and surrounding structures.
- **All cases of epiglottitis should be considered a respiratory emergency,** as inflammation of the epiglottis can lead to **airway obstruction.**
- Although historically a disease primarily of children, the advent of *Haemophilus influenzae* type b (Hib) vaccination has reduced childhood risk significantly.[4]
- Pathogens originate from the posterior nasopharynx, and
- Bacteria (*H. influenzae*, *Staphylococcus aureus*, group A β-hemolytic Streptococcus, and *Streptococcus pneumoniae*) are the most common causes but viruses and fungi, especially in the immunocompromised host, can also cause epiglottitis.
- Epiglottitis results from either direct spread from adjacent structures or from seeding of the epiglottis following transient bacteremia. It is important to consider a possible primary source for infection elsewhere such as pneumonia.

DIAGNOSIS

Clinical Presentation

- Sore throat, odynophagia, dysphagia, muffled voice ("hot potato voice") and fever are the most common symptoms.
- Patients may have anterior cervical lymphadenopathy and tenderness to palpation. In adults, oropharyngeal examination may be normal.
- Drooling, tripod posture, and respiratory distress may also be present.
- **Inspiratory stridor** is a classic sign and late finding indicating impending respiratory failure.
- **Manipulation of a tenuous airway should only be performed by specialists, as it can precipitate airway compromise.**
- Direct laryngoscopy performed by a subspecialist can assist both in confirming the diagnosis and in assessing the airway.[4]

Differential Diagnosis

- The differential diagnosis includes mononucleosis, whopping cough, respiratory diptheria, croup, and pharyngeal abscesses such as Ludwig's angina.
- Noninfectious causes such as mechanical obstruction by foreign bodies or tumor, angioedema, airway irritants (heat or chemicals), amyloidosis, and sarcoidosis should also be considered.

Diagnostic Testing

- Blood cultures and throat cultures are often negative but should still be obtained.
- Neck radiographs are often normal and are not necessary to make the diagnosis. If performed, findings may include an enlarged epiglottis or "thumb print sign" and normal subglottic space.
- Bedside ultrasonography is rapid, noninvasive, and accurate when performed by a trained and experienced physician. The classical sign visualized is the "alphabet P sign" in a longitudinal view through thyrohyoid membrane.[5]
- Direct laryngoscopy is the preferred method used to assist in the diagnosis and categorize severity of disease.

TREATMENT

- **Airway stabilization** should be considered before all else in patients with epiglottitis, and treatment should be tailored to the severity of airway compromise (see Table 5-5).[6]

TABLE 5-5	FRIEDMAN EPIGLOTTITIS STAGING	
Stage	Signs and Symptoms	Airway Management
I	No respiratory distress Respiratory rate <20/min	Close intensive care unit observation
II	Mild respiratory distress Respiratory rate 20–30/min	Intubation by anesthesia or with bronchoscopy (with equipment for emergent tracheostomy at bedside) or formal tracheostomy in operating room
III	Moderate respiratory distress Respiratory rate >30/min Stridor, retractions, perioral cyanosis Pco_2 >45 mm Hg	Immediate intubation or cricothyroidotomy
IV	Severe respiratory distress Severe stridor, retractions Cyanosis, delirium, loss of consciousness, hypoxia Respiratory arrest	Immediate intubation or cricothyroidotomy

Adapted from Ng HL, Sin LM, Li MF, et al. Acute epiglottitis in adults: a retrospective review of 106 patients in Hong Kong. *Emerg Med J*. 2008;25:253-255.

- After airway stabilization, antibiotics should be initiated.
  - Empiric antibiotic coverage consists of a third-generation cephalosporin, such as ceftriaxone 2 g every 24 hours.
  - Vancomycin may be added if there is concern for methicillin-resistant *S. aureus* (MRSA).
  - Treatment duration is often 7 to 10 days but may need to be extended for patients with bacteremia, meningitis, or immunodeficiency.
  - If possible, antibiotic coverage should be narrowed based on culture results.
- Steroids are often given, but their utility and optimal dose are unknown.
- For known Hib exposure, rifampin (RIF) 600 mg PO once a day for 4 days is recommended as post exposure prophylaxis for unvaccinated close contacts (>4 h a day for >5 d preceding episode). This is not recommended if all household contacts <2 years old have completed Hib immunization.

Rhinosinusitis

GENERAL PRINCIPLES

- Rhinosinusitis results in inflammation of the mucosa of the nose and paranasal sinuses.
- Sinusitis can be classified by
  - Duration (acute ≤1 mo, chronic >12 wk)
  - Location (maxillary, sphenoid, ethmoid, and frontal)
  - Type of organism—viral, bacterial, fungal, and noninfectious
- Paranasal sinuses are outpouchings of the nasal mucosa. They are lined with mucoperiosteum and cilia, which sweep mucus toward the ostia.

- Acute rhinosinusitis (ARS) is a result of impaired mucociliary clearance and obstruction of the ostia.
- This results in stagnant secretions and decreased ventilation, creating an ideal culture medium for bacteria.
- **Viruses** (e.g., rhinoviruses, adenovirus) are the most common cause of acute sinusitis.
- Secondary bacterial infection complicates ARS infrequently (0.5%–2.0%).
- The most common **bacterial** etiologies (often secondary) in acute sinusitis include:
  - *S. pneumonia*
  - *H. influenza*
  - *Moraxella catarrhalis*
- *S. aureus*, coagulase-negative staphylococci, and anaerobic bacteria are more common in chronic rhinosinusitis (CRS) but **CRS is more often an inflammatory process.**
- *S. aureus* is increasing in prevalence in sinusitis patients with nasal polyps.
- *Pseudomonas aeruginosa* infection frequently occurs in patients with cystic fibrosis.
- Fungal causes include *Mucor*, *Rhizopus*, and *Aspergillus.*
  - Risk factors for fungal sinusitis include neutropenia, diabetes mellitus, HIV, and other immunocompromised states.
  - In immunocompetent hosts, the presence of fungi is more likely to represent an allergic reaction to environmental fungi rather than a true infection.
- Vasculitis is an uncommon noninfectious cause of rhinosinusitis.

DIAGNOSIS

Clinical Presentation

- The diagnosis of rhinosinusitis is usually entirely clinical and the differentiation between viral and bacterial infections can be difficult.
- Multiple studies regarding the utility of symptoms and signs for diagnosing acute sinusitis have sometimes reached differing conclusions. A few have used the true gold standard (i.e., sinus puncture and culture) but more have used a surrogate standard (e.g., sinus plain films and computed tomography [CT]). Radiography cannot differentiate viral from bacterial sinusitis.
- ARS symptoms within the first 7 to 10 days of illness typically indicate a viral rhinosinusitis.
- Acute bacterial sinusitis usually presents with symptoms that persist >10 days or worsen within the first 10 days.[7,8]
- **The prominent symptoms of acute bacterial rhinosinusitis are nasal congestion, purulent rhinorrhea, facial–dental pain, high fever (≥39°C),** postnasal drainage, headache, and cough.
- Signs of ARS include sinus tenderness, purulent nasal discharge, erythematous mucosa, pharyngeal secretions, and periorbital edema.
- Cough is more prominent in chronic sinusitis.

Diagnostic Testing

- Bacterial cultures of the nasal cavity or of purulent secretions are not helpful.
- When an atypical pathogen or intracranial extension is suspected, invasive sinus cultures may be performed by an otolaryngologist.
- Radiographic imaging is neither necessary nor recommended for the diagnosis in the majority of patients. When performed, **limited sinus CT** should be used. Findings consistent with sinusitis are:
  - Mucosal thickening >4 mm
  - Air-fluid level
  - Complete sinus opacification
  - Absence of all three has a high sensitivity in ruling out disease

TREATMENT

- **Most cases of ARS are caused by viruses and are expected to significantly improve without antibiotic treatment within 10 to 14 days.** Treatment should, therefore, focus on management of symptoms for most patients.
- Trials of the efficacy of antibiotics in ARS have been of variable quality and differing outcome measures. Most of the randomized trials did not limit enrollment to only subjects with bacterial infections. Nonetheless, taken together, there may be a **modest benefit from antibiotic treatment.**
- Uncomplicated acute bacterial rhinosinusitis may be treated with or without antibiotics, with cure rates as high as 60% with the later approach.
  - **Patients without severe or prolonged symptoms may be managed initially with symptomatic treatment alone** and followed for resolution. Worsening of symptoms during this time should prompt a reconsideration of antibiotic therapy.
  - Individual clinical judgment should be exercised when making the decision to forgo or prescribe antibiotic therapy.
- The **treatment of choice for uncomplicated acute bacterial rhinosinusitis is amoxicillin-clavulanate** for 5 to 7 days.[8]
- Doxycycline and levofloxacin may be considered for patients with beta-lactam allergy.
- Macrolides and trimethoprim-sulfamethoxazole are not recommended as alternative therapies due to high rate of resistance among *S. pneumonia and H. influenzae.*
- The optimal duration of antibiotic therapy is unclear, but systematic review has failed to show clear benefit with >10 day courses.[8]
- In patients who worsen or do not improve during the initial 3 to 5 days of antimicrobial therapy, cultures by direct sinus aspiration should be obtained.
- Although the evidence is somewhat limited, the addition of **intranasal steroids** and sinus irrigation may have modest positive benefit and is recommended in the treatment of both ARS and CRS.[9]
- Although a mild improvement of symptoms can occur with the use of systemic steroids, findings among studies are inconsistent and thus they are not routinely recommended.[10]
- **Analgesics** should be prescribed to those with significant pain.
- Data to support the use of decongestants, antihistamines, mucolytics/expectorants, are weak and not recommended for the treatment of ARS.[7,11]

COMPLICATIONS

- Orbital cellulitis, brain abscess, meningitis, cavernous thrombosis, osteomyelitis, and mucocele are all possible but quite uncommon.
- Colonizing rather than pathogenic bacteria typically causes CRS. Antibiotics are not recommended as patients often do not respond clinically to them and biofilms are frequent. Fungal pathogens are frequently found in cultures of patients with chronic sinusitis, but treatment is not recommended in immunocompetent patients.[8]

Acute Bronchitis

GENERAL PRINCIPLES

- Acute bronchitis is inflammation of the large and mid-sized airways characterized by the sudden onset of cough with or without production of phlegm and accompanying upper respiratory and constitutional symptoms.

- A specific etiology is found in a minority of patients. The most common pathogens are usually viruses (Table 5-1), and less than 10% of cases are due to bacteria.[12]
- The pathophysiology is mediated by direct invasion of epithelial cells of the tracheobronchial tree by pathogens, with resultant release of inflammatory mediators. Patients then develop airway hypersensitivity leading to cough and, occasionally, wheezing.

DIAGNOSIS

Clinical Presentation

- Cough for at least 5 days is necessary to diagnose acute bronchitis. **Coughing may last up to 3 weeks for an episode of acute bronchitis.** Purulent sputum production is also common (up to half of patients) and does not signify a more serious infection such as pneumonia.
- Listen for wheezes, rales, and rhonchi on physical examination.
- Evaluation should focus on ruling out pneumonia. The presence of abnormal vital signs (heart rate ≥100 beats/min, respiratory rate ≥24 breaths/min, or oral temperature ≥38°C) along with abnormal lung examination findings (focal consolidation, egophony, fremitus) is concerning for pneumonia and uncommon in bronchitis.

Differential Diagnosis

The differential diagnosis includes pneumonia, influenza, gastroesophageal reflux, postnasal drip, smoking, toxic inhalations, and angiotensin-converting enzyme inhibitors, asthma, chronic bronchitis, and chronic obstructive pulmonary disease exacerbation.

Diagnostic Testing

- **Routine sputum cultures are not recommended** as bacterial pathogens rarely cause acute bronchitis.
- Patients with severe paroxysmal cough or cough >2 weeks should have nasopharyngeal (NP) swab done for culture or polymerase chain reaction (PCR) testing to evaluate for pertussis.
- Influenza testing should be considered based on seasonal patterns of influenza and patient presentation.
- Chest radiography should not be performed routinely in the absence of abnormal vital signs or concerning physical examination findings.
- The diagnosis of tracheobronchitis in hospitalized patients can be challenging. Patients will often have signs of pneumonia with fever, leukocytosis, and purulent sputum production. However, they will have a clear chest radiograph.
- Quantitative or semiquantitative sputum cultures in symptomatic patients can be obtained to guide therapy.

TREATMENT

- **Multiple studies have shown no benefit in antimicrobial therapy for generally healthy patients with acute outpatient non–pertussis-related bronchitis.**[13]
- Symptom management is the cornerstone of therapy. This often includes nonsteroidal anti-inflammatory drugs, acetaminophen, dextromethorphan, or codeine.[13]
- If clinical suspicion for pertussis is high and a patient presents within the first 2 weeks of symptoms, consider azithromycin 500 mg PO once, then 250 mg PO daily for 4 days to reduce the risk of transmission.
- In cases of tracheobronchitis, treatment should be based on sputum culture results.

Community-Acquired Pneumonia

GENERAL PRINCIPLES

- Community-acquired pneumonia (CAP) is defined as infection of the pulmonary parenchyma in patients who have not spent any significant amount of time in the hospital, dialysis centers, nursing homes, or clinics recently.
- The rate of CAP is between 1.5 and 14 cases per 1000 persons per year and costs billions of US dollars per year.[14,15]
- Before antibiotics, Sir William Osler called it "the captain of the men of death." Even with antibiotics, pneumonia is the leading cause of hospitalization and death worldwide.[15]
- Common pneumonia associations and pathogens are listed in Table 5-6.[15]
- All patients should be offered the influenza vaccine annually and before discharge from the hospital.
- Patients aged 65 years or older, and those with certain medical conditions, should receive the pneumococcal vaccination with both the 23-valent and the 13-valent vaccine, as outlined by the Recommended Immunization Schedule for Adults Aged 19 Years or Older, United States, 2017.[16]

DIAGNOSIS

Clinical Presentation

- CAP is a clinical diagnosis requiring a combination of history, physical examination, and an infiltrate on chest radiograph.
- The presentation of CAP is extremely variable. Frequently, patients will present with productive cough, fever, dyspnea, and pleuritic chest pain. However, delirium, headache, myalgias, nausea, and vomiting can be seen in elderly individuals or in cases of atypical or "walking" pneumonia.
- Pneumonia can present with abnormalities in any or all of the vital signs. Extremes in vital signs portend a worse prognosis, as shown in the Pneumonia Severity Index (Table 5-7).[17]

TABLE 5-6	TYPICAL ASSOCIATED EXPOSURE IN PNEUMONIA
Association	**Organism**
Aspiration	Gram-negative, oral anaerobes
Lung abscess	Community-acquired methicillin-resistant *S. aureus*, oral anaerobes, fungal, *Mycobacterium tuberculosis*, atypical mycobacteria
Bat/bird droppings	*Histoplasma capsulatum*
Bird fanciers	*Chlamydophila psittaci*
Rabbit exposure	*Francisella tularensis*
Farm animals	*Coxiella burnetii*
HIV	*Pneumocystis jiroveci*, *Cryptococcus neoformans*, mycobacteria
Cruise ship	*Legionella* spp.
Bioterrorism	*Bacillus anthracis*, *Yersinia pestis*, *Francisella tularensis*

TABLE 5-7 PNEUMONIA SEVERITY INDEX

Characteristic	Points
Sex	
Male	0
Female	−10
Demographic Factors	
Age	1 per year
Nursing home resident	10
Comorbidities	
Neoplasia	30
Liver disease	20
Heart failure	10
Cerebrovascular disease	10
Renal disease	10
Physical Examination	
Altered mental status	20
Respiratory rate ≥30/min	20
Systolic blood pressure <90 mm Hg	20
Temperature <35°C (95°F) or ≥40°C (104°F)	15
Heart rate ≥125/min	10
Laboratories	
Arterial pH <7.35	30
Blood urea nitrogen ≥30 mg/dL	20
Sodium <130 mmol/L	20
Glucose ≥250 mg/dL	10
Hematocrit <30%	10
PO_2 <60 mm Hg	10
Radiographic Findings	
Pleural effusion	10

Total Points	Class	Mortality (%)	Management
0	I	0.1	Outpatient
<70	II	0.6	Outpatient
71–90	III	0.9	Brief inpatient
91–130	IV	9.3	Inpatient
>130	V	27.0	Inpatient

Adapted from Fine MJ, Auble TE, Yealy DM, et al. A prediction rule to identify low-risk patients with community-acquired pneumonia. *N Engl J Med*. 1997;336:243-250.

- Physical examination findings consistent with pneumonia are the same as lung consolidation such as tactile fremitus, dullness to percussion, decreased breath sounds, rales, and egophony.

Differential Diagnosis

The differential diagnosis for CAP includes heart failure, pneumonitis, pulmonary edema, septic emboli, malignancies, foreign body inhalation, and pulmonary infarction.

Diagnostic Testing

Laboratories

- Usually no workup is warranted for patients who will receive outpatient treatment.
- Sputum for Gram stain and culture should be strongly considered for all patients.
- Blood cultures are usually performed on hospitalized patients and should be obtained before empiric antibiotics if possible.
- Recent rapid multiorganism PCR-based testing has shown bacterial and viral detection rates as high as 86%.[18]
- Laboratories that may be helpful in selected patients include:
  ○ Urine *Legionella* antigen: Highly sensitive and specific, but only detects serogroup 1, which causes 80% to 90% of infections
  ○ Urine pneumococcal antigen (80% sensitive)
  ○ Multiorganism PCR NP swab
  ○ Sputum for acid-fast staining if there is a clinical suspicion for mycobacterial infection

Imaging

- Chest radiography should be performed on all patients suspected of having CAP.[15,19]
- The location of the infiltrate may help indicate the causative organism.
  ○ *S. pneumoniae* and *Legionella* pneumonia typically cause lobar infiltrates.
  ○ "Atypical" and viral pneumonias are typically diffuse or bilateral.
  ○ Aspiration pneumonia location depends on the position of the patient when they aspirated. It may present as a cavitary lesion if long-standing.
  ○ *Pneumocystis* pneumonia may have a negative chest radiograph but a CT scan will usually show evidence of disease diffuse interstitial disease.

Diagnostic Procedures

Bronchoscopy, CT scan, and thoracentesis are further diagnostic procedures and studies that are typically reserved for severe or nonresponding CAP.

TREATMENT

- The initial step in determining treatment is deciding whether a patient with CAP requires hospitalization or can be safely treated as an outpatient.
- There are two commonly used prediction tools to help assess risk of mortality.
  ○ The Pneumonia Severity Index, commonly known as the PORT score, was the first indicator used to evaluate for severity of CAP in patients presenting to the emergency department. It has been well validated but requires a lengthy number of laboratory tests (Table 5-7).[17]
  ○ The CURB-65 or the more simplified CRB-65, which requires no blood tests, is designed to help risk stratify patients presenting to the clinic to either outpatient or inpatient treatment (Table 5-8).[19]
- Other findings consistent with poor prognosis include thrombocytopenia, leukopenia, multilobar infiltrates, septic shock requiring vasopressors, and invasive mechanical ventilation.

TABLE 5-8	CURB-65 SCORE	
Characteristics	**Points**	
Confusion	1	
Urea nitrogen >20 mg/dL	1	
Respiratory rate >30/min	1	
Blood pressure, systolic <90 mm Hg	1	
Age ≥**65**	1	

Total Points	Mortality (%)	Management
0	0.7	Outpatient
1	3.2	Outpatient
2	3	Inpatient
3	17	Consider intensive care unit
4	41.5	Consider intensive care unit
5	57	Consider intensive care unit

Adapted from Lim WS, van der Eerden MM, Laing R, et al. Defining community acquired pneumonia severity on presentation to hospital: international derivation and validation study. *Thorax.* 2003;58:377-382.

- Antibiotics are the mainstay of therapy for CAP because most cases are caused by bacterial pathogens. However, it is important to consider that around 25% of cases are caused by viral pathogens and will not respond to antibiotic therapy.

Medication

- Treatment options for CAP are presented in Table 5-9.[20,21]
- Antibiotic changes should be made according to susceptibilities from your laboratory or culture data as soon as possible to provide the narrowest spectrum antibiotics for a particular pathogen.
- Changing from IV to PO antibiotics should also be constantly reevaluated. Patients can be switched from an IV to a PO regimen and discharged from the hospital when clinically stable or improving.
- Duration of therapy for CAP should be 5 days for low-severity pneumonia, provided that the patient has been afebrile for over 48 hours and has clinically improved, and 7 days for severe pneumonia that can be prolonged depending on the clinical course.[21]
- Several meta-analyses have evaluated the adjunctive use of corticosteroids in CAP. Although these analyses suggest that corticosteroids are safe and may even be beneficial in severe CAP, adequately powered studies are lacking to recommend their use in general patient populations.[22]
- **Antibiotics should be administered as soon as CAP is diagnosed, ideally within the first 4 hours of arrival to the hospital, as there is evidence that delay in antibiotic therapy leads to higher patient mortality.**[15,20]

TABLE 5-9	TREATMENT OF COMMUNITY-ACQUIRED PNEUMONIA	
Category	First Line Alternative	Antibiotic Selection
Outpatient, no comorbidities	Macrolide (azithromycin) **or** Doxycycline	Azithromycin is the preferred macrolide because of tolerability
Outpatient, with comorbidities	β-Lactam (amoxicillin/clavulanate or cefpodoxime) **PLUS** macrolide **or** Respiratory fluoroquinolone (FQ) (moxifloxacin/levofloxacin)	Respiratory FQs should be limited to situations in which other options cannot be prescribed or are ineffective
Inpatient, non-ICU	IV β-lactam (ceftriaxone) **PLUS** macrolide **or** Respiratory FQ	There are increasing rates of FQ resistance in certain communities
Inpatient, ICU	IV β-lactam (ceftriaxone, ampicillin–sulbactam) **PLUS** azithromycin **or** respiratory FQ If concern for MRSA, add vancomycin or linezolid If concern for *Pseudomonas*, change β-lactam to cefepime, meropenem, or piperacillin–tazobactam	For penicillin-allergic patients, use a respiratory FQ and aztreonam Daptomycin should never be used for MRSA pneumonia
Aspiration	Clindamycin **PLUS** respiratory FQ **or** amoxicillin/clavulanate **or** piperacillin–tazobactam	Anaerobe coverage is required for community-acquired aspiration pneumonia for oral anaerobes

Adapted from Mandell LA, Wunderink RG, Anzueto A, et al. Infectious Diseases Society of America/American Thoracic Society consensus guidelines on the management of community-acquired pneumonia in adults. *Clin Infect Dis.* 2007;44(suppl 2):S27-S72.
ICU, intensive care unit; MRSA, methicillin-resistant *Staphylococcus aureus.*

COMPLICATIONS

- **Lack of clinical response** is the most common complication of pneumonia. Causes may include the following:
  - **Wrong antibiotic** (e.g., resistant organism, incorrect choice, and/or insufficient dose)
  - **Wrong diagnosis** (e.g., drug fever, heart failure, pulmonary embolism, vasculitis, and malignancy)
  - **Complication** (e.g., empyema, acute respiratory distress syndrome [ARDS], secondary infection, superinfection, meningitis, and endocarditis)
- Consider further workup as follows:
  - Testing for mycobacteria, *Legionella*, varicella-zoster virus, herpes simplex virus, and CMV, especially in the immunocompromised patient.

TABLE 5-10	PLEURAL FLUID CHARACTERISTICS		
Characteristic	Transudate	Uncomplicated Parapneumonic Effusion	Complicated Parapneumonic Effusion
Appearance	Clear	Variable	Variable[a]
WBC count (cells/μL)	<1000	Variable	Variable
WBC differential	Variable	Predominately neutrophils	Predominately neutrophils
Protein (g/dL)	<3.0	>3.0	>3.0
Glucose (mg/dL)	Same as serum	>60	40–60
pH	Greater than serum	>7.2	7.0–7.2
LDH (units/mL)	<200	<1000	>1000
Bacteria	Absent	Absent	Absent[a]

Empyema may have bacteria present on Gram stain; the pleural fluid will appear grossly purulent.
LDH, lactate dehydrogenase; WBC, white blood cell.

- ○ Bronchoscopy, sometimes with biopsy, for routine, mycobacterial, and fungal staining and culture
- ○ Thoracentesis
- ○ CT scan with contrast
- **Parapneumonic effusions are common.** Typically, such effusions are relatively small and resolve with proper antibiotic treatment. Diagnostic thoracentesis is indicated if the effusion is free-flowing and layers >1 cm on a lateral decubitus film.
- The characteristics of pleural fluid are presented in Table 5-10.
  - ○ **Uncomplicated parapneumonic effusions** are exudative and usually sterile.
  - ○ **Complicated parapneumonic effusions** result from persistence of bacterial invasion of the pleural space, though cultures are often negative. Biochemical features include a pH < 7.2 and low glucose (<60 mg/dL) and high lactate dehydrogenase levels. Chest tube drainage is generally required.
  - ○ **Empyema** signifies gross purulence in the pleural space but cultures are sometimes still negative. Management of empyema requires chest tube placement and often, surgical decortication.

Hospital-Acquired and Ventilator-Associated Pneumonias

GENERAL PRINCIPLES

- Nosocomial pneumonias are more likely to be caused by resistant pathogens and therefore are treated differently than CAP.
- There are two categories of nosocomial pneumonias.[23]

○ **Hospital-acquired pneumonia (HAP)**: develops ≥48 hours after admission to a hospital.

○ **Ventilator-associated pneumonia (VAP)**: any pneumonia that develops >48 hours after endotracheal intubation.

Epidemiology

- Nosocomial pneumonia is the most common hospital-acquired infection.[24]
- HAP alone increases hospital stay by 7 to 9 days and costs an additional $40,000 per patient.
- 50% of all antibiotics prescribed in the intensive care unit are for HAP.
- Attributable mortality due to HAP is 33% to 50%.
- Patients with late-onset HAP/VAP (>4 d after hospitalization) and those who received IV antibiotics within 90 days are more likely to be infected with multidrug-resistant (MDR) organisms.

Etiology

- The organisms causing HAP and VAP are often drug-resistant pathogens including MRSA, *Escherichia coli*, *Klebsiella*, *Serratia*, *Stenotrophomonas*, *Burkholderia*, *Pseudomonas*, and *Acinetobacter*. However, community organisms such as *S. pneumoniae* and *Haemophilus* are not uncommon.
- Viruses, atypical bacteria, and fungal pathogens rarely cause nosocomial pneumonia in immunocompetent patients. However, these pathogens should be kept in the differential diagnosis in immunocompromised hosts, in patients who do not respond to therapy or are very ill, and during influenza season.

Pathophysiology

- For these infections to occur, pathogens must invade the lower respiratory tract, usually by aspiration or microaspiration.
- The oral flora dramatically changes within a few days of hospitalization to a predominately gram-negative spectrum, often with the drug-resistant pathogens mentioned above.

Risk Factors

- Conditions that increase the risk of aspiration
- Use of proton pump inhibitors or H2 blockers for stress ulcer prophylaxis
- Intubation increases the risk of microaspiration despite an inflated endotracheal tube cuff
- Heavily sedated and paralyzed patients have a higher risk of developing pneumonia
- Repeated intubation and extubation increase the risk of infection
- Poorly controlled hyperglycemia

Associated Conditions

- One important associated condition to consider is ARDS.
- ARDS patients should receive a low tidal volume, high positive end-expiratory pressure protocol to minimize additional barotrauma.

DIAGNOSIS

Clinical Presentation

- The diagnosis of nosocomial pneumonia is difficult because the findings are often nonspecific and extremely variable.
- Patients will frequently present with productive cough, fever, dyspnea, and pleuritic chest pain.

- The diagnosis should also be considered in patients with new or progressive infiltrates on chest radiography, fever or hypothermia, purulent sputum, leukocytosis, change in oxygenation, tachypnea, and hypotension.
- These finding are especially important in patients who may suffer from delirium and dementia or are currently intubated.

Differential Diagnosis

- The differential diagnosis of nosocomial pneumonia includes aspiration pneumonitis, ARDS, septic emboli, heart failure, pulmonary hemorrhage, vasculitis, malignancy, and tracheobronchitis.
- Tracheobronchitis and HAP may have a very similar presentation, but a new lung infiltrate is not expected in tracheobronchitis.

Diagnostic Testing

Laboratories

- The goal of diagnostic testing is twofold: (1) confirm pneumonia as the diagnosis and (2) isolate the organism to narrow the antibiotic spectrum.
- Blood cultures, although positive less than 25% of the time, may identify concomitant bacteremia. Noninvasive sampling through tracheal aspirate/sputum (76% sensitivity, 75% specificity) should be considered before invasive bronchoscopy sampling.[23]
- Bronchoscopy (69% sensitivity, 82% specificity) should be considered in patients unable to provide adequate sputum sample and should be strongly considered when diagnosis is in question.
- Other laboratories to consider include urine pneumococcal antigen, urine *Legionella* antigen (only detects serogroup 1), multiorganism PCR NP swab and urine *Histoplasma* antigen.

Imaging

- Chest radiography is required to differentiate between tracheobronchitis and pneumonia.
- CT scan of the chest should be considered if the diagnosis is in question.

Diagnostic Procedures

Bronchoscopy is the hallmark diagnostic procedure in pneumonia. Bronchoalveolar lavage, bronchial washings, and biopsy may be performed based on the clinical setting. These are often sent for fungal, bacterial, mycobacterial, and viral studies, plus histopathological examination.

TREATMENT

- The treatment of nosocomial pneumonia is presented in Table 5-11.[25]
- Treatment duration should be 7 days for most cases.
- *Pseudomonas* infection should be treated for 8 to 14 days with a single antipseudomonal agent, ideally based on culture susceptibilities. Combination therapy with two agents to which the isolate is susceptible should be considered if the patient is in septic shock, at high risk for death (>25%), or if local antibiogram shows that >10% gram-negative isolates are resistant to the agent being considered for monotherapy.
- Once patients are started on antibiotics, respiratory cultures should be monitored closely.
  - If negative, consider narrowing spectrum to the antibiotics recommended for those not at risk for MDR organisms (Table 5-11).
  - If positive, narrow antibiotic spectrum after 72 hours based on culture results.
- Procalcitonin may have a role in assisting treatment decisions by distinguishing between bacterial and nonbacterial causes of pneumonia. This test could reduce antibiotic exposure and/or side effects without negatively impacting mortality. However, the use of procalcitonin has not yet been included in clinical algorithms or become a standard of care.[25]

TABLE 5-11 TREATMENT OF NOSOCOMIAL PNEUMONIA[a]

Category	Other Factors[b]	Empiric Therapy
HAP	Low risk of MRSA[c]	Piperacillin–tazobactam 4.5 g IV q6h **or** Cefepime 2 g IV q8h **or** Levofloxacin 750 mg IV q24h **or** Meropenem 1 g IV q8h **or** Imipenem 500 mg IV q6h
	Risk of MRSA	**ADD** Vancomycin 15 mg/kg IV q8–12h **or** Linezolid 600 mg IV q12
	Septic shock or IVDU in the prior 90 d	**ADD** a second antipseudomonal antimicrobial (avoid 2 β-lactams) such as Aztreonam 2 g IV q8h **or** Amikacin 15 mg/kg IV daily
VAP[d]	Gram-positive antibiotic with MRSA activity	Vancomycin 15 mg/kg IV q8–12h **or** Linezolid 600 mg IV q12
	β-Lactam with gram-negative antibiotic with antipseudomonal activity	Piperacillin–tazobactam 4.5 g IV q6h **or** Cefepime 2 g IV q8h **or** Meropenem 1 g IV q8h **or** Imipenem 500 mg IV q6h
	Non-β-lactam with Gram-negative antibiotic with antipseudomonal activity	Aztreonam 2 g IV q8h **or** Amikacin 15 mg/kg IV daily **or** Levofloxacin 750 mg IV q24h

Adapted from Kalil AC, Metersky ML, Klompas M, et al. Management of adults with hospital-acquired and ventilator-associated pneumonia: 2016 clinical practice guidelines by the Infectious Diseases Society of America and the American Thoracic Society. *Clin Infect Dis.* 2016;63(5):e61-e111. doi:10.1093/cid/ciw353.

[a]Choice of agent should be based on pattern of causative organisms and susceptibilities in each health care setting.

[b]Azithromycin should be considered for patients with a high suspicion for atypical organisms or *Legionella* and are not on respiratory fluoroquinolone (FQ). For patients allergic to penicillin consider a FQ and aminoglycoside or aztreonam or meropenem (<1% cross-reactivity). Inhaled antibiotics (e.g., colistin and aminoglycosides) have been used in selected populations and should be used only after consultation with an infectious disease specialist.

[c]Indications for MRSA coverage include intravenous antibiotic treatment during the prior 90 days, and treatment in a unit where the prevalence of MRSA among *S. aureus* isolates is not known or is >20%. Before detection of MRSA by culture or nonculture screening may also increase the risk of MRSA.

[d]Choose 1 g-positive option, one β-lactam gram-negative option, and one non-β-lactam gram-negative option as initial empirical therapy.

ESBL, extended spectrum β-lactamase; FQ, fluoroquinolone; HAP, hospital-acquired pneumonia; MDR, multidrug resistant; MRSA, methicillin-resistant *Staphylococcus aureus*; VAP, ventilator-associated pneumonia.

Lung Abscess

GENERAL PRINCIPLES

- A lung abscess consists of a collection of necrotic lung tissue contained within a cavity occurring as a result of progressive infection of the lung parenchyma.
- Organisms associated with lung abscesses are listed in Table 5-12.[26]
- Aspiration is a key event in many cases of lung abscess. Predisposing conditions that should be considered include alcohol and sedative use, seizures, strokes, and neuromuscular disease.

DIAGNOSIS

Clinical Presentation

- Patients may present with fever, productive cough, putrid sputum, or chest pain. They may also have weight loss, night sweats, and hemoptysis. These symptoms may also be concerning for malignancy or tuberculosis (TB).
- Decreased breath sounds and hyper-resonance in the area of the cavitation may be appreciated. Poor dentition, malodorous breath, and purulent sputum are classic findings on physical examination but are often not present.

TABLE 5-12	CAUSES OF LUNG ABSCESS
Bacterial	**Fungal**
Gram-positive anaerobic cocci from oral mucosa such as *Peptostreptococcus*	*Histoplasma*
	Coccidioides
	Blastomyces
Pigmented gram-negative bacilli (*Prevotella, Porphyromonas, and Bacteroides*)	*Cryptococcus*
	Aspergillus
	Rhizopus
Fusobacterium spp. (Lemierre syndrome)	**Parasitic**
Staphylococcus aureus (from both necrotizing pneumonia and hematogenous spread from septic emboli)	*Entamoeba*
	Echinococcus
Pseudomonas	**Noninfectious**
Klebsiella	Bronchogenic carcinoma
Legionella	Granulomatosis with polyangiitis (formerly known as Wegener)
Nocardia	Rheumatoid nodules
Burkholderia	Sarcoidosis
Streptococcus milleri	Pulmonary infarction
Mycobacterium	Congenital pulmonary cysts
Rhodococcus	
Actinomyces	
Polymicrobial	

Diagnostic Testing

Laboratories
- Blood cultures are rarely positive in classic aspiration pneumonia, particularly in the case of suspected anaerobic infection.
- Respiratory isolation and sputum testing for TB should be performed in all patients with cavitary lung lesions.
- Sputum cultures should be obtained as they may grow more common aerobic sources of infection. Be aware that oral contamination is common and culture results may be misleading.

Imaging
- Chest radiography is obviously necessary in diagnosis. The lower lobes are usually involved if the aspiration occurred while in an upright position, but can be seen in the upper lobes if supine at the time of aspiration. Cavitation is usually solitary. Multiple cavitary lesions suggest a different process or necrotizing pneumonia rather than lung abscess.
- CT scan is not required for the diagnosis of lung abscess; however, the improved resolution may assist in ruling out malignancies or processes affecting the pulmonary parenchyma. CT scan will also help to diagnose an associated empyema, a common complication of lung abscess.

Diagnostic Procedures
Bronchoscopy is rarely performed in classic lung abscess, as it is unlikely to yield positive results for anaerobic organisms. It may be helpful if atypical organisms including fungi, parasites, mycobacteria, or malignancy are suspected.

TREATMENT

Medications
- Recommended antibiotic regimens for lung abscess include:
  - Clindamycin 600 mg IV q8h
  - Ampicillin–sulbactam 3 g IV q6h
- Alternative regimens:
  - Piperacillin-tazobactam 3.375 mg IV q6h
  - Meropenem 1 g IV q8h
- Clindamycin is more efficacious than penicillin (PCN) because of increasing PCN resistance.
- Metronidazole monotherapy is not effective due to the presence of microaerophilic nonculturable organisms.
- For suspected resistant organisms consider using
  - Meropenem or piperacillin–tazobactam for gram-negative coverage
  - Vancomycin or linezolid for MRSA coverage
- Treatment duration is controversial.
  - IV antibiotics can be converted to PO as patients clinically improve and are able to tolerate PO.
  - Imaging may be obtained at regular intervals to monitor for treatment and duration. Experts recommend continuing oral antibiotics until a follow-up chest radiograph is clear (usually achieved after 2–3 mo of therapy).
  - Oral options for consolidation phase commonly include amoxicillin-clavulanate 875 mg PO twice daily and clindamycin 300 mg four times daily.
- Anaerobic coverage should be continued in all cases of lung abscess regardless of culture results.

- Aspiration pneumonia in patients who have been hospitalized more than a few days is much more likely to be due to resistant gram-negative organisms than oral anaerobes because of a change in colonized oral flora. These patients often do not need anaerobic coverage.

Other Nonpharmacologic Therapies

- Drainage is important to resolve lung abscess. Postural drainage and chest physiotherapy are used.
- Barium swallow study should be considered to evaluate for aspiration if no clear cause is identified.

Surgical Management

- Rarely, surgical resection is required to treat lung abscesses that do not resolve despite antibiotic therapy.
- Percutaneous catheter drainage is an alternative to resection and may be used in severe or difficult-to-treat cases. Bronchopleural fistula and pneumothorax are complications that may occur with a percutaneous approach.

COMPLICATIONS

- Complications include pleural effusion/empyema and hemoptysis.
- Any persistent fluid accumulation with lung abscess or layering >1 cm on decubitus radiograph on the involved side should be aspirated to evaluate for empyema.
  - Most patients with complicated pleural effusions should have a chest tube placed.
  - All patients with empyema require chest tube drainage and may benefit from other surgical procedures.
  - Antibiotic therapy is the same as lung abscess.

Influenza

GENERAL PRINCIPLES

Definition

Influenza is an acute febrile respiratory illness caused by the influenza viruses.

Classification

- Influenza A: severe illness and associated with pandemics
- Influenza B: severe illness in immunocompromised or elderly
- Influenza C: mild illness

Epidemiology

- Most persons with influenza will recover without sequelae. However, it can cause serious illness and death, particularly in young children, pregnant, immunocompromised patients, and the elderly.
- Influenza causes between 250,000 and 500,000 deaths globally every year.
- Influenza is predominantly seasonal:
  - Northern hemisphere: November to April
  - Southern hemisphere: May to September
- Antigenic drift:
  - Caused by point mutations in hemagglutinin or neuraminidase of circulating strains
  - Can lead to epidemics
  - Vaccine changed annually to account for antigenic drift

- Antigenic shifts:
  - Caused by complete change in hemagglutinin and/or neuraminidase
  - Can lead to pandemics
- Spread person to person by contact with respiratory secretions. Infection and replication occur solely in the respiratory tract.

Prevention

- Vaccination:
  - Since 2010, CDC's Advisory Committee on Immunization Practices (ACIP) has recommended annual influenza vaccination for all people aged ≥6 months without contraindications.
  - Efficacy of vaccination is 50% to 90% depending on the outbreak and circulating strains and varies yearly.[27]
  - They are four major types available in the United States: trivalent (IIV3), quadrivalent (IIV4), recombinant (RIV3), and live attenuated (LAIV4).
  - High-risk patients should be prioritized:
    - Nursing home residents, health care workers, and those >65 years old
    - Those with active pulmonary, cardiovascular, liver, renal, or neurologic disease
    - Immunocompromised individuals: diabetes, malignancy, HIV, transplant, on immunosuppressants, pregnant
  - Contraindications to vaccination:
    - History of severe allergy to vaccine components
    - Guillain–Barré syndrome within 6 weeks of prior influenza immunization
    - In acute febrile illness (fever >40°C) wait until fever resolves
- Patients with severe egg allergy (i.e., anaphylaxis) should receive the RIV3 vaccine.
- High-dose vaccine in adults >65 years old has been shown to elicit a higher hemagglutination antibody titers against all three influenza viruses and appears to be more efficacious compared with the standard dose.[27]
- Droplet precautions and routine hand-washing for hospitalized patients.
- Chemoprophylaxis after exposure should be administered to the following groups:
  - High-risk individuals within 2 weeks of vaccine administration or unable to receive vaccine.
  - Close contact with people at high risk for influenza complications.
  - Residents of institutions experiencing influenza outbreaks.

DIAGNOSIS

Clinical Presentation

- High-grade fever, cough, coryza, and headache are common presenting symptoms. Systemic symptoms are common in influenza and rare in other upper respiratory tract viral infections. Systemic symptoms may last up to 2 weeks.
- High temperature is suggestive of influenza. Abnormalities such as hypoxia and tachypnea are uncommon and could be signs of another illness or a complication of influenza such as bacterial pneumonia.
- Viral culture is the gold standard but very slow.
- Rapid testing is readily available and commonly used.
  - Rapid antigen testing (lower sensitivity)
  - Immunofluorescence microscopy (direct or indirect) has variable sensitivity and specificity based on manufacturers
  - PCR

TREATMENT

- **Medications are only effective if administered within 24 to 48 hours of onset of symptoms** and may be beneficial in hospitalized patients suffering from complications or severe influenza.
- **Neuraminidase inhibitors are the treatment of choice.** Oseltamivir 75 mg PO twice daily, inhaled Zanamivir 10 mg twice daily, both for 5 days, or Peramivir 600 mg IV single, are currently FDA approved.
- M2 inhibitors (amantadine and rimantadine) are not recommended due to widespread high levels of resistance in influenza A and lack of efficacy in influenza B.
- Resistance evolves rapidly and updated recommendations can be found annually at the Centers for Disease Control and Prevention influenza web site.

Tuberculosis

GENERAL PRINCIPLES

Epidemiology

- TB is now the most common infectious cause of death worldwide. About one-third of the world's population is infected with latent TB.
- Only a small fraction of immunocompetent patients with latent TB will progress to active TB. The **lifetime** risk of progression is 10%.
- In poorly controlled HIV and other patients with impaired immune systems, the **annual** progression rate from latent to active TB is 10%.

Pathophysiology

- TB is spread by aerosolized droplets from patients with active pulmonary disease.
- Mycobacteria proliferate in alveolar macrophages, transported to hilar lymph nodes, and subsequently spread to almost any other part of the body, especially the upper lobes of the lung, the pleura, lymph nodes, bones, and genitourinary and central nervous systems.

Risk Factors and Associated Conditions

- Patients at high risk of TB exposure include immigrants from high-prevalence countries, the homeless, IV drug users, migrant farm workers, and prisoners.
- If infected, risk of progression to active TB includes HIV/AIDS patients, alcoholics, immunocompromised patients, diabetics, and patients who have received antitumor necrosis factor agents.

DIAGNOSIS

Clinical Presentation

- In active pulmonary TB, patients frequently present with nonproductive chronic cough (3 wk or more in duration), fevers, chills, night sweats, and weight loss. Hemoptysis may also occur.
- Patients with latent TB are often asymptomatic.
- Physical examination findings are often nonspecific in TB.

Diagnostic Criteria

- The diagnosis of active pulmonary TB is made with laboratory findings of acid-fast organisms on sputum and/or a positive nucleic acid amplification test for *Mycobacterium tuberculosis* complex, plus culture growing *M. tuberculosis.*
- Culture-negative pulmonary TB is diagnosed with active TB symptoms, no alternative diagnosis, and improvement on TB therapy. TB skin testing (PPD) cannot be used to rule out TB in active infection.
- Latent TB is diagnosed with a positive PPD (Table 5-13) or interferon-γ release assay (preferred in patients who have had bacillus Calmette–Guérin vaccine).[28]

Differential Diagnosis

The differential diagnosis includes nontuberculous mycobacterial infections, fungal infections, malignancies, lung abscess, septic emboli, and antineutrophil cytoplasmic antibody–associated vasculitis, which can all cause cavitary pulmonary lesions and symptoms suggestive of TB.

Diagnostic Testing

Laboratories
- Sputum via natural cough, induction, or bronchoscopy is the gold standard to diagnose pulmonary TB.[28]
- Samples should ideally be cultured in both solid and liquid mycobacterial cultures.
- A nucleic acid amplification test should be performed on all patients if available. On smear-negative samples, sensitivity of these assays can be up to 90% if three sputum samples are tested.
- Respiratory isolation can be removed under the following circumstances
  - Rule out:
    - Three consecutive negative acid-fast bacillus (AFB) sputum smears collected 8 to 24 hours apart, with at least one specimen obtained in the early morning **and** alternate diagnosis.
  - Treatment for TB:
    - Treatment for TB for at leas 2 weeks **and** symptomatic response to therapy.[29]

TABLE 5-13	TUBERCULIN SKIN TEST INTERPRETATION
Reaction Size (mm)	**Risk Group**
≥5	HIV, close contact with active TB case, CXR consistent with TB, immunosuppressed, receiving anti-TNF agents
≥10	Dialysis, diabetes, <90% IBW, IVDU, lymphoma, leukemia, head/neck cancer, children ≤4 y old, foreign born from countries of higher incidence, high-risk patients, i.e., health care workers, incarcerated, homeless
≥15	Otherwise healthy persons without risk factors for TB

CXR, chest radiograph; IBW, ideal body weight; IVDU, intravenous drug use; TB, tuberculosis; TNF, tumor necrosis factor.

- Sputum for AFB smear and culture should be obtained every 2 weeks until a smear-negative specimen is obtained and then daily until three negative specimens are obtained. Thereafter, sputum specimens for AFB smear and culture should be obtained monthly until culture-negative.
- All patients with confirmed or suspected TB should have HIV testing.
- Baseline laboratories for liver transaminases, alkaline phosphatase, creatinine, and platelet count should be obtained. These do not need to be reassessed unless abnormalities are detected or patients are at high risk for subsequent abnormalities.
- Baseline visual acuity and color differentiation should be performed and monitored monthly for all patients treated with ethambutol (EMB).

TREATMENT

- Directly observed therapy is considered the standard of care.[30]
- Drug-susceptible pulmonary TB treatment regimens are listed in Table 5-14
- Radiographic evidence of improvement should be seen on chest radiography by 2 months.
- Please see Figure 5-1
- Monthly clinical evaluation should be performed to assess adherence and adverse effects including visual disturbances for EMB.

TABLE 5-14	TUBERCULOSIS TREATMENT REGIMENS			
Regimen	Intensive Phase (8 wk)		Continuation Phase (18 wk)	
	Drugs	Interval and Dose	Drugs	Interval and Dose
1	INH 5 mg/kg (max 300 mg)	7 d/wk for 56 doses	INH	7 d/wk for 126 doses
	RIF 10 mg/kg (max 600 mg)	OR 5 d/wk for 40 doses	RIF	OR 5 d/wk for 90 doses
2	PZA 20–25 mg/ kg (max 2 g)			3 times a week for 54 doses
3		3 times a week for 24 doses		
	EMB 15–20 mg/kg (max 1.6 g)			
4		7 d/wk for 14 doses, then 2 times a week for 12 doses		2 times a week for 36 doses

Adapted from Nahid P, Dorman SE, Alipanah N, et al. Official American Thoracic Society/ centers for disease control and prevention/infectious diseases society of America clinical practice guidelines: treatment of drug-susceptible tuberculosis. *Clin Infect Dis.* 2016;63:147-195. doi:10.1093/cid/ciw376.

Comments: Regimen 1 is preferred and the most effective regimen. Patients with HIV, immunosuppressed, with cavitary disease, positive smear cultures after completing intensive phase, smoker or with poorly controlled diabetes, should have a continuation phase of 7 months. EMB, ethambutol; INH, isoniazid; PZA, pyrazinamide; RIF, rifampin.

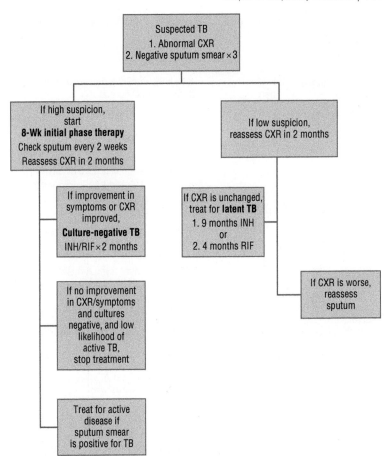

FIGURE 5-1 Management algorithm for suspected culture-negative tuberculosis. CXR, chest radiograph; INH, isoniazid; RIF, rifampin; TB, tuberculosis.

- All patients with HIV on antiretroviral therapy and suspected TB should have an experienced HIV clinician assess proper drug therapy, as there are complex drug reactions particularly with RIF and rifapentine.
- Extrapulmonary TB should be treated with 6- to 9-month regimens, which include isoniazid (INH)/RIF, except for meningitis, which requires 9 to 12 months of therapy. Steroids should also be added in patients with TB meningitis or pericarditis.
- Pyrazinamide and EMB dosing regimens must be modified in patients with end-stage renal disease on hemodialysis. TB regimens in patients with hepatic dysfunction should be carefully selected as well. Often patients without significant transaminitis can be on hepatotoxic drugs with close monitoring.
- Pyridoxine supplementation (25–50 mg daily) is recommended for patients on INH.
- Side effects from medications are not uncommon. Common side effects are listed in Table 5-15.[30]

TABLE 5-15	MANAGEMENT OF ANTITUBERCULOSIS THERAPY SIDE EFFECTS	
Side Effect	**Drug**	**Treatment**
Nausea/GI upset	RIF RPT	Check HFP. Continue meds and administer with food if HFP normal
Drug-induced hepatitis (AST 3 × ULN and symptoms or AST 5 × ULN without symptoms)	INH RIF **PZA**	Stop INH/RIF/PZA, substitute with second-line medications: EMB, SM, amikacin, kanamycin, capreomycin, FQ Consider hepatitis testing Obtain hepatotoxin exposure history Restart INH, RIF, and PZA in sequential order after transaminases improve
Fever, worsening radiographic findings, or symptoms in an HIV patient	HAART	Rule out secondary process Exacerbation likely from immune reconstitution inflammatory syndrome if HAART recently started Continue treatment, symptomatic relief For severe cases, prednisone has been used

Adapted from Centers for Disease Control and Prevention, American Thoracic Society, Infectious Diseases Society of America. Treatment of tuberculosis. *MMWR Recomm Rep.* 2003;52:1-77.

AST, aspartate aminotransferase; EMB, ethambutol; FQ, fluoroquinolone; GI, gastrointestinal; HAART, high-active antiretroviral therapy; HFP, hepatic function panel; INH, isoniazid; PZA, pyrazinamide; RIF, rifampin; RPT, rifapentine; SM, streptomycin; ULN, upper limit of normal.

REFERENCES

1. Shulman ST, Bisno AL, Clegg HW, et al. Clinical practice guideline for the diagnosis and management of group A streptococcal pharyngitis: 2012 update by the Infectious Diseases Society of America. *Clin Infect Dis.* 2012;55(10):1279-1282.
2. McIsaac WJ, Goel V, To T, Low DE. The validity of a sore throat score in family practice. *CMAJ.* 2000;163(7):811-815.
3. Centor RM, Witherspoon JM, Dalton HP, Brody CE, Link K. The diagnosis of strep throat in adults in the emergency room. *Med Decis Making.* 1981;1(3):239-246.
4. Guardiani E, Bliss M, Harley E. Supraglottitis in the era following widespread immunization against Haemophilus influenzae type B: evolving principles in diagnosis and management. *Laryngoscope.* 2010;120(11):2183-2188.
5. Hung TY, Li S, Chen PS, et al. Bedside ultrasonography as a safe and effective tool to diagnose acute epiglottitis. *Am J Emerg Med.* 2011;29(3):359.e351-e353.
6. Shah RK, Stocks C. Epiglottitis in the United States: national trends, variances, prognosis, and management. *Laryngoscope.* 2010;120(6):1256-1262.
7. Chow AW, Benninger MS, Brook I, et al. IDSA clinical practice guideline for acute bacterial rhinosinusitis in children and adults. *Clin Infect Dis.* 2012;54(8):e72-e112.
8. Ahovuo-Saloranta A, Rautakorpi UM, Borisenko OV, Liira H, Williams JW, Makela M. Antibiotics for acute maxillary sinusitis in adults. *Cochrane Database Syst Rev.* 2014(2):CD000243.
9. Chong LY, Head K, Hopkins C, Philpott C, Schilder AG, Burton MJ. Intranasal steroids versus placebo or no intervention for chronic rhinosinusitis. *Cochrane Database Syst Rev.* 2016;4:CD011996.

10. Venekamp RP, Thompson MJ, Hayward G, et al. Systemic corticosteroids for acute sinusitis. *Cochrane Database Syst Rev.* 2011(12):CD008115.

11. Chong LY, Head K, Hopkins C, et al. Saline irrigation for chronic rhinosinusitis. *Cochrane Database Syst Rev.* 2016;4:CD011995.

12. Braman SS. Chronic cough due to acute bronchitis: ACCP evidence-based clinical practice guidelines. *Chest.* 2006;129(suppl 1):95S-103S.

13. Smith SM, Fahey T, Smucny J, Becker LA. Antibiotics for acute bronchitis. *Cochrane Database Syst Rev.* 2017;6:CD000245.

14. Park H, Adeyemi AO, Rascati KL. Direct medical costs and utilization of health care services to treat pneumonia in the United States: an analysis of the 2007-2011 medical expenditure panel survey. *Clin Ther.* 2015;37(7):1466-1476.e1461.

15. Prina E, Ranzani OT, Torres A. Community-acquired pneumonia. *Lancet.* 2015;386(9998):1097-1108.

16. Kim DK, Riley LE, Harriman KH, Hunter P, Bridges CB; Advisory Committee on Immunization Practices. Recommended immunization schedule for adults aged 19 years or older, United States, 2017. *Ann Intern Med.* 2017;166(3):209-219.

17. Fine MJ, Auble TE, Yealy DM, et al. A prediction rule to identify low-risk patients with community-acquired pneumonia. *N Engl J Med.* 1997;336(4):243-250.

18. Baron EJ, Miller JM, Weinstein MP, et al. A guide to utilization of the microbiology laboratory for diagnosis of infectious diseases: 2013 recommendations by the Infectious Diseases Society of America (IDSA) and the American Society for Microbiology (ASM)(a). *Clin Infect Dis.* 2013;57(4):e22-e121.

19. Lim WS, van der Eerden MM, Laing R, et al. Defining community acquired pneumonia severity on presentation to hospital: an international derivation and validation study. *Thorax.* 2003;58(5):377-382.

20. Postma DF, van Werkhoven CH, van Elden LJ, et al. Antibiotic treatment strategies for community-acquired pneumonia in adults. *N Engl J Med.* 2015;372(14):1312-1323.

21. Dawson-Hahn EE, Mickan S, Onakpoya I, et al. Short-course versus long-course oral antibiotic treatment for infections treated in outpatient settings: a review of systematic reviews. *Fam Pract.* 2017;34(5):511-519.

22. Wan YD, Sun TW, Liu ZQ, Zhang SG, Wang LX, Kan QC. Efficacy and safety of corticosteroids for community-acquired pneumonia: a systematic review and meta-analysis. *Chest.* 2016;149(1):209-219.

23. Kalil AC, Metersky ML, Klompas M, et al. Executive summary: management of adults with hospital-acquired and ventilator-associated pneumonia: 2016 clinical practice guidelines by the Infectious Diseases Society of America and the American Thoracic Society. *Clin Infect Dis.* 2016;63(5):575-582.

24. Magill SS, Edwards JR, Bamberg W, et al. Multistate point-prevalence survey of health care-associated infections. *N Engl J Med.* 2014;370(13):1198-1208.

25. Schuetz P, Wirz Y, Sager R, et al. Effect of procalcitonin-guided antibiotic treatment on mortality in acute respiratory infections: a patient level meta-analysis. *Lancet Infect Dis.* 2018;18(1):95-107.

26. Mandell LA, Wunderink RG, Anzueto A, et al. Infectious Diseases Society of America/American Thoracic Society consensus guidelines on the management of community-acquired pneumonia in adults. *Clin Infect Dis.* 2007;44(suppl 2):S27-S72.

27. Jackson ML, Chung JR, Jackson LA, et al. Influenza vaccine effectiveness in the United States during the 2015–2016 season. *N Engl J Med.* 2017;377(6):534-543.

28. Lewinsohn DM, Leonard MK, LoBue PA, et al. Official American Thoracic Society/Infectious Diseases Society of America/centers for disease control and prevention clinical practice guidelines: diagnosis of tuberculosis in adults and children. *Clin Infect Dis.* 2017;64(2):111-115.

29. Jensen PA, Lambert LA, Iademarco MF, Ridzon R; Centers for Disease Control and Prevention. Guidelines for preventing the transmission of *Mycobacterium tuberculosis* in health-care settings, 2005. *MMWR Recomm Rep.* 2005;54(RR-17):1-141.

30. Nahid P, Dorman SE, Alipanah N, et al. Official American Thoracic Society/centers for disease control and prevention/infectious diseases society of America clinical practice guidelines: treatment of drug-susceptible tuberculosis. *Clin Infect Dis.* 2016;63(7):e147-e195.

31. Ng HL, Sin LM, Li MF, Que TL, Anandaciva S. Acute epiglottitis in adults: a retrospective review of 106 patients in Hong Kong. *Emerg Med J.* 2008;25(5):253-255.

32. American Thoracic Soceity, CDC, Infectious Diseases Society of America. Treatment of tuberculosis. *MMWR Recomm Rep.* 2003;52(RR-11):1-77.

Infections of the Gastrointestinal and Hepatobiliary Tract

Lemuel B. Non and Jennie H. Kwon

6

Infections of the Oral Cavity

Herpetic Gingivostomatitis

GENERAL PRINCIPLES

- Herpetic gingivostomatitis is caused by herpes simplex virus (HSV)-1 and occasionally by HSV-2.
- It is a disease of children and adults, especially in immunocompromised patients.

DIAGNOSIS

Clinical Presentation[1]

- The clinical presentation ranges from a few painful ulcers without systemic manifestations to fever, sore throat, malaise, and regional lymphadenopathy.
- Primary infection is more severe than recurrent disease.
- Pain occurs 1 to 2 days before the onset of oral lesions, which are 2- to 4-mm small ulcers with an erythematous base. Symptoms persist for 2 to 3 days, although the vesicles may take 1 to 2 weeks to resolve.

Differential Diagnosis

The differential diagnosis includes herpangina, varicella, herpes zoster, hand-foot-and-mouth disease, aphthous ulcers, Behçet syndrome, cyclical neutropenia, and erythema multiforme.

Diagnostic Testing

- Diagnosis is made clinically based on presentation and physical examination findings.
- Direct immunofluorescence, polymerase chain reaction (PCR), or viral culture may be performed on samples from the ulcers.

TREATMENT

- Treatment is usually supportive with hydration and pain relief.
- For severe symptoms, acyclovir 15 mg/kg fives times a day for 5 to 7 days may be given for immunocompetent children who present within the first 72 to 96 hours. Immunocompromised patients should receive intravenous acyclovir 30 mg/kg per day in three divided doses or oral acyclovir 1000 mg/d in three to five divided doses. Dose adjustments based on renal function may be necessary.

Salivary Gland Infections

GENERAL PRINCIPLES

- Salivary gland infections are usually caused by viruses, including mumps virus, parainfluenza, coxsackievirus, echovirus, Epstein–Barr virus (EBV), and HIV, although bacterial infections also occur.
- Risk factors for bacterial or suppurative parotitis include advanced age, diabetes, dehydration, anticholinergic medication or diuretic use, and poor oral hygiene.
- Bacterial parotitis is usually polymicrobial; *Staphylococcus aureus*, *Streptococcus pyogenes*, viridans streptococci, *Haemophilus influenzae*, gram-negative bacteria (particularly *Klebsiella* spp.), anaerobes, and, rarely, mycobacteria are involved.

DIAGNOSIS

Clinical Manifestations

- Viral parotitis is associated with gradual onset of painful swelling of the parotid glands, which could be either unilateral or bilateral.
- Mumps is sometimes associated with orchitis and/or meningoencephalitis.
- Bacterial parotitis usually begins with rapid onset of pain, swelling, and induration.
- Manual palpation is painful and can result in discharge of pus from the duct.

Diagnostic Testing

- Diagnosis of mumps is based on clinical characteristics and exposure history. Detection of mumps IgM in serum, a rise in convalescent antibody titers, or detection of virus by RT-PCR or viral culture helps establish the diagnosis.
- Purulent drainage from the Stensen duct may be sent for culture, or fluid for culture can be obtained extraorally by needle aspiration.

TREATMENT

- Viral parotitis is managed symptomatically.
- Suppurative parotitis may be empirically covered by ampicillin/sulbactam, or oxacillin (or vancomycin if high risk for methicillin-resistant *S. aureus* [MRSA]) plus metronidazole. Antibiotics should be narrowed based on culture results.
- Drainage of the duct should be assisted by manual massage.

Esophageal Infections

Viral Esophagitis

GENERAL PRINCIPLES

- HSV-1 and cytomegalovirus (CMV) are common viral causes. HSV-2 and varicella-zoster virus (VZV) are rarely encountered.
- Viral esophagitis usually occurs in immunocompromised patients, but HSV-1 can sometimes occur in immunocompetent hosts.

DIAGNOSIS

Clinical Presentation

- Abrupt onset of severe odynophagia is a common presenting symptom. Patients may also present with nausea, vomiting, and persistent retrosternal pain. Herpes labialis or skin involvement may precede or occur concurrently with esophageal infection.[2]
- Symptoms are more gradual in CMV esophagitis. Nausea, vomiting, fever, epigastric pain, diarrhea, and weight loss may be present; dysphagia and odynophagia are less common.[3]
- Early HSV lesions are vesicular and are found in the mid- to distal esophagus; the vesicles then slough off and leave discrete, circumscribed ulcers with raised edges.
- CMV is associated with extensive, large, shallow ulcers in the distal esophagus.
- VZV esophagitis is extremely rare. Concurrent shingles is helpful in diagnosis.

Differential Diagnosis

- Less common infections include cryptococcosis, histoplasmosis, tuberculosis, and cryptosporidiosis.
- Noninfectious causes include lymphoma, Kaposi sarcoma, squamous cell carcinoma, peptic esophagitis, aphthous ulcers, tablet mucositis, corrosive ingestion, mucositis from chemotherapy, and idiopathic ulcerative esophagitis in AIDS.

Diagnostic Testing

Diagnosis is made by visualization on endoscopy and confirmed by histopathological examination of brushings and biopsy from ulcer edge (HSV) and ulcer base (CMV). Samples should be sent for viral culture or PCR.

TREATMENT

- Immunocompromised patients with HSV should be treated with acyclovir 400 mg PO five times a day, famciclovir 250 mg PO three times daily or valacyclovir 500 mg PO three times daily for 14 to 21 days. IV acyclovir 5 mg/kg q8h should be used if swallowing is a problem. Immunocompetent patients may be treated to shorten symptom duration.
- CMV is treated with ganciclovir at an induction dose of 5 mg/kg IV q12h for 21 to 28 days or until signs and symptoms have resolved. Oral valganciclovir 900 mg twice daily can be used when tolerated. Foscarnet is an alternative for ganciclovir-resistant CMV esophagitis.
- VZV esophagitis can be treated with acyclovir or famciclovir.

Infections of the Stomach

Helicobacter pylori Infection

GENERAL PRINCIPLES

- *Helicobacter pylori* is a spiral, gram-negative, urease-producing bacillus that causes chronic infection of the gastric mucus layer.
- Transmission is unclear but is usually acquired during childhood.
- Infection is associated with being born outside of North America and low socioeconomic status.

DIAGNOSIS

Clinical Presentation

- *H. pylori* infection is associated with peptic ulcer disease (PUD), low-grade gastric mucosa-associated lymphoid tissue (MALT) lymphoma, and gastric adenocarcinoma.
- Symptoms include epigastric discomfort with a burning sensation. Less commonly, nausea, vomiting, and anorexia occur. Bleeding may occur, leading to signs and symptoms of anemia. Most patients are asymptomatic.

Diagnostic Testing

- Testing for *H. pylori* should be performed only if treatment is planned.
- Testing should be offered to patients with active PUD, history of PUD (except those with documented *H. pylori* clearance), low-grade gastric MALT lymphoma, and early gastric cancer.
- Although evidence is weak, testing may also be offered to patients with the following: uninvestigated dyspepsia in patients <60 years old and with no concerning alarm signs for malignancy, long-term aspirin use, long-term nonsteroidal anti-inflammatory drugs, unexplained iron-deficiency anemia, and idiopathic thrombocytopenic purpura.[4]
- Proton pump inhibitors (PPIs) should be stopped for at least 2 weeks and antibiotics for at least 4 weeks before all tests except serology.[4]
- Either noninvasive or invasive (endoscopic) testing may be pursued. Endoscopy is mandatory if the patient is over the age of 55 years, anemic, and has had weight loss, gastrointestinal (GI) bleeding, or a palpable mass.[4]
- Noninvasive tests include antibody tests, the urea breath test, and the stool antigen test.
- Endoscopy is performed to obtain mucosal biopsy specimens and to perform rapid urease testing, histology, and culture.

TREATMENT

- If clarithromycin resistance is <15%, clarithromycin-based triple therapy is recommended: a PPI, clarithromycin 500 mg twice daily, and amoxicillin 1 g twice daily or metronidazole 500 mg twice daily.[4]
- In patients with recent exposure to or resistance to macrolides and those with allergy to penicillin, bismuth quadruple therapy for 10 to 14 days with a PPI, bismuth subcitrate (120–300 mg) or subsalicylate (300 mg) mg PO four times a day, metronidazole 250 mg PO four times a day, and tetracycline 500 mg PO four times a day can be used.
- Other recommended regimens include clarithromycin with PPI, amoxicillin, and metronidazole × 10 to 14 days and levofloxacin, PPI, and amoxicillin × 10 to 14 days. Sequential therapy is also an option and could be pursued in consultation with a specialist.
- Test for eradication should be performed in all patients with urea breath test, fecal antigen rest, or by endoscopy with biopsy-based testing >4 weeks after treatment and after PPI has been stopped for 2 weeks.

Intestinal Infections

Acute Infectious Diarrhea

GENERAL PRINCIPLES

- Clinically significant diarrhea is defined as three or more loose or watery stools per day.
- Infectious diarrhea can be caused by viruses, bacteria, and less commonly protozoa.

- Acute diarrhea is an episode of ≤14 day duration and is usually of infectious etiology. Viruses, particularly noroviruses, are the principal cause of gastroenteritis in the United States.
- The most common bacterial causes of diarrhea in the United States include *Salmonella, Campylobacter, Escherichia coli, Vibrio, Yersinia, Shigella*, and *Clostridium difficile.*
- *Cryptosporidium* outbreaks have been associated with contaminated municipal water supplies and community swimming pools.

DIAGNOSIS

Clinical Manifestations

- A careful history and physical examination is important. History of antibiotic use, recent or remote travel, duration of diarrhea, amount of weight loss, water supply, hobbies or occupation, pets, drugs, family exposure, and diet should be elicited.
- The two main categories are: **watery diarrhea** and **dysenteric diarrhea**.[5]
- The majority of the cases are watery diarrhea, with no blood in the stool, suggesting an enterotoxic bacterial, viral, or noninvasive parasitic process. Pathogens include enterotoxigenic *E. coli*, enteroaggregative *E. coli*, enteroinvasive *E. coli*, *Vibrio cholerae*, and viruses.
- Dysenteric diarrhea involves the colon and occasionally the distal small intestine and is characterized by the passage of bloody stools. Symptoms may include fever, low-volume stools with blood and mucus, chills, abdominal cramping, and tenesmus.
  ○ The most common bacterial pathogens for dysenteric syndrome are *Campylobacter*, nontyphoid *Salmonella*, *Shigella*, and Shiga toxin–producing *E. coli*, such as O157:H7.
  ○ *Aeromonas* spp., non-*Vibrio cholerae*, and *Yersinia enterocolitica* are less common.

Differential Diagnosis

Noninfectious causes of diarrhea include drugs, food allergies, primary GI diseases such as inflammatory bowel disease and carcinoid syndrome.

Diagnostic Testing

- Indications for stool testing include dysentery, moderate-to-severe disease (defined as change in activities to total disability due to diarrhea), and symptoms >7 days.
- Patients with travel-associated diarrhea may be treated empirically without testing.
- When available, the following tests should be performed: examination for fecal leukocytes, stool culture, parasite examination, stool antigen testing, and stool toxin testing.
- Fecal leukocytes usually indicate an invasive enteric pathogen, such as *Shigella*, *Salmonella*, *Campylobacter*, *Y. enterocolitica*, *Aeromonas hydrophila*, *Vibrio parahaemolyticus*, enteroinvasive *E. coli*, or enterohemorrhagic *E. coli*. Mononuclear cells suggest typhoid fever or amebic dysentery. Previously, the finding of fecal leukocytes was an indication for stool culture, but this is imprecise. Culture should be obtained in suspected patients regardless of this finding.
- Stool examinations for ova and parasites are indicated in all patients who have had diarrhea for >2 weeks, have traveled to developing countries, drink well water, are HIV positive, or men who have sex with men.
- Special stains are needed for amebic trophozoites, *Cryptosporidium*, *Isospora*, and *Microsporidia*, so specify the organisms of interest.
- Stool antigen assays can detect *Isospora*, *Giardia*, *Cryptosporidium*, and *Entamoeba histolytica*.
- Stool toxin assays detect *C. difficile* toxin and Shiga-like toxin.
- Stool cultures identify common bacterial pathogens such as *Campylobacter* spp., *Salmonella* spp., and *Shigella* spp.

- ○ The "3-day rule" is applied by most microbiology laboratories. Patients who develop diarrhea after 3 days of hospitalization are less likely to have a non–*C. difficile* bacterial or parasitic cause of diarrhea, and stool for cultures and/or ova and parasites is not recommended.
- ○ Patients aged ≥65 years and those with comorbid diseases, neutropenia, or HIV infection are the exception to the "3-day rule," and warrant cultures even when onset of diarrhea is ≥3 days after hospitalization.
- Blood cultures should be obtained in severely ill patients or immunocompromised patients, or when salmonellosis is suspected.
- Endoscopy is useful in identifying amebiasis, in ruling out inflammatory bowel disease, and when no pathogen can be identified by other means.
- Several PCR-based multiplex molecular testing methods have been recently approved by the FDA. They offer a comprehensive and rapid way for diagnosis, but they do not distinguish between active infection and colonization. Preferably, these tests should be done with traditional testing as above.[5]

TREATMENT

- Fluid and electrolyte replacement is the mainstay of therapy.
- Dietary alteration is helpful and includes a lactose-free diet, starches and cereals, crackers, and soup.
- Symptomatic therapy with antimotility agents, such as loperamide and bismuth sulfate, may reduce the number of stools. **Antimotility agents alone should be avoided with dysentery symptoms** as they may worsen disease.
- Antimicrobial therapy can be given empirically in travel-associated watery or dysenteric diarrhea (see section Traveler's Diarrhea). Targeted therapy is recommended in non–travel-associated dysenteric diarrhea after microbiologic assessment. The following may be given[5]:
- ○ Ciprofloxacin 500 mg PO twice daily for 3 days or 750 mg as a single dose.
- ○ Levofloxacin 500 mg for 3 days or as a single dose.
- ○ Ofloxacin 400 mg for 3 days or as a single dose.
- ○ Azithromycin 1000 mg as a single dose or 500 mg daily for 3 days.
- ○ Rifaximin 200 mg 3x/d for 3 days.
- ○ Of note, fluoroquinolone-resistant *Campylobacter* species are prevalent in Southeast Asia and the Indian subcontinent. Azithromycin 1 g PO × 1 dose should be used in these regions.
- ○ **Antibiotics are contraindicated in diarrhea caused by enterohemorrhagic** *E. coli*, such as *E. coli* O157:H7, as they may increase the risk of hemolytic uremic syndrome (HUS) but do not reduce the duration of diarrhea.

CHRONIC INFECTIOUS DIARRHEA

Chronic diarrhea refers to diarrheal symptoms lasting ≥30 days. Most chronic diarrheas are noninfectious. Infectious causes are usually parasitic. See chapters below for discussion of specific etiologies, see Chapter 17 for discussion of giardiasis, and Chapter 13 for a discussion of cryptosporidiosis, microsporidiosis, cyclosporiasis.

Foodborne Illnesses

GENERAL PRINCIPLES

- Foodborne illnesses result from the ingestion of foods contaminated with pathogenic organisms, toxins, or chemicals (see Table 6-1).
- Most foodborne illness results in vomiting and/or diarrhea (food poisoning).

TABLE 6-1	COMMON ORGANISMS CAUSING FOODBORNE ILLNESS
Staphylococcus aureus	Ham, poultry, egg salad, pastries
Bacillus cereus	Fried rice, meats, vegetables
Clostridium perfringens	Beef, poultry, gravy, Mexican food
Escherichia coli O157:H7	Undercooked beef, raw milk
Salmonella	Poultry, beef, egg, dairy products
Shigella	Egg salads, potato salads, lettuce
Campylobacter jejuni	Raw milk, poultry (spring, summer)
Vibrio cholerae	Shellfish
Yersinia enterocolitica	Milk, tofu, pork
Enteroinvasive *E. coli*	Cheese
Enterotoxigenic *E. coli*	Salad, cheese, sausage, seafood, cheese, hamburger
Clostridium botulinum	Vegetables, fruits (especially home-canned), fish

DIAGNOSIS

Clinical Manifestations

- Timing of symptoms and food exposure is important.
- Foodborne illness with vomiting as the main symptom:
  - Nausea and vomiting within 1 to 6 hours of ingestion is suggestive of a preformed toxin, due to either *S. aureus* or *Bacillus cereus*. Both are self-limited, but *B. cereus* can rarely cause hepatic necrosis.
  - Noroviruses cause nausea, vomiting, and diarrhea. It has been associated with large outbreaks on cruise ships, restaurants, and long-term care facilities. Symptoms may last up to 48 to 72 hours.[6]
  - Anisakiasis causes nausea, vomiting, and epigastric pain. It is associated with consumption of raw fish infected with anisakid nematodes.
- Foodborne illness with diarrhea as the main symptom[7]:
  - Abdominal cramps and diarrhea without vomiting within 8 to 16 hours of ingestion are usually caused by toxins produced in vivo (*B. cereus* and *Clostridium perfringens*). *C. perfringens* rarely causes hemorrhagic necrosis of the jejunum (pigbel) and is associated with consumption of chitterlings.
  - Abdominal cramps and watery diarrhea within 1 to 3 days suggest enterotoxigenic *E. coli*, *V. parahaemolyticus*, *V. cholerae*, *Campylobacter jejuni*, *Salmonella* spp., and *Shigella* spp. Disease is enterotoxin- or cytotoxin-mediated. Symptoms usually resolve in 76 to 92 hours but may last >1 week.
  - Bloody diarrhea without fever 3 to 5 days after eating suggests noninvasive enterohemorrhagic *E. coli*, such as *E. coli* O157:H7. Infection is characterized by severe abdominal cramping and diarrhea, which is initially watery but subsequently grossly bloody. There is risk for the development of HUS.
  - *Cryptosporidium parvum* causes chronic infection in immunocompromised patients and water-related self-limited watery diarrhea in immunocompetent hosts. The incubation period is typically 1 week, but can be up to 4 weeks.
  - *Cyclospora cayetanensis* causes watery diarrhea 7 days after ingestion of contaminated food, usually imported berries.

- Foodborne illness with non-GI symptoms[7]:
  - Nausea, vomiting, and diarrhea within 1 hour of ingestion of seafood suggest scombroid poisoning, ciguatera fish poisoning, or shellfish poisoning.
  - Scombroid poisoning presents as a histamine release reaction 10 to 60 minutes after eating contaminated fish. Symptoms include flushing, headache, dizziness, urticaria along with GI symptoms and resolve within 12 hours.
  - Ciguatera fish poisoning presents with abdominal cramps and diarrhea 1 to 3 hours after eating contaminated reef fish. Neurologic symptoms of circumoral paresthesias occur 3 to 72 hours after the meal and may last from a few days to several weeks.
  - Shellfish poisoning, of which the most common type is paralytic, occurs 30 to 60 minutes after eating shellfish. Symptoms include numbness and tingling of the face, lips, tongue, and extremities.
  - Nausea, vomiting, diarrhea, and **descending paralysis** (beginning with cranial nerve weakness manifested as dysphonia, dysphagia, diplopia, and blurred vision, followed by muscle weakness and respiratory insufficiency) suggest *Clostridium botulinum* toxin ingestion. The sensory system is intact. The differential includes Guillain–Barré syndrome, which can develop 1 to 3 weeks after *Campylobacter* spp. infection.
  - Diarrhea followed by fever and systemic complaints such as headache, muscle aches, and stiff neck may suggest infection with *Listeria monocytogenes.*
  - *Yersinia* spp. cause watery diarrhea in children aged 1 to 5 years, but may mimic appendicitis in older children and adolescents.

Diagnostic Testing

- Obtain appropriate specimens from patients (see "Acute Infectious Diarrhea: Diagnosis").
- Botulism is diagnosed by the detection of toxin in food, serum, or stool of patients or *C. botulinum* spores in the stool by culture.

TREATMENT

- Supportive therapy is indicated for most foodborne illness.
- Treatment is instituted where appropriate (see "Acute Infectious Diarrhea: Treatment").
- State health departments should be notified.
- Antitoxin for botulism should be administered as soon as possible if botulism is suspected. The State Health Department should be contacted immediately for assistance and for obtaining the antitoxin.

Traveler's Diarrhea

GENERAL PRINCIPLES

- Traveler's diarrhea is defined as three or more unformed stools per day in a person traveling to a developing nation.
- Infection is acquired through ingestion of fecally contaminated food or water.
- **Enterotoxigenic *E. coli*** are the most common cause, contributing up to a third of cases.
- Other common pathogens include *Salmonella* spp., *Shigella* spp., *Campylobacter* spp., and enteroaggregative *E. coli.*
- Viral causes include noroviruses and rotavirus.
- Parasites are less common and are usually seen in long-term travelers.
- Prevention includes avoiding raw fruits, vegetables, water, and ice cubes. All water should be boiled or bottled. More information can be found at http://www.cdc.gov/travel/ or call 1-877-FYI-TRIP (1-877-394-8747). Antibiotic prophylaxis breeds resistance and is recommended only for patients at high risk for morbidity and mortality from diarrhea.

DIAGNOSIS

- Diarrhea, anorexia, nausea, vomiting, and cramping abdominal pain can occur.
- Patients may have low-grade fever.
- The illness is self-limited, usually lasting 3 to 5 days.
- Postinfectious irritable bowel syndrome may develop in some patients.

TREATMENT

- Treatment is usually empiric.
- See "Acute Infectious Diarrhea: Treatment."

Enteric Fever (Typhoid Fever)

GENERAL PRINCIPLES

- Several enteric infections characterized by abdominal pain and fever are distinct from acute infectious diarrhea. These include enteric fever, mesenteric adenitis (which can mimic appendicitis), and eosinophilia with abdominal cramps/diarrhea.
- Enteric fever, which refers to both typhoid fever and paratyphoid fever, is an acute systemic illness with fever, headache, and abdominal discomfort caused by *Salmonella enterica* Typhi (formerly *S. typhi*) and *S. enterica* Paratyphi.
- Typhoid fever is prevalent in Asia, Africa, and Latin America.
- Multidrug-resistant (MDR) strains of *S.* Typhi are increasingly prevalent globally.
- Risk factors for typhoid fever include gastrectomy, hypochlorhydria, altered intestinal motility, prior antibiotic therapy, sickle cell anemia, chronic liver disease, and CD4+ T-cell deficiency.
- Organisms are ingested, multiply in intestinal lymphoid tissue, and disseminate systemically via lymphatic or hematogenous routes. Incubation period is 5 to 21 days.
- Infection may be food- or waterborne.
- A live oral *S.* Typhi strain Ty21a and a parenteral Vi polysaccharide vaccine are available. Unfortunately, they are not completely effective and do not protect recipients from *S.* Paratyphi infection. Booster doses are given every 5 years.
- The oral Ty21a vaccine is taken every other day for 4 days at least 2 weeks before departure. It should not be given to pregnant women or patients with immunodeficiency.
- Parenteral Vi polysaccharide vaccine is administered as a single dose intramuscularly at least 2 weeks before potential exposure. The vaccine is safe for immunocompromised individuals, including HIV-infected patients. Efficacy is similar to oral vaccine. Booster doses are given every 2 to 3 years.
- Travelers should be advised about precautions regarding the foods and water they consume, even after they received the vaccine.

DIAGNOSIS

Clinical Manifestations

- Symptoms include insidious onset of fever, headache, and abdominal pain with cough, conjunctivitis, and constipation or diarrhea.
- Diarrhea is rare after the first few days.
- Physical examination may reveal abdominal tenderness, hepatosplenomegaly, rose spots (faint, maculopapular, salmon-colored blanching lesions predominately on the trunk), relative bradycardia, and mental status changes. Rales may be present.
- Complications include pneumonia, endocarditis, osteomyelitis, arthritis, and meningitis.

Differential Diagnosis

The differential includes infections with *Y. enterocolitica*, *Yersinia pseudotuberculosis*, and *Campylobacter fetus*, as well as typhoidal tularemia. Noninfectious etiologies can present similarly.

Diagnostic Testing

- Obtain multiple blood, stool, and urine cultures. Urine and stool cultures are positive in <50% of patients. Rose spots and duodenal contents may also be cultured. If cultures are negative, bone marrow can be cultured, as it may be positive even after antibiotics have been started.
- Serology is unreliable and should not be done in place of culture.

TREATMENT

- Resistance to antibiotics is increasing. MDR *S.* Typhi and *S.* Paratyphi are defined as strains resistant to ampicillin, chloramphenicol, and trimethoprim–sulfamethoxazole.
- A fluoroquinolone (e.g., **ciprofloxacin**, 500 mg PO twice daily for 10 d) may be used but should be avoided in travelers coming from South and Southeast Asia due to high rates of resistance (>80%).
- Third-generation cephalosporin can be used (**ceftriaxone**, 2 g IV daily for 1–2 wk.
- **Azithromycin** 1 g daily for 5 days is an alternative regimen, but resistance is also increasing.[8]

Antibiotic-Associated Diarrhea/Colitis

GENERAL PRINCIPLES

- *C. difficile* is a spore-forming, gram-positive obligate anaerobe.
- ***C. difficile* infection (CDI) should be suspected in any patient who has diarrhea in association with antibiotic exposure.**
- Asymptomatic colonization can occur in 10% to 30% of hospitalized patients; it is important to differentiate between colonization and CDI.
- Risk factors for CDI include advanced age, hospitalization, cancer chemotherapy, GI surgery, manipulation of the GI tract such as tube feeding, and acid-suppressing medications. **The most important modifiable risk factor is exposure to antimicrobial agents.**
- CDI results in acute inflammation of the colonic mucosa. Disease results from spore germination, overgrowth, and toxin production. Pathogenic strains produce toxin A and B or B alone. About 10% of *C. difficile* strains produce no toxin and are not pathogenic.
- During infection, only the epithelium and the superficial lamina propria are affected, although in more severe cases, deeper tissues are involved. Pseudomembranes may be found throughout the colon but are worst in the rectosigmoid region. The ileum is rarely involved unless there is a previous colostomy/ileostomy.

DIAGNOSIS

Clinical Manifestations

- Infection results in profuse watery or green mucoid, foul-smelling diarrhea with cramping abdominal pain usually beginning 4 to 10 days after starting antibiotic therapy (range 24 h to 8 wk).
- The stool may be positive for occult blood.
- Patients may develop toxic megacolon, perforation, and peritonitis.

Differential Diagnosis

- Osmotic diarrhea from antibiotic use is more common than CDI, but not associated with fever or leukocytosis.
- Other differential diagnoses include Crohn disease, ulcerative colitis, ischemic colitis, or infection with other intestinal pathogens, such as *E. coli*, *Salmonella* spp., *Campylobacter* spp., *Yersinia* spp., *E. histolytica*, or *Strongyloides*.

Diagnostic Testing[9]

- Testing should **only** be carried out in patients with new-onset ≥3 unformed stools in 24 hours.
- Multistep testing of stool is recommended. Detection of *C. difficile* glutamate dehydrogenase antigen using enzyme immunoassay (EIA) or detection of *C. difficile* nucleic acid using nucleic acid amplification testing (NAAT) is usually the first step. This must be followed by an EIA detecting toxin A and B or toxin B.
- Endoscopy may be useful, but pseudomembranous colitis is seen in only about half of patients with CDI.

TREATMENT

- Offending antibiotics should be stopped when possible.
- Antibiotic treatment of CDI is presented in Table 6-2.

Diverticulitis

GENERAL PRINCIPLES

- Infection of the diverticula, including extension into adjacent tissues, can result from obstruction from a fecalith.
- Inflammation or micropuncture of diverticula can lead to perforation with pericolic abscess formation, fistula formation, or, less commonly, peritonitis.
- Organisms usually include anaerobes and facultative gram-negative bacilli.

DIAGNOSIS

- Left lower quadrant pain and a change in bowel habits is the typical presentation.
- Fever, chills, nausea, and vomiting can occur.
- Microscopic rectal bleeding occurs in up to 25% of cases.
- Occasionally, shock and peritonitis can develop.
- Computed tomography (CT) scanning is helpful to evaluate for abscess formation.

TREATMENT

- Initial, uncomplicated diverticulitis is primarily a medical disease. Bowel rest (nothing by mouth), IV fluids, and IV antimicrobial therapy are the mainstay of treatment.
- IV antibiotic regimens are as follows:
  - β-Lactam/β-lactamase inhibitor such as ampicillin–sulbactam (3 g q6h) or piperacillin/tazobactam (3.375 g IV q6h)
  - A third-generation cephalosporin such as ceftriaxone (1 g IV q24h) **and** metronidazole (500 mg IV q8–12h)
  - A fluoroquinolone (e.g., ciprofloxacin 400 mg IV q12h **or** levofloxacin 500 mg or 750 mg IV daily) **and** metronidazole (500 mg IV q8h)

TABLE 6-2	*CLOSTRIDIUM DIFFICILE* INFECTION MANAGEMENT	
Type of CDI	**Criteria**	**Treatment**
Mild-to-moderate and first or second episode		Vancomycin 125 mg PO q6h for 10–14 d Fidaxomicin 200 mg PO q12h × 10 d Metronidazole 500 mg PO q8h for 10–14 d (only if first two options are not available)
≥Third episode		Vancomycin 125 mg PO q6h for 10–14 d, considering tapering[a] or pulsed regimen Fidaxomicin 200 mg PO q12h × 10 d, considering tapering regimen Fecal microbiota transplantation
Severe	Leukocytosis with >15,000 cells/μL or Creatinine ≥1.5 times the premorbid level	Vancomycin 125 mg PO q6h for 10–14 d Fidaxomicin 200 mg PO q12h × 10 d
Severe, complicated	Ileus, megacolon, pending perforation, hypotension, or shock	Vancomycin 125–500 mg PO q6h +/– vancomycin enema + metronidazole 500 mg IV q8h. Request surgical consult

[a]An example of tapering vancomycin regimen (after acute treatment): 125 mg PO q8h for 1 wk, 125 mg PO q12h for 1 wk, 125 mg PO daily for 1 wk, 125 mg PO every other day for 2 wk, then 125 mg PO three times a week for 2 to 8 wk.
CDI, *Clostridium difficile* infection.

- ○ A carbapenem, such as imipenem (500 mg q6h) or meropenem (1 g q8h) or ertapenem (1 g daily)
- ○ Dose adjustments for renal function may be necessary
- Regardless of the initial empiric regimen, the therapeutic regimen should be revisited once culture results are available.
- Patients who are not severely ill can be treated with oral antibiotics such as ciprofloxacin 500 mg PO q12h plus metronidazole 500 mg PO q8h, amoxicillin-clavulanate 875 mg PO q12h, or moxifloxacin 400 mg PO daily.
- The patient may need percutaneous drainage of an abscess.
- Surgical intervention is indicated if the patient does not respond in 48 to 72 hours and has recurrent attacks at the same location, as well as for fistula formation, obstruction, perforation, or if carcinoma is suspected.

Peritoneal Infections

Primary Peritonitis

GENERAL PRINCIPLES

- Primary peritonitis or spontaneous bacterial peritonitis (SBP) occurs mostly in patients with liver disease and ascites, although it can occur in patients with other causes of ascites (e.g., heart failure, nephrotic syndrome).[10]

- SBP is almost always monobacterial.
- The most common organisms are *E. coli*, *K. pneumonia*, and *Streptococci*, including *Streptococcus pneumoniae*.
- Rare etiologies include *Candida* spp., *Cryptococcus neoformans*, and *Aspergillus* spp. Infection with these organisms are more aptly referred to as spontaneous fungal peritonitis.

DIAGNOSIS

Clinical Manifestations

- New onset of abdominal pain with evidence of systemic sepsis in a patient with chronic ascites suggests SBP.
- Presentation can be subtle, with acute deterioration of renal function, unexplained encephalopathy, and borderline fever.
- **A low threshold for paracentesis is appropriate in patients with chronic ascites.**

Diagnostic Testing

- Diagnosis is made by paracentesis, with fluid sent for culture (in blood culture bottles to increase yield), cell count, and differential.
- Blood cultures should be obtained, as bacteremia occurs in up to 75% of patients.
- Definitive diagnosis is made by a positive culture combined with a neutrophil count in the peritoneal fluid >250 cells/µL.
- **Since cultures are not always positive, patients with chronic ascites with neutrophil count >250 cells/µL should be treated with antibiotics.**
- A polymicrobial infection plus ascitic fluid protein >1 g/dL, glucose <50 mg/dL, or lactate dehydrogenase (LDH) >serum level suggests secondary peritonitis and the need for emergent imaging to detect GI perforation.[10]

TREATMENT

- Initial therapy usually consists of a third-generation cephalosporin, such as ceftriaxone, 2 g IV daily or cefotaxime 2 g IV q8h, or levofloxacin, or a β-lactam/β-lactamase inhibitor. Therapy should be tailored to the results of cultures.
- Treatment should continue for 5 days. Extended courses may be used for resistant or harder-to-treat organisms (e.g., *P. aeruginosa*, Enterobacteriaceae)
- Albumin infusions (1.5 g/kg on day 1 and 1 g/kg on day 3) reduce acute renal failure.
- Poor prognosis is associated with renal failure, hyperbilirubinemia, hypoalbuminemia, and encephalopathy.
- Indications for prophylaxis include history of SBP and high risk for developing SBP (low ascitic fluid protein value of <1.5 g/dL). Norfloxacin 400 mg PO daily, ciprofloxacin 500 mg PO daily, or trimethoprim–sulfamethoxazole DS 1 tab PO daily are used.
- Short-course prophylaxis with a quinolone or a third-generation cephalosporin (ceftriaxone 1 g IV daily for 7 d) improves survival in patients with variceal hemorrhage, regardless of the presence of ascites.[10]

Secondary Peritonitis

GENERAL PRINCIPLES

- Infection results from perforation of the GI tract with spillage of intestinal contents into the peritoneum or from contiguous spread from a visceral infection or abscess.
- **Secondary peritonitis is typically a polymicrobial infection with enteric organisms.**

DIAGNOSIS

Clinical Manifestations

- Manifestations include severe abdominal pain, nausea, vomiting, anorexia, fever, chills, and abdominal distension.
- Patients may have abdominal tenderness, hypoactive or absent bowel sounds, rebound, guarding, and abdominal rigidity.

Diagnostic Testing

- Blood cultures are positive in 20% to 30% of cases.
- An abdominal series helps rule out free air and obstruction.
- An abdominal CT or ultrasound looking for the source of infection may be helpful.

TREATMENT

- Broad-spectrum antibiotics that cover both gram-negative aerobic and anaerobic organisms should be started, and treatment should continue for ≥5 to 7 days.
- Ampicillin–sulbactam, 3 g IV q6h, or a third-generation cephalosporin with metronidazole (e.g., ceftriaxone 1–2 g IV daily and metronidazole 500 mg IV q8h).
- Surgical management of the source, such as repair of perforations and removal of necrotic or infected material, is essential.

Peritonitis Associated With Chronic Ambulatory Peritoneal Dialysis

GENERAL PRINCIPLES

- Peritonitis associated with chronic ambulatory peritoneal dialysis occurs at an average rate of one infection per person per year.
- Recurrent infection may result in sclerosing peritonitis, which can lead to discontinuation of ambulatory peritoneal dialysis.
- Infections usually originate from contamination of the catheter by skin organisms, due to exit site infections or subcutaneous tunnel catheter infections.
- Transient bacteremia or contamination of the dialysate delivery system during bag exchanges can also occur.
- **Common causative organisms are gram-positive organisms,** such as *S. aureus, S. epidermidis, streptococcus species,* **gram-negative bacilli, anaerobes,** and, less commonly, *M. tuberculosis, Aspergillus, Nocardia,* and *Candida* spp.

DIAGNOSIS

- Symptoms include abdominal pain, tenderness, nausea, vomiting, fever, and diarrhea.
- Diagnosis is made by analysis and culture of the dialysate. Peritonitis is diagnosed when dialysate has a leukocyte count >100 cells/µL with >50% neutrophils.[11]
- Ascites cultures reveal the organisms >50% of the time.
- Blood cultures are rarely positive.

TREATMENT

- Intraperitoneal antibiotics that cover both gram-positive and gram-negative organisms should be used. The intraperitoneal route is preferred unless the patient has sepsis.
- First-generation cephalosporin such as cefazolin (vancomycin if there are high rates of MRSA) and an aminoglycoside or a third-generation cephalosporin should be used empirically.[11]

- Antibiotic therapy should be adjusted based on culture results.
- Intraperitoneal antibiotics can be given continuously or intermittently with once-daily exchange. Examples of continuous intraperitoneal antibiotic dosing are as follows[11]:
  - Vancomycin 1.0 g/L dialysate loading dose, then 25 mg/L dialysate maintenance dose
  - Gentamicin 8 mg/L loading, then 4 mg/L maintenance
  - Cefazolin 500 mg/L loading, then 125 mg/L maintenance
  - Cefepime 500 mg/L loading, then 125 mg/L maintenance
- Most patients improve in 2 to 4 days. If symptoms persist >96 hours, reevaluate to rule out a GI source.
- Depending on the organism and the severity of the illness, patients may need their catheters removed. This is especially true in the case of relapsing or refractory peritonitis, fungal peritonitis, and refractory catheter infections.

Biliary Infections

Cholecystitis

GENERAL PRINCIPLES

- In >90% of cases, cholecystitis is caused by impaired biliary drainage due to the impaction of gallstones in the cystic duct.
- Acalculous cholecystitis can occur in acutely ill patients following surgery or burns.
- Causative organisms usually consist of normal intestinal flora such as *E. coli*, *Klebsiella*, *Enterobacter*, *Proteus* spp., *Enterococcus* spp., and anaerobes.

DIAGNOSIS

Clinical Manifestations

- Patients usually describe right upper quadrant abdominal pain that radiates to the right shoulder and scapula, with or without fever.
- Patients may have Murphy sign, which is tenderness on the right upper quadrant of the abdomen on deep inspiration.
- Complications of cholecystitis may include gangrene of the gallbladder, perforation, emphysematous cholecystitis, cholecystoenteric fistula, pericholecystic abscess, intraperitoneal abscess, peritonitis, liver abscess, and bacteremia.

Differential Diagnosis

The differential diagnosis includes myocardial infarction, pancreatitis, perforated ulcer, right lower lobe pneumonia, intestinal obstruction, cholangitis, hepatitis, and right kidney disease.

Diagnostic Testing

- Hyperbilirubinemia and alkaline phosphatase elevation are usually not observed, and, if present, should warrant evaluation for cholangitis or choledocholithiasis.
- Imaging with ultrasound, CT, or technetium hepatoiminodiacetic acid (HIDA) scan is diagnostic.

- Ultrasound and CT may reveal stones, a thickened gallbladder wall, a dilated lumen, or pericholecystic fluid. Ultrasound is usually the preferred first choice. A sonographic Murphy sign, which is the same as produced by physical examination, with visualization of an inflamed gallbladder on ultrasound, may be elicited during the procedure and is also diagnostic.
- The HIDA scan may reveal an occluded cystic duct and nonvisualization of the gallbladder.

TREATMENT

- Treatment consists of IV fluid resuscitation, pain control, and, in high-risk patients, broad-spectrum antibiotic therapy covering gram-negative bacilli and anaerobes. Surgical options include laparoscopic cholecystectomy, open cholecystectomy, or percutaneous cholecystostomy.[12]
- Monotherapies include ampicillin/sulbactam 3 g IV q6h, piperacillin/tazobactam 3.375 g IV q6h, ertapenem 1 g IV q24h, or meropenem 1 g IV q8h.
- Combination therapies include metronidazole 500 mg IV q8h plus a third-generation cephalosporin, such as ceftriaxone 1 g IV q24h, or ciprofloxacin 400 mg IV q12h.
- Immediate surgery is indicated for emphysematous cholecystitis, perforation, and suspected pericholecystic abscess.
- The timing of surgery in uncomplicated cholecystitis is varied; surgery is usually performed within 6 days of onset of symptoms, but can be delayed for 6 weeks if the patient is responding to medical management. Earlier surgery is associated with fewer complications and hospitalizations.

Cholangitis

GENERAL PRINCIPLES

- Acute cholangitis is characterized by inflammation and bacterial infection involving the hepatic and common bile ducts as a result of biliary obstruction.
- Obstruction of the common bile duct results in congestion and necrosis of the walls of the biliary tree followed by proliferation of bacteria.
- Obstruction is often due to gallstones, but can be due to tumor, chronic pancreatitis, parasitic infection, or a complication of endoscopic retrograde cholangiopancreatography (ERCP).
- Organisms are similar to those associated with cholecystitis.

DIAGNOSIS

Clinical Manifestations

- Patients frequently have a history of gallbladder disease.
- The onset is usually acute.
- The classic presentation of Charcot triad is present in about 50% of patients and consists of fever, right upper quadrant pain, and jaundice. If confusion and hypotension (Reynold pentad) are also present, there is significant morbidity and mortality.
- Complications of cholangitis include bacteremia, shock, gallbladder perforation, hepatic abscess, and pancreatitis.

Differential Diagnosis

The differential includes cholecystitis, hepatic abscess, perforating ulcer, pancreatitis, intestinal obstruction, right lower lobe pneumonia, and myocardial infarction.

Diagnostic Testing

- Leukocytosis, hyperbilirubinemia, and elevated alkaline phosphatase and transaminases are seen; disseminated intravascular coagulation (DIC) may be present.
- Blood cultures are positive in >50% of patients.
- Ultrasound can be used to evaluate gallbladder size, the presence of stones, and the degree of bile duct dilatation.
- According to the Tokyo guidelines, acute cholangitis should be suspected in patients with at least fever (with or without chills) or laboratory evidence of inflammation (leukocytosis, elevated CRP, etc.) and jaundice or abnormal liver chemistry. It is definite when, in addition to fulfilling criteria for suspected cholangitis, the patient also has imaging findings of biliary dilatation and an underlying etiology (stone, stricture, recent stent, etc.).[13]

TREATMENT

- Treatment consists of IV fluid resuscitation and broad-spectrum antibiotics.
- Antibiotic regimens are similar to cholecystitis.
- Prompt decompression of the common bile duct is mandatory. ERCP serves as both a diagnostic and therapeutic modality in cholangitis. The standard approach is with endoscopic sphincterotomy with stone extraction and/or stent insertion. Decompression may also be carried out percutaneously or with an open surgical approach.

Viral Hepatitis

Acute Viral Hepatitis

GENERAL PRINCIPLES

- Acute viral hepatitis is a systemic infection that affects the liver predominantly. There are five major hepatotropic viruses (A, B, C, D, and E) that cause acute hepatitis.
- With the exception of hepatitis A infection, all the viral hepatitides can cause chronic infection, leading to chronic liver disease and cirrhosis. Hepatitis B and C are associated with hepatocellular carcinoma (Table 6-3).
- An HAV vaccine is available and is 85% to 100% effective in preventing disease. Vaccination doses should be given at 0 and 6 to 12 months (Havrix) or 0 and 6 to 18 months (Vaqta). Immunization against HAV should be given to:
  - Men who have sex with men
  - People traveling to high-risk areas
  - Patients with chronic liver disease
  - Military personnel
  - IV drug users
- Hepatitis B vaccine is given at 0, 1 to 2, and 4 to 6 months. Immunization is recommended for:
  - Sexual partners and household contacts of a person who is hepatitis B surface antigen (HBsAg) positive
  - Persons who are not in a long-term monogamous relationship
  - Persons seeking diagnosis or treatment for a sexually transmitted infection
  - Current or recent IV drug users
  - Staff and residents of care facilities for the developmentally disabled

TABLE 6-3	VIRAL HEPATITIS				
	Incubation Average (Range)	Main Route of Transmission	Chronic Phase	Diagnostic Tests	Vaccine
Hepatitis A	4 wk (2–8 wk)	Fecal–oral	No	Anti-HAV IgM: acute infection	Havrix 0 and 6–12 mo
				Anti-HAV IgG: resolved infection, immunity	Vaqta 0 and 6–18 mo
Hepatitis B	2–3 mo (1–6 mo)	Vertical, sexual, blood-borne such as intravenous drug use	Yes	See Table 6-4	0, 1–2, and 4–6 mo
Hepatitis C	6–8 wk (2–26 wk)	Blood-borne	Yes	Anti-HCV; HCV RNA: infection	Not available
Hepatitis D	2–8 wk	Blood-borne	Yes	Anti-HDV with anti-HBc IgM: coinfection with HBV	Vaccine for hepatitis B
				Anti-HDV with anti-HBc IgG: superinfection with HBV	
Hepatitis E	6 wk (2–8 wk)	Fecal–oral	Yes	Anti-HEV IgM:acute infection	Not commercially available
				Anti-HEV IgG: resolved infection	

- ○ Public safety and health care workers potentially exposed to blood or blood-contaminated body fluids
- ○ End-stage renal disease patients
- ○ Chronic liver disease patients
- ○ HIV-infected patients
- ○ International travelers to endemic regions (>2%)
- If combined hepatitis A and B vaccine (Twinrix) is used, the doses are given at 0, 1, and 6 months.
- No FDA-approved vaccines are available for HCV, HDV, or HEV.

DIAGNOSIS

Clinical Manifestations

- Symptoms range from asymptomatic illness to fulminant hepatic failure.
- A large proportion of infections with any of the hepatitis viruses are asymptomatic or anicteric.
  - Hepatitis A causes minor disease in childhood, with >80% of infections being asymptomatic. In adults, infection is more often symptomatic.
  - Infections with HBV, HCV, and HDV can also be asymptomatic.
- Clinically apparent acute hepatitis presents with jaundice or elevated liver enzymes.
- Common symptoms in the preicteric phase include fever, myalgia, nausea, vomiting, diarrhea, fatigue, malaise, and dull right upper quadrant pain.
- About 10% of patients with acute HBV infection and 5% to 10% patients with acute HCV infection present with a serum sickness–like illness, with fever, urticarial or maculopapular rash, and migratory arthritis. This diminishes rapidly after the onset of jaundice.
- Coryza, photophobia, headache, and cough are symptoms of hepatitis A.
- Fulminant hepatic failure typically presents with hepatic encephalopathy within 8 weeks of symptoms or within 2 weeks of onset of jaundice.
  - Fulminant hepatitis carries a high mortality.
  - Pregnant women with acute HEV infection have a 15% risk of fulminant liver failure and a mortality rate of 10% to 40%.
  - The risk of liver failure in HAV infection increases with age and with preexisting liver disease.
- There are very few specific physical findings in the preicteric phase.
  - Urticaria may be present if a serum sickness–like syndrome develops.
  - In the icteric phase, jaundice and a slightly enlarged and tender liver may be present.
  - A minority of patients may have a palpable spleen tip.
  - Signs of hepatic encephalopathy and asterixis may be present if fulminant hepatic failure develops.

Differential Diagnosis

- EBV, CMV, rubella, measles, mumps, and coxsackie B can cause mild liver enzyme abnormalities but rarely jaundice.
- Disseminated herpes virus infection with hepatic involvement can occur in immunocompromised hosts.
- Yellow fever is a cause of acute hepatitis in Central and South America.
- Elevated transaminases can be seen in rickettsial infection, bacterial sepsis, *Legionella* infection, syphilis, and disseminated mycobacterial and fungal infections.
- Q fever (*Coxiella burnetii*) is associated with jaundice in 5% of patients.
- Noninfectious causes may include many drugs that can cause hepatitis, including acetaminophen, isoniazid, and alcohol.
- Usually, the aspartate transaminase (AST) is elevated out of proportion to the alanine transaminase (ALT) in acute alcohol-related hepatitis.
- Anoxic liver injury can occur from hypotension, heart failure, or cardiopulmonary arrest.
- Cholestatic liver disease and other diseases (e.g., Wilson disease, sickle cell disease, acute Budd–Chiari syndrome, tumor infiltration of the liver, and Gilbert and Dubin–Johnson syndromes) can lead to acute hepatitis.

Diagnostic Testing

- Large elevations of AST and ALT (>eightfold normal) may occur.
- The degree of rise in transaminases does not correlate with risk of developing hepatic failure.

- Bilirubin, alkaline phosphatase, and LDH may be one to three times normal.
- DIC can develop with fulminant hepatic failure, along with prothrombin time (PT) elevation and hypoglycemia.

TREATMENT

- Treatment for acute hepatitis is supportive and includes bed rest, a high-calorie diet, avoidance of hepatotoxic medications, and abstinence from alcohol.
- Patients should be hospitalized for severe dehydration or hepatic failure if the bilirubin level is >15 to 20 mg/dL or if PT is prolonged; most patients can be managed at home.
- Transaminases, alkaline phosphatase, bilirubin, and PT should be monitored one to two times per week for 2 weeks and then every other week until normalized.
- Corticosteroids do not shorten disease course or lessen symptoms and may predispose to longer illness and more relapses.
- Patients with fulminant hepatic failure should be considered for liver transplantation.

ACUTE HEPATITIS A

- HAV is an acute, self-limited disease, but can cause fulminant hepatitis in adults. The incubation period ranges from 15 to 50 days (mean 30 d).
- Outbreaks of HAV occur worldwide.
- Infection at a younger age is less severe and leads to immunity.
- **Detection of anti-HAV IgM antibodies together with a typical clinical presentation is diagnostic** of acute hepatitis A infection. IgM is detectable up to 6 months after exposure, and IgG confers lifelong protective immunity.

ACUTE HEPATITIS B

- HBV is the most common cause of chronic viral hepatitis worldwide and a major cause of acute viral hepatitis.
- HBV infection is rare in developed countries, occurring in 2% of the population.
  - The incidence is 20% in high-risk areas of Southeast Asia and sub-Saharan Africa.
  - Vertical transmission is common in high-risk areas.
  - In low-risk countries, sexual or blood-borne transmission through IV drug use is the main mode of transmission.
- The incubation period is usually 28 to 160 days, averaging 2 to 3 months.
- HBV has a more insidious onset and a more prolonged course than HAV. The occurrence of the serum sickness–like syndrome favors the diagnosis of HBV infection.
- The diagnosis rests on serologic testing (Table 6-4).[14]
  - HBsAg: appears in serum 1 to 10 weeks after an acute exposure to HBV, before the onset of symptoms or elevation of serum ALT. In patients who subsequently recover, HBsAg becomes undetectable after 4 to 6 months. **Persistence of HBsAg for more than 6 months implies chronic infection.**
  - Hepatitis B surface antibody (HBsAb): appears when HBsAg declines in patients who mount a protective immune response. **It confers immunity** in patients with recovered hepatitis B or with previous vaccination. Please see Table 6-4.
  - Hepatitis B core antibody (HBcAb): suggests hepatitis B infection. IgM HBcAb could be the only positive antibody in the "window period" (the period of acute hepatitis B infection when both HBsAb and HBsAg may be negative).
  - Hepatitis B envelope antigen (HBeAg): serves as a marker for hepatitis B replication and infectivity. **The presence of HBeAg indicates high HBV DNA and high rates of transmission.**
  - Hepatitis B envelope antibody (HBeAb): a marker for low HBV DNA and lower rates of transmission in patients without protective immunity.

TABLE 6-4 SEROLOGIC MARKERS FOR HEPATITIS B INFECTION

HBsAg	HBsAb	IgM HBcAb	IgG HBcAb	HBeAg	HBeAb	Interpretation
+	−	+	−	−	−	Acute infection
−	−	+	−	−	−	Window period
−	+	−	−	−	−	Postvaccination: immune
−	+	−	+	−	+	Recovery: immune
+	−	−	+	+	−	High replicative phase
+	−	−	+	−	+	Low, nonreplicative phase

ACUTE HEPATITIS C

- HCV infection usually presents as a chronic hepatitis, but can be symptomatic in acute infections.
- The primary route of transmission is blood exposure, such as transfusion or IV drug use, but up to 20% of patients have no identifiable exposure. The incidence of HCV is also increasing in men who have sex with men, attributed to traumatic, insertive anal intercourse, and people who abuse opioids. Vertical transmission is rare.
- The incubation period is 2 to 26 weeks, with an average of 6 to 8 weeks.
- In patients with suspected acute HCV infection because of recent exposure, clinical symptoms, or elevated transaminases, both HCV ab and HCV RNA should be performed. **Acute HCV infection is likely in a patient with detectable HCV RNA and a negative HCV ab.**
- Because spontaneous clearance occurs in 15% to 25%, treatment is not recommended until chronic infection is established (see Chronic Hepatitis: Hepatitis C).

ACUTE HEPATITIS D

- HDV, also known as delta agent, is an incomplete RNA virus and requires HBsAg to enable replication and infection; **HDV always occurs in association with hepatitis B infection.**
- The primary route of transmission is parental, either via transfusion or IV drug use. The incubation period is variable.
- HDV is endemic to the Mediterranean Basin, the Middle East, and portions of South America.
- The two most common forms of infections are acute HBV and HDV coinfection and acute HDV infection superimposed on chronic HBV infection (superinfection).
- Clinically, HDV tends to be a severe illness with a high mortality (2%–20%). HDV often has a protracted course and frequently leads to cirrhosis.
- Anti-HDV antibody testing should be carried out only when evidence of HBV infection is found. Antibody is negative in the acute phase, but rises in the convalescent stage.
- Most patients with acute coinfection clear both infections.
- Superinfection results in chronic HDV infection along with chronic HBV infection. High titers of HDV antibody indicate ongoing infection.

ACUTE HEPATITIS E

- Epidemiologically, HEV resembles HAV, with fecal–oral transmission and both epidemic and sporadic cases.
- Most cases occur in developing countries, including India, Southeast Asia, Africa, and Mexico, in association with contaminated drinking water.
- Young adults are affected, with high mortality rates in pregnant women. US cases usually have a history of travel to endemic areas. HEV has an incubation period of 2 to 8 weeks, averaging approximately 6 weeks.
- Anti-HEV antibodies may be detected, but in the United States, serologic testing (HEV IgM and IgG) and PCR are available only through the Centers for Disease Control and Prevention. IgM is usually detectable by the onset of symptoms.
- Rarely, HEV infection can result in chronic infection in patients with immunocompromising conditions, such as receipt of organ transplantation, HIV infection, and hematologic malignancy.

Chronic Hepatitis

GENERAL PRINCIPLES

- Chronic viral hepatitis is defined as the presence of **liver inflammation persisting for ≥6 months and is associated with HBV, HCV, HDV, and HEV infection.**
- When cirrhosis is present, early referral to a hepatologist for evaluation is recommended.
- **The majority of patients with chronic viral hepatitis are asymptomatic.**
- Patients may complain of lethargy and right upper abdominal pain.
- Extrahepatic manifestations include polyarteritis nodosa (HBV), glomerulonephritis (HBV, HCV), mixed cryoglobulinemia (HCV), porphyria cutanea tarda (HCV), or membranous glomerulonephritis (HEV).
- Physical findings occur late in the course of viral infection and indicate the presence of cirrhosis. These include spider angiomata, hepatomegaly, splenomegaly, ascites, jaundice, gynecomastia, testicular atrophy, asterixis, and loss of body hair.
- Initial testing for HBsAg, anti-HBsAb, anti-HBcAb, HBeAg, anti-HBeAb, and anti-HCVAb should be carried out. HEV is rare in the United States, but when suspected, the blood sample can be sent to the CDC for HEV RNA.
- All patients should have complete blood count, metabolic panel, including AST, ALT, bilirubin, and albumin, as well as INR.

CHRONIC HEPATITIS B

GENERAL PRINCIPLES

- The risk of developing chronic HBV infection varies with age and is higher in children <5 years old than in immunocompetent adults.
- Risk factors for progression to cirrhosis include older age, HBV genotype C, high levels of HBV DNA, alcohol consumption, and concurrent infection with HCV, HDV, or HIV.

DIAGNOSIS

- In addition to the above laboratory evaluation, testing for coinfection with HCV, HDV, and HIV should be performed.
- Fibrosis and necroinflammation testing should also be obtained in all patients with chronic viral hepatitis as it helps determine the phase of the infection and affects treatment decisions. See Table 6-5. The gold standard is liver biopsy, but noninvasive testing, such as FibroSure/FibroTest, AST-to-platelet ratio index (APRI), FIB-4, transient elastography, etc., are also useful.

TABLE 6-5 PHASES OF CHRONIC HEPATITIS B VIRUS INFECTION

Phase	ALT Level	HBV DNA (IU/mL)	HBeAg	Histology	Treatment
Immune-tolerant	Normal	>1 million	+	Minimal inflammation and fibrosis	Not recommended, but ALT should be checked every 6 mo
HBeAg+ immune-active	Elevated	≥20,000	+	Moderate-severe inflammation or fibrosis	Recommended
Inactive	Normal	Undetectable	−	Minimal inflammation, variable fibrosis	Not recommended
HBeAg− Immune reactivation	Elevated	≥2000	−	Moderate-severe inflammation or fibrosis	Recommended

TREATMENT

- Treatment is recommended in patients in the immune-active phase. See Table 6-5 for details. The recommended treatment of chronic HBV infection is either with pegylated-interferon-2α (peg-IFN) 180 μg weekly or the nucleoside/nucleotide analogs (NAs). First-line NAs include entecavir 0.5 mg tab PO daily in treatment-naïve/noncirrhotic (1 mg daily for patients with decompensated cirrhosis), tenofovir disoproxil 300 mg tab PO daily, and tenofovir alafenamide 25 mg tab PO daily. Other approved therapies include lamivudine, telbivudine, and adefovir. Response is measured by loss of HBeAg, development of HBeAb and cessation of viral replication in HBeAg-positive patients, and viral suppression in HBeAg-negative patients.
- **Patients coinfected with HIV** should be treated with combined antiretroviral therapy that includes NAs active against HBV.[14] The preferred antiretroviral backbone therapy is the fixed-dose combination of tenofovir/emtricitabine, although tenofovir with lamivudine can also be used. If none of the preferred backbone can be used, treat the patient's HBV with entecavir; choose the 1 mg dose if treatment-experienced with lamivudine or telbivudine.

CHRONIC HEPATITIS C

General Principles

- In the United States, 70% of infections are caused by genotype 1, 15% to 20% by genotype 2, 10% by genotype 3, and 1% each by genotypes 4, 5, and 6. Of genotype 1 infections, approximately 60% are due to genotype 1a and 35% are genotype 1b.

Diagnosis

- The diagnostic screening test is serum HCV antibody. **The presence of HCV antibody suggests prior exposure to HCV but does not convey immunity.**
- Screening for chronic HCV is recommended in the following at-risk groups:
  - persons born between 1945 and 1965
  - injection drug users
  - intranasal illicit drug users
  - persons on hemodialysis
  - children born to HCV-infected mothers
  - persons who were ever incarcerated
  - patients with HIV
  - those who ever received blood products before July 1992 and those who received clotting factor concentrates produced before 1987
  - those with unexplained chronic liver disease or chronic hepatitis.
- A positive HCV ab should be followed up with HCV RNA. **Chronic HCV infection is defined as those with detectable HCV RNA for more than 6 months.**
- In addition to the workup for chronic viral hepatitis, HCV genotype should be performed in all patients with chronic HCV infection. Coinfection with HBV and HIV should be checked, and immunity to HAV and HBV should also be assessed with serology.
- Fibrosis testing should be obtained in all patients with chronic HCV to look for the level of fibrosis and/or presence of cirrhosis. The gold standard is liver biopsy, but noninvasive testing, such as FibroSure/FibroTest, APRI, FIB-4, transient elastography, etc., are also useful.
- In patients with cirrhosis, it is imperative to determine if they are decompensated or not. Decompensated cirrhosis is usually characterized by any of the presence of the following: jaundice, ascites, variceal hemorrhage, hepatic encephalopathy, or Child-Turcotte-Pugh class B or C. These patients should be referred to hepatology or to a liver transplant center.

Treatment

- The current treatment of chronic HCV involves a combination of all-oral direct-acting antivirals (DAAs) from the following drug classes: NS3/4a protease inhibitors, NS5a complex inhibitors, and NS5B polymerase inhibitor[15] (see Table 6-6).
- The goal of treatment is the achievement of sustained viral response at 12 weeks after treatment (SVR12). All the recommended regimens for chronic HCV have >90% SVR12 rates.
- Quantitative HCV RNA should be obtained at 4 weeks and at 12 weeks after therapy (SVR12).
- **All patients with HIV** should be screened for HCV, and treatment of HCV is usually recommended after suppressing HIV with antiretrovirals. The treatment of the HIV/ HCV coinfected patient is similar to HCV-monoinfected patient, but **drug–drug interactions** should be in mind while selecting the appropriate treatment.

CHRONIC HEPATITIS D

- Chronic HDV occurs only in the presence of chronic HBV.
- Diagnosis is made by persistence of HDV antigen in the liver or anti-HDV titers.
- The incidence of chronicity is <5% in coinfection but >50% in superinfection.
- IFN-α has limited efficacy, and the oral agents used for HBV are not effective for hepatitis D.

TABLE 6-6	LIST OF DIRECT-ACTING ANTIVIRALS FOR CHRONIC HCV INFECTION			
Treatment	HCV Genotype (GT)	Use in Noncirrhotic	Use in Compensated Cirrhosis	Use in Renal/Liver Disease
Elbasvir-Grazoprevir	1, 4	Test GT1a pts for NS5a resistance If with no resistance, once daily × 12 wk. If with resistance, give for 16 wk with RBV.	Yes	Avoid in Child-Turcotte-Pugh (CTP) class B or C
Glecaprevir-Pibrentasvir	1, 2, 3, 4, 5, 6	1 tab once daily × 8 wk	Yes, but given for 12 wk	Avoid in CTP class B or C
Ledipasvir-Sofosbuvir	1, 4, 5, 6	1 tab once daily × 12 wk 8-wk regimen may be given to tx-naïve, non-Black, noncirrhotics with HCV VL <6 M	Yes	Avoid CrCl <30
Sofosbuvir-Velpatasvir	1, 2, 3, 4, 5, 6	1 tab once daily × 12 wk	Yes	Avoid CrCl <30

(Continued)

| TABLE 6-6 | \| LIST OF DIRECT-ACTING ANTIVIRALS FOR CHRONIC HCV INFECTION (CONTINUED) |

Treatment	HCV Genotype (GT)	Use in Noncirrhotic	Use in Compensated Cirrhosis	Use in Renal/Liver Disease
(Ombitasvir-Paritaprevir-Ritonavir)	1, 4	For GT1a: given daily as extended release with Dasabuvir, plus weight-based Ribavirin (RBV) × 12 wk For GT1b: given daily as extended release with Dasabuvir × 12 wk For GT4: given with weight-based RBV × 12 wk	Alternative; given for 24 wk; there is risk for severe liver injury	Avoid in CTP class B or C
(Simeprevir) and (Sofosbuvir)	1	1 tab each once daily × 12 wk	Alternative; given for 24 wk; use only if no Q80k polymorphism.	Avoid in CTP class B or C
(Daclatasvir) and (Sofosbuvir)	1, 2, 3	1 tab each once daily × 12 wk Not approved in the US	Alternative only in GT2, and is given for 24 wk. Also an alternative in GT3, but given with or without RBV for 24 wk	Avoid CrCl <30

Other Hepatic Infections

Pyogenic Liver Abscess

GENERAL PRINCIPLES

- Pyogenic liver abscesses are the most common type of visceral abscess. The right lobe is most commonly involved.
- Liver abscesses result from the following:
  - Direct spread from biliary infection. Underlying biliary tract disease such as gallstones or malignant obstruction is present in about 40% to 60% of cases. Enteric gram-negative bacilli and *Enterococci* are predominant, and anaerobes are not generally involved.

- Spread from the portal circulation, usually related to bowel leakage and peritonitis. Mixed flora with aerobic and anaerobic species are often isolated.
- Hematogenous seeding, usually due to single organism such as *S. aureus* or *Streptococcus* species.
- *Klebsiella pneumoniae* is an important cause of primary liver abscess in Asia and is associated with metastatic infections, such as endophthalmitis, meningitis, and brain abscess.

DIAGNOSIS

Clinical Manifestations

- Fevers and chills along with right upper quadrant pain and possibly pleuritic symptoms (depending on the location of abscess) are usual presentations. Fatigue, malaise, and weight loss are common.
- Onset can be insidious; liver abscess was a common cause of fever of unknown origin before CT scanning.
- Over half of the patients have tender hepatomegaly.
- Jaundice is not present unless there is ascending cholangitis or extensive involvement with multiple hepatic abscesses.

Diagnostic Testing

- Elevated alkaline phosphatase, mild elevations in the transaminase levels, and leukocytosis are seen.
- Blood cultures are positive in about half of the patients.
- Cultures from liver abscesses are diagnostic.
- Ultrasound and CT are the imaging methods of choice.

TREATMENT

- Drainage of the abscess is important and may need to be repeated several times, particularly if there are multiple lesions.
  - Drainage can usually be carried out percutaneously.
  - Surgical drainage is needed for loculated abscesses, underlying disease requiring primary surgical management, and inadequate response to percutaneous drainage after 7 days of treatment.
- Patients should receive broad-spectrum antibiotics.
  - β-Lactam/β-lactamase inhibitor or third-generation cephalosporin and metronidazole are recommended.
  - Fluoroquinolone plus metronidazole or a carbapenem can also be used.
  - Duration of treatment is 4 to 6 weeks. Intravenous antibiotics can be switched to oral therapy (amoxicillin–clavulanate or fluoroquinolone plus metronidazole) after 2 to 4 weeks if the patient has a good response to drainage.
- Follow-up imaging is necessary only with prolonged clinical symptoms or when drainage is not making good progress. Radiologic abnormalities resolve much more slowly than clinical and biochemical markers—around 16 weeks for abscesses <10 cm, 22 weeks for abscesses >10 cm.

Amebic Liver Abscess

GENERAL PRINCIPLES

- Amebic liver abscesses are the most common extraintestinal manifestation of *E. histolytica*.
- Organisms ascend the portal venous system and establish infection.

- Amebic liver abscess occurs mainly in the developing world. Most cases in the United States are among travelers.
- Amebic liver abscesses typically occur within weeks after returning from an endemic area but can also occur years later.

DIAGNOSIS

Clinical Manifestations

- Clinical differentiation between amebic and pyogenic liver abscess is difficult.
- Patients with amebic abscess may have a history of diarrhea and may lack spiking fevers.
- Frequently, amebic abscesses are solitary and occur in the right lobe of the liver.

Diagnostic Testing

- The workup is the same as with pyogenic abscess; gallium scans do not show increased uptake.
- A definitive diagnosis is made by finding invasive trophozoites on microscopic examination from tissue or pus obtained from the abscess or culture, but the yield is low (about 20%–30%).
- Serologic testing for antibodies to *E. histolytica* is sensitive. A negative test rules out the diagnosis except in early infection (<1 wk).
- Percutaneous aspiration is not recommended except in cases where immediate exclusion of a pyogenic abscess is warranted. Typical amebic pus is described as anchovy paste and is thick, acellular, proteinaceous debris consisting of necrotic hepatocytes and a few leukocytes.

TREATMENT

- Treatment consists of metronidazole 500 to 750 mg PO q8h for 7 to 10 days or tinidazole 2 g daily for 5 days followed by the luminal agents paromomycin 10 mg/kg PO q8h for 10 days, or diiodohydroxyquin (iodoquinol) 650 mg PO q8h for 20 days.
- In contrast to pyogenic liver abscesses, drainage of amebic liver abscesses is not usually necessary. Aspiration is usually reserved for patients with extremely large abscesses to decrease the risk of rupture or no response to antibiotics after 3 to 5 days.
- Complete radiologic resolution may take up to 2 years and repeated imaging is not helpful.

REFERENCES

1. Kolokotronis A, Doumas S. Herpes simplex virus infection, with particular reference to the progression and complications of primary herpetic gingivostomatitis. *Clin Microbiol Infect.* 2006;12(3):202-211.
2. Wang H-W, Kuo C-J, Lin W-R, et al. Clinical characteristics and manifestation of herpes esophagitis. *Medicine (Baltimore).* 2016;95(14):e3187.
3. Baroco AL, Oldfield EC. Gastrointestinal cytomegalovirus disease in the immunocompromised patient. *Curr Gastroenterol Rep.* 2008;10(4):409-416. http://www.ncbi.nlm.nih.gov/pubmed/18627655. Accessed October 2, 2017.
4. Chey WD, Leontiadis GI, Howden CW, Moss SF. ACG clinical guideline: treatment of Helicobacter pylori infection. *Am J Gastroenterol.* 2017;112(2):212-239.
5. Riddle MS, DuPont HL, Connor BA. ACG clinical guideline: diagnosis, treatment, and prevention of acute diarrheal infections in adults. *Am J Gastroenterol.* 2016;111(5):602-622.
6. Lopman BA, Steele D, Kirkwood CD, Parashar UD. The vast and varied global burden of norovirus: prospects for prevention and control. *PLoS Med.* 2016;13(4):e1001999.

7. American Medical Association, American Nurses Association-American Nurses Foundation, Centers for Disease Control and Prevention, et al. Diagnosis and management of foodborne illnesses: a primer for physicians and other health care professionals. *MMWR Recomm Rep.* 2004;53(RR-4):1-33. http://www.ncbi.nlm.nih.gov/pubmed/15123984. Accessed October 2, 2017.

8. Judd M, Mintz E. Typhoid and paratyphoid fever. In: CDC Yellow Book. 2018. Retrieved from URL: https://wwwnc.cdc.gov/travel/yellowbook/2018/infectious-diseases-related-to-travel/typhoid-paratyphoid-fever.

9. McDonald LC, Gerding DN, Johnson S, et al. Clinical practice guidelines for Clostridium difficile infection in adults and children: 2017 update by the Infectious Diseases Society of America (IDSA) and Society for Healthcare Epidemiology of America (SHEA). *Clin Infect Dis.* 2018;66(7):987-994.

10. Runyon BA, AASLD Practice Guidelines Committee. Management of adult patients with ascites due to cirrhosis: an update. *Hepatology.* 2009;49(6):2087-2107.

11. Li PK, Szeto CC, Piraino B, et al. ISPD peritonitis recommendations: 2016 update on prevention and treatment. *Perit Dial Int.* 2016;36(5):481-508. doi:10.3747/pdi.2016.00078.

12. Mori Y, Itoi T, Baron TH, et al. TG18 management strategies for gallbladder drainage in patients with acute cholecystitis: updated Tokyo guidelines 2018 (with videos). *J Hepatobiliary Pancreat Sci.* 2018;25(1):87-95. doi:10.1002/jhbp.504.

13. Miura F, Okamoto K, Takada T, et al. Tokyo guidelines 2018: initial management of acute biliary infection and flowchart for acute cholangitis. *J Hepatobiliary Pancreat Sci.* 2018;25(1):31-40.

14. Terrault NA, Bzowej NH, Chang K-M, et al. AASLD guidelines for treatment of chronic hepatitis B. *Hepatology.* 2016;63(1):261-283.

15. AASLD/IDSA HCV Guidance Panel. Hepatitis C guidance: AASLD-IDSA recommendations for testing, managing, and treating adults infected with hepatitis C virus. *Hepatology.* 2015;62(3):932-954.

Urinary Tract Infections

Juan J. Calix and Jeffrey P. Henderson

7

GENERAL PRINCIPLES

- Approximately 40% to 50% of women and 5% of men will be diagnosed with a urinary tract infection (UTI) during their lifetimes, with an annual self-reported incidence of about 12% in women and 3% in men in the United States.[1-4]
- The high incidence of UTIs results in significant morbidity across populations and a heavy burden on the health care system.
- An emerging challenge in UTI management is the alarming increase in incidence of multidrug-resistant (MDR) UTIs. MDR infections have been repeatedly linked to inappropriate antimicrobial use.
- One of the leading causes of inappropriate antimicrobial use is antibiotic treatment of asymptomatic bacteriuria (ASB; see below). **Medical care providers must place special emphasis on distinguishing UTIs from asymptomatic bacteriuria, as the latter does NOT merit antimicrobial treatment in most cases.**
- A UTI is considered **complicated if it is associated with an underlying condition that predisposes to antimicrobial failure, e.g., pregnancy, uncontrolled diabetes, anatomic abnormalities, presence of urinary catheter, immunocompromising conditions, hospital-associated infection, etc.** In the absence of these factors, a UTI is considered uncomplicated
  - Although many UTIs can be diagnosed by clinical presentation alone, urinalysis (UA) and urine culture are mainstays of UTI diagnosis, management, and monitoring.
  - Ideally, urinalyses should be performed on midstream, clean-catch urine samples and promptly refrigerated or plated for culture within 2 hours of collection.
  - Urine dipstick testing for nitrites or leukocyte esterase is a readily available and an inexpensive screening method for UTIs. The sensitivity of a positive nitrite or leukocyte esterase on urine dipstick is ~75%; therefore, negative results should not preclude treatment in symptomatic patients.[2]
  - UTI diagnosis can also be made by microscopic examination or urine. This method is less sensitive, but more specific than dipstick testing. Either pyuria (>8 leukocytes/ high-power field [HPF]) or bacteriuria (>1 organism per oil-immersion field) is suggestive of UTI.
  - **A high number of epithelial cells per HPF on microscopic examination likely indicates collection of an inadequate urine sample.** Culture, dipstick, and microscopic results obtained from these samples can be misleading, and a UTI diagnosis should not rely solely on an inadequate urine sample. Repeat analysis of a fresh urine collection should be considered.

Asymptomatic Bacteriuria

GENERAL PRINCIPLES

Definition

ASB is defined as the presence of colonizing bacteria in the urine culture of patients WITHOUT other signs or symptoms of infection and/or without pyuria detected on UA.

Etiology

- Uropathogenic bacteria are often associated with ASB.
- In women, *Escherichia coli* is the most common cause of ASB.
- Men have a lower incidence of ASB but often harbor other gram negatives, enterococci, and coagulase-negative staphylococci.
- Stents, urinary catheters, and other indwelling devices can be colonized by multiple organisms, including urease-producing organisms and *Pseudomonas.*

Risk Factors

- ASB prevalence increases with age and is associated with sexual activity.
- Prevalence is 6% among sexually active nonpregnant young women.[2]
- It is uncommon in young men, but frequency increases with age and the onset of prostatic hypertrophy.
- A history of voiding dysfunction, diabetes, hemodialysis, immunosuppression, and the presence of an indwelling urinary catheter are independent risk factors for developing ASB.

DIAGNOSIS

- In women without UTI symptoms (see below), ASB is diagnosed with the isolation of ≥10^5 colony forming units (cfu)/mL of the same bacterial strain in two consecutive clean-voided urine samples. In asymptomatic men, a single clean-catch specimen with ≥10^5 cfu/mL of a single bacterial species is sufficient for diagnosis. If straight catheterization is used to obtain a specimen, bacteriuria can be diagnosed if ≥10^2 cfu/mL of a single bacterial species is isolated.[5]
- **Screening for ASB is only indicated for select populations:**
  ○ **Pregnant women** should be screened between 12 and 16 weeks gestation for ASB because of an increased risk of pyelonephritis, premature labor, and an association with lower infant birth weights. **Screening for pyuria is not sufficient, and a urine culture is always indicated.** Rescreening later in pregnancy should be considered for individual cases, such as women with urinary tract anomalies, sickle cell syndromes, or a history of preterm labor. Women treated for bacteriuria should be retested periodically throughout pregnancy.
  ○ **Patients undergoing any urologic procedures that are expected to cause mucosal bleeding, including transurethral resection of the prostate, should be screened for bacteriuria.** If present, treatment should be started shortly before the procedure. Antibiotics do not need to be continued afterward unless an indwelling catheter is continued postoperatively.
- **Screening should NOT be performed in the absence of signs or symptoms of infection in the following populations:** healthy men, nonpregnant women, diabetic patients, elderly patients, patients with a history of spinal cord injury, or patients with indwelling urinary catheters.

TREATMENT

- **Pregnant women with a positive ASB screen should be treated**, but the optimum length of treatment has not been established. A 5- to 7-day course of nitrofurantoin is considered first-line therapy (see Table 7-1).[4-9] Trimethoprim, a folic acid antagonist, should be avoided, especially early in pregnancy. Fluoroquinolones should also be avoided.

TABLE 7-1	EMPIRIC THERAPY FOR URINARY TRACT INFECTIONS	
Disease	**Empiric Therapy (Follow Culture Susceptibility When Available)**	**Notes**
Simple cystitis[6]	*First line:* Nitrofurantoin sustained release 100 mg PO twice daily × 5 d OR TMP-SMX DS mg PO twice daily × 3 d OR TMP (if sulfa allergic) 100 mg PO twice daily × 3 d *Alternate:* Fosfomycin 3 g PO × 1 d OR pivmecillinam 400 mg PO twice daily × 5 d (not available in the United States) *Second line:* Ciprofloxacin 250 mg PO twice daily × 3 d OR levofloxacin 250 mg PO twice daily × 3 d	Avoid TMP-SMX if local resistance is >20% or if used within the prior 3 mo. Consider alternatives to TMP/SMX in older women. Avoid FQs if local resistance is >10% Most non-*Escherichia coli*, non-*Citrobacter* Gram-negative bacteria, e.g., *Klebsiella, Proteus, Pseudomonas*, etc., are nitrofurantoin resistant
Cystitis in men[7]	*Initial episode:* TMP-SMX for at least 7 d *Recurrent episode:* ciprofloxacin 500 mg PO twice daily OR levofloxacin 500 mg PO qday for x10–21 d.	Consider urologic referral for recurrent disease or pyelonephritis
Recurrent cystitis in women[4]	*Postcoital prophylaxis:* TMP-SMX SS × 1 dose OR nitrofurantoin 100 mg × 1 dose OR cephalexin 250 mg × 1 dose. *Continuous prophylaxis:* TMP-SMX SS qday OR every other day OR nitrofurantoin 50 mg qday OR cephalexin 125 mg qday OR fosfomycin 3 g every 10 d	Cranberry juice and topical vaginal estrogen in postmenopausal women *may* have a role in preventing recurrent UTI.
Pregnancy[8]	Nitrofurantoin 100 mg PO four times a day × 7 d OR cephalexin 200–500 mg PO four times a day × 7 d OR cefuroxime axetil 250 mg PO four times a day × 7 d	Treat all asymptomatic bacteriuria in pregnancy. Screen pregnant women near the end of the first trimester with urine culture[5]

(Continued)

TABLE 7-1	EMPIRIC THERAPY FOR URINARY TRACT INFECTIONS (CONTINUED)	
Disease	**Empiric Therapy (Follow Culture Susceptibility When Available)**	**Notes**
Complicated UTI,[7] i.e., presence of underlying condition that predisposes to antimicrobial failure (see text)	*Mild–moderate disease:* second-generation FQ.[a] *Severe disease, recent FQ, or institutionalized:* cefepime 2 g IV q12h *OR* third-generation cephalosporin[b] OR carbapenem[c] OR piperacillin–tazobactam 3.375–4.5 g IV q6h. Consider adding vancomycin empirically if gram-positive cocci are seen on urine Gram stain	Base empiric coverage on local sensitivity patterns and narrow therapy according to culture results. Typically treat for 10–14 d, but consider shortening course if underlying condition is resolved (e.g., removal of indwelling device or stone, etc.)
Candiduria[9]	*Candida albicans:* Fluconazole 100–200 mg PO qd × 5 d. *Critically ill or non-albicans species:* amphotericin B.	Remove catheter if present. Indications to treat: symptoms with pyuria, hardware, pregnancy, before GU surgery, or risk of dissemination
Pyelonephritis[6]	*Outpatient:* (consider only in patients with uncomplicated UTI who can tolerate oral medications) Ciprofloxacin 500 mg PO twice daily × 7 d *OR* ciprofloxacin ER 1000 mg PO qd × 7 d *OR* levofloxacin 750 mg PO daily × 5 d *Inpatient:* second-generation IV FQ[a] OR aminoglycoside[d] OR ampicillin–sulbactam 1–2 g IV q6h *OR* third-generation cephalosporin.[b] *Pregnancy:* Cefazolin 1 g IV q8h *OR* ceftriaxone 1 g IV *OR* IM q24h *OR* piperacillin 4 g IV q8h	If susceptibility is confirmed, can use TMP-SMX DS PO twice daily × 14 d for outpatient therapy Consider ceftriaxone 1000 mg × 1 dose OR a single 24-h dose of an aminoglycoside, followed by outpatient oral therapy, especially if local FQ resistance >10% or if TMP-SMX is used empirically. Use IV antibiotics until the patient is afebrile × 48 h, then change to PO to complete 14 d. Avoid FQs during pregnancy. Do not use nitrofurantoin or fosfomycin.

[a]Oral: ciprofloxacin 500 mg PO twice daily; ofloxacin 200 mg PO twice daily; levofloxacin 500 mg PO qd; norfloxacin 400 mg PO twice daily. Parenteral: levofloxacin 500 mg IV qd; ciprofloxacin 400 mg IV q12h.
[b]Cefotaxime 1 or 2 g IV q8h; ceftriaxone 1 g IV qd; ceftazidime 1–2 g IV q8–12h.
[c]Imipenem 500 mg IV q6h; meropenem 1 g IV q8h.
[d]Gentamicin or tobramycin 2 mg/kg loading dose IV, then 1.5–3 mg/kg/d or divided dose.
FQ, fluoroquinolone; GU, genitourinary; TMP-SMX, trimethoprim–sulfamethoxazole.

- **Treatment is NOT recommended in the following groups:**
  - ○ ASB in **premenopausal, nonpregnant women** is associated with an increased risk of symptomatic UTI, but is NOT associated with long-term adverse outcomes. Although antibiotics may lead to bacterial clearance, treatment does not decrease the frequency of symptomatic UTI and may paradoxically increase the incidence of a recurrent UTI[10]; therefore, treatment is not recommended.
  - ○ There is no benefit of treating ASB in **elderly patients** in nursing homes or in the community. In fact, inappropriate use of antibiotics in nursing home patients, of which the majority is prescribed for suspected UTIs, has been linked to adverse outcomes in residents receiving antibiotics and in their untreated coresidents.[11]
  - ○ **Patients with diabetes** are routinely screened for proteinuria, and ASB is often an incidental finding. Although diabetic patients are at a higher risk of acute cystitis and complications from UTIs, treatment does not change the frequency of these events or improve renal function outcomes. Recolonization is common after therapy is stopped.
  - ○ **Patients with spinal cord injury or chronic indwelling catheters** experience a high rate of asymptomatic bacterial colonization, though little evidence supports antibiotic treatment of ASB in this population. Further, these patients are at high risk of developing resistant organisms with repeated courses of unnecessary antibiotics.

Uncomplicated Cystitis in Women

GENERAL PRINCIPLES

- Uncomplicated bacterial cystitis is one of the most common causes of physician office visits and antibiotic use in women.
- Most episodes of cystitis are uncomplicated and self-limited; however, some cases can be complicated by pyelonephritis and bacteremia.

Epidemiology

The estimated incidence of uncomplicated UTI in the United States depends greatly on the population studied. For college-age women, it is estimated to be 0.7 episodes per person-year[4]; 25% to 50% of women have recurrent infection within 1 year of the initial infection.[2]

Etiology

- Most uncomplicated UTIs originate when vaginal and bowel flora ascend the urethra. Emerging research suggests some uropathogens may be able to persist within bladder tissue and can cause chronic or recurrent cystitis.[12]
- 75% to 95% of uncomplicated cystitis cases are caused by *E. coli*.[3,4] Less commonly, cystitis is associated with *Staphylococcus saprophyticus*, *Enterococcus*, *Klebsiella pneumoniae*, *Proteus mirabilis*, or *Pseudomonas*.
- Typical uropathogens, especially uropathogenic *E. coli*, have acquired specialized virulence factors that enable them to adhere to host tissue, survive and acquire nutrients in urinary environments, and evade host defenses.
- Atypical pathogens for UTI, such as tuberculosis, candida and non-*saprophyticus* staphylococci (including MRSA), typically spread hematogenously to the urinary tract. UTIs originating from hematogenous or lymphatic spread of infection are much less frequent.

Risk Factors

- Prior UTI history
- Recent or frequent vaginal intercourse
- Spermicide use, especially when used with a diaphragm
- A childhood or maternal UTI history is associated with recurrent UTI

DIAGNOSIS

- Uncomplicated UTI is often clinically diagnosed, based on the classic symptoms of dysuria, increased urinary frequency, urinary urgency, malodorous urine, suprapubic pain, and occasionally hematuria.
- For low-risk women with recurrent UTIs and the cluster of classic symptoms, an office visit is not necessary for the diagnosis and treatment of uncomplicated cystitis.
- UA is not essential for diagnosis of uncomplicated UTI when typical symptoms are present.
- A patient with dipstick-positive pyuria in the setting of the recent onset of typical symptoms does not need a urine culture and may be treated empirically. The absence of pyuria should prompt a search for alternative causes of clinical signs and symptoms.
- Women with concurrent vaginal discharge or irritation should be evaluated for causes of vaginitis and cervicitis. Sexually active women with dysuria in the absence of pyuria should be evaluated for sexually transmitted infections (STIs; see Chapter 11).
- Urine microscopic analysis and culture are warranted in women who have had symptoms for >7 days, persistent symptoms despite empiric antibiotics, or recurrent symptoms within a month of treatment. Using a threshold of $>10^2$ bacteria/mL of urine increases the sensitivity of testing in symptomatic patients, with little effect on specificity.
- Patients with fever, complicating predisposing factors or signs/symptoms of upper urinary tract involvement, should be evaluated for complicated forms of UTI (see below).
- Patients with symptoms that are not responsive to typical short-course antibiotic therapy and whose urine samples repeatedly show the absence of bacteriuria may be evaluated for interstitial cystitis or the painful bladder syndrome spectrum of disease.

TREATMENT

- Current guidelines recommend a **5-day course of nitrofurantoin**, a 3-day course of trimethoprim–sulfamethoxazole (TMP-SMX) or trimethoprim alone, or a single dose of fosfomycin as empiric treatments for uncomplicated cystitis, as long as local resistance rates to these antibiotics ≤20% among uncomplicated cystitis uropathogens.[6] Longer courses of antibiotics have not been shown to increase bacterial clearance, though recurrence rates may be lower.
- **Fluoroquinolones should not be used as first-line treatment for uncomplicated UTIs** because of increasing resistance rates to these important broad-spectrum agents. They should only be used if first-line medications are unavailable or if there is a patient history of drug intolerance.
- Other than pivmecillinam (which is not available in the United States), β-lactams are generally inferior to the UTI antibiotics listed above and should be considered second-line agents.
- Empiric coverage for MRSA is not recommended.
- Even in the setting of high incidence of TMP-SMX resistance among local uropathogens, cure rates using trimethoprim exceed 85%.[4]
- Phenazopyridine, a urinary analgesic, may be used for 1 to 2 days to relieve dysuria. Providers should be aware of the relative and absolute contraindications of this medication (renal insufficiency, liver disease, glucose-6-phosphate dehydrogenase deficiency).
- Refer to Table 7-1 for further details.[4-9]
- If symptoms do not improve within 48 hours of initiating antibiotics, clinical evaluation and urine culture should be performed. **Otherwise, posttreatment urine cultures are not a part of routine UTI treatment and should not be obtained.**
- Patients with persistent symptoms after 48 to 72 hours of appropriate antibiotics (per culture susceptibilities) or with multiple recurrent incidences of UTI should be considered for evaluation for nephrolithiasis or anatomical abnormalities, with CT or ultrasound imaging or possible referral for cystoscopy or urodynamic tests.

PREVENTION

- As diaphragm use and spermicide use are strongly associated with UTIs, patients with recurrent UTIs may benefit from alternative forms of contraception.
- A Cochrane review of 24 studies concluded that the use of cranberry products had no statistically significant effect on preventing UTIs, compared with placebo or no treatment.[13] Notably, cranberry extract may interact with other medications, including warfarin.
- Pre- or postcoital micturition, "front-to-back" wiping patterns, and the avoidance of douching have not been proven to prevent UTIs, but are commonly recommended, low-risk interventions.
- Antibiotic prophylaxis with daily low-dose TMP-SMX or nitrofurantoin may be considered in women with three or more UTIs per year, i.e., recurrent cystitis. Postcoital antibiotics are another option for patients with recurrent UTIs related to sexual activity.[4] Refer to Table 7-1 for more detail.[4-9]

Pyelonephritis

GENERAL PRINCIPLES

Pyelonephritis is the infection and inflammation of the kidney, typically secondary to an ascending urinary infection. Classically, patients with pyelonephritis present with flank pain, fever/chills, and nausea/vomiting, often in the presence of cystitis symptoms and bacteriuria. Health care providers should have a high index of suspicion in patients presenting with these red-flag symptoms, as pyelonephritis can be an organ- and life-threatening infection.

DIAGNOSIS

- Examination findings include unilateral or bilateral costovertebral tenderness.
- UA testing usually reveals significant pyuria, hematuria, and bacteriuria. Observation of leukocyte casts is of questionable value in discriminating pyelonephritis from cystitis.
- Urine cultures should be collected from all patients with signs and symptoms suggestive of pyelonephritis, preferably before starting antibiotics.
- Hospitalized patients should also have blood cultures drawn; bacteremia is detected in 15% to 20% of hospitalized patients with pyelonephritis.
- Although CT studies with contrast may reveal evidence of renal inflammation associated with pyelonephritis, imaging is not recommended as part of routine management. CT or ultrasound studies may be indicated in select patients, however (see below).

TREATMENT

- **Urine sample should be obtained for culture before initiating any antimicrobial therapy.** Initiate empiric antibiotic treatment and consider modifying based on culture results.
- Outpatient therapy can be considered in select patients with uncomplicated acute pyelonephritis and who can tolerate oral medications.
- If local prevalence of fluoroquinolone resistance is <10%, it is reasonable to consider a 7-day course of oral ciprofloxacin (500 mg twice daily, or 1000 mg extended release daily) or a 5-day course of levofloxacin (750 mg daily).
- If local prevalence of fluoroquinolone resistance is >10%, an initial one-time IV dose of 1 g ceftriaxone or a 24-hour consolidated dose of an aminoglycoside is recommended while awaiting culture and susceptibility information.

- If the causative organism is susceptible, 14 days of TMP-SMX 1 double strength tablet twice daily can be used.[6]
- Patients requiring hospitalization can be treated with an intravenous fluoroquinolone, a third- or fourth-generation cephalosporin (and/or an aminoglycoside), an aminoglycoside (and/or ampicillin), an extended-spectrum penicillin (and/or an aminoglycoside), or a carbapenem. These patients should be transitioned to an oral regimen once stable. Adjust antibiotics per culture results.
- Patients who do not respond to treatment within 48 hours should be evaluated for obstruction, intrarenal or perinephric abscesses, and renal calculi by ultrasonography or CT scan.

Urinary Tract Infections in Men

GENERAL PRINCIPLES

- UTIs and ASB are less common in men than women.
- Cystitis in men can be uncomplicated. However, **recurrent UTIs should prompt evaluation for anatomic abnormalities.** Conversely, >50% of recurrent UTIs in men are caused by **prostatitis.**

Etiology

- More than 50% of UTIs in men are caused by *E. coli.*
- Other pathogens include *Klebsiella, Proteus, Providencia, Pseudomonas,* enterococci, and other gram-negative enterics.

Risk Factors

- Sexual intercourse with a partner colonized with uropathogens[14]
- Insertive anal sex without using a condom
- Lack of circumcision
- Prostatic hypertrophy contributes to a higher incidence of UTI in older men

DIAGNOSIS

- As in women, UTIs in men present with dysuria, increased urinary frequency, urgency, and suprapubic pain. Symptoms are often subtle in elderly men. Sexually active men should also be evaluated for STIs.
- Other causes of dysuria in men include urethritis, prostatitis, and epididymitis.

TREATMENT

- See Table 7-1 for summary of treatments.
- **All men presenting with urinary symptoms should be evaluated with a pretreatment UA and midstream urine culture.**
- On initial presentation for UTI, otherwise healthy, young men can be treated empirically with TMP-SMX for 7 days, with adjustments according to culture data.
- Men with recurrent UTIs or anatomic abnormalities should be treated empirically with a urinary fluoroquinolone. Based on susceptibility testing, continue treatment with a quinolone or TMP-SMX for 10 to 21 days.
- Prophylactic antibiotic use has not been well-studied in men.
- Further evaluation with imaging and/or urologic referral should be considered for male patients with recurrent UTI associated with upper urinary tract symptoms (e.g., fever, flank pain) or with symptoms that do not respond within 48 hours of starting antibiotics.

Acute Bacterial Prostatitis

GENERAL PRINCIPLES

- Acute bacterial prostatitis (ABP) usually presents with urinary symptoms; fever; chills; pelvic, perineal, or rectal pain; and obstructive symptoms (dribbling, hesitancy). Patients may also present with sepsis without associated urinary symptoms.
- ABP is most often caused by *E. coli* or other gram-negative enterics.[15]
- Complications include urinary retention and prostatic abscess.

Epidemiology

- ABP accounts for 5% of total prostatitis cases.
- Most patients are <65 years old and have a history of recent urinary tract manipulation.

Pathophysiology

- Bacteria associated with prostatitis are typically also found among the intestinal flora.
- Bacteria may reach the prostate following urethral ascension by urinary reflux through the prostatic ducts.
- Bacteria may also reach the prostate through direct inoculation (following instrumentation) or bacteremic seeding.

Risk Factors

- Indwelling catheters, urinary instrumentation, and receptive anal intercourse.
- Patients with HIV or diabetes are at a higher risk of developing prostatic abscesses.

DIAGNOSIS

- Male patients with UTIs potentially have prostatic involvement, but diagnosis of ABP can be challenging.
- Diagnosis is usually based on the presence of systemic symptoms of infection (e.g., fever, chills, etc.), bacteriuria and pyuria on urine dipstick, and presence of prostate tenderness on rectal examination. Warmth and swelling may also be noted.
- Prostatic massage is contraindicated in patient with suspected ABP, as the maneuver may lead to translocation of bacteria into the bloodstream.
- UA of midstream urine should reveal pyuria and bacteriuria. **Consider alternative diagnoses if UA is negative.**
- Blood leukocytosis is common.
- Prostate-specific antigen levels can be markedly elevated for up to a month following an episode of ABP.

TREATMENT

- Refer to Table 7-2 for recommended antibiotic regimens.[7,16]
- Pretreatment urine and blood cultures should also be drawn whenever possible.
- Prostate inflammation facilitates tissue penetration by antibiotics.
- If bladder outlet obstruction develops, patients may require catheterization.
- Pain control, hydration, and a promotility bowel regimen are recommended adjunctive therapies.
- Ultrasound or pelvic CT should be obtained only if prostatic abscess is suspected, such as in cases where there is incomplete response to culture-directed or broad-spectrum antibiotics.
- ABP with prostatic abscess should be evaluated by surgical service for drainage.

TABLE 7-2	DIAGNOSIS AND TREATMENT OF PROSTATITIS BY NATIONAL INSTITUTES OF HEALTH CLASSIFICATION		
Disease	**Diagnosis**	**Treatment**	**Alternative Treatments**
Acute Bacterial Prostatitis[7]	1. Presents typical signs or symptoms (see text) 2. UA/UCx with bacteriuria, pyuria 3. Prostate tenderness, warmth, and/or swelling on examination 4. +/− leukocytosis	*Outpatient:* TMP-SMX 1 tab PO twice daily × 6 wk *OR* ciprofloxacin 500 mg PO q12h × 6 wk *Inpatient:* Ampicillin 2 g IV q6h *PLUS* gentamicin 5 mg/kg q8h until afebrile, then switch to PO therapy	If no improvement on susceptibility-guided abx, consider pelvic CT or u/s to evaluate for abscess
Chronic Bacterial Prostatitis (CBP)[16]	1. Recurrent or persistent urinary signs and symptoms for >3 mo 2. Treat any acute UTI 3. Perform Mears–Stamey test, i.e., obtain urine and prostatic fluid cultures 4. If prostate fluid culture (+), then CBP	**Obtain culture results before starting abx** Ciprofloxacin 500 mg PO twice daily × 4 wk *OR* levofloxacin 500 mg PO qday × 4 wk *OR* norfloxacin 400 mg PO twice daily × 4 wk *OR* TMP-SMX 1 tab PO twice daily × 4 wk	Doxycycline 100 mg PO twice daily × 4 wk Patient should be evaluated for anatomical/neurologic abnormalities and for malignancies.
Chronic prostatitis/ chronic pelvic pain syndrome[7]	Same as CBP, but no bacterial etiology is identified on repeated cultures	**Urology referral is often necessary** Reassurance, stress management, analgesics.	α-blockers (alfuzosin, terazosin), 5α-reductase inhibitors (finasteride) 4-wk trial of an FQ may be considered
Asymptomatic prostatitis	Incidentally discovered inflammation on prostate biopsy or semen analysis	Refer for urologic evaluation	

abx, antibiotics; FQ, fluoroquinolone; TMP-SMX, trimethoprim–sulfamethoxazole; UA, urinalysis; UCx, urine culture; UTI, urinary tract infection.

Chronic Bacterial Prostatitis

GENERAL PRINCIPLES

- Chronic prostatitis (CP), defined as chronic or recurrent urinary symptoms for over 3 months, is a common problem, affecting approximately 8% of men and accounts for approximately 2 million outpatient visits annually in the United States.[16]
- Almost all cases of CP are associated with urinary inflammation, but many cases are noninfectious. CP/chronic pelvic pain syndrome (CP/CPPS) is a spectrum of disease diagnosed with the presence of inflammatory urinary symptoms, but the absence of a clear bacterial cause. **The role of antibiotics in treatment of CP/CPPS remains unclear.**
- Chronic bacterial prostatitis (CBP) is defined as presence of inflammatory urinary symptoms for over 3 months, with a clear bacterial cause identified on UA or culture.
- CBP may result from acute prostatitis, but it commonly occurs in men with no prior prostatitis history. It has a variable clinical course and is often difficult to cure.
- If a male patient has recurrent UTIs with no anatomic abnormalities or long-term urinary catheterization, CBP is the most likely underlying cause.

Etiology

- As with ABP, *E. coli* is also the most common etiologic agent in CBP. Other associated organisms include enterococci, *Ureaplasma*, fungi, and tuberculosis.
- Patients with HIV are at risk of CP from atypical organisms.

Risk Factors

- Risk factors are largely shared with ABP.
- Older men are at higher risk of developing CP as a complication of prostatic hypertrophy and associated urinary stasis.
- Prostatic calculi can harbor colonizing bacteria and may be a source for chronic infection.

DIAGNOSIS

- Male patients with urinary symptoms lasting longer than 3 months should undergo evaluation for CP.
- UA and urine cultures should be obtained while the patient is symptomatic.
- Postvoid residual volumes should be measured if urinary obstruction is suspected.
- The prostate should be evaluated for symmetry and consistency. Irregularities should be further investigated for possible malignancy.
- Before further diagnostic evaluation, coexisting UTIs should be treated with nitrofurantoin or a β-lactam antibiotic, which does not penetrate prostate tissue.
- The Meares–Stamey test is the preferred method of diagnosing CBP.
  ○ Ideally, testing should be postponed until a month after all antibiotic use.
  ○ Ejaculation should be avoided within 2 days of the test.
  ○ For the 4-glass Meares–Stamey test, first-void urine, midstream urine, elicited prostatic fluid, and postmassage urine samples are collected and cultured.
  ○ A 2-glass method culturing midstream urine before massage and elicited prostatic fluid has been shown to correlate with the 4-glass method and is easier to perform.
  ○ If cultures are positive only in prostatic fluid, or if bacteria counts are more than 10 times higher in prostatic fluid compared with premassage urine, then CBP can be definitively diagnosed.
  ○ This is a complex method often requiring referral to urology or other dedicated service.

TREATMENT

- CBP treatment is challenging because many antibiotics poorly penetrate prostatic tissue. Thus, CBP requires at least 4 weeks of treatment based on susceptibility testing.[16]
- Patients should be reevaluated after treatment. If symptoms are still present or recur, then a further 3 months of therapy is warranted.
- Repeat urine and prostatic fluid cultures should be collected at 6 months.
- Refer to Table 7-2 for details.[7,16]

Epididymitis and Orchitis

GENERAL PRINCIPLES

- Epididymitis results from retrograde spread of pathogens in the urethra. Orchitis (infection of the testicle) is almost always an extension of epididymitis.
- Epididymitis and orchitis most commonly occur in young, sexually active men but can also be seen in older men with a recent history of urinary tract manipulation.
- **The most common etiologies in sexually active men are *Neisseria gonorrhoeae* and *Chlamydia trachomatis*. *E. coli* and other gram-negative enterics are the most common pathogens in men >35 years old and those with a history of urinary tract instrumentation.**
- Given widespread vaccination, mumps virus infection is a rare cause of orchitis. However, it should be suspected in patients with orchitis and other classical signs (e.g., concurrent parotitis).
- Potential complications include abscess formation, testicular infarction, testicular atrophy, and infertility.

DIAGNOSIS

- The most common presenting symptom is a dull unilateral ache in the scrotum, which may radiate to the flank. Concomitant urinary symptoms and/or urethral discharge may be present.
- On examination, the epididymis is typically swollen and very tender. Lifting the ipsilateral testicle may elicit extreme pain.
- UA, urine culture, and gonorrhea/chlamydia nucleic acid amplification testing (NAAT) should be obtained before starting treatment.
- In patients with active sexual history, other concomitant STI testing should be considered.
- If there is any suspicion of testicular torsion, a testicular ultrasound should be obtained emergently. Testicular neoplasm is usually not painful but should also be considered in the differential.

TREATMENT

- Sexually active men should be treated empirically for chlamydia and gonorrhea (see Chapter 11 and Table 7-2). Regardless, NAAT testing should be obtained before treatment, for tracking recurrent infections.
- If an enteric bacterial etiology is suspected, treat with levofloxacin 500 mg PO daily or ofloxacin (not available in the United States) 300 mg PO twice daily for 10 days.
- Bed rest, scrotal support, and analgesics may offer symptomatic relief.
- If abscess or infarction is suspected/diagnosed, the patient should be referred to urology for further evaluation.

Catheter-Associated Urinary Tract Infections

GENERAL PRINCIPLES

- Catheter-associated infections are the most common health care–associated infection, affecting 900,000 inpatients in the United States annually. However, they are often preventable.
- Up to 25% of inpatients have urethral catheters inserted during their hospital stay. Health care providers should be judicious about the use of indwelling urinary catheters and **avoid their use whenever possible.**
- The indication for an existing indwelling catheter should be regularly and frequently reviewed, and catheters should be removed as soon as they are no longer needed.
- As urinary stents carry many of the same risks as urinary catheters, stents should also be removed when no longer needed.

Definition

- Diagnosis of catheter-associated urinary tract infections (CA-UTIs) requires the presence of the following[17]:
  - The signs or symptoms of UTI
  - $\geq 10^3$ cfu/mL of a single uropathogen or ≥ 1 species of bacteria identified in cultures of urine collected from a suprapubic or urethral catheter or from a midstream collection if a catheter has been removed within the past 48 hours.
- In the absence of signs or symptoms of UTI, the patient is considered to have catheter-associated asymptomatic bacteriuria (CA-ASB).[17] **The vast majority of bacteriuria associated with catheters is CA-ASB.**

Epidemiology

- An estimated 20% to 30% of patients with CA-ASB eventually develop a CA-UTI.
- The urinary tract is the most common source of nosocomial gram-negative bacteremia; however, bacteremia only develops in 1% to 4% of bacteriuric patients.

Etiology

- *E. coli*, other gram-negative enterics, *Pseudomonas aeruginosa*, gram-positives (staphylococci, enterococci), and yeast are the organisms most commonly isolated from catheterized urine.
- Presence of a catheter facilitates the formation of biofilms by these organisms. In turn, biofilm formation promotes polymicrobial infections and increased antibiotic resistance.
- CA-UTI is associated with health care settings and biofilms; thus, **MDR organisms are of particular concern in these infections.**

Pathophysiology

- Infection can result from bacteria introduced into the urethra from nonsterile catheter insertion or uropathogen intra- or extraluminal migration upward across breaks in the closed catheter system.
- Catheterization also disrupts the uroepithelium, facilitating bacterial adhesion.
- Once attached to the catheter surface or uroepithelium, uropathogens produce extracellular polysaccharides that trap other bacteria, Tamm–Horsfall proteins, urinary salts, and other nutrients. These mature into biofilms where pathogens can resist host clearance and exchange genes promoting antibiotic resistance.
- Urease-producing organisms (e.g., *Proteus* and some *Pseudomonas*, *Klebsiella*, and *Providencia*) facilitate catheter encrustations that can obstruct the catheter.

Risk Factors

- **All patients with an indwelling catheter are expected to develop bacteriuria within 30 days of catheter insertion.**
- Risk factors for developing CA-UTI include diabetes, advanced age, female sex, elevated serum creatinine at the time of insertion, and catheter insertion outside of the operating room.[17]

DIAGNOSIS

- The signs and symptoms of CA-UTI are often nonspecific and may include fever, rigors, flank pain, and altered mental status. Patients with spinal cord injury may have a sense of foreboding, increased spasticity, and autonomic dysfunction.
  - During the 48 hours after catheter removal, CA-UTI may present as dysuria, urgency, increased urinary frequency, or suprapubic pain.
- As no benefit of antibiotic treatment for CA-ASB has been established, **patients with urinary catheters should not be screened for CA-ASB.**
  - If CA-UTI is suspected, UA and urine culture should be performed before starting antibiotics. Diagnosis of CA-UTI requires identification of $\geq 10^3$ cfu/mL of a single uropathogen or ≥ 1 species of bacteria in urine cultures obtained from patients with indwelling catheters or from a midstream collection if a catheter has been removed within the past 48 hours.
- Urine cultures from patients with condom catheters are often contaminated with skin flora; therefore, the threshold for significant bacteriuria is $\geq 10^5$ cfu/mL. Contamination is minimized by collecting midstream urine specimen or a specimen from a new catheter and after cleaning the glans.
- The presence or absence of pyuria should not be used to diagnose or rule out CA-ASB or CA-UTI; however, in symptomatic patients without pyuria, diagnoses other than UTI should be considered.

TREATMENT

- **Removal of the infected catheter is the cornerstone of CA-UTI treatment.** If medically necessary, a new catheter can be placed after starting antibiotic treatment.
- Treatment of CA-ASB is only indicated for women who are pregnant, patients who are immunocompromised, and patients who will be undergoing urologic procedures. **However, regular screening for CA-ASB in these populations is not indicated and may lead to unnecessary antibiotic usage.**
- CA-UTI with mild illness can be treated with levofloxacin 500 mg PO daily for 5 days or ciprofloxacin 500 mg PO q12h for 10 days. A 3-day regimen may be considered for women ≤ 65 years old if the catheter has been removed and no upper tract symptoms are present.
- Moderate to severe CA-UTI should be treated for ≥ 7 days. Because CA-UTI is often associated with drug-resistant organisms, empiric therapy with an intravenous antipseudomonal cephalosporin, carbapenem, or penicillin with β-lactamase inhibitor is appropriate until susceptibilities are available.
- If there is a delayed response to antibiotic treatment, continue treatment for 10 to 14 days.
- In most cases, catheter removal is sufficient for treatment of candiduria. Antifungal therapy should be initiated **only in cases** of symptomatic pyuria with no bacterial source identified **and** if the patient is immunocompromised or at high risk for candidemia.

PREVENTION

- **Indwelling catheters should not be used to manage incontinence, except to promote healing of open decubitus or perineal ulcers.**
- Alternatives to urinary catheterization should be considered, especially for female, elderly, and immunocompromised patients.[9,17]
  - A condom catheter is a reasonable alternative for men, especially for short-term catheterization, but does not eliminate the risk of CA-UTI.
  - Intermittent straight catheterization is a good alternative for both short- and long-term catheterization.
  - There is no consensus on the risk of long-term suprapubic catheters versus long-term urethral catheterization.
  - Consider noninvasive methods (e.g., portable bladder ultrasound) to evaluate residual urine volume rather than timed, repeated catheterization.
- Indwelling catheters should be inserted using sterile technique and frequently monitored to ensure that the catheter remains patent. In the nonacute care setting, clean conditions are considered sufficient for intermittent catheterization.
- Re-evaluate the need for a urinary catheter daily while a patient is in the hospital.
- Other strategies to prevent or delay infection include the use of antimicrobial-coated catheters and the use of closed catheter drainage systems.
- Cranberry extract, daily urethral meatal disinfection, catheter irrigation, and routine catheter exchanges **have not** shown to effectively prevent CA-UTI.
- **There is no role for antibiotic prophylaxis for CA-UTI prevention.**
- **Screening for CA-ASB is not recommended in patients with long-term catheters or those who intermittently straight-catheterize.**

Special Cases in Urinary Tract Infections

GENERAL PRINCIPLES

UTIs in patients who have urinary tract abnormalities (i.e., anatomical, functional, foreign bodies) or are immunocompromised are considered to have complicated UTIs.

Funguria

- Almost all cases in which fungi are isolated in urine culture are due to fungal colonization of the urinary tract. Funguria is most commonly caused by *Candida albicans* but can be caused by non-*albicans* Candida species and other fungi.
- Most patients with asymptomatic funguria do not require antimicrobial treatment. Urinary catheters should be removed, if present.
- Treatment for asymptomatic funguria should take into account the risk of invasive fungemia. Therefore, treatment is indicated only for patients who are neutropenic, have a history of a renal transplant, or are scheduled to have a urologic procedure.
- In almost all cases of UTI where both bacteria and fungi are identified on culture, treatment of the bacterial agent, only, is sufficient.
- Treat azole-sensitive *Candida* with fluconazole 200 mg daily for 7 to 14 days. If resistant, treat with amphotericin B or flucytosine.[18]
- Providers should have a low threshold for imaging the kidney and urinary tract for abnormalities (e.g., fungus balls, abscess) in patients with persistent funguria, especially in diabetics.

Diabetes

- Incidence of ASB, UTI, and complications from UTI is higher among patients with diabetes. Impaired host immunity and autonomic neuropathy may be contributing factors.

- Proteinuria, advanced age, and history of recurrent UTIs are risk factors for UTIs in diabetic patients.
- ASB is often incidentally found in diabetics due to regular UA in this population. **Treatment of ASB does not improve clinical outcomes; and patients with diabetes should not be screened for bacteriuria.**
- Diabetes is a risk factor for funguria, which often resolves with tighter glucose control alone. Antifungal treatment is rarely indicated for asymptomatic funguria in diabetics.
- Pyelonephritis and other severe complications, such as perinephric abscess, renal papillary necrosis, renal cortical abscess, and emphysematous pyelonephritis, may present insidiously in diabetic patients. Emphysematous pyelonephritis is a surgical emergency, whereas emphysematous cystitis can be treated with antibiotics.

Anatomic Abnormalities and Urinary Stones

- Patients with adult polycystic kidney disease (APKD), vesicoureteric reflux, or obstructive uropathy are at higher risk of developing upper urinary tract disease and subsequent renal failure.
- Antibiotic prophylaxis or treatment of ASB has **not** been shown to delay renal impairment.
- Infected cysts or pyelonephritis in the setting of APKD requires a long course of an IV fluoroquinolone followed by prophylaxis.
- Urinary tract stones should be removed whenever possible to minimize the need for antibiotics. Stone removal should strongly be considered in patients with persistent or recurrent UTI, as urinary stones can remain chronically colonized despite antimicrobial treatment.

Renal Transplant

- UTIs are common among renal transplant recipients and are associated with graft dysfunction and rejection in this population.
- Recipients should be treated before transplant if UTI is present. All patients should receive perioperative antibiotic prophylaxis.
- A course of at least 6 months of low-dose TMP-SMX has been shown to reduce UTIs after renal transplantation.[19] Ciprofloxacin and norfloxacin are alternatives. Prophylaxis may need to be extended indefinitely for patients with anatomical or functional urinary tract abnormalities or those who have recurrent UTIs.
- Transplant recipients with urinary symptoms should receive empiric treatment with a fluoroquinolone or TMP-SMX for 10 to 14 days. Obtain urine cultures before starting treatment, and adjust antibiotics to susceptibilities.

REFERENCES

1. Foxman B. Epidemiology of urinary tract infections: incidence, morbidity, and economic costs. *Am J Med.* 2002;113(suppl 1A):5S-13S.
2. American College of Obstetricians and Gynecologists. ACOG practice bulletin no. 91: treatment of urinary tract infections in nonpregnant women. *Obstet Gynecol.* 2008;111:785-794.
3. Foxman B. The epidemiology of urinary tract infection. *Nat Rev Urol.* 2010;7:653-660.
4. Hooton TM. Uncomplicated urinary tract infection. *N Engl J Med.* 2012;366:1028-1037.
5. Nicolle LE, Bradley S, Colgan R, et al. Infectious Diseases Society of America guidelines for the diagnosis and treatment of asymptomatic bacteriuria in adults. *Clin Infect Dis.* 2005;40:643-654.
6. Gupta K, Hooton TM, Naber KG, et al. International clinical practice guidelines for the treatment of acute uncomplicated cystitis and pyelonephritis in women: a 2010 update by the Infectious Diseases Society of America and the European Society for Microbiology and Infectious Diseases. *Clin Infect Dis.* 2011;52:e103-e120.

7. Bonkat G, Pickard R, Bartoletti R, et al. European Association of Urology Guidelines on Urological Infections. 2018. Available at https://uroweb.org/guideline/urological-infections/#1. Accessed January 27, 2019.

8. Fihn SD. Acute uncomplicated urinary tract infection in women. *N Engl J Med*. 2003;349:259-266.

9. Gould CV, Umscheid CA, Agarwal RK, et al. Guideline for prevention of catheter-associated urinary tract infections 2009. *Infect Control Hosp Epidemiol*. 2010;31:319-326.

10. Cai T, Mazzoli S, Mondaini N, et al. The role of asymptomatic bacteriuria in young women with recurrent urinary tract infections: to treat or not to treat? *Clin Infect Dis*. 2012;55(6):771-777.

11. Daneman N, Bronskill SE, Gruneir A, et al. Variability in antibiotic use across nursing homes and the risk of antibiotic-related adverse outcomes for individual residents. *JAMA Intern Med*. 2015;175:1331-1339.

12. Rosen DA, Hooton TM, Stamm WE, Humphrey PA, Hultgren SJ. Detection of intracellular bacterial communities in human urinary tract infection. *PLoS Med*. 2007;4(12):e329.

13. Jepson RG, Williams G, Craig JC. Cranberries for preventing urinary tract infections. *Cochrane Database of Syst Rev*. 2012;10.

14. Grabe M, Bishop MC, Bjerklund-Johansen TE, et al. *Guidelines on the Management of Urinary and Male Genital Tract Infections*. Arnhem, The Netherlands: European Association of Urology (EAU); 2008:79-88.

15. Etienne M, Chavanet P, Sibert L, et al. Acute bacterial prostatitis: heterogeneity in diagnostic criteria and management. Retrospective multicentric analysis of 371 patients diagnosed with acute prostatitis. *BMC Infect Dis*. 2008;8:12.

16. Schaeffer AJ. Chronic prostatitis and the chronic pain syndrome. *N Engl J Med*. 2006;355:1690-1698.

17. Hooton TM, Bradley SF, Cardenas DD, et al. Diagnosis, prevention and treatment of catheter associated urinary tract infection in adults: 2009 international clinical practice guidelines from the Infectious Diseases Society of America. *Clin Infect Dis*. 2010;50:625-663.

18. Pappas PG, Kauffman CA, Andes D, et al. Clinical practice guidelines for the management of candidiasis: 2009 update by the Infectious Diseases Society of America. *Clin Infect Dis*. 2009;48:503-535.

19. Fox BC, Sollinger HW, Belzer FO, et al. A prospective, randomized, double-blind study of trimethoprim-sulfamethoxazole for prophylaxis of infection in renal transplantation: clinical efficacy, absorption of trimethoprim-sulfamethoxazole, effects on the microflora, and the cost-benefit of prophylaxis. *Am J Med*. 1990;89:255-274.

Infections of the Bone and Joint

8

Shadi Parsaei and Stephen Y. Liang

Acute and Chronic Osteomyelitis

- Osteomyelitis is an inflammatory process of the bone due to an infecting microorganism(s).
- Classification can be based on: duration, location, and origin/etiology:
  - Infection can develop over days to weeks (acute) or months to years (chronic).
  - Any bone can be affected, although certain bones are more commonly involved than others (e.g., vertebrae, extremities with vascular compromise).
  - Mechanisms of pathogenesis include hematogenous seeding, direct traumatic inoculation, or contiguous spread from a neighboring site of infection.
  - See Table 8-1 for specific clinical scenarios associated with less common pathogens.
- Various bacterial virulence factors facilitate bone infection (e.g., *Staphylococcus aureus* has the ability to block inhibitive proteolysis and adheres well to bone).[1,2]
- Local inflammation, with the release of cytokines, toxic oxygen radicals, and proteolytic enzymes, damages bone and tissue, leading to abscess formation.
- In chronic osteomyelitis, invasion of vascular channels by pus eventually leads to ischemic necrosis and devascularized bone fragments ("sequestra").
- Three categories of osteomyelitis will be discussed in detail: (1) hematogenous osteomyelitis, (2) diabetes- and peripheral vascular disease–associated osteomyelitis, and (3) traumatic and other types of contiguous osteomyelitis

TABLE 8-1	UNUSUAL ORGANISMS ASSOCIATED WITH BONE AND JOINT INFECTIONS	
Organism	**Clinical Scenario**	**Special Considerations**
Mycobacterium tuberculosis	Exposure to an endemic area or known tuberculosis contact	Most common site of bone involvement is spine (Pott disease). Check for concurrent HIV infection
Brucella spp.	Exposure to an endemic area; may have history of ingestion of unpasteurized dairy products or animal exposure	Commonly causes sacroiliitis or vertebral osteomyelitis
Salmonella	Sickle cell disease	Infection usually occurs in the long bones
Candida spp.	Intravenous drug use	

(Continued)

TABLE 8-1	UNUSUAL ORGANISMS ASSOCIATED WITH BONE AND JOINT INFECTIONS (CONTINUED)	
Organism	**Clinical Scenario**	**Special Considerations**
Human oral flora (*Eikenella corrodens*, *Peptostreptococcus*, *Fusobacterium*)	Bone inoculation by human bite (e.g., hand injury while punching person's face), licking needle before injection drug use	Human bites carry a high rate of infection and often require surgical debridement
Group B streptococci	Diabetes, underlying malignancy	
Animal oral flora (*Pasteurella multocida*, *Capnocytophaga* spp., anaerobes)	Cat or dog bite	In setting of deep tissue injury, start empiric antibiotics. Rabies prophylaxis should be considered
Mycoplasma hominis	Septic arthritis in post-partum period or immu-nocompromised patient	May be associated with urinary tract instrumentation
Aeromonas spp.	Water contaminating an open fracture or wound	*Pseudomonas* is also a common pathogen seen with water contamination

Hematogenous Osteomyelitis

GENERAL PRINCIPLES

Epidemiology

- Hematogenous osteomyelitis commonly affects vertebral bodies and adjacent disc spaces (lumbar > thoracic > cervical) in older adults.[3,4]
- Increasing incidence of vertebral osteomyelitis is due in part to a rise in special patient populations with IDU (injection drug use), indwelling vascular access, and immunocompromise.[4]
- Oftentimes, bones and joints are concurrently affected. Sacroiliac and sternoclavicular joint infections are more commonly encountered in the setting of IDU.

Etiology

- Bone infection occurs because of bacteremia and hematogenous seeding from distant foci.[4]
- Infection is often monomicrobial:
  - *S. aureus* and gram-negative rods (including *Pseudomonas*) are most common.[3]
  - Methicillin-resistant *S. aureus* (MRSA) remains an important pathogen.[5]
  - Other organisms can include *Streptococcus* spp. and coagulase-negative staphylococci or enterococcus.

Risk Factors

- Older age and male sex.[6]
- Conditions predisposing to bacteremia: IDU, urinary tract infection, and presence of indwelling vascular access (e.g., central venous or dialysis catheter).
- Preexisting degenerative joint disease or prosthetic hardware.

DIAGNOSIS

Clinical Presentation

History
- History should focus on identifying risk factors for bacteremia and establishing the presence of localized symptoms such as pain, swelling, and drainage. Systemic symptoms, such as fever, may or may not be present.
- Prior recent antibiotic use should be queried as this may affect organism recovery with microbiological culture.

Physical Examination
- Examination should include inspection for erythema, tenderness, or fluctuance.
- The presence of a draining sinus tract is indicative of chronic osteomyelitis.
- Neurologic complications may occur in up to a third of patients with vertebral osteomyelitis.[7]

Differential Diagnosis

Erosive osteochondrosis, malignancy, gout, amyloidosis, soft tissue infection, bursitis, Modic-type degenerative changes, and fractures can all mimic osteomyelitis.

Diagnostic Testing

Laboratories
- Baseline testing, including a complete blood count and renal function and liver function tests, should be performed.
- WBC count may be normal or elevated.
- Elevated inflammatory markers such as erythrocyte sedimentation rate (ESR) and C-reactive protein (CRP) correlate with the degree of bone involvement, but are nonspecific and can be normal in some cases.
- **Blood cultures should be obtained and are positive in 58% (range: 30%–78%) of the patients.**[2]
- Invasive diagnostic procedures may be avoidable if a causative organism is recovered from blood culture.

Imaging
- MRI is more sensitive and specific (96% and 93%, respectively) than CT, radionuclide studies, or plain radiography.[8]
- Plain radiography can demonstrate soft tissue swelling, narrowing or widening of joint space, periosteal reaction, and bone destruction.
- MRI and CT can detect complications including paraspinal abscess formation.
- MRI is the test of choice for vertebral osteomyelitis in the presence of neurologic symptoms. Discitis with involvement of the adjacent vertebrae is a clue to the diagnosis.

Diagnostic Procedures
- Tissue sampling is necessary in most cases of hematogenous osteomyelitis in the setting of negative blood cultures.
- If the patient is clinically stable, efforts to obtain a microbiological diagnosis before antibiotic administration should be undertaken.
- Bone samples obtained through CT-guided needle or open biopsy should be sent for aerobic and anaerobic bacterial, fungal, and mycobacterial culture, as well as histopathologic examination.
- A causative organism is identified in 77% (reported range 44%–100%) of patients undergoing CT-guided percutaneous or open biopsy, but varies depending on sampling strategy.[3]

TREATMENT

Medications

- **Whenever possible, antibiotic administration should be delayed in the stable patient until tissue can be sampled and sent for culture and histopathology.**
- Antibiotics should be tailored to the causative organism and are generally administered intravenously (see Table 8-2).
- Length of treatment should be 6 to 8 weeks, counting from the date of the last surgical debridement or from the date of the first negative blood culture (if initial blood cultures were positive), whichever occurs the latest.

Other Nonpharmacologic Therapies

- A fitted thoracolumbosacral orthosis brace may be needed when vertebral destruction is extensive.
- Physical therapy is useful for improving functionality once neurologic stability is ensured.

TABLE 8-2	ORGANISM-DIRECTED THERAPY IN BONE AND JOINT INFECTIONS		
Microorganism	**General Considerations**	**First Choice**	**Alternative Choice**
Methicillin-sensitive *Staphylococcus aureus*	At time of discharge, preference is generally given to antibiotics administered once daily or via continuous infusion due to ease of home infusion	β-Lactam (oxacillin 2 g intravenously every 6 h or 12 g over 24 h via continuous infusion; cefazolin 2 g intravenously every 8 h)	Ceftriaxone 2 g intravenously every 24 h (may be preferred over cefazolin for outpatient administration)
Methicillin-resistant *S. aureus* or coagulase-negative staphylococci	Goal vancomycin troughs are 15–20 µg/mL and twice-daily administration is preferred to once daily	Vancomycin 15–20 mg/kg intravenously every 12 h	Daptomycin 6 g/kg intravenously every 24 h
Vancomycin-intermediate *S. aureus* (VISA)	Data for VISA treatment in bone and joint infections are limited.	Daptomycin 6 g/kg intravenously every 24 h	Linezolid 600 mg orally every 12 h
Streptococcal species	At time of discharge, preference is generally given to antibiotics administered once daily or via continuous infusion due to ease of home infusion	Penicillin G 3–4 million units intravenously every 4 h or 12–18 million units over 24 h via continuous infusion pump	Ceftriaxone 2 g intravenously every 24 h

TABLE 8-2	ORGANISM-DIRECTED THERAPY IN BONE AND JOINT INFECTIONS (CONTINUED)		
Microorganism	General Considerations	First Choice	Alternative Choice
Enteric gram-negative bacilli (i.e., *Escherichia coli*, *Klebsiella*, and *Proteus* spp.)	Treatment must be based on antibiotic susceptibility testing. Until susceptibility results are available, therapy should be guided by the individual hospital's antibiogram	Fluoroquinolone (ciprofloxacin 750 mg orally every 12 h), third-generation cephalosporin (ceftriaxone 2 g intravenously every 24 h), carbapenem (ertapenem 1 g intravenously every 24 h)	Cefepime 2 g intravenously every 12 h
Pseudomonas aeruginosa	Higher or more frequent doses of antibiotic therapy are needed for adequate coverage	Fluoroquinolone (ciprofloxacin 750 mg orally every 12 h); cefepime or ceftazidime intravenously 2 g every 8 h	Piperacillin–tazobactam 4.5 g intravenously every 6 h
Anaerobes	Carbapenems and piperacillin–tazobactam possess activity against anaerobes; additional anaerobic coverage is not necessary when these antibiotics are used	Metronidazole 500 mg by mouth every 8 h	Clindamycin 300–600 mg by mouth every 6–8 h is preferred in cases where oral flora is suspected

Surgical Management

- Surgery is often not necessary in cases of acute, uncomplicated hematogenous osteomyelitis.
- Surgical intervention is required in the setting of neurologic compromise and/or for drainage of a large abscess or spinal stabilization. Intraoperative cultures and histopathology can aid diagnosis.

SPECIAL CONSIDERATIONS

- **Culture-Negative Osteomyelitis**
  - Inability to identify a causative organism despite bone biopsy is most commonly due to previous antibiotic exposure and/or sampling error.
  - If the initial bone culture is negative, repeat percutaneous or open biopsy for culture and potentially molecular diagnostics while withholding antibiotics should be considered.

TABLE 8-3	ANTIBIOTIC DOSING IN HEMODIALYSIS PATIENTS FOR BONE AND JOINT INFECTIONS
Antibiotic	Dosing
Vancomycin	20 mg/kg loading dose during the last hour of the dialysis session, then 500 mg during the last 30 min of each subsequent dialysis session
Cefepime	2 g after each weekday dialysis session, 3 g after the weekend dialysis session
Cefazolin	2 g after each dialysis session, 3 g after the weekend dialysis session
Daptomycin	6 mg/kg after each dialysis session

- ○ If culture results are not obtained, empiric coverage of the most likely causative organism(s) is appropriate.
- ○ A combination of vancomycin and a third- or fourth-generation cephalosporin is reasonable empiric coverage for culture-negative hematogenous osteomyelitis.
- **Dialysis Patients:** Care should be taken to choose an antibiotic regimen that can be easily administered to patients requiring hemodialysis (see Table 8-3).

COMPLICATIONS

- Spinal instability and neurologic compromise can occur in vertebral osteomyelitis.
- Associated abscess (psoas, epidural, or paraspinal abscess in vertebral osteomyelitis) can necessitate percutaneous or open surgical drainage.
- Up to 12% of cases of lumbar vertebral osteomyelitis are complicated by an epidural abscess, with higher rates reported in thoracic and cervical vertebral osteomyelitis.[9]
- Long-term antibiotic therapy can be complicated by line-related infections; *C. difficile* infection; hematologic, renal, or liver toxicity; and other antibiotic-specific adverse events.

MONITORING/FOLLOW-UP

- Clinical reassessment is indicated after 3 to 6 weeks of antibiotic therapy.
- Concern for treatment failure is warranted if symptoms fail to improve and inflammatory markers (CRP and ESR) remain persistently elevated.
- Repeat imaging is not routinely indicated as it does not correlate well with clinical healing. However, imaging is warranted in the setting of clinical deterioration, failure to improve, or to ensure resolution of a large abscess.[10]

OUTCOME/PROGNOSIS

- Acute osteomyelitis is generally easier to cure than chronic infection.
- Cure rates for vertebral osteomyelitis approach 90%, with mortality <5%.[3]
- Back pain and neurologic symptoms persist in a minority of patients with vertebral osteomyelitis; functional limitations may persist in up to one-third of survivors.[9]

Osteomyelitis Associated With Diabetes and Peripheral Vascular Disease

GENERAL PRINCIPLES

- This type of osteomyelitis develops almost exclusively in the feet of patients at risk, often originating from a non-healing ulcer.
- Infection is polymicrobial in nature, with common organisms including *S. aureus*, other gram-positive cocci (e.g., streptococci), various gram-negative bacteria, and anaerobes.[11]
- Risk factors for foot infections in the setting of diabetes mellitus and/or peripheral vascular disease include vascular compromise, poor glycemic control, diabetic end-organ damage, poorly fitted footwear, and trauma.
- Preventive strategies include:
  ○ Optimization of glycemic control
  ○ Smoking cessation
  ○ Preventative foot care (e.g., appropriate footwear, avoidance of foot trauma, daily foot examination)
  ○ Early aggressive management of foot ulcers

DIAGNOSIS

Clinical Presentation

History
- Determine the duration of the ulcer and history of prior foot osteomyelitis. Long-standing foot ulceration (>2 wk) over a bony prominence increases the likelihood of osteomyelitis.
- Ask about associated local (e.g., wound drainage, erythema, and tenderness) and systemic (e.g., fevers and chills) symptoms.
- Trauma may suggest fracture or presence of a foreign body.

Physical Examination
- Measure the size and depth of the ulcer. Ulcers >2 cm^3 in size and >3 mm in depth increase the probability of underlying bone infection.[12]
- Check pedal pulses to assess vascular supply.
- Visible bone or a positive probe-to-bone test indicates a presumptive diagnosis of osteomyelitis.

Differential Diagnosis

An infected diabetic foot ulcer without bone involvement and diabetic neuropathic arthropathy (i.e., Charcot arthropathy) can mimic diabetic foot osteomyelitis.

Diagnostic Testing

Laboratories
- Baseline testing, including a complete blood count and renal function and liver function tests, is indicated.
- WBC count may be normal or elevated.
- Elevated inflammatory markers such as ESR and CRP correlate with the presence of bone involvement, but are nonspecific. ESR elevation above 70 mm/h increases the likelihood of osteomyelitis by a factor of 11.[12]
- Blood cultures should be obtained if signs of systemic infection are present.

Imaging
- Plain radiography may demonstrate local osteopenia with bone lucency or periosteal reaction, but may take up to 2 or 4 weeks to become apparent.
- MRI is more useful than CT or radionuclide imaging and remains the test of choice in most cases with a sensitivity of 90% to 100%.[13] Indium-111 scans can be useful in distinguishing between osteomyelitis and Charcot arthropathy in select patients.[13,14]

Diagnostic Procedures
- Microbiological discordance between superficial and deep tissue/bone cultures is common.
- Routine use of superficial cultures, especially in the setting of non-debrided wounds, is not recommended due to the frequent presence of organisms that colonize the skin surface.[15]
- A superficial culture can be used to identify drug-resistant organisms such as MRSA, which may correlate well with bone culture (40%).[16]
- Percutaneous bone biopsy for histopathology and microbiologic culture is useful in establishing the presence and etiology of underlying osteomyelitis.
- Vascular supply should be assessed (usually first by measuring ankle-brachial indices) to determine the need for revascularization procedures.

TREATMENT

Medications
- Medical therapy to achieve cure without surgical intervention or with minimal debridement may be possible in cases without extensive gangrene, necrosis, or limb-threatening infection.[17]
- Antibiotics are generally administered for 4 to 6 weeks and may be extended when chronically infected bone remains. Duration of therapy may be shortened significantly when all of the infected bone and tissue has been resected and surgical margins are deemed to be free of infection or amputation has occurred far proximal to the site of osteomyelitis.
- Oral antibiotics with high bioavailability (e.g., metronidazole, clindamycin, and fluoroquinolones) can be used, but parenteral antibiotics are preferable in most cases.
- No single regimen has been shown to be superior and few head-to-head trials comparing antibiotic regimens exist to guide treatment.
- If deep culture results are available, antibiotic therapy directed at isolated organisms should be used (Table 8-2).
- If deep culture results are not available, empiric polymicrobial antibiotic coverage, including anaerobes, is appropriate and should be guided by the following considerations:
  - Ease of outpatient administration
  - Risk factors for resistant gram-negative bacilli including *Pseudomonas* (prior antibiotic therapy, long-standing ulceration, ulcer with significant water exposure)
  - Existence of superficial culture growing drug-resistant organisms (e.g., MRSA)
- Empiric therapy should cover gram-positive (including MRSA), gram-negative, and anaerobic organisms.

Nonpharmacologic Therapies
- Optimal glycemic control is important to promote healing in diabetic patients.
- Local wound care with ongoing debridement of devitalized tissue is crucial.
- Use of adjunctive hyperbaric oxygen remains controversial.

Surgical Management
- Orthopedic surgery or podiatry consultation is usually indicated.
- Debridement and/or amputation is often necessary for cure, especially when chronically infected bone (sequestrum) is present.

- Revascularization may be necessary in the setting of vascular insufficiency to promote healing and ensure antibiotic delivery.

SPECIAL CONSIDERATIONS

Care should be taken to choose an antibiotic regimen that can be easily administered to patients requiring hemodialysis (Table 8-3).

COMPLICATIONS

- Amputation of an infected foot/limb carries high morbidity.
- Complications of long-term antibiotic therapy (e.g., line-related infections; hematologic, renal, or liver toxicity; and other antibiotic-specific adverse events) can occur (see Table 8-4).

MONITORING/FOLLOW-UP

- Clinical reassessment for worsening of infection or poor wound healing should occur within the first 3 to 6 weeks of treatment.
- Concern for treatment failure is warranted if symptoms fail to improve and inflammatory markers (CRP and ESR) remain persistently elevated.
- Reimaging is not routinely indicated.

OUTCOME/PROGNOSIS

More than a third of patients require some level of amputation within the first 1 to 3 years following treatment.[18]

TABLE 8-4	LABORATORY MONITORING FOR OUTPATIENT ANTIBIOTIC THERAPY FOR COMMONLY USED ANTIBIOTICS
Antibiotic	**Suggested Labs/Frequency**
Vancomycin	CBC once weekly BMP twice weekly Vancomycin trough twice weekly (goal 15–20 mg/L)
Penicillin	CBC and BMP once weekly
Oxacillin or nafcillin	CBC and CMP once weekly
Cefazolin	CBC and BMP once weekly
Ceftriaxone	CBC and CMP once weekly
Carbapenems	CBC and CMP once weekly
Daptomycin	CBC, BMP, and CPK once weekly

BMP, basic metabolic profile; CBC, complete blood count; CMP, complete metabolic profile; CPK, creatine phosphokinase.

Traumatic and Other Contiguous Osteomyelitis

GENERAL PRINCIPLES

Epidemiology

Traumatic osteomyelitis with direct inoculation of bone often occurs in the setting of an open fracture. Contiguous osteomyelitis other than that associated with diabetes mellitus or peripheral vascular disease can extend from neighboring hardware or foreign body or from a decubitus ulcer.

Etiology

- *S. aureus* is common in all types of traumatic and contiguous osteomyelitis. Organisms associated with traumatic osteomyelitis can vary depending on the environment in which the open fracture was sustained, and may include unusual organisms (e.g., mycobacteria, fungi).
- Coagulase-negative staphylococci and *Propionibacterium* are associated with foreign body or hardware in subacute infection.
- Decubitus ulcer–associated osteomyelitis is often polymicrobial, with fecal organisms being common.

Risk Factors

- Open fracture with gross contamination
- Presence of hardware or foreign body
- Non-healing stage IV decubitus ulcer

DIAGNOSIS

Clinical Presentation

History
- Systemic symptoms, such as fever, are often absent in subacute or chronic osteomyelitis.
- Local symptoms such as increased pain, redness, or drainage are often present. Pain alone may be the only symptom in patients with hardware-associated infection.
- Prior recent antibiotic use should be queried as this may impact organism recovery during microbiologic culture.
- In the case of open fractures, the mechanism of injury and the degree and type of contamination can provide clues to the causative organisms.
- Local signs of infection such as foul smelling, drainage, erythema, tenderness, poor wound healing, or exposed bone suggest infection.

Physical Examination
- Inspect the wound for signs of infection (e.g., drainage, erythema, and swelling).
- A draining sinus tract is often indicative of chronic osteomyelitis.
- Clinical diagnosis of osteomyelitis, even the presence of visible bone, is unreliable in decubitus ulcers.[19]

Differential Diagnosis

Osteomyelitis can be confused with soft tissue infection without bone involvement in all types of contiguous osteomyelitis and mechanical failure in hardware-associated osteomyelitis.

Diagnostic Testing

Laboratories
- Baseline testing, including a complete blood count and renal function and liver function tests, is indicated.
- WBC count may be normal or elevated.

- Elevated inflammatory markers such as ESR and CRP correlate with the presence of bone involvement, but are nonspecific and may be normal.
- Blood cultures should be obtained if signs of systemic infection are present.

Imaging
- Plain radiography may demonstrate soft tissue swelling. Bone destruction can be difficult to interpret in the setting of fractures, post-surgical changes, or decubitus ulcers.[20] Hardware loosening or fracture nonunion may also be seen.
- CT, MRI, or nuclear medicine studies can also be used to aid in diagnosis of decubitus ulcer–associated osteomyelitis.
- MRI has the highest sensitivity (98%) and specificity (89%).[21]
- Definitive diagnosis of trauma- or hardware-associated osteomyelitis is often made during surgery, rather than radiographically.

Diagnostic Procedures
- Superficial culture of decubitus ulcers often yields colonizing rather than causative organisms and is generally not recommended.[19]
- Deep tissue intraoperative specimens in trauma- or hardware-associated infection can be invaluable in guiding choice of antibiotic therapy.
- Bone biopsy with histopathology and culture is useful in cases of suspected decubitus ulcer–associated osteomyelitis for both diagnostic and therapeutic purposes.

TREATMENT

A combined medical and surgical approach is almost always necessary for cure in these types of infections. In the case of decubitus ulcer-associated chronic osteomyelitis where resection of infected bone is not pursued or feasible, it may be reasonable to treat clinically apparent infectious "flares" with brief courses of antibiotics.

Medications
- Antibiotics are generally administered intravenously for 6 weeks.
- If only soft tissue infection is suspected (no osteomyelitis or progression of disease), 2 weeks of antibiotic therapy may be sufficient.
- If microbiologic culture results are available, therapy directed at isolated organisms should be used (Table 8-2).
- Empiric therapy should be reserved for culture-negative traumatic or hardware-associated osteomyelitis.
- Empiric therapy for decubitus ulcer–associated osteomyelitis should cover gram-positive (including MRSA), gram-negative, and anaerobic organisms.

Nonpharmacologic Therapies
Local wound care and ongoing debridement of devitalized tissue and unloading of pressure are useful in long-term management of decubitus ulcers.

Surgical Management
- Debridement and hardware removal, if present, is often necessary for cure.
- Suppressive oral antibiotic therapy is useful when hardware cannot be removed.
- Wound coverage through grafting or flaps may be necessary for complete wound closure.
- Diverting colostomy to prevent wound contamination in the setting of a sacral decubitus ulcer may help promote healing in some cases.

SPECIAL CONSIDERATIONS

Care should be taken to choose an antibiotic regimen that can be easily administered to patients requiring hemodialysis (Table 8-3).

COMPLICATIONS

- Loss of the functional limb (hardware- or trauma-associated osteomyelitis).
- Chronic osteomyelitis in decubitus ulcer–associated infection can result in difficult-to-cure infection.

MONITORING/FOLLOW-UP

- Clinical reassessment for worsening of infection or poor wound healing is indicated within the first 3 to 6 weeks of treatment.
- Concern for treatment failure is indicated if symptoms fail to improve and inflammatory markers (CRP and ESR) remain persistently elevated.
- Reimaging is not routinely indicated.

OUTCOME/PROGNOSIS

- Prognosis is variable and depends on many factors including age, comorbidities, causative organism, and type of contiguous osteomyelitis.
- Bacteremia due to decubitus ulcers is associated with a high mortality rate in the elderly (up to 50%).[22]

Septic Arthritis of the Native Joints

Gonococcal Arthritis

GENERAL PRINCIPLES

- Disseminated gonococcal infection (DGI) arises from hematogenous spread of *Neisseria gonorrhoeae* from a distant focus of infection.
- DGI presents in one of two ways:
  ○ Tenosynovitis, pustular acral skin lesions, and arthralgia (without obvious purulent arthritis), commonly referred to as "arthritis-dermatitis" syndrome
  ○ Purulent mono- or oligoarthritis without skin involvement
- *N. gonorrhoeae* produces many virulence factors that allow it to disseminate from sites of mucosal colonization. Pili facilitate attachment to the synovium.[23]
- DGI is most commonly seen in young, sexually active adults. Other risk factors include female gender, recent menstruation, pregnancy (including the immediate postpartum period), and complement deficiency.[23]
- Gonococcal arthritis is the most common bacterial arthritis in young adults.
- Septic arthritis complicates DGI in half of cases and is less likely to be associated with classic skin findings or tenosynovitis.

DIAGNOSIS

Clinical Presentation

History
- The classic DGI triad of migratory polyarthralgias, tenosynovitis (mainly of the fingers, hands, and wrists) and acral dermatitis is less likely in the setting of septic arthritis.
- With septic arthritis, mono- or oligoarthritis and fever may be the only clinical complaints.

- DGI has a predilection for the knee and wrist joints; symmetric joint involvement is uncommon.
- Obtain a thorough travel and sexual history (particularly given increasing rates of drug-resistant gonorrhea worldwide)

Physical Examination
- Examine the skin for characteristic, painless macules and pustular papules on the arms, legs, or trunk; often <10 lesions are seen, >40 lesions are uncommon.
- Examine the joints and tendons of the hands, wrists, and ankles for signs of tenosynovitis (e.g., erythema, tenderness to palpation, painful range of motion).

Differential Diagnosis

Other causes of infectious and noninfectious arthritis (bacterial septic arthritis, gouty arthritis, and reactive arthritis), meningococcemia, secondary syphilis, and connective tissue disease can be confused with DGI.

Diagnostic Testing

Diagnosis is usually based on clinical and epidemiologic features due to the low yield of diagnostic procedures.

Laboratories
- WBC count and inflammatory markers (ESR and CRP) may be elevated, but are nonspecific.
- Skin cultures, synovial cultures, and blood cultures are rarely positive, but genitourinary cultures are positive in more than 80% of patients.[23]
- DNA probes and nucleic acid amplification tests are FDA-approved for urethral and endocervical specimens and are highly sensitive and specific.[24]
- Screening for other sexually transmitted diseases, including HIV, should be performed.

Imaging
- Plain films may demonstrate effusion.
- MRI or CT can be used to detect septic arthritis, effusions, abscesses, or tissue edema.

Diagnostic Procedures
- Arthrocentesis is the test of choice.
- Purulent effusion (>50,000 WBCs) should be present.
- Gram stain is positive in <25% of cases and synovial fluid culture in only 50%; polymerase chain reaction can detect *N. gonorrhoeae* with a high degree of sensitivity.[25]

TREATMENT

Medications

- In the appropriate clinical setting (a young adult who is sexually active), dual empiric treatment for DGI should be initiated:
  - Ceftriaxone 1 g intravenously every 24 hours or cefotaxime 1 g intravenously every 8 hours used for initial therapy **plus** azithromycin 1 g by mouth as a single dose **or** doxycycline 100 mg by mouth twice daily for 7 days.
  - Can switch to oral therapy with cefixime 400 mg by mouth twice daily 24 to 48 hours after clinical improvement.[26]
  - Given the concern for decreasing susceptibility to cefixime internationally and tetracyclines among *N. gonorrhoeae* isolates in the United States, de-escalation and tailoring of antibiotic therapy based on susceptibility testing is encouraged, if available.[26]
  - Treat for a total of 7 to 14 days.

○ Patients should also receive treatment for chlamydial infection even if testing is negative (azithromycin 1 g by mouth as a single dose or doxycycline 100 mg PO twice daily for 7 d is one option).

Surgical Management

Drainage by repeated needle aspiration or arthroscopy is needed for purulent arthritis due to DGI.

SPECIAL CONSIDERATIONS

Sexual contacts should be treated for *Neisseria* and *Chlamydia* infection. Abstinence from intercourse is recommended for 7 days after both the patient and partner have completed treatment.[26]

COMPLICATIONS

Complications are rare, but can include joint damage, osteomyelitis, perihepatitis, meningitis, and endocarditis.

MONITORING/FOLLOW-UP

Patients with recurrent *Neisseria* infection should be screened for complement deficiency.

OUTCOME/PROGNOSIS

Prognosis is good, with return to normal joint function in the vast majority of patients.

Nongonococcal Arthritis

GENERAL PRINCIPLES

- Bacteria enter the joint space, triggering an acute inflammatory response with acute and chronic inflammatory cells. Cytokines and proteases degrade the cartilage and then progress to subchondral bone loss.[27]
- Nongonococcal septic arthritis is the most rapidly destructive joint disease.
- There are 10 to 20 cases per 100,000 in the general population.[27]
- Large joints are affected more often than small joints and up to 60% of cases occur in the hip or knee.[28]
- Joint infection occurs most commonly from hematogenous seeding due to transient bacteremia or endocarditis or less commonly from direct inoculation (joint surgery, arthrocentesis, and puncture wound).
- The most common cause of bacterial septic arthritis is *S. aureus*, including MRSA.[29]
- Other common bacterial causes include group B streptococci in diabetics, gram-negative bacilli in elderly or debilitated patients, and coagulase-negative staphylococci following medical procedures.
- Risk factors include older age, rheumatoid arthritis, diabetes mellitus, malignancy, risk factors for bacteremia (e.g., vascular catheter and IDU), and joint injection.

DIAGNOSIS

Clinical Presentation

- Patients present with acute onset of monoarticular arthritis manifesting as pain, swelling, and limited motion of the affected joint, often accompanied by fever.

- Examination usually reveals a warm, tender joint with effusion and decreased active and passive range of motion; however, examination of the shoulder and hip joint may be difficult and unrevealing.

Differential Diagnosis

Nongonococcal septic arthritis must be differentiated from other causes of infectious and noninfectious arthritis (e.g., gonococcal arthritis, gout, pseudogout, and reactive arthritis), Lyme disease, and connective tissue disease.

Diagnostic Testing

Laboratories
- WBC count and inflammatory markers (ESR and CRP) may be elevated, but are nonspecific.
- Blood cultures should be performed.

Imaging
- Plain films may demonstrate effusion.
- MRI or CT can be used to detect septic arthritis, effusions, abscesses, or tissue edema.

Diagnostic Procedures
- **Arthrocentesis is the test of choice.**
- Fluoroscopic guidance may be necessary to access certain joints (e.g., hip).
- Fluid should be sent for examination for cell count and differential (>50,000 WBCs is typical for septic arthritis), crystal examination, Gram stain, and culture.
- Gram stain is positive in 50% of cases and synovial fluid cultures are positive in >80%.[30]

TREATMENT

Medications

- Empiric therapy should be based on the Gram stain and clinical scenario and may include treatment directed at *S. aureus* and streptococci. Vancomycin 15 to 20 mg/kg intravenously every 8 to 12 hours **plus** ceftriaxone 2 g intravenously every 24 hours is a reasonable empiric regimen and can be continued for culture-negative cases.
- Targeted therapy is similar to that of other bone infections (Table 8-2).
- Treatment for 4 to 6 weeks is recommended, with longer durations favored in the setting of infection due to *S. aureus*.

Surgical Management

- Drainage by repeated needle aspiration (daily drainage may be required) or arthroscopy may be necessary for purulent arthritis.
- If adequate drainage cannot be maintained by less invasive methods or the hip joint is involved, open surgical drainage is indicated.

SPECIAL CONSIDERATIONS

- Other causes of infectious septic arthritis include the following:
  - Mycobacteria and fungi (often indolent and chronic in nature)
  - Lyme arthritis (chronic monoarthritis commonly involving the knees)
- Care should be taken to choose an antibiotic regimen that can be easily administered to patients requiring hemodialysis (Table 8-3).

COMPLICATIONS

- Complications include joint damage (50% of cases), osteomyelitis, and sequelae of prolonged bacteremia (endocarditis and seeding of other organs).
- Mortality rate is significant (5%–15%).[31]

MONITORING/FOLLOW-UP

- Clinical reassessment for monitoring of infection is indicated within the first 4 weeks of treatment.
- Prompt repeat arthrocentesis or surgical drainage is indicated if symptoms worsen or fail to improve with appropriate therapy.

OUTCOME/PROGNOSIS

Prognosis is fair, but high rates of permanent joint damage (>40% of adults in one series had a poor joint outcome) and unchanged mortality rates are discouraging.[31]

Prosthetic Joint Infections

GENERAL PRINCIPLES

- Microorganisms are introduced at the time of surgery or through transient or persistent bacteremia.
- Bacteria adhere to the prosthesis and biofilm formation protects organisms from the host immune response and limits antimicrobial penetration.[29]
- Prosthetic joint infections are mainly a disease of older adults due to the need for joint replacement surgery in advanced osteoarthritis.
- Infection rates are 1.5% in hip replacement and 2.5% in knee replacement.[32]
- **Early infection** (<3 mo after surgery) and **delayed infection** (3–24 mo after surgery) are mainly due to organisms introduced at the time of surgery.
- **Late infection** (>24 mo after surgery) is usually due to hematogenous seeding of organisms from the skin, respiratory tract, oropharynx, or urinary tract.
- The most commonly isolated organisms are coagulase-negative staphylococci (30%–43%), *S. aureus* (12%–23%), mixed flora (10%–11%), streptococci (9%–10%), gram-negative bacilli (3%–6%), enterococci (3%–7%), and anaerobes (2%–4%).[33]
- Risk factors include the following:
  - Older age
  - Comorbidities including rheumatoid arthritis, psoriasis, diabetes mellitus, immunocompromised state, malignancy, obesity, or poor nutritional status
  - Prior surgery at the prosthesis site
  - First 2 years following joint replacement

DIAGNOSIS

Clinical Presentation

- Early infection often presents with acute onset of joint pain, effusion, erythema and warmth at the prosthesis site, and fever.
- Delayed infection has a more insidious onset of symptoms such as loosening of the implant or pain with absence of systemic symptoms. Presentation of delayed infections depends on the virulence of the causative organism.
- Careful examination of the joint and incision site may reveal erythema and cellulitis, discharge, wound dehiscence, sinus tract formation, or pain with passive or active motion.

Differential Diagnosis

Aseptic mechanical problems (gout, pseudogout, hemarthrosis, metallosis, or prosthesis loosening) can present similarly.

Diagnostic Testing

Differentiation of infection from mechanical problems is mainly accomplished through sampling of deep tissue or fluid by joint aspiration or surgical exploration.

Laboratories
- WBC count and inflammatory markers (ESR and CRP) may be elevated, but are nonspecific.
- Blood cultures should be performed, although yield is low.
- Synovial fluid should be sent for cell count, differential, crystal analysis, Gram stain, and culture.
- Additional investigation for PJI with α-defensin protein testing appears promising[34] but may not be routinely available in many institutions.
- Sonication, an intraoperative technique used to dislodge bacteria from the surface of prostheses, may be subject to contamination or false positives[35] and may not be routinely available in many institutions.

Imaging
- Plain radiography may detect loosening of the prosthesis or osteomyelitis.
- MRI and CT can be limited by hardware artifact.

Diagnostic Procedures
- Joint aspiration can demonstrate increased WBCs (lower threshold than that of septic arthritis) and organisms on Gram stain or culture consistent with infection, but patients often proceed directly to surgical exploration if suspicion of infection is high or prosthesis replacement or repair is required.
- Multiple specimens (a minimum of 3, optimally between 5 and 6) should be sent from all operative procedures to increase culture yield.[35]

TREATMENT

Medical Management

- Empiric therapy should be based on the Gram stain and should be withheld until deep cultures are obtained if the patient is clinically stable.
- If empiric therapy is warranted, it should cover the most common causative organisms including *S. aureus*, coagulase-negative staphylococci, and gram-negative bacilli.
- Targeted therapy is similar to that for other bone infections (Table 8-2), with an exception being the addition of rifampin when staphylococcal infection is present.
- **Rifampin 300 to 450 mg by mouth twice daily should be added to cases of retained hardware (i.e., early infection with retained hardware or late infection when hardware cannot be removed) in staphylococcal infections due to its activity against biofilms.**
- Treatment is recommended for 6 to 8 weeks.
- Optimal treatment of proven PJI combines medical and surgical management.

Surgical Management

- Early infection (<3 mo postsurgery) with <3 weeks of symptoms, stable prosthesis, and minimally damaged soft tissue can be treated with debridement and retention of the prosthesis with a >70% cure rate.[33] Infections with *S. aureus* may have a higher failure rate.[36]

• Late infections (>3 wk) are optimally treated with a two-stage procedure where the implant is removed and antibiotic therapy is administered for 6 weeks followed by reimplantation of the prosthesis after an antibiotic-free window, resulting in a >90% cure rate.[37]

SPECIAL CONSIDERATIONS

• **Dialysis Patients:** Care should be taken to choose an antibiotic regimen that can be easily administered to patients requiring hemodialysis (Table 8-3).
• Retained hardware when removal is indicated.
  ○ In cases where prosthesis removal is not possible, acute therapy targeted at causative organisms plus rifampin if staphylococci are cultured followed by chronic oral antibiotic suppression therapy is common practice.
  ○ Chronic suppression is most successful for infections with streptococci or coagulase-negative staphylococci. Higher failure rates have been demonstrated for *S. aureus*.[38]
  ○ An oral antibiotic should be chosen based on bacterial susceptibility, ease of administration, and least likelihood of adverse events.
  ○ Commonly used antibiotics for chronic suppression include **trimethoprim–sulfamethoxazole or doxycycline**.

COMPLICATIONS

• Functional impairment of the joint is a feared complication.
• Severe systemic infection with systemic shock can occur with more virulent organisms.

MONITORING/FOLLOW-UP

• Clinical reassessment for worsening of infection or poor wound healing should occur within the first 3 to 6 weeks of treatment.
• Persistent or worsening symptoms or continued presence of elevated inflammatory markers should prompt further evaluation for continued infection.

OUTCOME/PROGNOSIS

Prognosis depends on the location, time since surgery, host factors, and infecting organism, but >90% of two-stage procedures and >70% of early infection treated with retained prosthesis result in a cure, generally with good prosthesis function.

Septic Bursitis

GENERAL PRINCIPLES

• Septic bursitis is a bacterial infection of the bursa overlying a joint.
• The olecranon, prepatellar, and infrapatellar bursae are common sites of infection.
• Bacteria are introduced through trauma, percutaneous inoculation, or rarely, hematogenous spread.
• Septic bursitis is due to *S. aureus* in >80% of cases.[39]
• Other causes include streptococci, gram-negative bacilli, mycobacteria, and fungi.
• Traumatic injury to the bursa is the most significant risk factor for infection.

DIAGNOSIS

- Patients note pain, redness, and warmth over affected bursa, with or without systemic symptoms.
- Evidence of trauma or puncture wound is often evident over the affected bursa.
- Septic arthritis of the joint, gout, traumatic bursitis, and rheumatic bursitis can all present similarly.
- **Aspiration of the bursa is the test of choice,** with fluid sent for cell count and differential, crystals, Gram stain, and culture.
- Aspiration of joint space may be necessary to rule out septic arthritis.

TREATMENT

- Antibiotic therapy targeting the offending organism is indicated for a 10- to 14-day course (Table 8-2).
- Oral regimens are reasonable in mild cases in otherwise healthy patients.[39]
- Daily aspiration should be performed until sterile fluid is obtained.

OUTCOME/PROGNOSIS

- Prognosis is generally good, but bursitis can recur.
- Recurrent bursitis may require bursectomy.

Viral Arthritis

GENERAL PRINCIPLES

- Viral arthritis is a syndrome of acute polyarthritis, fever, and rash due to viral infection.
- The pathophysiology of viral arthritis is poorly understood, but may result from direct infection of the synovium or the host's immune response to infection.
- Up to 60% of parvovirus infections,[40] and 20% of acute hepatitis B or chronic hepatitis C infections are complicated by viral arthritis.[41]
- Rubella virus is a common cause of arthritis in the developing world. Other viruses that cause arthritis include HIV, Epstein–Barr virus, enterovirus, mumps, adenovirus, and alphaviruses.
- Risk of viral arthritis is dependent on risk factors for the individual viral infections.
- Women are more likely than men to experience arthritis following parvovirus infection (60% vs. 30%).[40]

DIAGNOSIS

Clinical Presentation

History
- Parvovirus infection often presents with symmetric polyarthritis of the hands, wrists, and ankles accompanied by facial erythema ("slapped cheek") and fever.
- A symmetric polyarthritis of the hands, wrists, knees, and ankles in acute hepatitis B infection often precedes the development of jaundice during the febrile prodrome.
- Chronic hepatitis C virus is often associated with arthralgias. Frank arthritis resembling rheumatoid arthritis develops in a smaller number of patients.[41]
- Rubella causes arthritis most commonly in the small joints of the hands and is associated with onset of a rash.

Physical Examination
- Careful examination of the joints with attention to the hands, wrists, and ankles should demonstrate joint involvement.
- Skin examination may reveal a characteristic rash consistent with rubella or parvovirus.

Differential Diagnosis

Other causes of polyarthritis include rheumatoid arthritis, acute rheumatic fever, endocarditis, and DGI.

Diagnostic Testing
- Viral serology is generally most useful for diagnosis.
- Imaging is often unremarkable.
- Joint aspiration is rarely useful except to rule out other causes of arthritis as organisms are not generally recovered from the synovium.

TREATMENT

- Supportive care is the only treatment indicated for most cases of viral arthritis.
- Nonsteroidal anti-inflammatory drugs (NSAIDs) are useful for symptom management.
- Treatment of hepatitis C or chronic hepatitis B may serve to improve joint symptoms.

SPECIAL CONSIDERATIONS

Returning travelers with polyarthralgias should have a careful travel history performed to gauge risk for alphaviruses such as Chikungunya virus or flaviviruses (e.g., dengue virus).

OUTCOME/PROGNOSIS

- Viral arthritis rarely leads to significant long-term disability and is mostly self-limited.
- Parvovirus infections may have a relapsing course in a third of patients or a chronic course lasting months in up to 20% of patients.[40]
- Joint symptoms with chronic hepatitis B or C infection may persist, but permanent joint damage is rare.

Reactive Arthritis

GENERAL PRINCIPLES

- Reactive arthritis is defined as **sterile inflammation of joints** that may be related to a distant infection.
- Reactive arthritis is hypothesized to be due to poor clearance of the organism and/or dysregulatory immune response.
- There is an association with other seronegative spondyloarthropathies and HLA-B27.[42] However, the relation to HLA-B27 is weaker than that of ankylosing spondylitis.
- Reactive arthritis is an uncommon disease that mainly occurs in young adults. The male-to-female ratio is equal for reactive arthritis following gastroenteritis but much more common in males following genitourinary infection.
- Reactive arthritis can occur in outbreaks from a single source of infection.
- Numerous microbial infections can cause reactive arthritis:
  - Enteric bacteria include *Yersinia, Salmonella, Shigella, Campylobacter*, and *C. difficile*.
  - *Chlamydia trachomatis* (following urethritis).
  - *Chlamydophila pneumoniae* (following a respiratory tract infection).

DIAGNOSIS

Clinical Presentation

- Antecedent respiratory, genitourinary, or gastrointestinal infection can often be elicited, but in other cases the initiating infection may be asymptomatic or not reported.
- There is usually a 1- to 2-week lag (up to 4 wk with *Chlamydia*) between initial infection and joint symptoms.[42]
- It commonly presents as asymmetric oligoarthritis of the large joints of the lower extremities, along with extra-articular complaints. Back pain occurs in about half of the cases. Enthesopathy (e.g., Achilles tendinitis, plantar fasciitis, and dactylitis) is not uncommon.
- Evidence of joint redness, swelling, and pain with range of motion is characteristic.
- Extra-articular symptoms including conjunctivitis, acute anterior uveitis, and skin findings (e.g., circinate balanitis, keratoderma blenorrhagicum, and erythema nodosum) may be seen.

Differential Diagnosis

Reactive arthritis must be differentiated from other causes of acute poly- or oligoarthritis, including infectious and noninfectious causes.

Diagnostic Testing

- Reactive arthritis is a diagnosis of exclusion that should be considered in the appropriate clinical scenario when other causes of arthritis have been ruled.
- At the time of arthritis, cultures for triggering infection are often negative. An exception is *C. trachomatis*, which can often be identified in the urine via nucleic acid amplification tests or cultured from the urethra.[43]
- Serologic tests, when available, may support the diagnosis.

TREATMENT

- Symptomatic treatment with NSAIDs and local steroid injections are useful.
- No significant evidence exists to support antibiotic treatment for reactive arthritis per se, although culture-positive *C. trachomatis* should be treated.

OUTCOME/PROGNOSIS

Fifty percent of patients recover in the first 6 months of treatment, but a minority develop chronic or recurrent symptoms.[42]

REFERENCES

1. Foster TJ, Hook M. Surface protein adhesins of *Staphylococcus aureus*. *Trends Microbiol.* 1998;6:484-488.
2. Schmitt SK. Osteomyelitis. *Infect Dis Clin North Am.* 2017;31:325-338.
3. Mylona E, Samarkos M, Kakalou E, et al. Pyogenic vertebral osteomyelitis: a systematic review of clinical characteristics. *Semin Arthritis Rheum.* 2009;39:10-17.
4. Berbari EF, Kanj SS, Kowalski TJ, et al. 2015 Infectious Diseases Society of America (IDSA) clinical practice guidelines for the diagnosis and treatment of native vertebral osteomyelitis in adults. *Clin Infect Dis.* 2015;61:e26-e46.
5. Bhavan K, Marschall J, Olsen M, et al. The epidemiology of hematogenous vertebral osteomyelitis: a cohort study in a tertiary care hospital. *BMC Infect Dis.* 2010;10:158.
6. Sapico FL, Montgomerie JZ. Pyogenic vertebral osteomyelitis: report of nine cases and review of the literature. *Rev Infect Dis.* 1979;1:754-776.

7. Pigrau C, Almirante B, Flores X, et al. Spontaneous pyogenic vertebral osteomyelitis and endocarditis: incidence, risk factors, and outcome. *Am J Med*. 2005;118:1287.

8. Modic MT, Feiglin DH, Piraino DW, et al. Vertebral osteomyelitis: assessment using MR. *Radiology*. 1985;157:157-166.

9. McHenry MC, Easley KA, Locker GA. Vertebral osteomyelitis: long-term outcome for 253 patients from 7 Cleveland-area hospitals. *Clin Infect Dis*. 2002;34:1342-1350.

10. Kowalski TJ, Berbari EF, Huddleston PM, et al. Do follow-up imaging examinations provide useful prognostic information in patients with spine infection? *Clin Infect Dis*. 2006;43:172-179.

11. Hartemann-Heurtier A, Senneville E. Diabetic foot osteomyelitis. *Diabetes Metab*. 2008;34:87-95.

12. Butalia S, Palda VA, Sargeant RJ, et al. Does this patient with diabetes have osteomyelitis of the lower extremity? *JAMA*. 2008;299:806-813.

13. Jeffcoate WJ, Lipsky BA. Controversies in diagnosing and managing osteomyelitis of the foot in diabetes. *Clin Infect Dis*. 2004;39:S115-S122.

14. Newman LG, Waller J, Palestro CJ, et al. Unsuspected osteomyelitis in diabetic foot ulcers. *JAMA*. 1991;266:1246-1251.

15. Lipsky BA, Berendt AR, Cornia PB, et al. 2012 Infectious Diseases Society of America clinical practice guideline for the diagnosis and treatment of diabetic foot infections. *Clin Infect Dis*. 2012;54:e132-173.

16. Senneville E, Melliez H, Beltrand E, et al. Culture of percutaneous bone biopsy specimens for diagnosis of diabetic foot osteomyelitis: concordance with ulcer swab cultures. *Clin Infect Dis*. 2006;42:57-62.

17. Shank CF, Feibel JB. Osteomyelitis in the diabetic foot: diagnosis and management. *Foot Ankle Clin*. 2006;11:775-789.

18. Apelqvist J, Larsson J, Agardh CD. Long-term prognosis for diabetic patients with foot ulcers. *J Intern Med*. 1993;233:485-491.

19. Darouiche RO, Landon GC, Klima M, et al. Osteomyelitis associated with pressure sores. *Arch Intern Med*. 1994;154:753-758.

20. Sugarman B. Pressure sores and underlying bone infection. *Arch Intern Med*. 1987;147:553-555.

21. Huang AB, Schweitzer ME, Hume E, et al. Osteomyelitis of the pelvis/hips in paralyzed patients: accuracy and clinical utility of MRI. *J Comput Assist Tomogr*. 1998;22:437-443.

22. Bryan CS, Dew CE, Reynolds KL. Bacteremia associated with decubitus ulcers. *Arch Intern Med*. 1983;143:2093-2095.

23. Cucurull E, Espinoza LR. Gonococcal arthritis. *Rheum Dis Clin North Am*. 1998;24:305-322.

24. Stary A, Ching SF, Teodorowicz L, Lee H. Comparison of ligase chain reaction and culture for detection of Neisseria gonorrhoeae in genital and extragenital specimens. *J Clin Microbiol*. 1997;35:239-242.

25. Liebling MR, Arkfeld DG, Michelini GA, et al. Identification of Neisseria gonorrhoeae in synovial fluid using the polymerase chain reaction. *Arthritis Rheum*. 1994;37:702-709.

26. Workowski KA, Bolen GA; Centers for Disease Control and Prevention (CDC). Sexually transmitted diseases treatment guidelines, 2015. *MMWR Recomm Rep*. 2015;64:1-137.

27. Goldenberg DL. Septic arthritis. *Lancet*. 1998;351:197-202.

28. Mathews CJ, Coakley G. Septic arthritis: current diagnostic and therapeutic algorithm. *Curr Opin Rheumatol*. 2008;20:457-462.

29. Gupta MN, Sturrock RD, Field M. A prospective 2-year study of 75 patients with adult-onset septic arthritis. *Rheumatology*. 2001;40(1):24-30.

30. Weston VC, Jones AC, Bradbury N, et al. Clinical features and outcome of septic arthritis in a single UK Health District 1982–1991. *Ann Rheum Dis*. 1999;58(4):214-219.

31. Kaandorp CJ, Krijnen P, Moens HJ, et al. The outcome of bacterial arthritis: a prospective community-based study. *Arthritis Rheum*. 1997;40:884-892.

32. Lentino JR. Prosthetic joint infections: bane of orthopedists, challenge for the infectious disease specialists. *Clin Infect Dis*. 2003;36:1157-1161.

33. Zimmerli W, Trampuz A, Oschsner PE. Prosthetic joint infections. *N Engl J Med*. 2004;351:1645-1654.

34. Berger P, Van Cauter M, Driesen R, et al. Diagnosis of prosthetic joint infection with alpha-defensin using a lateral flow device: a multicentre study. *Bone Joint J*. 2017;99:1176-1182.

35. Osmon DR, Berbari EF, Berendt AR, et al. Diagnosis and management of prosthetic joint infection: clinical practice guidelines by the Infectious Diseases Society of America. *Clin Infect Dis*. 2013;56:e1-e25.

36. Byren I, Bejon P, Atkins BL, et al. One hundred and twelve infected arthroplasties treated with "DAIR" (debridement, antibiotics and implant retention): antibiotic duration and outcome. *J Antimicrob Chemother*. 2009;63:1264-1271.
37. Trampuz A, Zimmerli W. Prosthetic joint infections: update in diagnosis and treatment. *Swiss Med Wkly*. 2005;135:243-251.
38. Segreti J, Nelson JA, Gordon MT. Prolonged suppressive antibiotic therapy for infected orthopedic prostheses. *Clin Infect Dis*. 1998;27:711-713.
39. Zimmermann B, Mikolich DJ, Ho G. Septic bursitis. *Semin Arthritis Rheum*. 1995;24:391-410.
40. Moore TL. Parvovirus-associated arthritis. *Curr Opin Rheumatol*. 2000;12:289-294.
41. Ohl C. Infectious arthritis of native joint. In: Mandell GL, Bennett JE, Dolin R, eds. *Mandell, Douglas, and Bennett's Principles and Practice of Infectious Diseases*. 7th ed. Philadelphia, PA: Churchill Livingstone, Elsevier; 2009:1443-1456.
42. Leirisalo-Repo M. Reactive arthritis. *Scand J Rheumatol*. 2005;34:251-259.
43. Galadari I, Galadari H. Nonspecific urethritis and reactive arthritis. *Clin Dermatol*. 2004;22:469-475.

Skin and Soft Tissue Infections

Darrell McBride and Stephen Y. Liang

9

Impetigo

GENERAL PRINCIPLES

Definition

Impetigo is a contagious superficial infection of the epidermis caused by *Staphylococcus aureus* or β-hemolytic streptococci. It can be divided into bullous and nonbullous forms.

Epidemiology

- Nonbullous impetigo is more common.
- Impetigo usually affects young children (ages 2–5) but can occur in any age group.[1]
- Incidence is highest in tropical climates or during the summer months in temperate areas.[2]
- Infection is easily spread to others via contact with exposed skin.

Etiology

- **S. aureus is the most common cause of both forms of impetigo.**[2]
- β-hemolytic streptococci (primarily *Streptococcus pyogenes*) may cause nonbullous impetigo, either alone or as a coinfection with *S. aureus*.
- Bullous impetigo is caused by *S. aureus* strains that produce **exfoliative toxin A**.[3]
  - Cases caused by community-acquired methicillin-resistant *S. aureus* (CA-MRSA) are increasing, although the majority of cases are caused by methicillin-sensitive strains.[3]
  - Many CA-MRSA isolates do not possess the gene encoding for this virulence factor.[4]

Pathophysiology

- Streptococcal impetigo begins with skin colonization, followed by inoculation of the organisms via minor skin trauma. Staphylococcal impetigo is usually preceded by nasal colonization.
- *S. aureus* produces exfoliative toxin A, which causes disruption of the adhesive junctions in the superficial epidermis in bullous impetigo.

Risk Factors

- Poverty, poor hygiene, and crowded living conditions increase the likelihood of transmission.
- Minor trauma, insect bites, and inflammatory dermatoses also increase the risk of acquisition.[1]

DIAGNOSIS

Clinical Presentation

- Characteristic painful skin lesions are generally the only presenting complaint.
- Systemic symptoms are rare, but local lymphadenitis may be present.
- The lesions of nonbullous impetigo usually occur on the exposed areas of the face or extremities, whereas bullous impetigo is more commonly found on the trunk.

- Nonbullous impetigo begins with papules that develop into vesicles on a bed of erythema. These lesions enlarge to form pustules that rupture and become coated in a characteristic **thick golden crust** over the course of 4 to 6 days.
- Bullous impetigo begins with fragile vesicles that rapidly enlarge into flaccid fluid-filled bullae. These bullae frequently rupture and leave a thin brown crust.

Differential Diagnosis

The differential diagnosis includes contact dermatitis, bullous pemphigoid, and Stevens–Johnson syndrome.

Diagnostic Testing

- An appropriate history and clinical appearance are diagnostic.
- Lesions that fail to respond to appropriate therapy should be cultured and alternative diagnoses considered.

TREATMENT

- Topical therapy is as effective as oral systemic antibiotics in patients with few lesions.
  - **Topical mupirocin** (2% applied three times daily) is the first-line topical agent.[1] Resistance to this agent among staphylococcal strains is increasing, and treatment should be reassessed if there is no clinical improvement within 3 to 5 days.
  - **Topical retapamulin** (1% applied twice daily) has been FDA approved for treatment and has comparable efficacy to mupirocin.[5]
- Oral systemic antibiotics should be used in cases of widespread disease or if lesions are present in an area where topical therapy is not practical.
  - A penicillinase-resistant penicillin (dicloxacillin), β-lactam/β-lactamase inhibitor combination (amoxicillin/clavulanate), or first-generation cephalosporin (cephalexin) can be used as these agents are active against streptococci and β-lactamase-producing strains of *S. aureus* (see Table 9-1).[1]
  - Clindamycin should be used when MRSA is suspected or in cases of serious β-lactam allergy. Linezolid should be considered if there is a high rate of inducible clindamycin resistance in the area (see Table 9-2).
- Duration of therapy should be based on clinical response but is generally 7 to 10 days.[1]
- Hand-washing should be promoted, and patients and family members should be educated in ways to improve personal hygiene when applicable.

COMPLICATIONS

Poststreptococcal glomerulonephritis may rarely follow streptococcal impetigo, but acute rheumatic fever has not been reported following streptococcal impetigo.

Abscesses, Furuncles, and Carbuncles

GENERAL PRINCIPLES

Classification

- Skin abscesses are purulent infections that involve the dermis and deeper cutaneous tissue.
- Furuncles ("boils") are similar to skin abscesses but involve the hair follicles with small subcutaneous abscesses.
- A carbuncle is a collection of furuncles that form a single suppurative lesion that drains through multiple hair follicles.

TABLE 9-1	ANTIBIOTIC DOSING AND ROUTES OF ADMINISTRATION FOR SELECTED ANTIBIOTICS COMMONLY USED IN SKIN AND SOFT TISSUE INFECTIONS

Antibiotic	Dosage and Administration	
	Adults	**Children**
Oral Options		
Penicillin V	500 mg four times daily	<12 y: 25–50 mg/kg/d divided three to four times daily (max 3 g/d)
		≥12 y: 500 mg four times daily
Dicloxacillin	500 mg four times daily	<40 kg: 25–50 mg/kg/d divided four times daily (max 2 g/d)
		≥40 kg: 500 mg four times daily
Cephalexin	500 mg four times daily	25–50 mg/kg/d divided four times daily (max 4 g/d)
Clindamycin	300–450 mg three to four times daily	30–40 mg/kg/d divided three to four times daily (max 1.8 g/d)
Amoxicillin–clavulanate	875 mg twice daily	<16 y and <40 kg: 25–45 mg amoxicillin component/kg/d divided every 12 h
		≥16 y or ≥40 kg: 875 mg twice daily
Intravenous Options		
Penicillin G	3–4 million units intravenously every 4 h	100,000–400,000 units/kg/d divided every 4–6 h (max 24 million units/d)
Oxacillin	1–2 g every 4 h	100–200 mg/kg/d divided every 4–6 h (max 12 g/d)
Ampicillin–sulbactam	1.5–3 g every 6 h	100–200 mg ampicillin/kg/d divided every 6 h (max 12 g/d)
Cefazolin	1–1.5 g every 8 h	25–100 mg/kg/d divided every 6–8 h (max 6 g/d)
Cefepime	1 g every 12 h (increase to 2 g for treatment of *Pseudomonas aeruginosa*)	50 mg/kg/dose every 12 h (max 2 g/dose)
Piperacillin–tazobactam	4.5 g every 8 h (increase to every 6 h for treatment of *P. aeruginosa*)	240 mg piperacillin/kg/d divided every 8 h (increase to 300–400 mg piperacillin/kg/d divided every 6 h for treatment of *P. aeruginosa*, max 16 g/d)
Meropenem	500 mg every 8 h	10 mg/kg/dose every 8 h (max 500 mg/dose)
Clindamycin	600–900 mg every 8 h	25–40 mg/kg/d divided every 6–8 h (max 2.7 g/d)
Vancomycin	15–20 mg/kg every 12 h	15–20 mg/kg/dose every 6–8 h

TABLE 9-2	ANTIBIOTIC THERAPY FOR COMMUNITY-ACQUIRED METHICILLIN-RESISTANT *STAPHYLOCOCCUS AUREUS*	

Antibiotic Name	Dosage and Administration	
	Adults	Children
Oral Options		
Trimethoprim–sulfamethoxazole	Two double-strength tablets twice daily	Age >2 mo: 8–12 mg TMP/kg/d divided twice daily (max 320 mg TMP/d)
Clindamycin	300–450 mg three to four times daily	30–40 mg/kg/d divided three to four times daily (max 1.8 g/d)
Doxycycline	100 mg twice daily	Avoid use in children <8 y of age 2–4 mg/kg/d divided twice daily (max 200 mg/d)
Linezolid	600 mg twice daily	<12 y: 30 mg/kg/d divided three times daily ≥12 y: 20 mg/kg/d divided twice daily (max 1200 mg/d)
Tedizolid	200 mg daily	Not FDA approved in children, insufficient data
Intravenous Options		
Clindamycin	600–900 mg every 8 h	25–40 mg/kg/d divided every 6–8 h (max 2.7 g/d)
Vancomycin	15–20 mg/kg every 12 h	15–20 mg/kg/dose every 6–8 h
Daptomycin	6 mg/kg every 24 h	Not FDA approved in children 6 mg/kg every 24 h
Ceftaroline	600 mg every 12 h	Not FDA approved in children
Linezolid	600 mg every 12 h	<12 y: 30 mg/kg/d divided every 8 h ≥12 y: 20 mg/kg/d divided every 12 h (max 1200 mg/d)
Tedizolid	200 mg 24 h	Not FDA approved in children
Telavancin	10 mg/kg every 24 h	Not FDA approved in children
Tigecycline[a]	100 mg × 1 dose, then 50 mg every 12 h	Not FDA approved ≥12 y: 1.5 mg/kg × 1 dose (max 100 mg), then 1 mg/kg/dose every 12 h (max 50 mg)
Dalbavancin	1000 mg × 1 then 500 mg 1 wk later	Not FDA approved in children
Oritavancin	1200 mg IV × 1	Not FDA approved in children

[a]There may be an increased risk of mortality when using tigecycline in comparison with other antibiotics when treating serious infections.

Epidemiology

- Skin abscesses are very common and account for more than 3 million emergency center visits each year.[6] Furuncles and carbuncles are also common.
- Outbreaks of cutaneous abscesses and furunculosis, usually caused by *S. aureus*, can occur with close contact.[1]

Etiology

- **S. aureus is the predominant cause of skin abscesses, furuncles, and carbuncles.** CA-MRSA causes up to 75% of these infections in some centers.[7]
- Other organisms less frequently cause these infections, depending on environmental and host factors.
  - ○ Lesions adjacent to a mucous membrane (perioral, vulvovaginal, or perirectal) or associated with injection drug use may be polymicrobial.
  - ○ Furuncles may also be caused by other organisms in skin flora, including *Candida* species.
  - ○ *Pseudomonas aeruginosa* or atypical mycobacteria are seen with a history of water exposure.

Pathophysiology

- Inoculation of bacteria through nonintact skin is the most frequent cause of skin abscesses, although bacteremic seeding of the skin can occur.
- Furuncles can result as a progression of folliculitis. These infections may occur anywhere on hairy skin but are usually found in areas exposed to friction or maceration (e.g., neck, axilla, and buttocks).
- Carbuncles are more likely to occur in the back of the neck and lower extremities.[1]
- Panton–Valentine leukocidin, a cytotoxin causing leukocyte destruction and tissue necrosis, is found in some strains of *S. aureus* and has been associated with necrotic skin lesions.[8]

Risk Factors

- Risk factors for cutaneous MRSA infections are presented in Table 9-3.
- Conditions leading to minor breaches in the skin (intravenous or subcutaneous drug use, dermatological conditions, and abrasions).

TABLE 9-3	RISK FACTORS ASSOCIATED WITH COMMUNITY-ACQUIRED METHICILLIN-RESISTANT *STAPHYLOCOCCUS AUREUS* (CA-MRSA) SKIN AND SOFT TISSUE INFECTIONS

Household or day-care contacts of a patient with proven community-associated MRSA infection

Children

Men who have sex with men

Military personnel

Incarcerated persons

Athletes, particularly in contact sports

Native Americans or Pacific Islanders

History of MRSA infection

Intravenous drug users

Hemodialysis

DIAGNOSIS

Clinical Presentation

- The presence of characteristic skin lesions is generally the only complaint.
- There may be a history of skin infections in close contacts or in the patient's past history.
- Skin abscesses appear as painful, erythematous, fluctuant nodules that often have an overlying pustule.
- Furuncles have a similar appearance, with a hair emerging through the pustule.
- Carbuncles present as a fluctuant mass with purulent drainage from multiple hair follicles.
- Scarring may occur, especially after multiple recurrences.

Differential Diagnosis

- Folliculitis is more superficial and without purulent drainage.
- Hidradenitis suppurativa is similar but has a more chronic course.
- Epidermoid cysts can be confused with skin abscesses.
- Skin lesions secondary to systemic infections with *Pseudomonas*, *Aspergillus*, *Nocardia*, or *Cryptococcus* can be seen in immunocompromised patients.

Diagnostic Testing

- Culture and Gram stain are helpful, especially with changing resistance profiles of CA-MRSA.
- In appropriate settings, stains and cultures for fungi and mycobacteria may be beneficial.

TREATMENT

- **Skin abscesses, large furuncles, and carbuncles should be incised and drained.**
- **Antibiotic therapy is often not necessary.** It should be considered in patients with extensive disease, surrounding cellulitis, systemic symptoms, abscesses in areas that are difficult to drain (i.e., face) and immunocompromise.
- Therapy should be directed against *S. aureus*, including MRSA. Oral antibiotics can be used for uncomplicated cases; patients that require hospital admission should receive intravenous antibiotics (see Table 9-2 for treatment options for CA-MRSA). Antibiotic duration is based on clinical response, typically 5 to 10 days.
- Small furuncles can be treated with warm compresses.
- Patients should be educated on ways to improve personal hygiene and wound care when appropriate.

SPECIAL CONSIDERATIONS

- Antibiotic prophylaxis is given before incision and drainage of skin and soft tissue infections in patients with underlying cardiac conditions associated with the highest risk of adverse outcome from infective endocarditis. More than 20% of patients with *S. aureus* skin infection who require incision and drainage will suffer at least one recurrence.[9]
- Recurrent skin infections are associated with *S. aureus* colonization of the nares or skin, and eradication of *S. aureus* in those with positive nasal swabs may decrease infection rates. **Decolonization may be considered if patients have recurrent infection despite appropriate hygiene interventions** (see Table 9-4 for decolonization regimen).

TABLE 9-4	OUTPATIENT REGIMEN FOR ERADICATION OF NASAL CARRIAGE OF *STAPHYLOCOCCUS AUREUS*

- Careful attention to personal hygiene.
- Avoid sharing personal items (i.e., razors, soaps, lotions, linens) and discard or launder all potentially contaminated personal items midway through decolonization regimen.
- Thoroughly clean household surfaces with cleaning solution active against methicillin-resistant *S. aureus* (i.e., bleach solution).
- Mupirocin 2% ointment should be applied to nares twice daily for 5–10 d.
- 4% chlorhexidine whole-body wash once daily for 5–14 d. May substitute dilute bleach baths twice weekly for 3 mo.
- Oral regimens should be reserved for cases of recurrence despite the above measures and may include oral rifampin plus trimethoprim–sulfamethoxazole or clindamycin.

Cellulitis and Erysipelas

GENERAL PRINCIPLES

Classification

- Cellulitis involves the deeper dermis and subcutaneous fat.
- Erysipelas is a more superficial infection that involves the upper layers of the dermis and superficial lymphatics.

Epidemiology

- Cellulitis is a relatively common condition with an estimated incidence rate of 25/1000 person-years. The incidence is greatest in the middle-aged and elderly.
- The estimated incidence of erysipelas is about 0.1/1000 person-years. Erysipelas has a bimodal age distribution.

Etiology

- Any breakdown in the cutaneous barrier allows the entry and spread of organisms colonizing the skin surface.
- **The majority of cases are caused by gram-positive bacteria, with β-hemolytic streptococci, particularly *S. pyogenes,* accounting for as much as 80%.**
- *S. aureus* (both methicillin-sensitive and methicillin-resistant strains) is a common cause of cellulitis in some regions of the United States.
- Other organisms can cause cellulitis depending on host and environmental factors (see Table 9-5).

Risk Factors

- Surgical incisions, trauma, ulcerations, inflammatory dermatoses, and fissures secondary to tinea pedis are common predisposing skin disruptions.[10,11]
- Obesity, venous insufficiency, disruption of lymphatic drainage, and other conditions that cause chronic edema increase the risk of skin infection and may contribute to recurrent disease.
- Risk factors for CA-MRSA infections are outlined in Table 9-3.

TABLE 9-5	UNUSUAL ORGANISMS IN SKIN AND SOFT TISSUE INFECTIONS	

Organism	Clues to Diagnosis	Other Considerations
Water Exposure		
Vibrio vulnificus	Saltwater exposure	Treatment of choice for mild infections is doxycycline
Aeromonas hydrophila	Freshwater exposure	Treatment of choice for mild infections is ciprofloxacin
Mycobacterium marinum	Saltwater or freshwater exposure (lesions often begin as a papule)	Treatment should include two active agents (clarithromycin plus either ethambutol or rifampin is preferred) Duration of therapy is typically 3–4 mo
Streptococcus iniae	Aquaculture workers (usually a localized infection of the hands)	Susceptible to penicillin
Occupational Exposure		
Erysipelothrix rhusiopathiae	Occupational animal exposure (fishermen, butchers, veterinarians) (usually a localized infection of the hands)	Susceptible to penicillin
Bites and Injuries		
Human oral flora (peptostreptococci, Eikenella corrodens, Viridans streptococci)	Human bite	Treatment of choice for mild infections is amoxicillin–clavulanate
Pasteurella multocida and Capnocytophaga canimorsus	Dog or cat bite	Cat bites warrant prophylactic antibiotics because of high rate of infection. Treatment of choice is amoxicillin–clavulanate
Clostridium tetani	Devitalized tissue (e.g., crush injury) or wound contamination with soil or rust	Can progress to generalized tetanus characterized most often by trismus ("lockjaw"). Age-appropriate tetanus vaccine should be given if ≥10 y since last vaccine in minor, clean wounds or if ≥5 y since last vaccine for all other wounds. Tetanus immunoglobulin should be given to patients with unknown or incomplete vaccination status in all but minor, clean wounds.

TABLE 9-5	UNUSUAL ORGANISMS IN SKIN AND SOFT TISSUE INFECTIONS (CONTINUED)	
Organism	**Clues to Diagnosis**	**Other Considerations**
Immunosuppression		
Cryptococcus neoformans	Impairment of cell-mediated immunity	Represents disseminated disease. Fluconazole is the treatment of choice.
Helicobacter cinaedi	HIV infection; multifocal cellulitis	Represents disseminated infection with bacteremia. Treatment is not well-defined.
Candida species	Impairment of cell-mediated immunity	Represents disseminated infection. Treatment with echinocandins (e.g., micafungin). If *Candida parapsilosis*, use lipid formulation amphotericin B.
Aspergillus species	Impairment of cell-mediated immunity	Can be either disseminated infection or local infection. Treatment with voriconazole is recommended.
Fusarium species	Impairment of cell-mediated immunity	Generally localized infection but can become disseminated. Treatment with high-dose IV voriconazole or posaconazole.
Mucor/Rhizopus	Impairment of cell-mediated immunity	Generally localized infection but can be disseminated. Treatment with lipid formulation amphotericin B or posaconazole.

DIAGNOSIS

Clinical Presentation

History
- Both cellulitis and erysipelas present as a **spreading area of cutaneous erythema, warmth, edema, and pain**.
- Systemic symptoms, such as fever and chills, are more common with erysipelas.
- Careful assessment of risk factors for unusual pathogens or CA-MRSA (see Tables 9-3 and 9-5) should be performed.

Physical Examination
- Both infections mainly occur on the lower extremities, although any body site may be affected. Erysipelas has been associated with a butterfly distribution on the face.
- They present as areas of skin warmth, edema, and erythema without an underlying focus of infection.
- Erysipelas appears as a raised lesion with clearly demarcated borders, whereas the borders in cellulitis are less distinct.[1]
- Skin may have an orange peel appearance (peau d'orange) due to superficial edema surrounding tethered hair follicles. There may be associated lymphangitis.
- Vesicles, bullae, petechiae, and ecchymoses may also occur.

Differential Diagnosis

- Differentiation from necrotizing fasciitis (NF) is essential (see section "Necrotizing Fasciitis").
- Deeper foci of infection, such as osteomyelitis, septic arthritis, and bursitis, may present with overlying cutaneous inflammation.
- Herpes zoster, erythema migrans, and viral exanthems may present with erythema.
- Cutaneous malignancies, contact dermatitis, insect bites, gout, drug reactions, vasculitis, thrombophlebitis, and lipodermatosclerosis may mimic the appearance of cellulitis.

Diagnostic Testing

- Signs of inflammation such as elevated white blood cell (WBC) count or elevated erythrocyte sedimentation rate and C-reactive protein (CRP) may be present.
- Blood cultures are positive in <5% of cases and are usually performed only when signs of systemic toxicity are present.
- Cultures of intact skin are usually not helpful, but cultures of purulent discharge, unroofed vesicles, or bullae may be beneficial in cases where unusual or drug-resistant pathogens are suspected.

TREATMENT

Oral antibiotics are appropriate in mild infection, but intravenous administration should be used in patients with systemic symptoms or those that cannot tolerate oral intake (see Tables 9-1 or 9-2).

- **Erysipelas:**
  - If there is any uncertainty regarding the diagnosis, the patient should be treated as per the cellulitis recommendations.
  - **As the majority of cases of erysipelas are caused by streptococci, penicillin or amoxicillin remains the treatment of choice.**
    - Patients with penicillin allergy may be treated with cephalosporins, in the absence of severe reactions, or clindamycin.
    - If suspicion of *S. aureus* is high, an antistaphylococcal penicillin (i.e., dicloxacillin) or first-generation cephalosporin (i.e., cephalexin) should be used.
- **Cellulitis**
  - Empiric therapy should be directed toward β-hemolytic streptococci and *S. aureus*.
    - Appropriate oral options include **dicloxacillin, amoxicillin/clavulanate, or cephalexin**. Clindamycin may be used in patients with severe β-lactam allergies.
    - Parental antibiotic options include oxacillin or cefazolin. Clindamycin or vancomycin may be used in patients with severe β-lactam allergies.
  - Patients with risk factors for MRSA infections (Table 9-3), from a community with a prevalence of MRSA >30%, with evidence of systemic toxicity, or with failure to respond to treatment, should be treated with empiric antimicrobials effective against MRSA (see Table 9-2).
    - Vancomycin is the most appropriate initial intravenous agent. Daptomycin, linezolid, tedizolid, telavancin, ceftaroline, oritavancin, and dalbavancin can be considered in patients unable to tolerate vancomycin or with a known history of vancomycin-intermediate or vancomycin-resistant *S. aureus*. Clindamycin may also be considered if the cellulitis is community-acquired and the local resistance rates among CA-MRSA strains are low.
    - Linezolid is an appropriate choice for oral therapy. Clindamycin may also be given orally if local resistance rates are low. Trimethoprim–sulfamethoxazole should be avoided unless it is certain that the infection is not due to streptococci.

○ Treatment duration should be based on clinical response. Uncomplicated cases require only a 5-day course of antibiotic treatment[1]; however, longer treatment durations, usually 7 to 14 days, are necessary for complicated infections or those caused by drug-resistant pathogens such as MRSA.

○ Patients with clinical presentations or risk factors for more unusual pathogens (Table 9-5) should be treated with empiric therapy directed toward these organisms.

○ Elevation of the affected area reduces edema and may prevent lymphedema.[1]

○ Treatment of underlying conditions (edema, ulcerations, dermatoses, and tinea infection) will reduce the risk of recurrence.[1]

COMPLICATIONS

• Acute complications include thrombophlebitis, NF, abscess formation, bacteremia, and toxic shock syndrome (TSS).

• Symptoms usually worsen in the first 24 hours of treatment because of exacerbation of inflammation.

OUTCOME/PROGNOSIS

• Most cases of cellulitis and erysipelas resolve with treatment.

• Recurrence is common, occurring in 15% to 30% of patients.

• Recurrent episodes of cellulitis can lead to cumulative lymphatic damage and lymphedema.

Necrotizing Fasciitis, Including Fournier Gangrene

GENERAL PRINCIPLES

Definition

NF is a life-threatening infection characterized by necrosis of the subcutaneous tissues with progression along superficial and deep fascia.[12]

Epidemiology

• NF is rare, occurring in less than 0.5 per 100,000 population.

• **NF type 1** is often associated with surgical wounds in immunocompromised patients.

• **NF type 2** is usually a spontaneous community-acquired infection that may occur in healthy individuals.

Etiology

• **In NF type 1, an average of five organisms are involved**, including mixed obligate anaerobes (*Bacteroides* or *Peptostreptococcus*), facultative anaerobes (streptococcal species or *S. aureus*), and aerobic coliforms (*Escherichia coli* or *Klebsiella*).[1]

• **NF type 2 is usually due to *S. pyogenes***, but mixed infection with *S. pyogenes* and *S. aureus* has been reported. *S. aureus* (MRSA), *Vibrio vulnificus*, *Aeromonas hydrophila*, and other streptococci have also been reported in patients with risk factors for these organisms.[1]

Pathophysiology

• NF type 1 occurs following surgery, dental disease or oral trauma (cervical NF), urethral or lower gastrointestinal (GI) trauma (Fournier gangrene), or decubitus or lower extremity ulcerations.

- NF type 2 results from infection of a minor skin lesion, but 20% of cases have no apparent skin breakdown.
  - Once *S. pyogenes* gains access to deep tissues, secreted proteases degrade extracellular matrix.
  - Streptococcal virulence proteins prevent phagocytosis, inhibit neutrophil function, and cause neutrophil apoptosis.
  - Production of superantigens results in excessive immune response and triggers release of cytokines, leading to severe tissue damage, ischemia, and shock.
  - This necrotizing process spreads along superficial facial planes, causing a rapidly progressive and severe illness.

Risk Factors
- NF type 1 is most frequently associated with surgical procedure or trauma.
- NF type 2 may be associated with diabetes or peripheral vascular disease but can occur as a sequelae of varicella or trauma.

DIAGNOSIS

Clinical Presentation
- NF is an infectious disease and surgical emergency, and early diagnosis is crucial.
- NF can be difficult to differentiate from cellulitis or other soft tissue infections, but several characteristic features should cause the clinician to consider the diagnosis.
  - Pain out of proportion to physical findings
  - Induration that extends beyond the area of visual skin involvement
  - Crepitus or subcutaneous gas
  - Rapid progression of skin findings
  - Systemic toxicity out of proportion to clinical findings
  - Failure to respond to appropriate medical therapy
- Patients may complain of exquisite pain early in the course of illness. This is followed by anesthesia as NF progresses.
- Findings may initially be quite subtle or indistinguishable from cellulitis. A dusky appearance to the skin, the presence of bullae, and/or crepitus are relatively specific findings for NF.

Differential Diagnosis
NF is most commonly mistaken for cellulitis, clostridial myonecrosis (CM), or pyomyositis.

Diagnostic Testing
- The Laboratory Risk Indicator for Necrotizing Fasciitis (LRINEC) includes several common laboratory findings. When severe skin infection is present, a score of ≥6 has a positive predictive value of 92% for NF.[13]
  - Elevated CRP >150 mg/L (4 points)
  - Leukocytosis with WBCs 15,000 to 25,000/μL (1 point) or >25,000/μL (2 points)
  - Anemia with hemoglobin 11 to 13.5 g/dL (1 point) or <11 g/dL (2 points)
  - Hyponatremia with Na <135 mmol/L (2 points)
  - Renal insufficiency with serum creatinine >1.6 mg/dL (2 points)
  - Serum glucose >180 mg/dL (1 point)
- Blood cultures are positive in 60% of cases of NF type 2 but are only positive in 20% of NF type 1 cases.
- Intraoperative cultures are most reliable and should be used to guide antibiotic therapy.
- Soft tissue plain radiographs, CT, or MRI may show subcutaneous gas or fascial edema.

TREATMENT

- **Treatment is both surgical and medical and should proceed rapidly.**
- Early surgical intervention with aggressive debridement is crucial and has been shown to decrease mortality.[1,14]
- Repeat evaluation in the operating room 24 to 36 hours after the initial debridement and daily thereafter until debridement is complete is usually required.[1]
- **Broad-spectrum antibiotics** should be initially directed at the likely causative organisms and modified as Gram stain and culture data are available.[1,14]
- Empiric broad-spectrum coverage to treat NF can be achieved with a **carbapenem** (meropenem), **extended-spectrum penicillin with a β-lactamase** inhibitor (piperacillin–tazobactam), or **cefepime in combination with metronidazole** (see Table 9-1), **plus:**
  ○ An **agent with activity against MRSA**, such as vancomycin, daptomycin, or linezolid (see Table 9-2), **plus.**
  ○ **Clindamycin** (see Tables 9-1 or 9-2) to inhibit toxin production. If the infection is due to *S. pyogenes*, therapy may be narrowed to penicillin and clindamycin. Linezolid may have some antitoxin effects as well but should not replace clindamycin for this purpose.

OUTCOME/PROGNOSIS

- Mortality remains >20% and can approach 50% when associated with TSS.[15,16]
- Morbidity, including disfigurement and limb loss, is common even with appropriate intervention.

Pyomyositis

GENERAL PRINCIPLES

- Pyomyositis is a suppurative infection of the skeletal muscle.
- In tropical regions, pyomyositis is most common in otherwise healthy young children and adults.
- Pyomyositis in temperate regions is generally a disease of immunocompromised young adults.[1]
- *S. aureus* is the most common cause, accounting for over 90% of tropical cases and 70% of temperate cases. MRSA is emerging as a common pathogen.[17] *S. pyogenes* is second, followed by other streptococci, enteric gram-negative bacilli, or polymicrobial infections. *Bartonella*, mycobacteria, or anaerobes are rare causes.[17]
- Seeding of the skeletal muscle occurs during an episode of bacteremia.
- Muscle trauma, which may be clinically unapparent, forms a nidus for infection and abscess formation.
- **Around 50% of patients with pyomyositis in temperate areas have an underlying medical condition**, including HIV, diabetes mellitus, rheumatologic diseases, malignancies, or other immunocompromised states.[17]
- **About 50% of patients have a known history of trauma.** Strenuous exercise may lead to pyomyositis in young athletes.

DIAGNOSIS

Clinical Presentation

- Localized pain, swelling, and cramping in the involved muscle group occur.
- Systemic symptoms, such as fever and chills, are common.
- The lower extremity muscles, especially the thigh, are most commonly involved, but chest, abdominal, and gluteal muscle involvement has been reported.[17]

- Multiple muscle groups are infected in up to 20% of cases.
- Superficial signs of inflammation on examination may not be initially present.
- The overlying area is often indurated and has a woody or brawny appearance.

Differential Diagnosis

The differential diagnosis includes muscle hematoma, osteomyelitis, severe cellulitis, NF, neoplasms, deep vein thrombosis, and muscle strains.

Diagnostic Testing

Laboratories
- Although pyomyositis is an infection of skeletal muscle, creatine kinase levels are often normal or only mildly elevated.[17]
- Blood cultures are positive in up to 30% of cases.[1]
- *S. aureus* pyomyositis should prompt an evaluation for endocarditis.

Imaging
- Ultrasound (US) may show hyperechogenicity due to muscle edema and hypoechogenicity from muscle necrosis.
- CT can detect muscle edema and rim-enhancing fluid collections indicative of abscesses.
- MRI is most sensitive in early infections and helps localize and identify the extent of muscle damage.[18]

Diagnostic Procedures
- Cultures should be obtained under US or CT guidance before antibiotic administration when possible.
- Intraoperative specimens should also be sent for culture and antibiotic susceptibilities.

TREATMENT

- Drainage by interventional radiology, or surgical drainage and debridement, is essential.
- For immunocompetent patients, empiric antibiotic therapy with vancomycin (see Table 9-1) is an effective therapy for both MRSA and *S. pyogenes* (see Table 9-2 for alternative treatments of MRSA).
- Immunocompromised patients should receive vancomycin in combination with other broad-spectrum antibiotics such as meropenem or piperacillin–tazobactam (see Table 9-1).
- Antibiotic therapy should be adjusted as culture results become available.
- Duration of therapy should be guided by clinical response but is generally 3 to 4 weeks in the absence of endocarditis or osteomyelitis.

COMPLICATIONS

- Endocarditis or osteomyelitis may be present secondary to bacteremia.
- Compartment syndrome requiring fasciotomy may occur.

Clostridial Myonecrosis or Gas Gangrene

GENERAL PRINCIPLES

Definition
- CM is a necrotizing infection of the skeletal muscle secondary to *Clostridium*. It is also commonly known as "gas gangrene."[1,19]
- It can be spontaneous or traumatic, including postsurgical.

Epidemiology

- Traumatic CM occurs in wounds complicated by compromised vascular supply.
- Spontaneous CM is usually seen in patients with neutropenia or GI malignancy.[1]

Etiology

- *Clostridium* species are anaerobic, gram-positive, spore-forming bacilli that are found in the soil and human GI tract.
- Traumatic CM is most frequently caused by *Clostridium perfringens*.
- Spontaneous CM is usually caused by *Clostridium septicum*.[1]

Pathophysiology

- Inoculation of *Clostridium* into deep tissue via crush injuries, stab wounds, or gunshot wounds that have created an anaerobic environment (caused by interruption of vascular supply) leads to traumatic CM.
- Spontaneous CM results when disruption in the GI mucosa allows *Clostridium* to spread hematogenously and seed the muscle.
- Once the muscle is seeded, infection proceeds very rapidly, sometimes in less than 24 hours.
- Clostridia cause this disease through the production of at least 10 different exotoxins, although the α-toxin is the most important. α-toxin hydrolyzes cell membranes and leads to tissue necrosis, hemolysis, platelet aggregation, and leukocyte inactivation. α-toxin also has a direct cardiodepressive effect that causes profound shock.[19,20]

Risk Factors

- Peripartum complications (i.e., abortion, retained placenta, prolonged rupture of membranes, and retained fetal tissue), subcutaneous drug injection ("skin popping"), surgery of the GI tract, and intramuscular injections are all risk factors.
- Spontaneous CM occurs not only with GI malignancy but also in immunocompromised patients (e.g., neutropenia and hematologic malignancy).

DIAGNOSIS

Clinical Presentation

- Traumatic CM should be suspected in cases of severe pain at the site of the surgical incision or trauma within 24 hours of the event accompanied by signs of systemic toxicity.
- Spontaneous CM should be suspected in cases of abrupt onset of muscle pain and signs of systemic toxicity in the setting of known immunocompromise or GI disease, although these may not be immediately apparent.
- Overlying skin may initially appear pale, followed by a violaceous or erythematous discoloration and bullae.
- The area is extremely tender to palpation, and underlying crepitus may be present.
- Patients may progress rapidly to severe shock.

Differential Diagnosis

- NF or pyomyositis can mimic CM.
- Spontaneous CM may be confused initially with muscle strain, injury, or other conditions leading to myalgia, such as influenza.

Diagnostic Testing

- Complete blood count and complete metabolic panel may show leukocytosis and signs of multiorgan failure including coagulopathy, hemolytic anemia, and renal and liver failure. The hemolytic anemia can be severe and recalcitrant to transfusion.

- Blood cultures are positive for *C. perfringens* in about 15% of cases of traumatic CM.
- Large, gram-variable rods may be recovered from wounds, bullae, and surgical samples.
- Plain films, CT scan, or MRI may demonstrate gas within tissue.

TREATMENT

- **Immediate surgical consultation should be sought when CM is suspected.**
- Early surgical debridement, antibiotics, and intensive supportive measures are required.
- Surgical intervention is often needed for definitive diagnosis and emergent treatment.
  - Necrotic, edematous, pale/gray muscle tissue that does not bleed or contract is often seen at the time of surgery.
  - There is usually an obvious release of gas on surgically entering the infected muscle.
  - Pathology reveals gas, cell lysis, and absent inflammation.
- Multiple repeated surgical debridements are often necessary.
- The recommended antibiotic regimen is **penicillin and clindamycin** for clostridial infections (see Table 9-1). Infection due to *Clostridium tertium* is treated with vancomycin or metronidazole.
- Empiric broad-spectrum treatment with vancomycin plus either piperacillin/tazobactam, ampicillin/sulbactam, or a carbapenem is recommended until *Clostridium* is identified.
- Patients should be monitored in the intensive care unit with aggressive treatment of shock and multiorgan failure when indicated.
- The role of hyperbaric oxygen remains controversial.[1]

COMPLICATIONS

- Patients can progress quickly to septic shock and multiorgan failure.
- Intravascular hemolysis in the setting of CM can be severe and requires transfusion support.

OUTCOME/PROGNOSIS

- Mortality rates are extremely high for spontaneous CM (67%–100%). Survivors should be evaluated for GI malignancy.[21,22]
- Mortality for traumatic CM is roughly 20%.[23]

Surgical Site Infections

GENERAL PRINCIPLES

Definition

Surgical site infections (SSIs) are defined as the occurrence of infection at or near the site of a surgical procedure within 90 days if prosthetic material is placed at the time of surgery.

Classification

- SSIs are divided into categories based on the infected organ system, body space, or depth of tissue involvement.
- Superficial infections involve the skin or subcutaneous tissue, and deep infections involve the deep soft tissues, muscle, or fascia.

Epidemiology

- SSIs account for 17% of all nosocomial infections.[24]
- Around 3% of patients undergoing surgery will develop an SSI.[1]
- SSIs increase the average cost of a hospital stay by $3000 to $30,000 per case.[25]

Etiology

- *S. aureus*, including MRSA, coagulase-negative staphylococci, enterococci, enteric gram-negative bacilli, and *Pseudomonas* account for the majority of SSIs.[26]
- Multidrug-resistant organisms are common as infections are usually acquired in the hospital setting.[27]
- SSIs that are clinically evident within 48 hours after the procedure are usually due to *S. pyogenes* or *Clostridium* species.[1]
- Procedure site:
  - Genitourinary or GI tract SSIs are often caused by mixed aerobic and anaerobic organisms.
  - Axillary SSIs have a higher rate of gram-negative organisms.
  - Perineal SSIs are usually due to gram-negative organisms and anaerobes.
  - Head and neck SSIs are often caused by oral flora.

Pathophysiology

- SSIs can result from endogenous flora in proximity to the surgical incision, seeding from a distant focus of infection, or exogenous exposures (hands of medical personnel, surgical attire, operative equipment, or aerosolized via the ventilation system).
- Organisms gain access to deep tissues because of breach in the usual anatomic barriers, either through direct inoculation at the time of surgery or postoperatively.
- SSIs may lead to failure of wound healing, dehiscence, and increased scar formation.

Risk Factors

- Patient risk factors include older age, diabetes, poor nutritional status, smoking, obesity, preexisting infection at another body site, colonization with pathogens such as *S. aureus*, immunosuppression, and prolonged preoperative hospital stay.
- Procedure-related factors include longer procedure duration, presence of foreign bodies, contamination of the wound, and inappropriate preparatory measures (prophylactic antibiotic choice, skin preparation, sterilization of equipment, and scrub duration).
- The type of procedure also has a significant impact on the likelihood of SSI, with abdominal procedures carrying the greatest risk.
- The Center for Disease Control and Prevention's (CDC) National Healthcare Safety Network surgical patient risk index incorporates the anesthesiologist preoperative assessment score, cleanliness of the wound, and procedure duration to classify patients into different risk levels for SSIs.[28]

DIAGNOSIS

Clinical Presentation

- With the exception of infection due to *S. pyogenes* or *Clostridium* species, SSIs usually do not become clinically evident until at least 5 days after the operation, with 14 days being typical.[1]
- Examination of the incision usually shows tenderness, swelling, erythema, and purulent drainage.

Diagnostic Criteria

According to the CDC guidelines,[23] superficial SSIs must meet one of the following criteria:

- Purulent drainage from the surgical site
- Organisms isolated from an aseptically obtained culture of fluid or tissue from the incision site or spontaneous dehiscence of a deep incision
- Local signs of infection (pain, edema, erythema, or warmth) in superficial SSIs or the presence of an abscess in deep infections
- Diagnosis of the SSI by the surgeon or attending physician (although practically, the diagnosis is made by a wide variety of health care professionals)

Differential Diagnosis

Organ/space infection should be suspected if superficial SSIs fail to improve despite adequate treatment.

Diagnostic Testing

- Gram stain of drainage is helpful with suspected infection <48 hours after surgery to identify clostridial or streptococcal species.
- Infected surgical sites should be cultured.

TREATMENT

- Early surgical intervention to open the infected wound and to debride necrotic tissue is the hallmark of treatment.
- The role of antibiotics is controversial in patients with minimal signs of systemic toxicity and less impressive wound findings.
- In patients with superficial SSI and fever, tachycardia, >5 cm of erythema surrounding wound, or any wound necrosis, a short course of antibiotics is indicated.[1]
- In deep tissue or organ/space SSIs, choice of empiric therapy and duration of treatment should be guided by the location of the infection and adequacy of the surgical debridement/drainage.
  - Empiric therapy to cover MRSA and streptococcal species with vancomycin (see Tables 9-1 or 9-2) is reasonable for cases where gram-negative and anaerobic organisms are not suspected.
  - Piperacillin–tazobactam, meropenem, or cefepime plus metronidazole may be used when gram-negative and anaerobic treatment is warranted.
  - Antibiotic choice should be modified as Gram stain and culture results become available.

OUTCOME/PROGNOSIS

- Significant morbidity can occur if incision does not heal promptly.
- Deep space and organ infections carry higher morbidity and mortality.

Toxic Shock Syndrome

GENERAL PRINCIPLES

Definition

TSS is a bacterial toxin–mediated illness characterized by acute onset of fever, hypotension, and multiorgan failure.[29]

Classification

TSS is classified based on the causal organism: staphylococcal TSS, which may be menstrual or nonmenstrual, and streptococcal TSS.

Epidemiology

- The overall incidence of staphylococcal TSS is estimated to be 1 to 3.4 per 100,000 women.
  - 90% of staphylococcal TSS cases occur in women, with roughly half of these being associated with menstruation.
  - The incidence of menstrual-associated staphylococcal TSS has significantly declined since the mid-1980s when most superabsorbency tampons were removed from the market.
- Invasive streptococcal diseases occur in an estimated 5 cases per 100,000 patients per year and up to 15% of these patients will develop streptococcal TSS.
- Half of the patients with NF will have associated TSS.

Etiology

- The majority of cases of staphylococcal TSS are caused by methicillin-sensitive strains of *S. aureus*. There are several case reports of TSS due to MRSA.
- Streptococcal TSS is caused by *S. pyogenes*.

Pathophysiology

- Bacterial superantigen production is a crucial component of the pathogenesis. Superantigens bind directly to MHC class II molecules and to T-cell receptors, which trigger excessive **unregulated T-cell activation** in which up to 30% of T cells begin releasing cytokines. This results in an **exaggerated systemic inflammatory response** that causes shock and multiorgan failure.[29]
- Menstrual staphylococcal TSS occurs because of vaginal colonization with a toxin-producing strain of *S. aureus*. **TSS toxin 1** (TSST1) is the superantigen in these cases and is capable of crossing mucosal barriers.
- Nonmenstrual staphylococcal TSS occurs when a toxin-producing *S. aureus* infects a wound or colonizes another mucosal surface. Only about 50% of nonmenstrual cases are caused by organisms that produce TSST1. **Staphylococcal enterotoxin B** can act as an alternative superantigen in TSST1-negative strains.
- Streptococcal TSS is usually associated with invasive diseases such as cellulitis, NF, or pyomyositis. *S. pyogenes* produces multiple virulence proteins that may function as superantigens, such as **streptococcal pyrogenic exotoxins** (SpeA, SpeB).

Risk Factors

- High-absorbency tampons for menstrual staphylococcal TSS
- Disruption of skin or mucous membranes (abscess, surgical procedures, and burns) in patients colonized or infected with the toxin-producing strains of *S. aureus*
- Trauma, surgery, older age, chronic illness, varicella infection, and nonsteroidal anti-inflammatory use predispose patients to invasive streptococcal disease

DIAGNOSIS

Clinical Presentation

History

- Patients with TSS may present with an acute influenza-like illness that rapidly progresses to shock and multiorgan failure within 8 to 12 hours after symptom onset.
- A history of menstruation with tampon use suggests staphylococcal TSS.

- Patients may report a history of trauma or severe pain at the site of infection that can mimic peritonitis or myocardial infarction.

Physical Examination
- Tachycardia, respiratory distress, petechiae, ecchymoses, or jaundice may appear shortly after initial presentation.
- The rash associated with TSS is a **diffuse macular erythema** that may resemble sunburn. It often involves both the skin and mucous membranes, includes the palms and soles, and may be transitory.
- Female patients should undergo vaginal examination, which may reveal hyperemia. Tampons or other foreign bodies should be removed.
- Patients with streptococcal TSS will often have an identifiable focus on examination.

Diagnostic Criteria
- Diagnostic criteria for staphylococcal TSS are presented in Table 9-6.
- Diagnostic criteria for streptococcal TSS are presented in Table 9-7.

Differential Diagnosis

The differential for TSS is broad and includes systemic infections such as gram-negative sepsis (including meningococcemia), Rocky Mountain spotted fever, and leptospirosis in previously healthy individuals.

Diagnostic Testing
- Blood cultures are positive in <5% of cases of staphylococcal TSS, but are positive in roughly 60% of cases of streptococcal TSS.

TABLE 9-6	DIAGNOSTIC CRITERIA FOR STAPHYLOCOCCAL TOXIC SHOCK SYNDROME

1. Fever: ≥38.9°C (°F)
2. Rash: diffuse macular erythroderma
3. Desquamation: occurs 1–2 wk after onset of illness, especially palms and soles
4. Hypotension: systolic blood pressure (BP) ≤90 mm Hg, orthostatic decrease in diastolic BP ≥5 mm Hg
5. Multisystem involvement (≥3 systems):
   a. GI: vomiting or diarrhea
   b. Muscular: severe myalgia or creatine kinase >2× normal
   c. Mucous membranes: vaginal, oropharyngeal, conjunctival hyperemia
   d. Renal: BUN or creatinine >2× normal, pyuria
   e. Hepatic: total bilirubin >2× normal
   f. Hematologic: platelets ≤100,000/μL
   g. CNS: disorientation or alteration of consciousness without focal neurologic signs
6. Negative results of blood, throat, or CSF cultures (blood cultures may be *Staphylococcus aureus* positive) and no rise in antibody titers against *Rickettsia rickettsii*, *Leptospira* spp., and rubeola

Confirmed case satisfies all six criteria.
Probable case satisfies five of six criteria.
BUN, blood urea nitrogen; CNS, central nervous system; CSF, cerebrospinal fluid.

TABLE 9-7	DIAGNOSTIC CRITERIA FOR STREPTOCOCCAL TOXIC SHOCK SYNDROME

1. Hypotension: systolic blood pressure ≤90 mm Hg
2. Two or more of the following:
   a. Renal impairment: creatinine ≥2 mg/dL
   b. Coagulopathy: platelets ≤100,000/µL or disseminated intravascular coagulation
   c. Hepatic involvement: transaminases or bilirubin >2× normal
   d. Generalized, erythematous, macular rash that may desquamate
   e. Adult respiratory distress syndrome
   f. Soft tissue necrosis (necrotizing fasciitis, pyomyositis)

Confirmed case includes isolation of *Streptococcus pyogenes* from a normally sterile site (blood, cerebrospinal fluid, peritoneal fluid, and tissue biopsy) in addition to satisfying both criteria.
Probable case includes isolation of *S. pyogenes* from a nonsterile site (throat, skin, and vagina) in addition to satisfying both criteria.

- Mucosal or wound cultures are positive in up to 90% of patients with staphylococcal TSS.
- Laboratory studies will show signs of multiorgan failure (see Tables 9-6 and 9-7).

TREATMENT

- Staphylococcal and streptococcal TSS should be treated with an appropriate **cell wall–acting antibiotic in combination with clindamycin**.
- Empiric choice of cell wall–acting antibiotic for staphylococcal TSS should include an agent that is effective against MRSA.
  - **Vancomycin** is the typical first-line choice, but linezolid, daptomycin, and telavancin are possible alternatives (see Table 9-2).
  - If *S. aureus* is found to be methicillin sensitive, the patient should be treated with **oxacillin or nafcillin**.
  - **Penicillin** is the most appropriate cell wall–acting antibiotic for the treatment of streptococcal TSS (see Table 9-1).
- As clindamycin binds to the 50S ribosomal subunits and prevents peptide bond formation, it is used to halt toxin production and arrest disease progression. In cases where clindamycin cannot be used, linezolid is an alternative that also arrests toxin production in vitro.
- **Intravenous immunoglobulin** (IVIG) may be considered for the treatment of both streptococcal and staphylococcal TSS with consideration of the following:
  - IVIG contains neutralizing antibodies against many of the superantigens implicated in causing both syndromes.
  - Studies have failed to show statistically significant improvement in patients treated with IVIG due to small samples sizes, but it is generally used, especially if patients are not responding to therapy.[29-31]
- Duration of antibiotic treatment is usually at least 14 days but depends on clinical response, the presence or absence of a focus of infection, and associated bacteremia.
- **Extensive fluid resuscitation is often required.**
- Vasopressors and mechanical ventilation may also be necessary.
- Aggressive debridement of any focus of infection, including SSIs, is important.
- Multiorgan failure is common (see Tables 9-6 and 9-7).

OUTCOME/PROGNOSIS

- Menstrual staphylococcal TSS has the best prognosis with a mortality rate of less than 2%.[32]
- Nonmenstrual staphylococcal TSS has a mortality rate of up to 5%.[32]
- The mortality rate for streptococcal TSS remains high, approximately 40% to 60%.[16,33,34]
- Recurrences of TSS are possible and can occur in one-third of patients with menstrual TSS. Recurrent episodes tend to be less severe.

REFERENCES

1. Stevens DL, Bisno AL, Chambers HF, et al. Practice guidelines for the diagnosis and management of skin and soft tissue infections. *Clin Infect Dis.* 2014;59:1373-1406.
2. Rørtveit S, Rørtveit G. Impetigo in epidemic and nonepidemic phases: an incidence study over 4(½) years in a general population. *Br J Dermatol.* 2007;157:100-105.
3. Durupt F, Mayor L, Bes M, et al. Prevalence of *Staphylococcus aureus* toxins and nasal carriage in furuncles and impetigo. *Br J Dermatol.* 2007;157:1161-1167.
4. Tristan A, Bes M, Meugnier H, et al. Global distribution of Panton-Valentine leukocidin-positive methicillin-resistant *Staphylococcus aureus*, 2006. *Emerg Infect Dis.* 2007;13:594-600.
5. Oranje AP, Chosidow O, Sacchidanand S, et al. Topical retapamulin ointment, 1%, versus sodium fusidate ointment, 2%, for impetigo: a randomized, observer-blinded, noninferiority study. *Dermatology.* 2007;215:331-340.
6. Taira BR, Singer AJ, Thode HC, Lee CC. National epidemiology of cutaneous abscesses: 1996 to 2005. *Am J Emerg Med.* 2009;27:289-292.
7. Moran GJ, Krishnadasan A, Gorwitz RJ, et al. Methicillin-resistant *S. aureus* infections among patients in the emergency department. *N Engl J Med.* 2006;355:666-674.
8. Lina G, Piémont Y, Godail-Gamot F, et al. Involvement of Panton-Valentine leukocidin-producing *Staphylococcus aureus* in primary skin infections and pneumonia. *Clin Infect Dis.* 1999;29:1128-1132.
9. Liu C, Bayer A, Cosgrove SE, et al. Clinical practice guidelines by the Infectious Diseases Society of America for the treatment of methicillin-resistant Staphylococcus aureus infections in adults and children: executive summary. *Clin Infect Dis.* 2011;52:285-292.
10. Björnsdóttir S, Gottfredsson M, Thórisdóttir AS, et al. Risk factors for acute cellulitis of the lower limb: a prospective case-control study. *Clin Infect Dis.* 2005;41:1416-1422.
11. Dupuy A, Benchikhi H, Roujeau J-C, et al. Risk factors for erysipelas of the leg (cellulitis): case-control study. *BMJ.* 1999;318:1591-1594.
12. Brook I, Frazier EH. Clinical and microbiological features of necrotizing fasciitis. *J Clin Microbiol.* 1995;33:2382-2387.
13. Wong CH, Khin LW. Clinical relevance of the LRINEC (Laboratory Risk Indicator for Necrotizing Fasciitis) score for assessment of early necrotizing fasciitis. *Crit Care Med.* 2005;33:1677.
14. Anaya DA, Dellinger EP. Clinical practices: necrotizing soft-tissue infection: diagnosis and management. *Clin Infect Dis.* 2007;44:705-710.
15. Wong CH, Chang HC, Pasupathy S, et al. Necrotizing fasciitis: clinical presentation, microbiology, and determinants of mortality. *J Bone Joint Surg Am.* 2003;85-A:1454-1460.
16. Darenberg J, Luca-Harari G, Jasir A, et al. Molecular and clinical characteristics of invasive group A streptococcal infection in Sweden. *Clin Infect Dis.* 2007;45:450-488.
17. Crum NF. Bacterial pyomyositis in the United States. *Am J Med.* 2004;117:420-428.
18. Turecki MB, Taljanovic MS, Stubbs AY, et al. Imaging of musculoskeletal soft tissue infections. *Skeletal Radiol.* 2010;39:957-971.
19. Stevens DL, Bryant AE. The role of clostridial toxins in the pathogenesis of gas gangrene. *Clin Infect Dis.* 2002;35:S93-S100.
20. Sakurai J, Nagahama M, Oda M. Clostridium perfringens alpha-toxin: characterization and mode of action. *J Biochem.* 2004;136:569-574.
21. Nordkild P, Crone P. Spontaneous clostridial myonecrosis. A collective review and report of a case. *Ann Chir Gynaecol.* 1986;75:274-279.
22. Bodey GP, Rodriquez S, Fainstein V, Elting LS. Clostridial bacteremia in cancer patients. A 12-year experience.*Cancer.* 1991;67:1928-1942.

23. Hart GB, Lamb RC, Strauss MB. Gas gangrene. *J Trauma*. 1983;23:991-1000.
24. Perencevich EN, Sands KE, Cosgrove SE, et al. Health and economic impact of surgical site infections diagnosed after hospital discharge. *Emerg Infect Dis*. 2003;9:196-203.
25. Urban JA. Cost analysis of surgical site infections. *Surg Infect*. 2006;7:S19-S22.
26. Mangram AJ, Horan TC, Pearson ML, et al. Guideline for prevention of surgical site infection, 1999. Hospital Practice Advisory Committee. *Infect Control Hosp Epidemiol*. 1999;20:250-278.
27. Hidron AI, Edwards JR, Patel J, et al. NHSN annual update: antimicrobial-resistant pathogens associated with healthcare-associated infections: annual summary of data reported to the Nation Healthcare Safety Network at the Centers for Disease Control and Prevention, 2006–2007. *Infect Control Hosp Epidemiol*. 2008;29:996-1011.
28. Haley R, Culver DH, Morgan WM, et al. Identifying patients at high risk of surgical wound infection. A simple multivariate index of patient susceptibility and wound contamination. *Am J Epidemiol*. 1985;121:206-215.
29. Lappin E, Ferguson AJ. Gram-positive toxic shock syndromes. *Lancet Infect Dis*. 2009;9:281-290.
30. Darenberg J, Ihendyane N, Sjölin J, et al. Intravenous immunoglobulin G therapy in streptococcal toxic shock syndrome: a European randomized, double-blind, placebo-controlled trial. *Clin Infect Dis*. 2003;37:333-340.
31. Shah SS, Hall M, Srivastava R, et al. Intravenous immunoglobulin in children with streptococcal toxic shock syndrome. *Clin Infect Dis*. 2009;49:1369-1376.
32. Hajjeh RA, Reingold A, Weil A, et al. Toxic shock syndrome in the United States: surveillance update, 1979–1996. *Emerg Infect Dis*. 1999;5:807-810.
33. Hasegawa T, Hashikawa SN, Nakamura T, et al. Factors determining prognosis in streptococcal toxic shock-like syndrome: results of a nationwide investigation in Japan. *Microbes Infect*. 2004;6:1073-1077.
34. Ekelund K, Skinhøj P, Madsen J, Konradsen HB. Reemergence of emm1 and a changed superantigen profile for group A streptococci causing invasive infections: results from a nationwide study. *J Clin Microbiol*. 2005;43:1789-1796.

Central Nervous System Infections

Abdullah Aljorayid and Robyn S. Klein

10

INTRODUCTION

- Central nervous system (CNS) infections can be associated with high morbidity and mortality. A high level of suspicion is necessary to diagnose and treat them as soon as possible.
- The clinical presentation depends on the CNS compartment involved and the pathogen. Infection should be suspected whenever a patient presents with fever, headache, and a change in mental status or focal neurologic involvement.

Meningitis

- Inflammation of the meninges, which usually presents with headache, fever, meningismus, and an elevated number of white blood cells (pleocytosis) in the cerebrospinal fluid (CSF).
- It can be **acute** (hours to days) or **chronic** (symptoms lasting over 4 wk).
- It is classified as bacterial, fungal, parasitic, or aseptic, the latter of which can be infectious (usually viral) or noninfectious, such as drug induced.
- Possible complications of meningitis include brain abscess, hydrocephalus, seizures, respiratory failure, coma, brain stem herniation due to intracranial hypertension, cortical vein phlebitis, sagittal sinus thrombosis, deafness, blindness, and developmental delay.

Acute Meningitis

GENERAL PRINCIPLES

Etiology

- Etiologies vary according to age group and risk factor (see Table 10-1[1]), and empiric therapy is based on these. The cause can be inferred from the cell count and characteristics of the CSF.
  - If there are >1000 neutrophils/mL, the predominant therapy should be directed against bacteria.
  - Lymphocytic pleocytosis, with <100 lymphocytes, would suggest an alternative etiology (see Table 10-2).
- **Bacterial:** The most common organism causing acute meningitis in adults in developed countries is *Streptococcus pneumoniae*, followed by *Neisseria meningitidis*. Type B *Haemophilus influenzae* in industrialized countries has decreased with the introduction of immunization (see below), but it is still an important cause in developing countries. Other etiologies include group B streptococci, enterococci, and gram-negative rods.
  - *Listeria monocytogenes* is an important pathogen in the elderly and immunosuppressed.
  - Coagulase-negative staphylococci and other skin flora are more common in patients with intraventricular shunts. Also, gram-negative rods and group B streptococci are more common in these patients.
  - *Treponema pallidum* (syphilis) can present as acute meningitis in primary syphilis.

TABLE 10-1	MOST COMMON ETIOLOGIES OF ACUTE BACTERIAL MENINGITIS BY AGE AND RISK FACTOR
Age/Risk Factor	**Common Bacterial Pathogens**
<1 mo	*Streptococcus agalactiae, Escherichia coli, Listeria monocytogenes, Klebsiella* spp.
1–23 mo	*Streptococcus pneumoniae, S. agalactiae, Haemophilus influenzae, E. coli, Neisseria meningitidis*
2–50 y	*N. meningitidis, S. pneumoniae*
>50 y	*S. pneumoniae, N. meningitidis, L. monocytogenes,* Gram-negative bacilli
Immunocompromised	*S. pneumoniae, N. meningitidis, L. monocytogenes,* Gram-negative bacilli
Basilar skull fracture	*S. pneumoniae, H. influenzae,* group A β-hemolytic streptococci
Penetrating head trauma	*Staphylococcus aureus,* coagulase-negative *Staphylococcus,* Gram-negative bacilli (including *Pseudomonas aeruginosa*)
Postneurosurgery	*S. aureus,* coagulase-negative staphylococci, Gram-negative bacilli (incl. *P. aeruginosa*)
Cerebrospinal fluid shunt	*Staphylococcus epidermidis* (coagulase-negative staphylococci), *S. aureus,* Gram-negative bacilli, *Propionibacterium acnes*

Adapted from Tunkel AR, Hartman BJ, Kaplan SL, et al. Practice guidelines for the management of bacterial meningitis. *Clin Infectious Dis.* 2004;39(9):1267-1284.

- **Viral: Enteroviruses** account for >85% of viral meningitis. Other viruses include arboviruses (West Nile virus [WNV], Zika virus, St. Louis encephalitis virus), mumps, herpes simplex virus (HSV)-2 (Mollaret meningitis), HSV-1, lymphocytic choriomeningitis virus, and HIV.
- **Fungal:** Usually chronic. In the immunosuppressed, *Histoplasma, Aspergillus,* and *Cryptococcus* can present as acute meningitis.
- **Parasitic:** *Naegleria fowleri, Acanthamoeba* spp., and *Balamuthia mandrillaris* are free-living amebas causing meningoencephalitis, usually fatal. *Angiostrongylus cantonensis* is the most common cause of eosinophilic meningitis outside Europe and North America, predominantly in Southeast Asia, the Pacific Islands, and the Caribbean.[2]
- **Noninfectious: Drugs** (e.g., nonsteroidal anti-inflammatory drugs, trimethoprim–sulfamethoxazole, OKT3 monoclonal antibodies, and carbamazepine) are the most common noninfectious causes of aseptic meningitis. IVIG has also been associated with aseptic meningitis.
- **Posttrauma or surgery:** Skin flora, especially staphylococci and streptococci, are the most common cause of acute meningitis following trauma or manipulation of CNS, followed by oropharyngeal bacteria and Gram-negative rods.

Pathophysiology

- Bacteremia (from nasopharyngeal source or other infected sites) precedes CNS invasion and replication in subarachnoid space. Blood cultures may be helpful in diagnosis.

TABLE 10-2	TYPICAL CEREBROSPINAL FLUID FINDING IN MENINGITIS IN ADULTS				
	Opening Pressure (mm H$_2$O)	White cells/µL	Glucose (mg/dL)	Protein (mg/dL)	Laboratory Diagnosis
Normal	180	0–5	50–75	15–40	None
Bacterial meningitis	⇑	100–5000 neutrophils	<40	100–500	Gram stain, culture
Tuberculous meningitis	⇑	<500 lymphocytes	<50	100–200	Acid-fast bacilli smear, culture, polymerase chain reaction (*PCR; M. tuberculosis*)
Cryptococcal meningitis	⇑	10–200 lymphocytes	<40	50–200	Cryptococcal antigen, India ink stain, fungal culture
Viral meningitis	⇑	10–1000 lymphocytes	Normal	50–100	Virus-specific PCR

- Contiguous spread from adjacent infection (e.g., otitis media, sinusitis, mastoiditis) can also cause meningitis.
- The polysaccharide capsules of *S. pneumoniae* and *H. influenzae* are important virulence factors; patients with hypocomplementemia or splenectomy are at increased risk (due to decreased opsonization).
- Viral invasion may follow viremia, but may also occur via the olfactory nerve and afferent nerve axons (e.g., HSV and arboviruses).
- Enteroviruses are transmitted via the fecal–oral route, and systemic invasion occurs via lymphoid tissues in the gut.

Risk Factors

- Age, lack of vaccination, immunosuppression (drugs, HIV, malignancy), asplenia, alcoholism, disruption of the blood–brain barrier, history of trauma, and presence of intraventricular shunt are major risk factors.
- Enteroviral meningitis is more common in the summer/fall.
- Sharing cups, eating utensil, kissing, hugging with people who are sick.
- Travel to endemic area can be a risk for certain pathogens (bacterial, fungal or parasites).
- Water-related activities are relevant if fungal or parasitic etiologies are considered.
- *L. monocytogenes* can be transmitted via unpasteurized dairy products, deli, or any raw food item.

Prevention

- **Vaccination:** Vaccines are available for *H. influenzae* type B, most strains of meningococcus and pneumococcus.
  - ○ *H. Influenzae*
    - ■ Vaccination against *H. influenzae* type B has led to >90% decreased incidence in developed countries; decreased rates of nasopharyngeal colonization has contributed to herd immunity.

- Current recommendations by the Advisory Committee on Immunization Practices (ACIP) include doses at 2, 4, and 6 months of age, with a booster at 12 to 15 months of age. The vaccine is also recommended for those with asplenia or sickle cell disease if they have not previously received the vaccine. Furthermore, adults with a hematopoietic stem cell transplant should be revaccinated with 3 doses of Hib in at least 4-week intervals 6 to 12 months after transplant regardless of their Hib history.[3]
  - *N. meningitidis*
    - The ACIP recommends one dose of quadrivalent meningococcal vaccine (covers serogroup A, C, W135, Y) for all those within ages 11 to 18 years, as transmission is highest in high schools and colleges.
    - Children between ages 2 and 10 years with risk factors such as asplenia or hypocomplementemia, adults who are splenectomized, and military recruits or travelers to endemic areas, such as sub-Saharan Africa and Saudi Arabia (participants in Hajj), should also be vaccinated. Two doses of quadrivalent vaccine should be given for the special population (e.g., HIV, patient with asplenia).[3]
    - Adults with anatomical or functional asplenia or persistent complement component deficiencies should also receive a series of serogroup B meningococcal vaccine.[3]
  - *S. pneumoniae*: Conjugate pneumococcal vaccines have decreased the rates of invasive pneumococcal disease in children and adults. Recently, invasive disease by serogroups not covered by vaccine has increased.
- **Chemoprophylaxis:**
  - *H. influenzae.* Controversial. ACIP recommends rifampin chemoprophylaxis for the following[4]:
    - Household contacts if one is <4 years and unimmunized.
    - Household contacts of an immunocompromised child regardless of immunization status.
    - All school contacts regardless of age when 2 or more cases occur in <60 days.
    - Index case <2 years or member of household with a susceptible contact treated with regimen other than ceftriaxone or cefotaxime.
  - *N. meningitidis*
    - **Prophylaxis is recommended for close contacts of a patient with meningococcal meningitis.**
    - Close contact is defined as exposure to oral secretions (e.g., kissing, mouth-to-mouth resuscitations, and unprotected endotracheal intubation) or prolonged contact within 3 feet or less, within 1 week before the onset of symptoms until 24 hours after initiation of appropriate antibiotic therapy.
    - **Household contacts, day care contacts, and health care personnel who were exposed to the patient's oral secretions need prophylaxis,** but NOT all health care personnel who are exposed to the patient.
    - The current recommendations for prophylaxis include the following[5]:
      - **Ciprofloxacin.** Only in adults, 500 mg orally once.
      - **Rifampin.** 600 mg PO q12h for 2 days for adults; 10 mg/kg PO q12h for 2 days for children >1 month of age; 5 mg/kg PO q12h for 2 days for infants <1 month of age.
      - **Ceftriaxone.** 250 mg **IM** once in adults and 125 mg **IM** once in children.
    - Chemoprophylaxis is indicated **even in individuals who received meningococcal vaccination in the past,** as it does not protect against serotype B.

DIAGNOSIS

Clinical Presentation

History

- Age, risk factors, exposures, vaccinations, and seasonality should be elicited.
- The patient may complain of acute onset of headache, neck stiffness/pain, and fever.

Physical Examination
- Fever is usually present in all forms of meningitis.
- Meningeal signs include nuchal rigidity and Kernig and Brudzinski signs. However, the absence of these findings does not exclude the diagnosis of meningitis.
- Altered mental status or even coma can be present in patients with prolonged course of symptoms and patients.
- Evidence of intracranial hypertension such as anisocoria, papilledema, nausea, vomiting, or cranial nerve paralysis provides information regarding severity and following diagnostic steps.
- Skin examination for exanthema, enanthem, vesicles.
- Parotitis (e.g., mumps).
- Lymphadenopathy (e.g., Epstein–Barr virus [EBV], HIV, cytomegalovirus [CMV]).

Differential Diagnosis
- Noninfectious causes of similar symptoms include subarachnoid hemorrhage, tumors, cysts, illicit drug or alcohol intoxications, aseptic meningitis, seizures, and migraine headache.
- HSV-2 can present as recurrent meningitis (Mollaret meningitis), which is self-limited and usually resolves spontaneously and needs no treatment.

Diagnostic Testing
Laboratories
- Peripheral blood should be obtained for cell count with differential looking for leukocytosis as well as a complete metabolic panel.
- Blood cultures may provide the etiology, especially important if the lumbar puncture (LP) cannot be performed.
- CSF studies are discussed under the section "Diagnostic Procedures."

Imaging
Computed tomography or magnetic resonance is indicated in patients with suspected mass lesion or risk of herniation, as indicated by the presence of focal signs or papilledema. Also, imaging is indicated for immunocompromised patients and those with a history of CNS disease.

Diagnostic Procedures
- Analysis of the CSF is essential. **An LP should be performed promptly unless clearly contraindicated.**
- **Signs of increased intracranial pressure should prompt studies to rule out a mass before an LP.**
- CSF should be sent for cell count with differential, protein, glucose, Gram stain, and culture in all patients. Specific tests such as enterovirus polymerase chain reaction (PCR) or WNV IgM will depend on risk factors, initial CSF analysis, and seasonality.
- Opening pressure should be obtained when performing LP (normal 50–200 mm H_2O).
- Bacterial meningitis presents with higher pleocytosis (up to the range of several thousand), with neutrophil predominance, low glucose (<40 mg/dL, CSF/serum ratio <0.4), and elevated protein. Gram stain is positive in 60% to 90% of patients with bacterial meningitis with pleocytosis.
- If there is concern for CSF shunt/drain infection, it is recommended to culture the shunt components. It is also recommended to hold the culture for at least 10 days in an attempt to identify organism such as *Propionibacterium acnes*.[6]
- A management algorithm is presented in Figure 10-1.

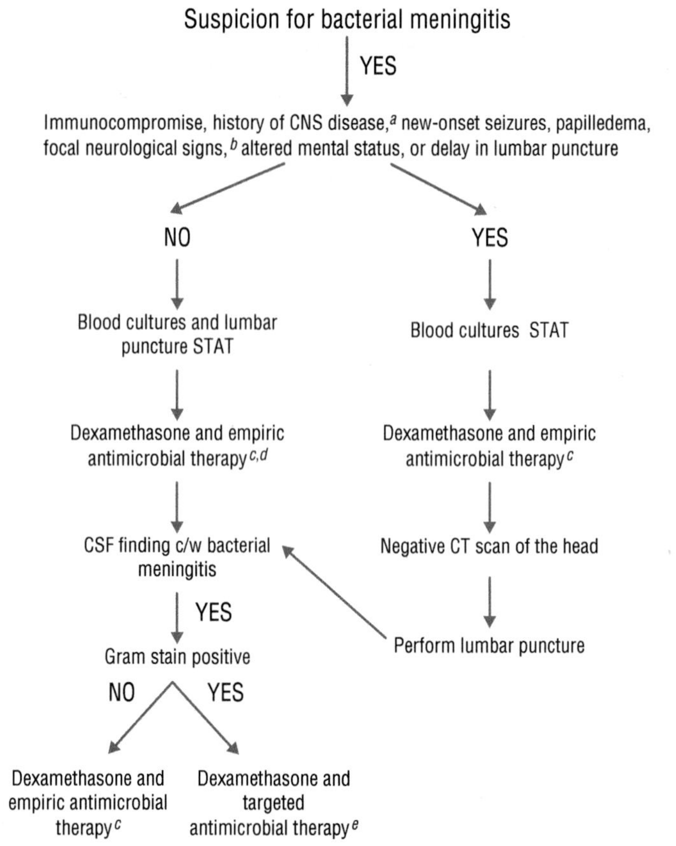

FIGURE 10-1 Algorithm for the management of acute bacterial meningitis in adults, from the guidelines of the Infectious Diseases Society of America.

[a]Mass lesion, stroke, or abscess; [b]dilated nonreactive pupil, gaze palsy, abnormal visual fields or ocular mobility, leg or arm drift; [c]see Table 10-3; [d]administer immediately after lumbar puncture; [e]see Table 10-4.

Adapted from Tunkel AR, Hartman BJ, Kaplan SL, et al. Practice guidelines for the management of bacterial meningitis. *Clin Infect Dis*. 2004;39:1267-1284.

TREATMENT

- **Bacterial meningitis is a medical emergency, and treatment should not be delayed** (Figure 10-1).[1]
- Administration of systemic antibiotics does not affect CSF findings for 24 hours. Recommendations for empiric treatment are given according to age groups and identified risk factors (see Table 10-3).[1]
- It is important to carefully manage fluids and electrolyte balance, as both hypervolemia and hypovolemia are associated with worse outcomes.
- In case of CSF shunt/drain infection, complete removal of the shunt/drain is recommended.[6]

TABLE 10-3	EMPIRIC ANTIBIOTIC RECOMMENDATIONS FOR ACUTE BACTERIAL MENINGITIS
Age/Risk Factor	**Empiric Antimicrobial Therapy**
<1 mo	Ampicillin plus cefotaxime or ampicillin plus aminoglycoside
1–23 mo	Vancomycin plus third-generation cephalosporin (ceftriaxone or cefotaxime)
2–50 y	Vancomycin plus ceftriaxone
>50 y	Vancomycin plus ceftriaxone (or cefotaxime) plus ampicillin
Immunocompromised	Vancomycin plus ampicillin plus cefepime or meropenem
Basilar skull fracture	Vancomycin plus ceftriaxone or cefotaxime
Penetrating head trauma	Vancomycin plus ceftazidime, cefepime, or meropenem
Postneurosurgery	Vancomycin plus ceftazidime, cefepime, or meropenem
Cerebrospinal fluid shunt	Vancomycin plus ceftazidime, cefepime, or meropenem

Adapted from Tunkel AR, Hartman BJ, Kaplan SL, et al. Practice guidelines for the management of bacterial meningitis. *Clin Infectious Dis.* 2004;39(9):1267-1284.

Medications

- **Corticosteroids**
  - In adults, evidence supports the use of adjunctive steroids for suspected acute bacterial meningitis due to pneumococcus.[1,7]
  - In children, the use of concomitant steroids is indicated for meningitis due to *H. influenzae* type B.
  - Dexamethasone at 0.15 mg/kg q6h should be started **with the first dose of antibiotics**.
  - In adults, steroids should be discontinued if further studies do not support the diagnosis of bacterial meningitis, specifically if no evidence of pneumococcal infection is found.
  - The use of dexamethasone before or with the first dose of antimicrobials has decreased the rates of hearing loss and short-term mortality in high-income countries.
- **Antimicrobials:** Antimicrobial treatment for acute meningitis is presented in Table 10-4.[1]

PROGNOSIS/OUTCOME

- Delay in treatment is a strong predictor for death.
- Hearing loss, seizures, cognitive impairment are the most common sequelae among survivors.

TABLE 10-4	SPECIFIC ANTIMICROBIAL THERAPY FOR ACUTE BACTERIAL MENINGITIS IN ADULTS ONCE PRESUMPTIVE ORGANISM IS IDENTIFIED	
Microorganism	**Recommended Therapy**	**Alternative Therapies**
Streptococcus pneumoniae	Vancomycin (30–45 mg/kg/d in 2–3 doses) plus third-generation cephalosporin (cefotaxime or ceftriaxone)	Cefepime, meropenem, fluoroquinolone Vancomycin continued only if MIC >1 µg/mL Penicillin or ampicillin if MIC <0.1 µg/mL
Neisseria meningitidis	Ceftriaxone (2 g q12h)	Chloramphenicol, meropenem
Haemophilus influenzae type B	Third-generation cephalosporin	Cefepime, chloramphenicol, fluoroquinolone
Listeria monocytogenes	Ampicillin or penicillin G	Meropenem, trimethoprim–sulfamethoxazole
Streptococcus agalactiae	Ampicillin or penicillin G	Third-generation cephalosporin
Pseudomonas aeruginosa	Cefepime or ceftazidime	Carbapenem (except ertapenem)

Adapted from Tunkel AR, Hartman BJ, Kaplan SL, et al. Practice guidelines for the management of bacterial meningitis. *Clin Infectious Dis.* 2004;39(9):1267-1284.

Chronic Meningitis

GENERAL PRINCIPLES

Definition

Chronic meningitis is defined as signs and symptoms suggestive of meningeal disease with CSF pleocytosis lasting 4 weeks or more.

Etiology

- **The most common infectious cause of chronic meningitis worldwide is tuberculosis, especially in the developing world.**
- **Fungi are the second most common causes**, including *Cryptococcus neoformans, Coccidioides immitis, Histoplasma capsulatum, Blastomyces hominis,* and *Candida* spp.
- Parasitic causes include *Acanthamoeba* spp. and neurocysticercosis (*Taenia solium*).
- Other bacterial causes include *T. pallidum, Borrelia burgdorferi, Brucella* spp., and *Tropheryma whippelii.*
- Potential noninfectious causes include meningeal carcinomatosis, collagen vascular disease (e.g., lupus and other forms of vasculitis), sarcoidosis, and toxin/drug induced.
- A significant minority of cases are idiopathic.

Pathophysiology

Depending on the infectious agent, the manifestations can be due to granuloma formation irritating the meninges, perivascular inflammation, or rupture of a parameningeal site, including an abscess or cyst with leakage into the meningeal space.[8]

Risk Factors

- Travel (for even short periods) to the Southwest United States and Mexico should raise the suspicion of coccidioidomycosis.
- Tuberculous meningitis should be suspected in immigrants from tropical or developing countries and if immunosuppressed patients travel to an endemic country.
- Histoplasmosis and blastomycosis should be suspected in patients from endemic areas.
- Immunosuppression. HIV-infected patients, transplant recipients, and patients on immunosuppressive drugs are at increased risk of cryptococcal meningitis, *Mycobacterium tuberculosis*, endemic mycosis and Whipple disease.
- Opportunistic fungal infection, burns, and total parenteral nutrition can increase the risk of candida meningitis.
- Exposures: Sexual behavior (neurosyphilis) and unpasteurized milk or contact with cows, goat or sheep from endemic countries (*Brucella*).
- Iatrogenic, e.g., outbreak of fungal meningitis after injections with contaminated steroids.[9]

DIAGNOSIS

Clinical Presentation

History
- Symptoms can wax and wane over a period of time, making the diagnosis difficult.
- Headaches, nausea, memory loss, and confusion are the most common symptoms.
- Fever may be absent.
- With progression of disease and possible development of hydrocephalus, other symptoms such as diplopia, ataxia, and dementia may occur.
- History of exposures, travel and immunosuppression, and occupational activities should be obtained.
- Associated symptoms such as weight loss, night sweats, tumors, or skin lesions may lead toward a certain etiology such as tuberculosis, malignancy, or fungal infection.
- History of sexually transmitted diseases and genital lesions suggests neurosyphilis as a possibility.
- Presence of oral ulcers, visual problems, and uveitis is suggestive of noninfectious causes such as Behçet disease.

Physical Examination
- A detailed neurologic examination is essential.
- Cranial nerve abnormalities can be seen due to chronic meningeal inflammation, without intracranial hypertension.
- Skin lesions may be present in fungal infections such as blastomycosis or cryptococcosis.
- Lymphadenopathy should raise suspicion of hematologic malignancy, sarcoidosis, tuberculosis, or histoplasmosis.

Differential Diagnosis

Other causes of headache, focal neurologic signs, dementia, and delirium should be considered when appropriate.

Diagnostic Testing

Laboratories
- Peripheral blood should be obtained for cell count with differential looking for leukocytosis as well as a complete metabolic panel.
- Serologies may be useful for coccidioidomycosis (serum complement fixation), cryptococcosis, Lyme disease, syphilis, and brucellosis.
- CSF studies are discussed under the section "Diagnostic Procedures."

Imaging
- MRI is the imaging method of choice. It may show blunting of sulci as evidence of edema, hydrocephalus, and meningeal enhancement.
- Granulomas may be seen in tuberculosis or cryptococcosis, especially if disseminated hematogenously (miliary tuberculosis).
- Intraparenchymal or intraventricular lesions may be seen in neurocysticercosis.

Diagnostic Procedures
- **CSF evaluation is essential.**
- Cell count with differential, glucose, protein, Gram stain, aerobic, mycobacterial, and fungal cultures should be sent. Larger volumes are needed for mycobacterial and fungal cultures.
- Pleocytosis is usually lymphocytic.
- Low-glucose concentrations are more typical of tuberculosis and fungal infections.
- If lymphocytic carcinomatosis is suspected, flow cytometry should be ordered.
- For the most common specific etiologies, the following CSF tests should be ordered:
  - *M. tuberculosis.* Acid-fast stains are not sensitive. At least 3 to 5 mL should be sent for culture. Nucleic acid amplification tests have varied sensitivity and specificity depending on the laboratory. Measurement of adenosine deaminase level may be a useful adjunctive test for diagnosis of tuberculous meningitis.[10,11]
  - **Cryptococcal meningitis.** CSF cryptococcal antigen has very high sensitivity but can remain positive even in treated patients. If unable to obtain CSF, a positive serum cryptococcal antigen correlates well in immunosuppressed patients.
  - *C. immitis.* CSF complement fixation antibody.
  - *H. capsulatum. Histoplasma* antigen in CSF. Urine *Histoplasma* antigen is not useful unless the patient has evidence of disseminated infection.
  - **Syphilis.** CSF VDRL or RPR. Indicate high suspicion for neurosyphilis on laboratory requisition.
  - PCR is available for some infections, like Whipple disease.
- Opening pressure should always be checked when LP is performed.
- Meningeal biopsy may be required in cases when the diagnosis is unclear. The presence of granulomas or the evidence of malignancy or vascular inflammation can help establish the diagnosis.
- Tuberculosis skin test (PPD) can be placed in patients. However, a negative PPD does not rule out tuberculosis. In patients with known history of negative PPD, **a new positive test should prompt treatment even if CSF studies are negative.**[12]

TREATMENT

May need to treat empirically if suspicion is high for an etiologic agent (e.g., *M. tuberculosis*), in immunosuppressed patients, or if the patient decompensates quickly and action is required.[12]

Medications
- *M. tuberculosis*[12]:
  - Four-drug therapy is recommended (i.e., isoniazid, rifampin, ethambutol, and pyrazinamide) for 2 months followed by consolidation with isoniazid and rifampin for 7 to 12 months.
  - Corticosteroids (dexamethasone or prednisone) have been shown to improve outcomes, especially in HIV-negative patients. Taper steroids over 6 to 8 weeks.
- **Cryptococcal meningitis**
  - See Chapter 13.

○ Induction phase: liposomal amphotericin B IV, 3 to 4 mg/kg/d (alternative: Amphotericin B deoxycholate 0.7 to 1.0 mg/kg/d IV), with flucytosine orally, 25 mg/kg every 6 hours.
○ Consolidation phase: high-dose fluconazole orally, 400 to 800 mg daily for 8 weeks
○ Maintenance phase: Fluconazole orally, 200 to 400 mg daily for almost a year.
- **Coccidioidomycosis**: Fluconazole is the mainstay of treatment for *C. immitis* meningitis.

Other Nonpharmacologic Therapies

Persistent intracranial hypertension in cryptococcal meningitis may require serial LPs, lumbar drain, or CSF shunts if there is hydrocephalus.

COMPLICATIONS

- Hydrocephalus, especially in cryptococcal meningitis.
- Tuberculous meningitis may result in cerebral ischemia/infarction, growth of a tuberculoma, seizures, hyponatremia, and death.

PROGNOSIS/OUTCOME

- Prognosis depends on the specific etiology, age, immunocompromised status and severity of disease at presentation, and time to initiation of treatment.
- Despite long-term treatment, the mortality rate of Tuberculous meningitis remains high. Sequelae include cranial nerve palsies, blindness, deafness, psychiatric disorders, and seizures.
- Similar sequelae can occur in all forms of fungal meningitis.

Encephalitis

GENERAL PRINCIPLES

Definition

- Encephalitis is an inflammation of the brain parenchyma, which usually presents as altered mental status or personality changes.
- It can be associated with meningitis and is referred to as meningoencephalitis.

Etiology

- Most infectious encephalitis is of viral origin, but the etiology is unknown in many patients.[13,14]
- **The most common cause of sporadic encephalitis is HSV,** which has a high morbidity and mortality if untreated.
- Viral etiologies depend on the epidemiology, geography, time of the year, and exposures. In the United States, WNV has emerged as a common cause, followed by **enteroviruses**. Rabies is a fatal yet preventable cause of encephalitis.
- Nonviral causes include *M. tuberculosis*, *Mycoplasma pneumoniae*, *Bartonella* spp., syphilis, fungi, and parasitic infections such as free-living amebas.
- Encephalitis may also be postinfectious, such as postimmunization or acute demyelinating encephalomyelitis (ADEM). *M. pneumoniae* and streptococcal disease may be associated with ADEM.
- JC virus causes progressive multiple leukoencephalopathy, seen in immunosuppressed patients, HIV infection, sarcoidosis, and patients on steroids and other immunosuppressed medications.
- Varicella zoster virus (VZV) as a complication of chicken pox (primary infection) or disseminated herpes zoster, particularly in the immunosuppressed.

- CMV, particularly in HIV and solid organ or bone marrow transplant patients.
- EBV and adenovirus are less common etiologies of encephalitis.
- Etiology based on epidemiology and risk factors shown in (Table 10-5).[15]

TABLE 10-5	CAUSES OF ENCEPHALITIS BASED ON EPIDEMIOLOGY AND RISK FACTORS	
Epidemiology or Risk Factor		**Possible Infectious Agent(s)**
Agammaglobulinemia		Enteroviruses, *Mycoplasma pneumoniae*
Age	Neonates	Herpes simplex virus type 2, cytomegalovirus, rubella virus, *Listeria monocytogenes, Treponema pallidum, Toxoplasma gondii*
	Infants and children	Eastern equine encephalitis virus, Japanese encephalitis virus (JEV), Murray Valley encephalitis virus (rapid in infants), influenza virus, La Crosse virus
	Elderly persons	Eastern equine encephalitis virus, St. Louis encephalitis virus, West Nile virus (WNV), sporadic CJD, *L. monocytogenes*
Animal contact	Bats	Rabies virus, Nipah virus
	Birds	WNV, Eastern equine encephalitis virus, Western equine encephalitis virus, Venezuelan equine encephalitis virus, St. Louis encephalitis virus, Murray Valley encephalitis virus, JEV, *Cryptococcus neoformans* (bird droppings)
	Cats	Rabies virus, *Coxiella burnetii, Bartonella henselae, T. gondii*
	Dogs	Rabies virus
	Horses	Eastern equine encephalitis virus, Western equine encephalitis virus, Venezuelan equine encephalitis virus, Hendra virus
	Old World primates	B virus
	Raccoons	Rabies virus, *Baylisascaris procyonis*
	Rodents	Eastern equine encephalitis virus (South America), Venezuelan equine encephalitis virus, tick-borne encephalitis virus, Powassan virus (woodchucks), La Crosse virus (chipmunks and squirrels), *Bartonella quintana*
	Sheep and goats	*C. burnetii*
	Skunks	Rabies virus
	Swine	JEV, Nipah virus
	White-tailed deer	*Borrelia burgdorferi*

TABLE 10-5	CAUSES OF ENCEPHALITIS BASED ON EPIDEMIOLOGY AND RISK FACTORS (CONTINUED)
Epidemiology or Risk Factor	**Possible Infectious Agent(s)**
Immunocompromised persons`	Varicella zoster virus (VZV), cytomegalovirus, human herpesvirus 6, WNV, HIV, JC virus, *L. monocytogenes, Mycobacterium tuberculosis, C. neoformans, Coccidioides* species, *Histoplasma capsulatum, T. gondii*

Ingestion items	Raw or partially cooked meat	*T. gondii*
	Raw meat, fish, or reptiles	*Gnathostoma* species
	Unpasteurized milk	Tick-borne encephalitis virus, *L. monocytogenes, C. burnetii*
Insect contact	Mosquitoes	Eastern equine encephalitis virus, Western equine encephalitis virus, Venezuelan equine encephalitis virus, St. Louis encephalitis virus, Murray Valley encephalitis virus, JEV, WNV, La Crosse virus, *Plasmodium falciparum*
	Sandflies	*Bartonella bacilliformis*
	Ticks	Tick-borne encephalitis virus, Powassan virus, *Rickettsia rickettsii, Ehrlichia chaffeensis, Anaplasma phagocytophilum, C. burnetii* (rare), *B.burgdorferi*
	Tsetse flies	*Trypanosoma brucei gambiense, Trypanosoma brucei rhodesiense*
Occupation	Exposure to animals	Rabies virus, *C. burnetii, Bartonella* species
	Exposure to horses	Hendra virus
	Laboratory workers	WNV, HIV, *C. burnetii, Coccidioides* species
	Physicians and health care workers	VZV, HIV, influenza virus, measles virus, *M. tuberculosis*
	Veterinarians	Rabies virus, *Bartonella* species, *C. burnetii*
Person-to-person transmission		Herpes simplex virus (neonatal), VZV, Venezuelan equine encephalitis virus (rare), poliovirus, nonpolio enteroviruses, measles virus, Nipah virus, mumps virus, rubella virus, Epstein–Barr virus, human herpesvirus 6, B virus, WNV (transfusion, transplantation, breast feeding), HIV, rabies virus (transplantation), influenza virus, *M. pneumoniae, M. tuberculosis, T. pallidum*

(Continued)

TABLE 10-5	CAUSES OF ENCEPHALITIS BASED ON EPIDEMIOLOGY AND RISK FACTORS (CONTINUED)	
Epidemiology or Risk Factor		**Possible Infectious Agent(s)**
Recent vaccination		Acute disseminated encephalomyelitis
Recreational activities	Camping/hunting	All agents transmitted by mosquitoes and ticks (see above)
	Sexual contact	HIV, *T. pallidum*
	Spelunking	Rabies virus, *H. capsulatum*
	Swimming	Enteroviruses, *Naegleria fowleri*
Season	Late summer/ early fall	All agents transmitted by mosquitoes and ticks (see above), enteroviruses
	Winter	Influenza virus
Transfusion and transplantation		Cytomegalovirus, Epstein–Barr virus, WNV, HIV, tick-borne encephalitis virus, rabies virus, iatrogenic CJD, *T. pallidum*, *A. phago-cytophilum*, *R. rickettsii*, *C. neoformans*, *Coccidioides* species, *H.capsulatum*, *T. gondii*
Travel	Africa	Rabies virus, WNV, *P. falciparum*, *T. brucei gambiense*, *T. brucei rhodesiense*
	Australia	Murray Valley encephalitis virus, JEV, Hendra virus
	Central America	Rabies virus, Eastern equine encephalitis virus, Western equine encephalitis virus, Venezuelan equine encephalitis virus, St. Louis encephalitis virus, *R. rickettsii*, *P. falciparum*, *Taenia solium*
	Europe	WNV, tick-borne encephalitis virus, *A. phagocytophilum*, *B. burgdorferi*
	India, Nepal	Rabies virus, JEV, *P. falciparum*
	Middle East	WNV, *P. falciparum*
	Russia	Tick-borne encephalitis virus
	South America	Rabies virus, Eastern equine encephalitis virus, Western equine encephalitis virus, Venezuelan equine encephalitis virus, St. Louis encephalitis virus, *R. rickettsii*, *B. bacilliformis* (Andes mountains), *P. falciparum*, *T. solium*
	Southeast Asia, China, Pacific Rim	JEV, tick-borne encephalitis virus, Nipah virus, *P. falciparum*, *Gnathostoma* species, *T. solium*
Unvaccinated status		VZV, JEV, poliovirus, measles virus, mumps virus, rubella virus

Adapted from Tunkel AR, Glaser CA, Bloch KC. The management of encephalitis: clinical practice guidelines by the Infectious Diseases Society of America. *Clini Infect Dis.* 2008;47(3):303-327.

Pathophysiology

- The cardinal pathological feature is inflammation of the brain parenchyma. Damage may be caused by direct pathogen invasion or by an immune-mediated mechanism causing demyelination and vasculitis.
- Herpes simplex encephalitis
  - **The most common herpes encephalitis in adults is HSV-1.**[15]
  - Direct invasion from the trigeminal or olfactory nerve may occur.
  - This may follow an acute oropharyngeal infection, reactivation, or recurrent HSV-1. In approximately one-third of patients, it can reactivate within the CNS without a known primary or recurrent HSV-1 infection.
- Arboviral encephalitis
  - In the United States, the most common arboviral infection is **WNV.**
  - Worldwide, other arboviral infections include Zika Virus (South and Central America), Japanese encephalitis virus (JEV) (Southeast Asia and China), chikungunya virus (India, sub-Saharan Africa, Pakistan, and Italy), and tick-borne encephalitis (Western Europe, Russia, and China).
  - After a mosquito (*Aedes* spp. or *Culex* spp.) or tick bite (*Ixodes*), there is virus replication, which results in viremia and subsequent dissemination to the CNS.
- Rabies
  - Rabies is transmitted to humans through the saliva of an infected animal following a bite. It can be transmitted by bats, raccoons, foxes, and dogs.
  - The incubation period can be long, up to 7 years, with a median of 2 months.
- Table 10-5 presents more details regarding etiologies and exposures.

Risk Factors

- Travel to endemic areas: China (JEV), the United States and Europe (WNV in summer months), and the East coast (eastern equine encephalitis)
- Mosquito or tick exposure
- Exposure to wild animals: dogs, raccoons, and bats (rabies)
- Seasonality: Summer months (WNV and ehrlichiosis/anaplasmosis)
- Activities: Camping (insect exposure), swimming (free-living amebas and enterovirus), and sexual contact (HIV)
- Immunocompromised: VZV, CMV, and JC virus
- Recent vaccination: ADEM
- Primary HSV infection in those <18 years old
- Ingestion of unpasteurized milk or other dairy products (*Listeria*) and raw meat (*Toxoplasm*a)

Prevention

- Avoid exposures as above.
- Rabies vaccine as well as rabies immunoglobulin should be administered to anyone who has been bitten by a wild animal or unimmunized dog or bats.
- A JEV vaccine is approved for travelers to endemic areas.

DIAGNOSIS

Clinical Presentation

History
- Risk factors should be assessed.
- **Altered mental status is the hallmark of encephalitis** and may precede other symptoms.
- HSV-1 should always be considered in patients with meningoencephalitis, even without a recent outbreak of herpes.

- Personality change and auditory hallucinations suggestive of temporal involvement should raise suspicion of HSV-1 infection.
- The patient may not be able to provide a history; so if unable to obtain any information, immediate action should be taken for diagnosis and management.
- Prodromal symptoms and exposures to sick people (e.g., *Mycoplasma*).
- Fever, altered consciousness, behavioral changes, headache, seizures, and/or focal neurological signs may occur.
- Meningeal signs and symptoms may be present in cases of meningoencephalitis.

Physical Examination
- Fever and altered mental status are the most common findings.
- Meningismus is usually absent, but can present in cases of meningoencephalitis.
- Focal neurologic signs, including aphasia and personality changes, ataxia, and cranial nerve palsies (tuberculosis and syphilis), may be seen.
- Generalized or focal seizures may be present.
- Movement disorders may suggest a flavivirus infection, such as WNV or JEV, or a postinfectious syndrome, such as ADEM or poststreptococcal chorea.
- Various rashes and animal/arthropod bites may provide useful clues.

Differential Diagnosis

- Possibilities include glioblastoma or meningioma, brain abscesses, meningitis, sarcoidosis, systemic lupus erythematosus, vasculitis, drugs, alcohol or other toxic encephalopathies, and delirium.
- In children with a history of recent immunization or recent viral infection, ADEM should be considered.

Diagnostic Testing

Imaging
- MRI is the most sensitive neuroimaging study.
- If MRI is unavailable or contraindicated, then a CT (with and without contrast) should be obtained.
- Findings may include temporal involvement (HSV-1), white matter lesions (demyelinating diseases), hemorrhages (VZV), lack of enhancement (JC virus), periventricular lesions, or mass lesions including tuberculomas and free-living amebiasis.

Diagnostic Procedures
- **All patients with a suspicion of encephalitis should undergo an LP unless clearly contraindicated**.
- The most common finding is a mild-to-moderate pleocytosis with lymphocytic predominance; glucose is usually normal and protein elevated.
- **A normal CSF in a patient with a history suggestive of HSV encephalitis should not delay treatment and specific testing.**
- Nucleic acid amplification tests (e.g., PCR):
  - **HSV PCR should be sent in all patients with encephalitis**.
  - The sensitivity of HSV PCR is 98% and specificity 96%, although this varies according to the laboratory.
  - Note that HSV PCR may be negative on day 1 or day 2 of the disease, so if the clinical picture and imaging suggest HSV, a PCR should be repeated later.[15]
  - Other PCRs are available for enterovirus, adenovirus, influenza, JC, EBV, CMV, VZV, rabies, *Ehrlichia*, *Bartonella*, and *Mycoplasma*.
- Antibodies:
  - The diagnosis of WNV is made by the presence of IgM antibodies in the CSF or serum. There is cross-reactivity with other flaviviruses, such as St. Louis encephalitis virus or JEV.

- ○ CSF and serum antibodies should be sent if rabies is suspected.
- ○ Blood PCR must also be available at CDC to check for Zika virus if suspected.
- If rabies is suspected, a skin biopsy from the nape of the neck can be performed; fluorescent antibody staining may reveal rabies antigen in cutaneous nerve fibers. PCR testing can also be carried out on saliva.

TREATMENT

- The treatment of HSV encephalitis is intravenous acyclovir at 10 mg/kg every 8 hours for 14 to 21 days.
- **Acyclovir should be started empirically on every patient who presents with a picture consistent with encephalitis.**
- For other viral etiologies, the treatment is mainly supportive.

PROGNOSIS/OUTCOME

- If untreated, mortality due to herpes simplex encephalitis can be as high as 70%; morbidity is high (>28%), and most survivors have some type of sequelae including severe cognitive impairment and disability.[15]
- WNV encephalitis can be severe in patients aged >50 years. Residual neurologic findings may include a poliomyelitis-like syndrome, persistent headaches and fatigue, and focal signs that can persist for months.

Brain Abscess

GENERAL PRINCIPLES

Etiology

The etiologic agent is usually determined by the location of the abscess or the predisposing factor (Table 10-6).[16] Most are caused by bacteria; fungi and parasites are less common causes.

Pathophysiology

- There are four distinct phases of development in a brain abscess[17]
- Early cerebritis with focal inflammation and edema (first few days)
- Late cerebritis with increasing size and development of a necrotic center
- Early capsular stage when a ring-enhancing capsule develops (1–2 wk)
- In the late capsular phase, a well-formed collagenous capsule develops and walls off the abscess (after about 2 wk)

Risk Factors

- **Pyogenic brain abscess**
  - ○ **Contiguous source: This is the most common source** including chronic otitis media, mastoiditis, cholesteatoma, chronic sinusitis, odontogenic fistulas/caries/abscesses, and cavernous sinus thrombosis.[17,18]
  - ○ **Hematogenous**: dissemination of infectious agent from an intrathoracic or intraperitoneal source to the brain including endocarditis, pulmonary arteriovenous malformation (e.g., as in hereditary hemorrhagic telangiectasia [HHT]), ventricular septal defects, and patent ductus arteriosus.
  - ○ **Trauma**: gunshot wounds, patients in combat.
  - ○ **Open brain surgery**.

TABLE 10-6	BRAIN ABSCESS: SOURCE, LOCATION, AND PATHOGENS	
Underlying Condition	**Probable Site of Abscess**	**Probable Pathogens**
Paranasal sinus disease	Frontal lobe	*Streptococci* (especially *S. milleri* group), *S. aureus*, *Haemophilus* spp., *Bacteroides* species
Otogenic source	Temporal lobe, cerebellum	Enterobacteriaceae, *Pseudomonas* species, *Streptococcus* species., *Bacteroides* species, *S. aureus*
Odontogenic source	Frontal lobe	*Streptococci*, *Staphylococci*, *Actinomyces* species, *Actinobacillus* species, *Bacteroides* species, *Fusobacterium* species
Pulmonary infection	Any lobe, possible multiple lobe involvement	*Streptococci*, *Staphylococci*, *Bacteroides* species, *Fusobacterium* species, Enterobacteriaceae
Bacterial endocarditis	Multiple lobe involvement, usually multiple abscesses in vascularized areas	*S. aureus*, *S. viridians*
Penetrating head trauma or postoperative	Depends on site of wound	*S. aureus* (methicillin sensitive and resistant), *Staphylococcus epidermidis*, *Streptococci*, Enterobacteriaceae, *Clostridium Staphylococci*
Right-to-left shunt (congenital cyanotic heart disease, pulmonary arteriovenous malformations)	Multiple abscesses, multiple lobes	*Streptococci*, *Staphylococci*, *Peptostreptococcus* species, *Haemophilus* species
Immunosuppressed patients (transplant recipients, immunosuppressant drugs)	Multiple abscesses, multiple lobes	*Aspergillus* species, *Nocardia* species., *Candida* species, *Toxoplasma gondii*, *Listeria monocytogenes*, mucormycosis, *Mycobacterium* species, *Cryptococcus* spp.
HIV infection	Multiple abscesses, any lobe	*T. gondii*, *Mycobacterium* species, *Cryptococcus neoformans*, *Aspergillus* species, *Nocardia* species

Adapted from Klein M, Pfister H-W, Tunkel AR, Scheld WM. Brain abscess. In: Scheld MW, Whitley RJ, Marra CM, eds. *Infections of the Central Nervous System*. Lippincott Williams & Wilkins; 2014.

- **Fungal:** Fungal brain abscesses occur in immunocompromised patients, such as bone marrow and solid organ transplant patients, patients on corticosteroids, uncontrolled diabetics with ketoacidosis (mucormycosis), and HIV-infected patients.
- **Parasitic:** Toxoplasmosis occurs in HIV-infected patients; neurocysticercosis in immigrants from endemic areas.

DIAGNOSIS

Clinical Presentation

History
- Presentation is usually indolent, especially if there is a contiguous source focus.
- Presentation varies according to location and if there are single or multiple abscesses.
- The most common symptom is headache, followed by fever, mental status changes, and focal neurologic deficits.[17,18]
- Fever, hemiparesis, and symptoms of increased intracranial pressure should heighten suspicion for brain abscess.
- Seizures can be the only presenting symptom.
- Look for predisposing conditions, immunosuppressed status, previous surgeries, or dental procedures.
- Family history of arteriovenous malformations or HHT may be helpful.

Physical Examination
- Fever may not be present.
- Focal signs and deficits and signs of increased intracranial pressure may be present.

Differential Diagnosis

The differential diagnosis is broad and includes brain tumors (primary or metastatic), epidural or subdural empyema, subdural hematoma, CNS lymphoma (difficult to distinguish from toxoplasmosis), cerebrovascular accident, venous sinus thrombosis (which may present with associated abscess), and sarcoidosis.

Diagnostic Testing

Laboratories
- The absence of leukocytosis does not rule out a brain abscess.
- Blood cultures should be obtained before administration of antibiotics.

Imaging
- Both CT with contrast and MRI with gadolinium can be used for diagnosis. MRI is more sensitive.[18]
- CT scan findings include the following:
  - Early cerebritis. Hypodense irregular area without enhancement
  - Abscess. Hypodense lesion with ring enhancement. Edema can be seen around lesion
  - A contiguous focus of infection may be identified
- MRI findings include the following:
  - T1: Hypointense lesion with ring enhancement
  - T2: Hyperintense central area with hypointense surrounding capsule and surrounding hyperintense edema
  - Diffusion-weighted imaging may be helpful in differentiating from malignancies

Diagnostic Procedures
- LP is generally contraindicated due to the risk of herniation.
- The only way to obtain definitive diagnosis is through examination of the contents of abscess.[17,19]

- Stereotactic biopsy with needle aspiration is the method of choice (CT guided) if the abscess is accessible.
- If the abscess is in a deep part of the brain, then surgical excision may be needed.
- Aspirate should be sent for histopathology, Gram stain, aerobic and anaerobic cultures, and fungal or mycobacterial cultures if indicated.
- To identify a potential source, other diagnostic tests may include echocardiography, panorex, chest plain radiograph, and CT pulmonary angiography.

TREATMENT

Medications

- Empiric **antibiotic treatment** should be initiated if abscesses are small (<2.5 cm), when diagnostic sample cannot be obtained, while awaiting results, or if studies fail to identify etiology.[19]
  - Empiric therapy should include an antibiotic with activity against anaerobes (e.g., metronidazole) until a specific etiology is found.
  - Recommendations are given based on presumed source of the abscess (see Table 10-7).
  - Intravenous antibiotic treatment should be prolonged (6–8 wk) and tailored to the specific etiology if possible.
- **Corticosteroids.** Dexamethasone 10 mg as loading dose, followed by 4 mg every 6 hours is recommended if there is significant edema and life-threatening mass effect.[19]

TABLE 10-7	RECOMMENDED EMPIRIC ANTIMICROBIAL TREATMENT BASED ON PRESUMED SOURCE OF ABSCESS
Source of Abscess	Empiric Antimicrobial Treatment
Paranasal sinus	Metronidazole plus either third-generation cephalosporin (plus vancomycin if methicillin-resistant *S. aureus* suspected)
Otogenic infection	Metronidazole plus ceftazidime or cefepime
Dental infection	Penicillin plus metronidazole
Bacterial endocarditis	Vancomycin plus metronidazole plus third-generation cephalosporin
Pulmonary infection	Penicillin plus metronidazole plus trimethoprim–sulfamethoxazole (if *Nocardia* is suspected)
Penetrating trauma	Vancomycin plus third-generation cephalosporin (may use fourth generation if *Pseudomonas* suspected)
Postoperative	Vancomycin plus cefepime, ceftazidime, or meropenem
Unknown	Vancomycin plus metronidazole plus third-generation cephalosporin

Doses: Vancomycin IV 30 to 45 mg/kg/d divided into 2 to 3 doses/d; metronidazole 500 mg IV q6–8h; ceftriaxone 2 g q12h, cefotaxime 2 g IV q4–6h.

Surgical Treatment

- Drainage, either via burr hole aspiration or surgical excision, should be performed on all abscesses >2.5 cm.[19]
- Open craniotomy with excision is indicated if abscesses fail to respond to antibiotics, for fungal abscesses, and if a foreign body is present.

COMPLICATIONS

Complications include seizures, obstructive hydrocephalus, and intraventricular rupture.

PROGNOSIS/OUTCOME

- Mortality used to be very high in the preantibiotic and pre-CT era.
- Mortality rate declined substantially in the past 60 years and was approximately 10% in studies since 2000.[18]
- Long-term sequelae (20%–70%) include seizures and focal deficits such as aphasia, ataxia, and cranial nerve palsies.
- There may be up to a 25% rate of recurrence.

REFERENCES

1. Tunkel AR, Hartman BJ, Kaplan SL, et al. Practice guidelines for the management of bacterial meningitis. *Clin Infect Dis.* 2004;39:1267-1284.
2. Slom TJ, Cortese MM, Gerber SI, et al. An outbreak of eosinophilic meningitis caused by *Angiostrongylus cantonensis* in travelers returning from the Caribbean. *N Engl J Med.* 2002;346:668-675.
3. Kim DK, Riley LE, Harriman KH, Hunter P, Bridges CB. Recommended immunization schedule for adults aged 19 years or older, United States, 2017. *Ann Inter Med.* 2017;166:209-219.
4. Briere EC, Rubin L, Moro PL, Cohn A, Clark T, Messonnier N. Prevention and control of Haemophilus influenzae type B disease: recommendations of the advisory committee on immunization practices (ACIP). *MMWR.* 2014;63:1-14.
5. Cohn AC, MacNeil JR, Clark TA, et al. Prevention and control of meningococcal disease: recommendations of the Advisory Committee on Immunization Practices (ACIP). *MMWR Recomm Rep.* 2013;62(RR-2):1-28.
6. Tunkel AR, Hasbun R, Bhimraj A, et al. 2017 Infectious Diseases Society of America's clinical practice guidelines for healthcare-associated ventriculitis and meningitis. *Clin Infect Dis.* 2017.
7. Brouwer MC, McIntyre P, Prasad K, van de Beek D. Corticosteroids for acute bacterial meningitis. *Cochrane Database Syst Rev.* 2015:Cd004405.
8. Helbok R, Broessner G, Pfausler B, Schmutzhard E. Chronic meningitis. *J Neurol.* 2009;256:168-175.
9. Kauffman CA, Pappas PG, Patterson TF. Fungal infections associated with contaminated methylprednisolone injections. *N Engl J Med.* 2013;368:2495-2500.
10. Thwaites G, Fisher M, Hemingway C, Scott G, Solomon T, Innes J. British infection society guidelines for the diagnosis and treatment of tuberculosis of the central nervous system in adults and children. *J Infect.* 2009;59:167-187.
11. Lewinsohn DM, Leonard MK, LoBue PA, et al. Official American Thoracic Society/Infectious Diseases Society of America/Centers for Disease Control and Prevention clinical practice guidelines: diagnosis of tuberculosis in adults and children. *Clin Infect Dis.* 2017;64:e1-e33.
12. Nahid P, Dorman SE, Alipanah N, et al. Official American Thoracic Society/Centers for Disease Control and Prevention/Infectious Diseases Society of America clinical practice guidelines: treatment of drug-susceptible tuberculosis. *Clin Infect Dis.* 2016;63:e147-e95.
13. Glaser CA, Gilliam S, Schnurr D, et al. In search of encephalitis etiologies: diagnostic challenges in the California Encephalitis Project, 1998–2000. *Clin Infect Dis.* 2003;36:731-742.
14. Glaser CA, Honarmand S, Anderson LJ, et al. Beyond viruses: clinical profiles and etiologies associated with encephalitis. *Clin Infect Dis.* 2006;43:1565-1577.
15. Tunkel AR, Glaser CA, Bloch KC, et al. The management of encephalitis: clinical practice guidelines by the Infectious Diseases Society of America. *Clin Infect Dis.* 2008;47:303-327.

16. cheld MW, Whitley RJ, Marra CM. *Infections of the Central Nervous System*. Lippincott Williams & Wilkins; 2014.
17. Mathisen GE, Johnson JP. Brain abscess. *Clin Infect Dis*. 1997;25:763-779; quiz 80-1.
18. Brouwer MC, Coutinho JM, van de Beek D. Clinical characteristics and outcome of brain abscess: systematic review and meta-analysis. *Neurology*. 2014;82:806-813.
19. Mamelak AN, Mampalam TJ, Obana WG, Rosenblum ML. Improved management of multiple brain abscesses: a combined surgical and medical approach. *Neurosurgery*. 1995;36:76-85; discussion-6.

Sexually Transmitted Infections

Matifadza Hlatshwayo and Hilary Reno

GENERAL PRINCIPLES

Sexually transmitted infections (STIs) are a significant cause of morbidity worldwide, with approximately 20 million new cases diagnosed annually in the United States alone. Half of all cases occur among the 15- to 24-year cohort. The standard clinical approach toward a patient at risk for STI is to match the clinical picture (a syndrome of typical symptoms in the setting of a corresponding history) with a diagnosis and then develop a complete differential diagnosis list to ensure consideration of other infections presenting atypically.

A thorough sexual history should be elicited, including the number and gender of partners, frequency of sexual contact, types of activity, consistency of correct condom use, and history of prior STIs. It is vital to ask these questions in a direct, nonjudgmental way, with consideration for the comfort of the patient. Studies have shown that primary care providers do not adequately assess their patients' risk for STIs.

Physical examination should focus on a detailed survey of the skin, oropharynx, external genitalia, lymph nodes, and anus; for women, a speculum and bimanual examination should be included. HIV screening and pretest counseling are warranted for all patients who present for STI evaluation as is consideration of pre-exposure prophylaxis to prevent HIV infection in patients at risk.

Prompt treatment of sex partners is a key component in controlling STIs. Local health departments can provide assistance in confidentially informing contacts, but traditionally, the responsibility has been placed on the patient to inform their sex partners of exposure.

Another option that is gaining acceptance is allowing patients to provide their partners with proper medications or a prescription without an examination by a health care provider, also known as **expedited partner therapy** (EPT).[1,2] This has been shown to be particularly effective in treating male partners of women with chlamydia or gonorrhea. Providers need to be aware of the laws specific to their jurisdiction concerning EPT, as it is only legislated in some states. Providers should also be aware of state-specific reporting guidelines and how to report to local health authorities. **Syphilis, gonorrhea, chlamydia, chancroid, and HIV/AIDS are reportable diseases in all states**.

Painful Genital Ulcer Diseases

- STIs that cause genital ulcers can be categorized by the presence of painful and painless ulcers.
- Lesions caused by genital herpes and chancroid tend to be painful, whereas those caused by syphilis, lymphogranuloma venereum (LGV), and granuloma inguinale tend to be painless.
- Genital ulcers may also be caused by noninfectious causes, such as Beçhet disease, malignancy, and trauma.

Genital Herpes

GENERAL PRINCIPLES

Epidemiology

- Painful ulceration is most likely caused by herpes simplex virus (HSV), a chronic, life-long infection.
- Traditionally, type 1 HSV (HSV-1) has been associated with oral lesions and type 2 HSV (HSV-2) with genital lesions. However, **either subtype may occur in either distribution.**
- 15.7% of people in the United States aged 14 to 49 years have genital HSV-2 infection, and it is estimated that 80% to 90% of people with HSV-2 are unaware that they are infected.
- Seroprevalence increases with age, and more women are affected than men.
- Genital HSV is of particular concern as it increases the risk of both acquiring and transmitting HIV.

Pathophysiology

- HSV is a double-stranded DNA virus that is spread by direct contact. Abraded skin or mucous membranes are more susceptible than intact skin.
- HSV-2 is typically transmitted through sexual contact and HSV-1 through nonsexual contact, although this rule is not absolute. Transmission of either HSV-1 or HSV-2 can occur perinatally.
- **Transmission can occur without active lesions**, as viral shedding continues even during asymptomatic periods.
- After entering the skin, the virus is transported along peripheral nerves to sensory and autonomic ganglia. Infection may spread by direct cell-to-cell invasion or by sensory nerve pathways. As replication involves nerve endings, the retrograde transport of virions occurs, which allows for infection to appear at other sites (e.g., thighs or buttocks). Central nervous system (CNS) disease may also occur as a result.
- **The virus can remain latent in ganglia indefinitely**, with periodic recurrences because of reactivation of latent virus. Viral latency and reactivation are not well understood, but often occur in the setting of recent trauma, illness, or emotional stress.

DIAGNOSIS

Clinical Presentation

- In symptomatic individuals, the incubation period is 2 to 12 days after infection.
- Virtually any genital lesion may be herpetic regardless of clinical characteristics.
- Typically, **small, painful grouped vesicles** develop in the genital and perianal regions which rapidly ulcerate and form shallow, tender lesions.
- Lesions are usually present for 2 to 3 weeks; viral shedding decreases with crusting.
- The first episode is usually the most severe and may be associated with inguinal adenopathy, fever, headache, myalgias, and aseptic meningitis.
- Cervicitis, proctitis, and urethritis may also occur.
- Less common manifestations include ocular disease, stomatitis, esophagitis, fulminant hepatitis, autonomic dysfunction, encephalitis, myelitis, and neuropathy.
- Owing to the severe manifestations that can result after the first episode, even in patients with initially mild clinical presentations, it is imperative to treat all first episodes.
- Recurrent episodes are commonly preceded by prodromal tingling or pain and are typically less severe and of shorter duration (4–6 d). Patients with a prolonged primary episode are more likely to experience a recurrence. In general, patients with HSV-1 genital infection have fewer recurrences and less asymptomatic viral shedding.

- Patients with immunocompromising conditions such as HIV, cancer, or solid or hematopoietic stem cell transplantation may experience prolonged or extensive outbreaks.
- Diagnosis is by recognition of the clinical syndrome on history and physical examination. Viral culture is the preferred method for making a diagnosis of genital HSV infection, but is only sensitive during the vesicular stage of the initial outbreak. Sensitivity declines rapidly as lesions heal. Vesicular fluid from an unroofed lesion should be placed in viral culture media and brought to the laboratory as soon as possible.
- Direct fluorescent antibody (DFA) staining of a scraped lesion or unroofed vesicle is another option, but is less sensitive than culture.
- Type-specific HSV antibodies appear weeks after infection. Assays are available and may be useful in determining seroprevalence for epidemiologic studies as well as counseling.
- HSV polymerase chain reaction (PCR) is more sensitive and is the preferred test at some centers, but commercial kits are neither readily available nor approved for genital HSV. PCR of the CSF with viral culture and typing are the tests of choice for suspected CNS infections.
- **Genital ulcers not classic for HSV infection should be evaluated for syphilis.**

TREATMENT

- Patients presenting with an initial episode of genital HSV should be treated. It is important to remember that **treatment decreases but does not eliminate viral shedding.** Recommended treatment regimens appear in Table 11-1.[3]
- For patients that have frequent episodes, suppressive therapy is known to reduce the frequency by 70% to 80%; treatment also decreases the rate of transmission between discordant couples (valacyclovir 500 mg PO daily).
- People with severe presentations, who require hospitalization, or have CNS manifestations should be treated with IV acyclovir.
- In patients who do not improve or who recur despite appropriate therapy, resistance should be suspected. Resistant virus does not respond to all three of the first-line therapies (acyclovir, valacyclovir, and famciclovir). Such patients should have an infectious diseases consultation to consider alternate regimens.
- All patients need to be counseled on the importance of informing their partners of their HSV status, avoiding sexual contact when lesions are present, using barrier methods even when lesions are not present, and recognizing the risk of vertical neonatal transmission.

Chancroid

GENERAL PRINCIPLES

- Chancroid is highly infectious and is caused by *Haemophilus ducreyi*, a fastidious gram-negative bacillus.
- The reported incidence of chancroid is low, but the true incidence is likely higher, as testing for *H. ducreyi* is infrequent and difficult.
- Some parts of Africa and the Caribbean probably have a higher incidence but epidemiologic data are sparse.
- Like HSV, infection with chancroid **increases the risk of HIV transmission and acquisition.**

DIAGNOSIS

Clinical Presentation

- The lesion is a **painful, nonindurated genital ulcer with a yellow-gray base, undermined edges, and a surrounding ring of erythema**. Multiple ulcers may be present.

TABLE 11-1	TREATMENT FOR HERPES SIMPLEX VIRUS INFECTIONS

Regimen

First episode		• **Acyclovir** 400 mg PO three times daily for 7–10 d OR 200 mg PO 5 times a day for 7–10 d **OR** • **Famciclovir** 250 mg PO three times daily for 7–10 d **OR** • **Valacyclovir** 1 g PO twice daily for 7–10 d
Recurrent or episodic episodes	HIV positive	• **Acyclovir** 400 mg PO three times daily × 5–10 d **OR** • **Famciclovir** 500 mg PO twice daily × 5–10 d **OR** • **Valacyclovir** 1 g PO **daily** × 5–10 d
	HIV negative	• **Acyclovir** 400 mg PO three times daily × 5 d, 800 mg PO twice daily × 5 d, or 800 mg three times daily × 2 d **OR** • **Famciclovir** 125 mg PO twice daily × 5 d, 1 g PO twice daily × 1 d, 500 mg PO once then 250 mg PO twice daily × 2 d, or 500 mg PO × 3 d **OR** • **Valacyclovir** 1 g PO twice daily × 5–10 d
Suppressive therapy (patients with >6 episodes/y)	HIV positive	• **Acyclovir** 400–800 mg twice to three times daily **OR** • **Famciclovir** 500 mg PO twice daily **OR** • **Valacyclovir** 500 mg PO twice daily
	HIV negative	• **Acyclovir** 400 mg PO twice daily **OR** • **Famciclovir** 250 mg PO twice daily **OR** • **Valacyclovir** 500 mg PO daily[a] **OR** 1 g PO daily

[a]May be less effective for patients with very frequent outbreaks (>10/y).

- Consider chancroid if the patient presents with typical manifestations, especially if there is a history of travel to an endemic area (Africa, Asia, and the Caribbean).
- It is often associated with **inguinal lymphadenopathy**, which is tender and may suppurate.
- Suppurative lymph nodes commonly develop secondary bacterial infections.

Diagnostic Testing

- **All ulcers suspicious for chancroid should be evaluated for HSV and syphilis.**
  - Isolating the organism on culture requires special media that are not widely available. Sensitivity is <80% even when cultured appropriately.[3]
  - PCR testing is rarely available.
  - Perform a dark-field examination for *Treponema pallidum* if ulcers have been present for <7 days. If ulcers have been present for >7 days, perform a serum rapid plasma reagent (RPR).
- Patients should be tested for HIV. If HIV-negative, retest in 3 months for HIV and syphilis.

TREATMENT

- **Azithromycin 1 g PO × 1 OR ceftriaxone 250 mg IM × 1** OR ciprofloxacin 500 mg PO twice daily × 3 days OR erythromycin base 500 mg PO three times daily × 7 days.[3]
- Lesions should be reexamined in 3 to 7 days and then weekly until healed (which may take as long as 2 wk).
- Treatment failures have been reported and are more common in patients with HIV. Longer regimens may be more appropriate for patients who have HIV or are unable to follow up.
- Large ulcers may not heal for several weeks and may result in permanent scarring.
- Inguinal buboes may require needle aspiration or incision and drainage.
- Partners should be treated if they had sexual contact with the patient up to 10 days before symptom onset.

Painless Genital Ulcer Diseases

In the United States, the most common STI-related cause of painless genital ulcers is syphilis. **The presence of any genital ulceration should prompt evaluation for syphilis.**

Syphilis

GENERAL PRINCIPLES

- Syphilis is a disease caused by the spirochete, *T. pallidum.*
- It follows a complex but predictable staged course of clinical manifestations interspersed with periods of latency.
- The systemic symptoms of syphilis are often nonspecific, thus earning its moniker "The Great Imitator."
- Treponemes enter the body through abrasions on skin or mucous membranes during sexual contact.
- Within hours, the organism spreads through the lymphatic system, to local lymph nodes, and into the bloodstream.
- The organism can also be spread vertically through transplacental transmission. Congenital syphilis rates are rising in the United States and are of great concern in public health.

DIAGNOSIS

Clinical Presentation

- See Table 11-2 for more detailed descriptions of the stages of syphilis.
- The incubation period between initial infection and the primary chancre is 10 to 90 days (average 21 d).

TABLE 11-2	CLINICAL MANIFESTATIONS, DIAGNOSTIC TESTS, AND TREATMENT FOR SYPHILIS			
Stage	Symptoms	Laboratory Diagnosis	Treatment	Alternative Regimen
Early—primary	Painless ulcer at inoculum site, local lymphadenopathy	DFA (if available) and serologic testing	**Benzathine PCN G** 2.4 million units IM × 1	If PCN-allergic: **Doxycycline** 100 mg PO twice daily × 14 d **OR** **Tetracycline** 500 mg PO four times daily × 14 d
Early—secondary	Macular or papular rash (palmar/plantar or generalized), mucous membrane lesions, constitutional symptoms (malaise, fever, headache, myalgias, arthralgias), generalized lymphadenopathy, patchy hair loss, condyloma lata, neurosyphilis (rare)	Nontreponemal serologic test (e.g., RPR), followed by treponemal-specific test for confirmation (e.g., TP-PA)	Same	Same
Early—nonprimary, nonsecondary syphilis (<1 y)	Generally asymptomatic		Same	Same
Unknown duration or late syphilis (>1 y or unknown)	Usually asymptomatic	Nontreponemal serologic test followed by treponemal-specific test for confirmation CSF VDRL if patient has HIV with low CD4, higher RPR, or neurologic symptoms; or in patients without HIV with symptoms of tertiary syphilis, or if evidence of neurologic/ophthalmic disease present	**Benzathine PCN G** 2.4 million units IM × 3 doses at 1-wk intervals	If PCN-allergic: **Doxycycline** 100 mg PO twice daily × 28 d **OR** **Tetracycline** 500 mg PO four times daily × 28 d

Tertiary	Cardiovascular involvement (aortic aneurysm, aortic insufficiency, coronary ostial stenosis); or gummatous disease	**Benzathine PCN G** 2.4 million units IM × 3 doses at 1-wk intervals. Some experts recommend treating cardiovascular syphilis with **IV PCN** (see Neurosyphilis)	If PCN-allergic: **Doxycycline** 100 mg PO twice daily × 28 d
Neurosyphilis	Often asymptomatic; involvement may be divided into categories: *Ocular*–Uveitis, interstitial keratitis, optic neuropathy, retinal vasculitis *Early*–Cranial nerve palsies, CVA, seizures *Late*–Tabes dorsalis (ataxia, lightning pains, pupillary abnormalities, wide-based gait); or general paresis (dementia, personality changes, tremor, reflex abnormalities)	**Aqueous crystalline PCN G** 3–4 million units IV every 4 hours × 10–14 d	If compliance ensured: **Procaine PCN** 2.4 million units IM daily + **probenecid** 500 mg PO four times daily × 10–14 d
Pregnancy	Same as for patients who are not pregnant	**PCN is the only recommended treatment— desensitize if necessary**	

CVA, cerebrovascular accident; DFA, direct fluorescent antibody; PCN, penicillin; RPR, rapid plasma reagent; TP-PA, *T. pallidum* particle agglutination assay.

- Primary lesions in the vagina or anus are often overlooked.
- The chancre usually lasts 1 to 6 weeks and resolves spontaneously with no scarring even without treatment.
- Secondary syphilis develops 4 to 10 weeks after the chancre resolves.
- Tertiary (symptomatic late latent) syphilis follows between 1 and 30 years after infection.
- These stages may overlap or present atypically in the setting of HIV coinfection.

Diagnostic Testing

- *T. pallidum* cannot be cultured in vitro, and the diagnosis relies on either **direct visualization of the organism or serologic testing.**
- In **primary syphilis**, the chancre should be evaluated for spirochetes with **dark-field microscopy or DFA testing.** Both are highly dependent on adequate sample collection and operator skill.
- Serologic testing and treatment for presumptive primary syphilis should be performed if a suspicious lesion is present.
- **Nontreponemal diagnostic tests** (e.g., RPR, Venereal Disease Research Laboratory [VDRL]) are **sensitive in immunocompetent patients, but are not specific**.
  - False-positive results may occur during pregnancy, in IV drug users, or in the presence of other diseases, such as other spirochete infections, tuberculosis, and autoimmune disorders.
  - False-negative results may occur very early in infection.
  - In advanced HIV disease, false-negative results or delayed appearance of seropositivity may be seen due to late antibody production.[3,4]
  - Very high antibody concentrations may interfere with RPR/VDRL testing and result in a false-negative test (prozone effect). The prozone effect is more common in patients with HIV.[5]
  - Titers tend to correspond to disease activity.
  - Patients with a history of treated syphilis may have low titers indefinitely. A fourfold increase in titer is indicative of reinfection.[3]
- **A positive RPR or VDRL should be followed by a confirmatory treponemal-specific test**, such as fluorescent treponemal antibody absorption (FTA-ABS), *T. pallidum* particle agglutination assay (TP-PA), or enzyme immunoassay (EIA).
- Some laboratories are conducting EIA for initial screening as part of a "reverse screening algorithm." A positive EIA should be followed with RPR with titer.
- **All patients with syphilis should be tested for HIV.**

TREATMENT

- Recommended treatment regimens are listed in Table 11-2.[3]
- All patients should have a clinical and serologic evaluation at least 6 and 12 months after treatment. Patients who are HIV positive, considered high risk, or are less likely to follow up should be re-evaluated sooner and more frequently.
- Partners should be treated if they had sexual contact with the patient up to 3 months before symptom onset. Patients with symptoms that persist or recur after appropriate treatment, and those with nontreponemal tests fourfold greater when repeated after appropriate treatment, should be considered for treatment failure or relapse by an experienced infectious diseases or STD provider.
- **Jarisch–Herxheimer reaction (i.e., fevers, headaches, and myalgias) is common** within 24 hours posttreatment, affecting up to 90% of patients treated with penicillin for early syphilis and up to 25% during later stages. Antipyretics can be used to alleviate symptoms. This reaction may precipitate early labor in pregnant women, but should not bar timely and appropriate treatment.

Lymphogranuloma Venereum

GENERAL PRINCIPLES

- LGV is caused by invasive *Chlamydia trachomatis* serovars L_1, L_2, and L_3.
- There are reports of increasing incidence in the United States, especially among men who have sex with men.

DIAGNOSIS

Clinical Presentation

- LGV is usually diagnosed clinically due to the lack of widespread serovar-specific testing.
- LGV initially manifests as a **painless, self-limited ulcer or papule at the inoculation site** 3 to 30 days after exposure. The ulcer is often missed and heals without scarring.
- The second stage is the development of **tender inguinal or femoral lymphadenopathy.** The enlarged nodes are usually unilateral and may become fluctuant and spontaneously drain. Constitutional symptoms and urethritis may also develop.
- The "groove sign" may be visible when the inguinal ligament forms a depression between enlarged inguinal and femoral lymph nodes. Its presence is suggestive of LGV, but is not frequently seen.
- Exposure through receptive anal intercourse can lead to proctocolitis similar to inflammatory bowel disease, which may progress to colorectal fistulas and strictures. Symptoms include anal discharge, rectal bleeding, and tenesmus.
- The third stage of the disease, which may not occur until years after exposure, is **hypertrophic granulomatous enlargement and ulceration of the external genitalia.** Elephantiasis of the genitalia may also occur by lymphatic obstruction.
- Genital and colorectal disease can be complicated by bacterial superinfections or coinfections with other STIs.

Diagnostic Testing

- A swab of a lesion or a bubo aspirate may be sent for culture, but this is not a sensitive method.
- **Nucleic acid amplification testing (NAAT) is the test of choice** for detecting all chlamydial serovars, but requires local laboratory validation of NAATs for extragenital samples.
- Genotyping to identify serovars is not widely available; if a patient has symptoms suspicious for LGV proctocolitis, a rectal swab should be sent to the state laboratory or the CDC for evaluation.
- Clinical evaluation, epidemiologic assessment, and exclusion of other possible causes remain the mainstay of diagnosis.

TREATMENT

- **Doxycycline 100 mg PO twice daily for 3 weeks OR erythromycin base 500 mg PO four times daily for 3 weeks.**[3]
- Pregnant women should be treated with erythromycin.
- Prolonged courses of azithromycin have been reportedly effective, but this has not been well-studied. A recent case of LGV with doxycycline failure was reportedly cured with moxifloxacin.[6]
- Patients should be reexamined to ensure response to treatment.
- Large, fluctuant buboes should be drained to speed resolution and prevent complications.

- Anyone who has had sexual contact with the patient during the 2 months before symptom onset should be examined and treated prophylactically with azithromycin 1 g PO × 1 dose or doxycycline 100 mg PO twice daily × 7 days.

Granuloma Inguinale (Donovanosis)

GENERAL PRINCIPLES

- Granuloma inguinale is caused by the intracellular gram-negative organism *Klebsiella granulomatis* (formerly *Calymmatobacterium granulomatis*).
- It is locally endemic in parts of the developing world and is uncommon in the United States.

DIAGNOSIS

Clinical Presentation

- The characteristic lesion is a **painless, beefy red vascular ulcerative lesion that tends to bleed when mechanically irritated**. Multiple lesions may be seen. There is typically no associated lymphadenopathy.
- The incubation period is thought to be 1 to 3 weeks.
- Rarely, extragenital infection can occur.

Diagnostic Testing

- *K. granulomatis* cannot be directly cultured.
- Tissue crush preparation or biopsy may show intracytoplasmic, bipolar-staining Donovan bodies. Tissue should also be evaluated for LGV, chancroid, and syphilis.
- Coinfection with other STIs is common.

TREATMENT

- **Doxycycline 100 mg PO twice daily × 3 weeks** OR azithromycin 1 g PO weekly × 3 weeks OR ciprofloxacin 750 mg PO twice daily × 3 weeks OR erythromycin base 500 mg PO four times daily × 3 weeks OR trimethoprim–sulfamethoxazole DS one tab PO twice daily for 3 weeks.[3]
- Longer treatment courses may be necessary, especially in immunocompromised patients. Addition of an aminoglycoside may speed resolution.

Other STIs

Gonorrhea, Mucopurulent Cervicitis, and Nongonococcal Urethritis

GENERAL PRINCIPLES

- **Cervicitis** presents as a symptom complex of mucopurulent vaginal discharge, abnormal vaginal bleeding, and/or dysuria. *Chlamydia*, gonorrhea, HSV, *Trichomonas vaginalis*, and human papilloma virus (HPV) can cause mucopurulent cervicitis.

- **Urethritis** is the corresponding symptom complex in men, causing mucopurulent penile discharge and dysuria. Urethritis is caused by gonorrhea or "nongonococcal urethritis" (NGU); the most common cause of NGU is *Chlamydia*, but *Mycoplasma genitalium* (15%–20%), *T. vaginalis, Ureaplasma urealyticum, Mycoplasma hominis*, HSV, and adenovirus may also cause infection.
- All patients presenting with cervicitis or urethritis should receive appropriate antibiotic treatment and safer sex counseling. Partners should also be tested and treated.

Epidemiology

- **Chlamydia is the most common reportable STI in the United States**, with over 1.5 million cases reported annually.
- **Gonorrhea is the second most common reportable bacterial STI in the United States**. It is estimated that only half of the cases are reported.
- Adolescents and young adults have the highest incidence of chlamydia and gonorrhea.

Pathophysiology

- *Neisseria gonorrhoeae* is a gram-negative intracellular diplococcus, visible within neutrophils on Gram stain.
- *C. trachomatis* is a gram-negative, obligate intracellular bacterium.
- *C. trachomatis* and *N. gonorrhoeae* infect columnar epithelial cells in the oropharynx, cervix, urethra, and rectum.
- Adolescent females are predisposed to chlamydia and gonorrhea because of the continued presence of columnar epithelium in the exocervix.

Risk Factors

Age ≤25 years, history of sexual contact with new or multiple partners, lack of barrier contraception use, drug use, and exchanging sex for drugs or money are significant risk factors for chlamydia and gonorrhea.

DIAGNOSIS

- **All sexually active women aged 25 years or younger should be screened for chlamydia and gonorrhea annually.**
- Pregnant women should be screened during the first prenatal visit and again in the third trimester if any risk factors are present.
- Older women with multiple or new sex partners should also be screened.
- **In high-prevalence settings, all sexually active men should be tested for chlamydia and gonorrhea.**
- Annual screening for urethral and rectal chlamydia and gonorrhea, as well as pharyngeal gonorrhea, is recommended for men who have sex with men while more frequent screening (every 3 mo) may be indicated in highest risk patients.

Clinical Presentation

- Asymptomatic chlamydial infection is common in both men and women. If symptoms of urethritis or cervicitis do develop, they will generally appear 7 to 21 days after exposure.
- Anorectal chlamydial infection may present as proctitis with anal irritation or itching, mucopurulent discharge, or tenesmus.
- Chlamydial conjunctivitis is associated with conjunctival hyperemia and eye discomfort; a mucoid discharge may be present.
- Left untreated, chlamydia can progress to pelvic inflammatory disease (PID), ectopic pregnancy, and infertility.

- Among men with urethral gonorrhea, 90% will develop mucopurulent discharge and dysuria 2 to 14 days after exposure.
- It is estimated that 50% of women with gonorrhea are asymptomatic, but nonspecific cervicitis symptoms may start in 1 to 2 weeks after exposure.
- Anorectal gonococcal infection may present as proctitis.
- Pharyngeal gonococcal infection is usually asymptomatic, but patients might develop a mild pharyngitis.
- Purulent ocular drainage can result from gonococcal conjunctivitis; gonococcal and chlamydial conjunctivitis in adults is usually a result of autoinoculation.
- *M. genitalium* is a known cause of urethritis in men and a likely etiology in persistent urethritis; it can be found in 10% to 30% of women with cervicitis.

Diagnostic Testing

- Mucopurulent urethral drainage in men should be evaluated with Gram stain and urinalysis.
  - Gram stain of secretions will show ≥2 leukocytes per high-power field (HPF) and, if gonorrhea is present, gram-negative intracellular diplococci.
  - A negative microscopic examination does not exclude infection in asymptomatic men.
- Gram staining of endocervical, anorectal, or pharyngeal secretion specimens for diagnostic purposes is not recommended.
- Patients with a history of multiple routes of exposure (i.e., vaginal, oral, and anal) should have all sites tested.
- Urinalysis may be positive for leukocyte esterase or demonstrate ≥10 leukocytes per HPF. Urine culture should be sent to evaluate for typical urinary tract infections.
- Culture has good specificity for both chlamydia and gonorrhea, but is less sensitive than other methods and is time consuming.
  - For gonorrhea, the swabbed specimen should be used to directly inoculate Thayer–Martin media and sent to the laboratory as soon as possible.
  - Diagnostic cultures are usually reserved for cases with an unclear diagnosis or, in the case of gonorrhea, unknown antibiotic susceptibility.
  - If gonorrhea resistance is suspected, clinicians should follow CDC recommendations and pursue culture if possible.
- NAAT is routinely used to test urine, vaginal, penile, and ocular discharge. While more sensitive than culture for pharyngeal and rectal specimens, extragenital NAAT use requires that laboratories perform validation.
- NAAT for *M. genitalium* detection is used in research settings as culture can take up to 6 months to grow. An FDA-approved NAAT is not currently available for clinical diagnosis.

TREATMENT

- **Because of the high coincidence of chlamydial infection and gonorrhea, treatment for both is recommended when there is suspicion for either.**
- Treatment for both can be accomplished with a **one-time, directly observed dose of azithromycin and ceftriaxone.** This is generally the best option, especially if follow-up is a concern.
- The preferred treatment for *M. genitalium* is azithromycin 1g PO once. Doxycycline is largely ineffective. Resistance is rapidly emerging, and in those cases moxifloxacin 400 mg PO daily for 10 to 14 days has been used. In cases complicated by PID, standard regimens are not effective, so a 7 to 14 day course of moxifloxacin 400 mg PO daily is recommended.
- Sex partners within the last 60 days should be evaluated and treated.
- Reinfection is very common. Partners need to be treated, and the patient should avoid all sexual contact until treatment is completed or 7 days following single-dose treatment.

- Test of cure is only indicated for pregnant women, if symptoms persist, or if there are concerns about antibiotic resistance or proper completion of therapy. All other patients should be encouraged to return for repeat testing in 3 to 4 months because of high rates of reinfection.
- See Table 11-3 for further detail.

COMPLICATIONS

- In women, bacterial cervicitis may progress to PID; see "Pelvic Inflammatory Disease" section.
- Bartholin or Skene gland infection may result in abscesses requiring drainage.
- Chlamydial urethritis can lead to epididymitis, prostatitis, or reactive arthritis in men.
- Gonorrhea can lead to epididymo-orchitis, prostatitis, and rarely urethral strictures.
- Disseminated gonococcal infection presents in one of two ways:
  - Tenosynovitis, papulopustular dermatitis, and arthralgia (without obvious purulent arthritis).
  - Purulent arthritis without skin involvement. Gonococcal arthritis is the most common cause of bacterial arthritis in young adults.
- Women within 7 days after the onset of menses or who are pregnant are at higher risk of developing disseminated infection.

Pelvic Inflammatory Disease

GENERAL PRINCIPLES

- Pelvic inflammatory disease is an ascending infection encompassing endometritis, salpingitis, tubo-ovarian abscess (TOA), and pelvic peritonitis.
- It is a known complication of chlamydial infection and gonorrhea, but other vaginal flora can also cause PID.
- Left untreated, 10% of women with PID can develop infertility. Other complications are ectopic pregnancy and chronic pelvic pain.

DIAGNOSIS

Clinical Presentation
History
- There is a wide range of clinical severity of PID, from asymptomatic infection to frank septic shock.
- Patients may have symptoms of cervicitis plus dyspareunia.
- Lower abdominal or pelvic pain suggests PID in a patient with cervicitis.

Physical Examination
- Fever is a common presenting sign of PID.[3]
- Cervicitis may be noted on a speculum examination.
- Bimanual examination will usually reveal uterine, adnexal, and/or cervical motion tenderness.
- Right upper quadrant pain and transaminitis suggest perihepatitis, or Fitz-Hugh–Curtis syndrome. Severe pain is caused by inflammation of Glisson capsule and the surrounding peritoneum.
- Consider another diagnosis (e.g., appendicitis and ectopic pregnancy) if mucopurulent discharge is not present and there are no leukocytes on wet prep examination.

TABLE 11-3	DIAGNOSIS AND TREATMENT OF SEXUALLY TRANSMITTED INFECTIONS ASSOCIATED WITH URETHRITIS OR CERVICITIS			
Disease	**Diagnostic Testing**	**Treatment**	**Alternative Treatment**	**Notes**
CT (*Chlamydia trachomatis*)	1. History and examination 2. Urinalysis and urine culture 3. NAAT of endocervical or urethral secretions 4. Culture if indicated and NAAT not available	Azithromycin 1 g PO × 1 OR Doxycycline 100 mg PO twice daily × 7 d	Erythromycin base 500 mg PO every 6 hours × 7 d OR Erythromycin ethylsuccinate 800 mg PO every 6 hours × 7 d OR Ofloxacin 300 mg PO twice daily × 7 d OR Levofloxacin 500 mg PO daily × 7 d	Doxycycline, erythromycin estolate, and FQs should be avoided during pregnancy
Uncomplicated GC ("the clap")	1. History and examination 2. Urinalysis and urine culture 3. Gram stain of urethral exudate, if present 4. NAAT of endocervical or urethral secretions 5. Culture if indicated and NAAT not available	Ceftriaxone 250 mg IM × 1 OR Cefixime 400 mg PO × 1 Plus concurrent treatment for CT **Gonococcal conjunctivitis:** Ceftriaxone 1 g IM × 1	History of severe cephalosporin allergy: best to desensitize, then treat with ceftriaxone OR Azithromycin 2 g PO × 1 (resistance reported, use only when no other option available); OR Spectinomycin 2 g IM × 1 (not available in the United States)	High levels of circulating FQ resistance now preclude the use of any FQ to treat any GC infections in the United States. Emerging macrolide resistance is also a concern

Disseminated gonococcal infection	1. History and examination 2. Culture and/or NAAT of all potential mucosal sites of infection 3. Blood cultures (often negative); 4. Arthrocentesis for cell count and culture in joints suspicious for septic arthritis	Ceftriaxone 1 g IV or IM daily OR Cefotaxime 1 g IV every 8 hours × 7 d OR Ceftizoxime 1 g IV every 8 hours Plus concurrent treatment for CT	Can switch to cefixime 400 mg PO twice daily 24–48 h after clinical improvement	If diagnosis is unclear, a trial of antibiotic therapy is warranted. If DGI, will usually improve rapidly. Higher doses and prolonged therapy are needed for meningitis or endocarditis
Trichomonas vaginalis ("trich")	1. In women: NAAT is preferred. Wet mount examination of vaginal secretion; rapid EIA is also available. 2. In men: NAAT is approved. Culture is available.	Metronidazole 2 g PO × 1 OR tinidazole 2 g PO × 1	Metronidazole 500 mg PO twice daily × 7 d	If pregnant, treatment is the same. If woman is HIV positive, the 7 d regimen is preferred.
NGU or MPC	1. History and examination 2. Test for CT and GC 3. In women: test for BV and trichomoniasis	Azithromycin 1 g PO × 1 OR Doxycycline 100 mg PO twice daily × 7 d Treat empirically for GC if local prevalence high or if patient is of high risk		If NGU persists after initial treatment: Metronidazole 2 g PO × 1 OR Tinidazole 2 g PO × 1

(Continued)

TABLE 11-3	DIAGNOSIS AND TREATMENT OF SEXUALLY TRANSMITTED INFECTIONS ASSOCIATED WITH URETHRITIS OR CERVICITIS (CONTINUED)			
Disease	Diagnostic Testing	Treatment	Alternative Treatment	Notes
PID	1. History and examination 2. Test for CT and GC 3. Wet prep examination for WBCs, clue cells, and trichomonads 4. Transvaginal ultrasound, laparoscopy, or endometrial biopsy reserved for difficult to diagnose cases	*IV Regimen A:* Doxycycline 100 mg PO or IV twice daily AND Cefotetan 2 g IV twice daily OR cefoxitin 2 g IV every 6 hours *IV Regimen B:* Clindamycin 900 mg IV every 8 hours PLUS Gentamicin 2 mg/kg IV loading dose, with 1.5 mg/kg IV every 8 hours for maintenance *PO Regimen B:* Cefoxitin 2 g IM × 1 with probenecid 1 g PO × 1 AND Doxycycline 100 mg PO twice daily × 14 d and/or Metronidazole 500 mg PO twice daily × 14 d *PO Regimen C:* IV third-generation cephalosporin AND Doxycycline 100 mg PO twice daily × 14 d and/or Metronidazole 500 mg PO twice daily × 14 d *PO Regimen A:* Ceftriaxone 250 mg IM × 1 AND Doxycycline 100 mg PO twice daily q14 d and/or Metronidazole 500 mg PO twice daily × 14 d	IV: Ampicillin/sulbactam 3 g IV every 6 hours PLUS Doxycycline 100 mg PO or IV twice daily PO: If unable to tolerate cephalosporins, consider treatment with levofloxacin 500 mg PO daily OR Ofloxacin 400 mg PO twice daily × 14 d if risk for GC is low Test for GC before treatment. If NAAT positive, will need to treat for GC as above. If culture positive, treatment based on susceptibilities	Can switch to PO therapy after 24 h of improvement. If no improvement after 72 h of PO regimen, reevaluate and switch to IV regimen

BV, bacterial vaginosis; CT, *Chlamydia trachomatis*; DGI, disseminated gonococcal infection; EIA, enzyme immunoassay; FQ, fluoroquinolone; GC, *Neisseria gonorrhoeae*; MPC, mucopurulent cervicitis; NAAT, nucleic acid amplification testing; NGU, nongonococcal urethritis; PID, pelvic inflammatory disease; WBC, white blood cells.

Diagnostic Testing

- All women with PID should be tested for chlamydia, gonorrhea, and HIV.
- Diagnosis of PID is supported by elevated erythrocyte sedimentation rate and/or C-reactive protein and documented infection with *C. trachomatis* and/or *N. gonorrhoeae.*
- More invasive studies, such as transvaginal ultrasonography, MRI, laparoscopy, or endometrial biopsy, are more specific tests for PID.

TREATMENT

- Antibiotic regimens are presented in Table 11-3.[3]
- Hospitalize patients who are acutely ill or have symptoms of an acute abdomen, are pregnant, are not tolerating or responding to outpatient antibiotics, or have a TOA.
- For women with mild or moderate PID, hospitalization is usually not necessary, and PO antibiotics provide effective treatment.
- If clinical improvement is seen on IV antibiotics, continue monitoring for another 24 hours before transitioning to PO antibiotics.
- If no improvement is seen within 72 hours, diagnostic laparoscopy may be necessary to further evaluate. If there has been no improvement after 72 hours of an outpatient PO regimen, reevaluate the patient and consider hospitalization with parenteral antibiotics.

Vulvovaginitis and Vaginosis

GENERAL PRINCIPLES

- Symptoms of vulvar or vaginal infection include abnormal vaginal discharge or odor, as well as vulvar itching and irritation.
- Trichomoniasis, bacterial vaginosis (BV), and candidiasis can cause these symptoms.
- BV represents shifting in the normal genital flora (especially *Lactobacillus*) toward anaerobes, *Gardnerella vaginalis*, and Mycoplasma species.
- Candidiasis is not generally sexually transmitted. Patients who are immunosuppressed are at higher risk of developing recurrent or severe vulvovaginal candidiasis and may benefit from longer courses of therapy.
- **Trichomoniasis is sexually transmitted. Men are almost always asymptomatic, but may have mild urethritis.**

DIAGNOSIS

- Trichomoniasis may cause diffuse cervical and vaginal erythema ("strawberry cervix") and a malodorous, frothy discharge with a pH ≥ 4.5.
  - NAATs are highly sensitive and recommended for diagnosis of trichomoniasis.
  - Wet mount examination will often show mobile trichomonads.
  - Culture is available in some locations.
- Point-of-care EIAs are also available. A wet mount examination should be performed on patients with suspected BV, which will demonstrate clue cells (i.e., vaginal epithelial cells with a stippled appearance due to adherent coccobacilli). Having three of the four following findings suggests BV: presence of clue cells, homogenous white vaginal discharge, vaginal discharge with pH ≥ 4.5, and a positive whiff test are suggestive of BV (Amsel criteria)
- Vulvovaginal candidiasis is diagnosed by a characteristic thick, curd-like vaginal discharge with intense vulvar inflammation, which will show fungal elements on 10% KOH preparation.

TREATMENT

- See Table 11-3 for treatment regimens for trichomoniasis.[3] Instruct patients to abstain from sexual activity until all partners are treated. Reinfection is very common.
- Treat BV with metronidazole 500 mg PO twice daily × 7 days OR metronidazole gel 0.75%, 5 g (1 applicator) intravaginally every night × 5 days OR clindamycin cream 2%, 5 g (1 applicator) intravaginally every night × 7 days.
  - BV is associated with adverse pregnancy outcomes. Symptomatic pregnant women should be tested and treated.
  - Clindamycin cream is associated with adverse outcomes during the second half of pregnancy and should be avoided.
  - Sex partners do not need to be treated.
- Vulvovaginal candidiasis is treated with over-the-counter intravaginal azole creams and suppositories or fluconazole 150 mg PO × 1 dose.

Genital Warts

GENERAL PRINCIPLES

- Genital warts are caused by HPV. Multiple subtypes exist. **Types 6 and 11** are associated with genital warts, whereas types 16, 18, 31, 33, and 35 are associated with cervical or anorectal neoplasias.
- Genital HPV is common, with an estimated 6.2 million new cases diagnosed annually in the United States. It is thought that 50% of sexually active adults will acquire genital HPV over their lifetimes.
- **Most cases are asymptomatic.**
- **Viral shedding occurs during and between symptomatic periods.** The incubation period is thought to be weeks to months.
- **Young adults and previously unvaccinated immunocompromised individuals (including HIV-positive individuals) should receive the HPV vaccine** to protect against certain high-risk subtypes of HPV.

DIAGNOSIS

- The appearance of HPV can vary considerably. Typically, verrucous papules are present, measuring approximately 1 cm in diameter, and can spontaneously remit and recur.
- **Visual inspection is usually sufficient for diagnosis.** Biopsy is only indicated if the diagnosis is uncertain, if the patient is immunocompromised, or if the lesions do not respond to treatment, have an unusual appearance (pigmented, fixed, or indurated), or persistently ulcerate or bleed.

TREATMENT

- Treatment is focused on the removal of visible warts and to induce as long a wart-free interval as possible.
- Treatment options are as follows[3]:
  - Imiquimod 5% cream. Patients should apply the cream to warts at night, three times a week for up to 16 weeks; 6 to 10 hours after application, the affected areas should be washed with soap and water.
  - Podofilox 0.5% solution or gel. Patients should be instructed to apply twice daily for 3 days, followed by 4 days of no therapy. This cycle may be repeated up to four times to treat visible warts. The total area treated should not exceed 10 cm^2.

- Cryotherapy. Treatment can be repeated every 1 to 2 weeks.
- Trichloroacetic acid (TCA), a small amount is applied weekly as needed.
- Surgical removal.
- Podofilox, imiquimod, and podophyllin are cytotoxins and should not be used during pregnancy.

Molluscum Contagiosum

GENERAL PRINCIPLES

- Molluscum contagiosum is a superficial skin infection caused by the molluscum contagiosum virus (MCV), a poxvirus.
- The incubation period ranges from 2 weeks to 6 months. Transmission is through direct skin contact or fomites, including sexual contact, shared clothes or towels, and contact sports.
- Patients with atopic dermatitis are at particular risk of autoinoculation and refractory infection.

DIAGNOSIS

- The diagnosis is usually made based on the appearance of the lesions. They usually measure 2 to 5 mm and are **waxy, painless, and umbilicated.** The central core of the lesion contains infectious viral particles.
- Patients who are immunocompromised may develop giant molluscum ($\geq$15 mm). Biopsy may be required to exclude fungal infections or malignancy.

TREATMENT

- Most cases resolve spontaneously within 6 to 12 months. Lesions may persist for years in patients who are immunocompromised. The lesions rarely scar but may become secondarily infected.
- No single treatment has been proven to be more effective than others in treating MCV.
  - In adults, lesions may be treated by **curettage or cryotherapy in the office setting, followed by patient-applied topical imiquimod**.
  - Imiquimod should be started three times weekly; if no irritation develops, applications should be increased to once daily.
  - Other treatments include salicylic acid, TCA, KOH, cantharidin, electrocauterization, and photodynamic therapy.
- Patients should be advised to keep lesions covered whenever possible and to avoid shaving over affected areas.
- Giant molluscum is very resistant to treatment. Lesions should be treated before they coalesce into giant lesions.
- In patients with HIV, lesions usually improve with antiretroviral therapy.

REFERENCES

1. Shiely F, Hayes K, Thomas KK, et al. Expedited partner therapy: a robust intervention. *Sex Transm Dis*. 2010;37:602-607.
2. Golden MR, Whittington WL, Handsfield HH, et al. Effect of expedited treatment of sex partners on recurrent or persistent gonorrhea or chlamydial infection. *N Engl J Med*. 2005;352:676-685.
3. Workowski KA, Berman S; Centers for Disease Control and Prevention (CDC). Sexually transmitted diseases treatment guidelines, 2015. *Clin Infect Dis*. 2015;61(suppl 8):S759-S762.

4. Kingston AA, Vujevich J, Shapiro M, et al. Seronegative secondary syphilis in 2 patients coinfected with human immunodeficiency virus. *Arch Dermatol.* 2005;141:431-433.

5. Jurado RL, Campbell J, Martin PD. Prozone phenomenon in secondary syphilis. Has its time arrived? *Arch Intern Med.* 1993;153:2496-2498.

6. Mcha F, de Barbeyrac B, Aoun O, et al. Doxycycline failure in lymphogranuloma venereum. *Sex Transm Infect.* 2010;86:278-279.

Human Immunodeficiency Virus Infection

12

Jane O'Halloran and Rachel Presti

GENERAL PRINCIPLES

- HIV, the causative organism of AIDS, was discovered in 1983, after an unusual cluster of opportunistic infections (OIs) associated with immunosuppression was observed in a group of men who have sex with men (MSM). HIV infects CD4 T cells, resulting in progressive immune deficiency and OIs.
- Mortality associated with untreated HIV is extremely high; however, highly active antiretroviral therapy (HAART) has rendered the disease a chronic illness. Studies have shown that life expectancy in patients who are diagnosed early in the course of infection, whose immune systems are intact and who commence HAART, is similar to that of HIV-negative counterparts.[1]
- Virologic suppression associated with successful HAART also dramatically decreases HIV transmission risk.[2]

Classification

- CDC classification is widely used for public health surveillance purposes. This classification uses clinical conditions (see Table 12-1) and CD4+ T cell count to group patients.
- Details are available at http://www.cdc.gov/hiv/resources/guidelines/

Epidemiology

- Since the beginning of the HIV epidemic around 70 million people have been infected. More than 36 million people worldwide are living with HIV, with the highest disease burden in sub-Saharan Africa. In 2016, approximately 50% of those infected with HIV were receiving HAART, and this number continues to increase with improved access.
- Heterosexual transmission is the most common mode of HIV acquisition worldwide, although MSM transmission accounts for more than a half of all new HIV infections each year in the United States and Europe.
- In the United States, more than a million people are living with HIV, although up to 15% of those are unaware of their diagnosis. African Americans are disproportionately affected by HIV, accounting for almost half of people living with HIV and almost half of new infections each year.
- Stigma associated with HIV infection and modes of transmission can hinder timely diagnosis and treatment.

Etiology

- HIV is a lentivirus that is part of the retrovirus family.
- There are two major types of HIV. HIV-1 is the most common type worldwide and likely originated from chimpanzee simian immunodeficiency virus. HIV-2 closely resembles HIV-1 but is characterized by a much slower progression to AIDS. It is endemic in West Africa and rare elsewhere.
- Different HIV-1 subtypes dominate various regions worldwide. HIV-1 infection in the United States is predominantly caused by subtype B.

243

TABLE 12-1	AIDS-DEFINING CONDITIONS (ADULTS AND ADOLESCENTS AGE ≥13 Y)

Candidiasis of bronchi, trachea, or lungs

Candidiasis of esophagus

Cervical cancer, invasive

Coccidioidomycosis, disseminated or extrapulmonary

Cryptococcosis, extrapulmonary

Cryptosporidiosis, chronic intestinal (>1 mo duration)

Cytomegalovirus disease (other than liver, spleen, or nodes)

Cytomegalovirus retinitis (with loss of vision)

Encephalopathy, HIV related

Herpes simplex: chronic ulcers (>1 mo duration) or bronchitis, pneumonitis, or esophagitis

Histoplasmosis, disseminated or extrapulmonary

Isosporiasis, chronic intestinal (>1 mo duration)

Kaposi sarcoma

Lymphoma, Burkitt (or equivalent term)

Lymphoma, immunoblastic (or equivalent term)

Lymphoma, primary, of brain

Mycobacterium avium complex or *Mycobacterium kansasii*, disseminated or extrapulmonary

Mycobacterium tuberculosis of any site, pulmonary, disseminated, or extrapulmonary

Mycobacterium, other species or unidentified species, disseminated or extrapulmonary

Pneumocystis jiroveci pneumonia

Pneumonia, recurrent

Progressive multifocal leukoencephalopathy

Salmonella septicemia, recurrent

Toxoplasmosis of brain

Wasting syndrome attributed to HIV

Pathophysiology

- Understanding the HIV life cycle played a critical role in developing successful HAART.
- Successful transmission of HIV infection at mucosal surfaces can occur with less than five HIV virions. Local replication and infection of draining lymph nodes occurs in the first 7 days following exposure and is undetectable by current assays.
- During the early stages of infection, there is massive replication of the virus in the gut lymphatic tissue accompanied by cytokine production and mucosal damage. Specific CD8 T-cell response is generated and determines control of the infection. Antibodies are robustly produced but cannot effectively neutralize the virus.

- Permanent viral reservoirs containing integrated proviral DNA are established predominantly in T cells and potentially macrophages. This integrated latent form of infection makes HIV-1 virus extremely difficult to eradicate. These reservoirs are the focus of much research aimed at HIV cure.
- The HIV viral envelope consists of a lipid bilayer with embedded gp120/gp41 complex. The viral capsid is made of p24; the core contains two single strands of RNA packaged with structural proteins and surrounded by the p17 matrix.
- The first step in the HIV replication cycle is the binding of the viral gp120 surface protein to CD4 receptor–containing cells.
- For viral fusion and entry to occur, coreceptor binding is necessary. HIV can use several chemokine receptors, but primarily uses CCR5, less often CXCR4. HIV can be tropic for either of the coreceptors or have a dual tropism. On binding to the chemokine coreceptor gp120/gp41 undergoes a conformational change, resulting in a hairpin-like structure that promotes fusion between the cell membrane and the virion.
  - **Fusion inhibitor.** Enfuvirtide (T-20) binds to gp41, preventing the fusion of the virion with the cell.
  - **Chemokine receptor inhibitor.** Maraviroc (MVC) binds the CCR5 receptor. An antagonist for a CXCR4 receptor is not clinically available.
- Once inside the cytoplasm, the viral RNA undergoes reverse transcription using a virally encoded reverse transcriptase. Viral RNA becomes double-stranded DNA that is later transported to the nucleus.
  - **Nucleoside reverse transcriptase inhibitors** (NRTIs) are structural analogs of normal nucleosides or nucleotides, which target the reverse transcriptase and terminate HIV DNA synthesis. Commonly used NRTIs include tenofovir disoproxil fumarate (TDF), tenofovir alafenamide (TAF), emtricitabine (FTC), lamivudine (3TC) and abacavir (ABC).
  - **Nonnucleoside reverse transcriptase inhibitors** (NNRTIs) bind to the reverse transcriptase and block polymerization of the viral DNA. Commonly used NNRTIs include efavirenz (EFV) and rilpivirine (RPV).
- After entering the nucleus, the double-stranded DNA integrates into the host chromosomal DNA, which is mediated by the HIV integrase. This process is referred to as DNA strand transfer. **Integrase strand transfer inhibitors** (INSTIs) bind to HIV integrase and prevent DNA strand transfer. Commonly used INSTIs include raltegravir (RAL), elvitegravir dolutegravir, and bictegravir.
- As viral RNA is produced, it gets packaged in a new virion with structural proteins and enzymes and then buds into the extracellular environment. The final infectious virion requires cleavage of structural proteins by HIV protease. **Protease inhibitors** (PIs) bind to HIV protease preventing the packaging of virion. PIs are frequently administered with a pharmacologic "boosting" agent. Ritonavir and cobicistat are the two agents currently used for boosting. Commonly used PIs include boosted darunavir or boosted atazanavir.

Risk Factors

- HIV transmission can occur via blood, semen, vaginal fluid, or breast milk that may contain cell-bound or free viral particles.
- Transmission occurs via unprotected sexual intercourse, contaminated blood (blood transfusion, sharing needles or equipment for illicit drugs, or occupational exposure), or perinatally from mother to child.
- The risk of transmission varies according to the type of sexual exposure (see Table 12-2).[3] The presence of genital ulcer disease and other STDs as well as high HIV viral loads in the source patient increases the risk of transmission.

TABLE 12-2	RISK OF HIV ACQUISITION ACCORDING TO TYPE OF SEXUAL EXPOSURE
Exposure Type	**Risk per 10,000 Exposures**
Receptive anal intercourse	138
Insertive anal intercourse	11
Receptive penile–vaginal intercourse	8
Insertive penile–vaginal intercourse	4
Receptive oral intercourse	Low
Insertive oral intercourse	Low

Adapted from https://www.cdc.gov/hiv/risk/estimates/riskbehaviors.html.

Prevention

Several approaches to HIV prevention currently exist including:

- **Treatment as prevention** (universal test and treat) is an important public health concept, which is based on the hypothesis that enhanced identification of HIV patients followed by rapid initiation of HAART regardless of CD4 T cell count or disease stage will reduce transmission and thus HIV infection rates at the population level. When the level of virus in the blood is undetectable, the risk of sexual transmission of HIV is negligible.
- Strategies to **prevent sexual transmission** of HIV include:
  - **Nonpharmacologic** methods including condom use, male circumcision, and testing for other sexually transmitted infections.
  - **Pharmacologic** methods can be divided into pre-exposure prophylaxis (PrEP) and postexposure prophylaxis (PEP).
    - **PrEP:** antiretroviral medications taken **before a potential exposure to HIV**. It is recommended as one option to prevent HIV acquisition in sexually active adults and intravenous drug users at substantial risk of infection. At present, TDF/FTC coformulated as Truvada taken daily or just before and after a sexual encounter is the only antiretroviral approved by the FDA for PrEP. The use of other oral antiretroviral agents including long-acting injectable antiretrovirals, microbicides, and antiretroviral topical formulations to prevent HIV transmission is in clinical trials.
    - **PEP** can be divided into two categories:
      - **Nonoccupational exposure:** nonoccupational postexposure prophylaxis (nPEP) is offered **for high-risk exposures (sexual or needle sharing) from a known HIV-positive source, presenting within 72 hours**. For nPEP, three-drug antiretroviral regimen is provided for 28 days. nPEP for a high-risk exposure from a source with an unknown HIV status has to be individualized. nPEP is not recommended if the exposed person presents after 72 hours.
      - **Occupational exposure:** Assess the source, volume of fluid, type, and timing of the exposure. HIV and hepatitis B (HBV) and C (HCV) testing is required. HIV testing of the exposed person should be performed at baseline, 6 weeks, 12 weeks, and 4 months provided a fourth-generation HIV Ag/Ab combination immunoassay is used. If not, testing should be extended to 6 months. Offer 28 days of antiretrovirals for exposures with increased transmission risk. A three-drug regimen of TDF, FTC, and RAL is currently recommended.

DIAGNOSIS

- **HIV screening tests:**
  - **CDC recommends routine HIV screening for all adolescents and adults (aged 13–64 y) in health care settings, as a part of routine medical care.** Separate consent is not required, but the patient should be informed of the HIV testing and a plan for linkage to care should be in place in the event of a positive test result.
  - Screening guidelines recommend the use of a fourth-generation HIV Ag/Ab combination immunoassay; however, this can be negative in the first 14 days after infection (window period).
  - The earliest positive test is the HIV viral load test with HIV RNA usually detectable approximately 7 days after infection.
  - Several rapid, tests are available for screening but only detect antibodies.
  - Confirmatory testing should follow any positive screening test.
  - All specimens reactive on screening assay should undergo additional testing with an immunoassay that differentiates HIV-1 from HIV-2 antibodies. The use of HIV Western blot as a confirmatory test is no longer the preferred assay as other immunoassays are more sensitive and specific.
  - Specimens that are reactive on screening test and nonreactive or indeterminate on the antibody differentiation assay should proceed to HIV-1 nucleic acid testing for confirmation. **If acute HIV is suspected, HIV-1 nucleic acid testing is the preferred screening test.**
  - **HIV screening of all pregnant women is recommended using an opt-out approach.** Repeat testing should be performed in the third trimester in women who tested negative at the initial screening.

Clinical Presentation

- **Acute HIV infection**
  - The symptoms of acute HIV infection resemble infectious mononucleosis or influenza-like illness with fever, pharyngitis, adenopathy, rash, myalgia or arthralgia, headaches, and fatigue. Oral ulcers and gastrointestinal symptoms (diarrhea, odynophagia, anorexia, abdominal pain, and vomiting) may also occur. Rarely neurologic symptoms may occur (meningitis, encephalitis, Guillain–Barre syndrome).
  - The severity of illness can vary, and patients may even be asymptomatic.
  - The time from exposure to clinical manifestations of the acute HIV is typically 2 to 4 weeks and lasts for about 3 weeks.
  - Massive depletion of CD4 T cells and rapid increase in HIV RNA is seen as the initial response to the infection. With evolution of HIV-specific immunity (primarily from HIV-specific CD8+ cytotoxic T lymphocytes), HIV RNA level falls by 2 to 3 logs and the symptoms of acute retroviral syndrome resolve. CD4 T cell counts rebound but remain below the baseline.
- **Chronic HIV infection**
  - The length of time from initial infection to clinical disease varies.
  - During the chronic phase of HIV infection, active virus replication is ongoing and progressive even if patients are asymptomatic. Persons with high levels of HIV RNA may progress to symptomatic disease faster than those with low HIV RNA levels.
  - Patients in this stage have chronic inflammation evidenced by increase in various inflammatory markers, likely from chronic immune activation caused by HIV infection. This increases the risk of non–AIDS-related comorbidities, such as cardiovascular disease, renal dysfunction, and non–AIDS-related malignancies. HAART reduces chronic immune activation, but not always to baseline.
  - The spectrum of disease changes as the CD4 cell depletion continues. **Life-threatening OIs classically occur when the CD4 cell count drops to <200 cells/μL.**

- There are several unique subsets of patients with different disease progression patterns compared with an average HIV-infected person.
  - **Long-term progressors.** These patients show little or no decline in CD4 cell count over an extended period of time and usually have only low-level viremia.
  - **Elite controllers.** Show slight or no decline in CD4 cell counts over an extended period of time and usually have extremely low HIV RNA, often <50 copies/mL.
  - **Rapid progressors.** Progress to AIDS rapidly. The mechanism of rapid progression is still unknown, but infection with CXCR4 tropic virus seems to accelerate the HIV disease.

History
- Initial evaluation of persons with HIV infection (either newly diagnosed or care transferred from another physician) should include a detailed history with particular focus on potential risk factors for HIV transmission and symptoms suggestive of OI.
- Routine screening for depression should also be performed as depression is prevalent in persons living with HIV. Patients should also be assessed for domestic violence and sexual abuse.
- Because of ongoing stigma associated with HIV infection, care should be taken to understand patients' desire for privacy and respect wishes about disclosure. Legal consequences regarding knowingly exposing others to HIV infection vary depending on local conditions and should be discussed.

Physical Examination
A comprehensive physical examination should be performed on initial and subsequent visits with particular focus placed on:

- **Skin:** conditions associated with HIV infection include seborrheic dermatitis, eosinophilic folliculitis, psoriasis, superficial fungal disease, molluscum contagiosum, and Kaposi sarcoma.
- **Oropharynx:** diseases including candida, hairy leukoplakia, mucosal Kaposi sarcoma, HSV infection, aphthous ulcers, and periodontal disease are associated with HIV infection.
- **Lymphatic:** generalized lymphadenopathy from follicular hyperplasia is well described in HIV infection, but considering the higher risk of malignancies (e.g., lymphoma) or disseminated infections, asymmetric, bulky, or rapidly enlarging adenopathy requires further evaluation.
- **Anogenital examination:** should be performed to evaluate for rectal masses, prostate size, external genital ulcers, or condylomatous lesions. Women should undergo pelvic examination to assess for abnormal vaginal discharge and cervical lesions.

Diagnostic Testing

Laboratories
- The following laboratory parameters should be performed at initial visit:
  - HIV antibody testing (if prior documentation is not available or if HIV RNA is below the assay's limit of detection)
  - CD4 T lymphocyte cell count
  - Plasma HIV RNA (viral load)
  - Complete blood count, chemistry profile, transaminase levels, blood urea nitrogen, and creatinine, urinalysis, and serologies for hepatitis A, B, and C viruses and syphilis.
  - Fasting blood glucose and serum lipids
  - Glucose-6-phosphate dehydrogenase (G6PD)
  - HLA B*5701 (if treatment with ABC is considered)
  - Serologic screening for CMV or toxoplasma may be considered if the baseline CD4 count is <200 and a delay in immune recovery or initiation of HAART is expected.
  - Genotypic resistance testing

- **HIV genotype testing**
  - It is important to be aware of the most commonly encountered HIV drug resistance mutations and their effect on the choice of HAART (see Table 12-3). Baseline genotype resistance testing for RT/PI mutations is recommended at the time of HIV diagnosis and before initiation of HAART. At present, baseline INSTI resistance testing is not recommended.
  - In persons failing ART, a genotype should be repeated to optimize further treatment options.
  - PIs and some INSTIs have high genetic barriers for drug resistance (need multiple mutations to confer resistance), whereas some NRTIs (such as lamivudine [3TC]) and most NNRTIs (EFV, nevirapine [NVP] and RPV) have low genetic barriers where a single mutation can result in resistance.

TABLE 12-3	IMPORTANT HIV RESISTANCE MUTATIONS

NRTI Resistance Mutation

M184V	Commonly seen as the first drug resistance mutation in patients who are failing treatment on 3TC- or FTC-containing regimens. It confers resistance to 3TC and FTC, decreased susceptibility to ABC and ddI. Conversely, it confers hypersusceptibility to AZT, d4T, and TDF. This mutation decreases HIV replication capacity.
K65R	Confers resistance to TDF and cross-resistance to ABC, 3TC, and ddI. Conversely, K65R induces hypersusceptibility to AZT. It also decreases the replication capacity, which may be additive when M184V is present.
L74V	Confers resistance to ddI and ABC. Conversely, it confers hypersusceptibility to AZT and TDF. L74V causes less replication capacity than wild-type virus.
TAMs	Occurs with exposure to AZT or d4T. There are two pathways: first pathway involves M41L, L210W, and T215Y, which confers high-level resistance to AZT/d4Tand has more NRTI cross-resistance; second pathway involves D67N, K70R, and K219Q/E, which confers low-level resistance to AZT/d4T and has less NRTI cross-resistance.

NNRTI Resistance Mutation

K103N	Commonly seen and confers resistance to EFV and NVP. ETR is still effective and should be considered as an alternative.

Note: Other NNRTI mutations may confer resistance to ETR; use of weighted score system is recommended when the use of ETR is considered in patients with NNRTI drug resistance.

PI Resistance Mutations

D30N	This is a signature NFV mutation that causes high level of resistance to NFV
I50L	Signature ATV mutation that causes high-level resistance to ATV but increased susceptibility to other PIs.

Note: When PI resistance occurs, it is usually as a result for cumulative mutations rather than a single point mutation.

(Continued)

TABLE 12-3	IMPORTANT HIV RESISTANCE MUTATIONS (CONTINUED)

INSTI Resistance Mutations

E138K/A	These mutations usually occur in combination with Q148 mutations. Alone they do not reduce INSTI susceptibility; however, in combination with Q148 they cause high-level resistance to RAL and EVG
Q148H	In combination with G140S, Q148H cause high-level resistance to RAL and EVG
N155H	Causes resistance to RAL and ETG. Virologic failure has occurred in patients treated with DTG who have N155H at baseline

3TC, lamivudine; ABC, abacavir; ATV, atazanavir; AZT, zidovudine; ddl, didanosine; DTG, dolutegravir; d4T, stavudine; EFV, efavirenz; ETG, elvitegravir; ETR, etravirine; FTC, emtricitabine; NFV, nelfinavir; NNRTI, non-nucleoside reverse transcriptase inhibitor; NRTI, nucleoside reverse transcriptase inhibitor; NVP, nevirapine; TAM, thymidine analog mutation; TDF, tenofovir; PI, protease inhibitor; RAL, raltegravir.

TREATMENT

- HAART has evolved over the past decade with easily tolerated and once-daily regimens widely available for treatment-naïve patients in resource-rich countries.
- **When to start:** Over the past few years there has been much debate related to the optimal timing of HAART in patients with intact immune systems. The Strategic Timing of Antiretroviral Treatment (START) trial that randomized subjects with CD4+ T cell counts >500 cells/μL to immediate or deferred (postpone until CD4+T cell count <350 cells/μL) showed higher rates of serious AIDS and non-AIDS events in those who deferred HAART.[4] As a result of this and the potential of treatment as prevention, current guidelines recommend **initiating HAART in all patients with HIV infection irrespective of CD4+ T cell count.**
- Once effective HAART is started, treatment interruption is strongly discouraged. Based on the SMART trial data, treatment interruption was associated with increased rates of OIs and death and increased rates of major cardiovascular, renal, and hepatic complications.[5]

Medications

- **What to start** (see Tables 12-4 through 12-10).
- Selection of an antiretroviral regimen is individually based, with consideration of toxicity, tolerability, pill burden, drug interactions, comorbidities, and baseline genotype.
- **The combination of dual NRTI backbone and a potent third agent from another class** is recommended and once-daily regimen is preferred.
- Recommended and alternative regimens:
  - In general, ART regimens for treatment-naïve patients should consist of two NRTIs combined with a third active antiretroviral from one of three classes including INSTI, NNRTI, or PI with a booster that can be cobicistat or ritonavir.
  - Current recommended and alternative regimes are outlined in Table 12-4.[6]
- Other regimens:
  - When compared with recommended and alternative regimens, other regimens may have decreased virologic efficacy, increased toxicity, increased pill burden, or limited data from clinical trials to support their use.

TABLE 12-4	RECOMMENDED INITIAL REGIMENS FOR ANTIRETROVIRAL-NAÏVE PERSONS

Recommended Regimens

INSTI plus two NRTIs:
    Dolutegravir/abacavir/lamivudine (HLA-B*5701 negative only)
    Dolutegravir plus tenofovir disoproxil fumarate/emtricitabine or tenofovir alafenamide/emtricitabine
    Elvitegravir/cobicistat/emtricitabine/tenofovir alafenamide or tenofovir disoproxil fumarate
    Raltegravir plus either tenofovir disoproxil fumarate/emtricitabine or tenofovir alafenamide/emtricitabine
Boosted PI plus two NRTIs:
    Darunavir/ritonavir plus either tenofovir disoproxil fumarate/emtricitabine or tenofovir alafenamide/emtricitabine

Alternative Regimens

NNRTI plus two NRTIs:
    Efavirenz/tenofovir disoproxil fumarate/emtricitabine
    Efavirenz/tenofovir alafenamide/emtricitabine
    Rilpivirine/tenofovir disoproxil fumarate/emtricitabine or tenofovir alafenamide/emtricitabine (if HIV RNA <100,000 copies/mL and CD4 >200 cells/µL)
Boosted PI plus two NRTIs:
    Atazanavir/cobicistat or atazanavir/ritonavir plus either tenofovir disoproxil fumarate/emtricitabine or tenofovir alafenamide/emtricitabine
    Darunavir/cobicistat or Darunavir/ritonavir plus abacavir/lamivudine (HLA-B*5701 negative only)
    Darunavir/cobicistat or Darunavir/ritonavir plus either tenofovir disoproxil fumarate/emtricitabine or tenofovir alafenamide/emtricitabine

INSTI, integrase strand transfer inhibitor; NNRTI, nonnucleoside reverse transcriptase inhibitor; NRTI, nucleoside reverse transcriptase inhibitor; PI, protease inhibitor.

TABLE 12-5	NUCLEOSIDE/NUCLEOTIDE REVERSE TRANSCRIPTASE INHIBITORS

	Dose	Food Restrictions	Side Effects	Comments
ABC	300 mg twice daily 600 mg once daily	None	Systemic hypersensitivity reaction Associated with increased cardiovascular risk in numerous cohort studies	Baseline HLA-B5701 needed before initiation; if positive do not initiate

(Continued)

TABLE 12-5	NUCLEOSIDE/NUCLEOTIDE REVERSE TRANSCRIPTASE INHIBITORS (CONTINUED)			
	Dose	Food Restrictions	Side Effects	Comments
ddl*	Preferred as an enteric-coated formula >60 kg: 400 mg once daily <60 kg: 250 mg once daily	On empty stomach	Pancreatitis, peripheral neuropathy, diarrhea	When coadministered with TDF adjust dose to 250 mg
FTC	200 mg once daily	None	Well tolerated	Clinically equivalent to 3TC.
3TC	150 mg twice daily 300 mg once daily	None	Well tolerated	As above, do not coadminister with FTC
d4T*	>60 kg: 40 mg twice daily <60 kg: 30 mg twice daily Extended release >60 kg: 100 mg once daily <60 kg: 75 mg once daily	None	Peripheral neuropathy, fat redistribution, lactic acidosis, pancreatitis; hyperlipidemia	
TDF	300 mg once daily	None	GI intolerance rare; renal toxicity, bone density loss	
TAF	25 mg once daily	None	Avoids the renal and bone density issues associated with TDF	Reduced dose when combined with cobicistat
AZT*or ZDV	300 mg twice daily	None	Bone marrow suppression, GI intolerance	

*no longer used in routine practice.
3TC, lamivudine; d4T, stavudine; ABC, abacavir; AZT or ZDV, zidovudine; ddl, didanosine; EFV, efavirenz; FTC, emtricitabine; GI, gastrointestinal; NRTI, nucleoside reverse transcriptase inhibitor; TAF, tenofovir alafenamide; TDF, tenofovir disoproxil fumarate.

TABLE 12-6   INTEGRASE STRAND TRANSFER INHIBITORS

	Dose	Food Restrictions	Side Effects	Comments
INSTI				
RAL	400 mg twice daily or 1200 mg once daily (HD)	No	Well tolerated, rarely rhabdomyolysis	Twice daily dosing recommended during pregnancy
ETG	150 mg boosted with 150 mg COBI	No	Tolerated well in general	Available as STR with TAF or TDF plus FTC.
DTG	50 mg once daily	No	Well tolerated, increased rates of insomnia	50 mg twice daily when used in the setting of baseline INSTI resistance
BIC	Fixed dose combination	No	Diarrhea, nausea	See coformulated ART

COBI, cobicistat; DTG, Dolutegravir; ETG, elvitegravir; HD, high dose; INSTI, integrase strand transfer inhibitor; RAL, raltegravir; STR, single table regimen.

TABLE 12-7   NON-NUCLEOSIDE REVERSE TRANSCRIPTASE INHIBITORS

	Dose	Food Restrictions	Side Effects	Comments
EFV	600 mg once daily	On empty stomach	CNS symptoms (dizziness, vivid dreams); false-positive cannabinoid test; hyperlipidemia	Take at night to reduce side effects
NVP	Start 200 mg once daily for 2 wk, then 200 mg twice daily	None	Rash, hepatotoxicity, hypersensitivity with liver failure	Avoid initiating in females with CD4 > 250 cells/µL and males with CD4 > 400 cells/µL

(Continued)

TABLE 12-7	NON-NUCLEOSIDE REVERSE TRANSCRIPTASE INHIBITORS (CONTINUED)			
	Dose	Food Restrictions	Side Effects	Comments
RPV	25 mg once daily	Taken with a meal of approximately 500 cal	CNS symptoms occur but less frequently than with EFV	Avoid in patients with CD4 cells/µL <200 or HIV RNA >100,000 copies/mL; Avoid concomitant use of PPIs
ETR	200 mg twice daily	After meal	Rash, Stevens–Johnson syndrome	Avoid concurrent use of all PIs except DRV
DLV	400 mg three times daily	None	Rash	Rarely used

CNS, central nervous system; DLV, delavirdine; DRV, darunavir; EFV, efavirenz; ETR, etravirine; NVP, nevirapine; PI, protease inhibitor; PPI, protein pump inhibitor; RPV, rilpivirine.

TABLE 12-8	PROTEASE INHIBITORS			
	Dose	Food Restrictions	Side Effects	Comments
ATV	300 mg with 100 mg RTV or 150 mg COBI once daily Unboosted: 400 mg once daily	Take with food	Benign elevation of indirect bilirubin	Must be boosted with concurrent use of TDF
DRV	800 mg with 100 mg RTV or 150 mg COBI once daily 600 mg with 100 mg RTV twice daily	Take with food	GI intolerance; headache, rash	Use twice a day during pregnancy
LPV/RTV/ fixed-dose combination	400 mg with 100 mg RTV twice daily	None	GI intolerance (dose dependent), dyslipidemia, hyperglycemia	

TABLE 12-8   PROTEASE INHIBITORS   (CONTINUED)

	Dose	Food Restrictions	Side Effects	Comments
FPV or fAPV	700 mg with 100 mg RTV twice daily 1400 mg with 200 mg RTV once daily Nonboosted: 1400 mg twice daily	None	Rash, GI intolerance	Rarely used
SQV	1000 mg with 100 mg RTV twice daily	Take with food	GI intolerance, headache; PR/QT interval prolongation	Requires RTV boosting Rarely used
NFV	Unboosted: 1250 mg twice daily	Take with food	Significant GI intolerance (diarrhea, nausea)	Does not require boosting Rarely used
IDV	800 mg with 100 mg RTV twice daily 800 mg three times daily	On empty stomach if taken without RTV	Nephrolithiasis, hyperbilirubin-emia	Needs adequate hydration Rarely used
TPV	500 mg with 200 mg RTV twice daily	Take with food	Hepatotoxicity, hyperlipidemia, GI intolerance, subarachnoid hemorrhage	Boosted with higher dose of RTV. Rarely used
RTV	Used as a boosting agent with other PIs (no longer used in full dose)	none	GI intolerance	Capsule form replaced by tablet not requiring refrigeration

ATV, atazanavir; COBI, cobicistat; DRV, darunavir; FPV or fAPV, fosamprenavir; GI, gastrointestinal; IDV, indinavir; LPV, lopinavir/r; NFV, nelfinavir; PI, protease inhibitor; RTV, ritonavir; SQV, saquinavir; TDF, tenofovir; TPV, tipranavir.

- In the event that TDF, TAF, or ABC cannot be used, some two-drug regimens are suggested including ritonavir-boosted DRV (DRVr) plus RAL or ritonavir-boosted lopinavir (LPVr) plus lamivudine (3TC).
- Future ART options
  - Changes in recommended and alternative regimens will likely occur in response to new HAART options becoming available.
  - Given the increased potency of some of the newer antiretrovirals, two-drug regimens may be feasible, decreasing cost and toxicity.

TABLE 12-9   OTHER ANTIRETROVIRAL CLASSES

	Dose	Food Restrictions	Side Effects	Comments
Fusion Inhibitor				
T-20	90 mg subcutaneous injection twice daily	No	Painful injection site reactions	Use of injection devices to reduce pain
CCR5 Receptor Antagonist				
MVC	300 mg twice daily	No	Generally well tolerated; hepatotoxicity	Baseline tropism testing is required before initiation
	150 mg twice daily with PIs (except TPV/r)			
	600 mg twice daily with EFV or ETR			Active against R5 using virus only
	150 mg twice daily with EFV or ETR and PI			

T-20, enfuvirtide; EFV, efavirenz; ETR, etravirine; MVC, maraviroc; PI, protease inhibitor; TPV, tipranavir.

TABLE 12-10   COMMONLY AVAILABLE COFORMULATED ART

Tenofovir disoproxil fumarate/emtricitabine	300/200 mg
Tenofovir alafenamide/emtricitabine	25/200 mg
Abacavir/lamivudine	600/300 mg
Zidovudine/lamivudine	300/150 mg
Efavirenz/tenofovir disoproxil fumarate/emtricitabine	600/300/200 mg
Rilpivirine/tenofovir disoproxil fumarate/emtricitabine	25/300/200 mg
Rilpivirine/tenofovir alafenamide/emtricitabine	25/25/200 mg
Elvitegravir/cobicistat/tenofovir disoproxil fumarate/emtricitabine	150/150/300/200 mg
Elvitegravir/cobicistat/tenofovir alafenamide/emtricitabine	150/150/10/200 mg
Dolutegravir/abacavir/lamivudine	50/600/300 mg
Bictegravir/emtricitabine/tenofovir alafenamide	50/200/25 mg
Atazanavir/cobicistat	300/150 mg
Darunavir/cobicistat	800/150 mg

- ○ Bictegravir is a potent INSTI with a side effect profile similar to existing INSTIs that is coformulated with TAF/FTC in a single tablet.
- ○ The first two drug single table regimen consisting of the NNRTI RPV and the INSTI dolutegravir will be a potential option for those requiring an NRTI sparing regimen.
- ○ Long-acting injectable INSTIs and NNRTIs will offer an alternative route of HAART administration.

Drug Interactions
- Many antiretrovirals use hepatic cytochrome P-450 pathway, particularly NNRTIs and PIs. Use of the pharmacologic boosters, ritonavir and cobicistat, will affect the CYP pathways.
  - ○ These can both inhibit and induce CYP isoenzymes. Therefore, drug interactions are common with other medication classes such as rifamycins, macrolides, statins, antifungals, anticonvulsants, and others.
  - ○ Owing to complexity of drug interactions and need for dose adjustment, it is best to refer to a drug interaction database or a specialized pharmacist. Some of the important drug interactions with antiretroviral medications are listed in Table 12-11.[6]
- NRTIs do not undergo hepatic transformation through the CYP metabolic pathway. In general INSTIs are metabolized by glucuronidation that is mediated by the UDP-glucuronosyltransferase (UGT1A1) enzymes. Strong inducers of UGT1A1 enzymes (e.g., rifampin) can decrease the concentration of INSTIs. Other inducers of UGT1A1 such as EFV, tipranavir (TPV)/r, or rifabutin may reduce INSTI concentration.
- CCR5 antagonist MVC is a substrate of CYP3A enzymes and P-glycoprotein. MVC is neither an inducer nor an inhibitor of the CYP3A system, but its concentration can increase with CPY3A inhibitors, such as RTV and other PIs. In this case, MVC dose requires adjustment.

TABLE 12-11	IMPORTANT DRUG INTERACTIONS WITH ANTIRETROVIRAL MEDICATIONS

Statins: Do not coadminister PIs with **simvastatin** and **lovastatin**; the statin levels significantly increase causing myopathy and rhabdomyolysis. Rosuvastatin, atorvastatin, and pravastatin can be administered at the lowest possible dose with close monitoring.

Atorvastatin	Start with lowest possible dose
Pravastatin	Avoid using with DRV/r, or start with lowest possible statin dose; other PIs do not require dose adjustment
Rosuvastatin	Coadministration with FPV/r does not require dose adjustment. For other PIs, start with lowest possible statin dose

Acid Reducers: ATV and RPV need acid environment (solubility depending on gastric pH), thus anything that may affect gastric pH should be avoided or used with caution.

PPIs	PPIs are not recommended in patients receiving ATV or RPV. Do not co-administer NFV and PPIs. DRV/r and TPV/r may reduce PPI level
H₂ receptor antagonists	H₂ receptor antagonist single dose should not exceed a dose equivalent of famotidine 20 mg daily or total daily dose equivalent of famotidine 20 mg twice daily in PI-naïve patients. When using with ATV/r or RPV, administer >10 h after the H₂ receptor antagonist

(Continued)

TABLE 12-11	IMPORTANT DRUG INTERACTIONS WITH ANTIRETROVIRAL MEDICATIONS (CONTINUED)

Benzodiazepines: PIs increase concentration of benzodiazepines, use with caution. Do not use midazolam or triazolam with PIs.

Antidepressants: Antidepressant response should be monitored and titrated based on clinical assessment.

Anticonvulsants

Phenytoin	Phenytoin level reduced with most of the PIs. Consider alternative anticonvulsant (typically lamotrigine). Do not coadminister with ETR
Carbamazepine	Coadministration with boosted PIs will increase carbamazepine level and decrease PI levels. Do not coadminister with ETR
Phenobarbital	PI levels reduced substantially; consider alternative. Do not coadminister with ETR
Lamotrigine	Lamotrigine level is decreased with concurrent use of PIs. Titrate lamotrigine dose to effect
VPA	VPA level decreased by LPV/r and conversely LPV/r level increased by VPA. Monitor VAP level and response.

Antifungals (Azoles): Azoles have significant interactions with PIs and NNRTIs.

Itraconazole	Coadministration of itraconazole and PIs may result in increased itraconazole or PI levels. Itraconazole level should be monitored for dose adjustments
Posaconazole	Posaconazole increases ATV level, monitor for adverse events
Voriconazole	Voriconazole level is reduced with concomitant use of RTV. Voriconazole is contraindicated to coadminister with EFV as standard dose. If coadministration is necessary, adjust dose to voriconazole 400 mg twice daily and EFV 300 mg once daily

Inhaled steroids

Concurrent use of RTV results in significant increased level of fluticasone (used in inhalers such as fluticasone/salmeterol or intranasal spray) causing systemic corticosteroid adverse effect. Avoid fluticasone, or give with caution. Similar side effects have been seen with inhaled budesonide.

Antimycobacterials

Do not coadminister rifampin and PIs. Rifabutin dose should be adjusted. Refer Chapter 13 for detailed dosing. Clarithromycin level may be increased with concurrent PIs; monitor for side effects. Clarithromycin level is reduced with concurrent use of NNRTIs; monitor for efficacy.

Hormonal Contraceptives

Boosted PIs significantly reduce the ethinyl estradiol level, thus alternatives or additional method of contraception should be used. ATV/r may be used if the oral contraceptives contain at least 35 µg of ethinyl estradiol. NVP decreases ethinyl estradiol level, thus alternative or additional method of contraception should be used. EFV may decrease ethinyl estradiol level. Depomedroxyprogesterone acetate is usually the common hormonal contraceptive choice.

Phosphodiesterase Type 5 Inhibitors: Concurrent use of PIs increases levels of medications in this class; start with lower dose and monitor for side effects.

TABLE 12-11	IMPORTANT DRUG INTERACTIONS WITH ANTIRETROVIRAL MEDICATIONS (CONTINUED)

Methadone: NNRTI decrease methadone levels and require titration of the dose to avoid opiate withdrawal, therefore they are best avoided with methadone

Herbals: St. John wort decreases the level of PIs and should not be coadministered.

Adapted from Panel on Antiretroviral Guidelines for Adults and Adolescents. *Guidelines for the Use of Antiretroviral Agents in HIV-1-Infected Adults and Adolescents*: Department of Health and Human Services; 2017. http://www.aidsinfo.nih.gov/ContentFiles/AdultandAdolescentGL.pdf.

ATV, atazanavir; DRV, darunavir; EFV, efavirenz; ETR, etravirine; FPV, fosamprenavir; LPV, lopinavir; NNRTI, nonnucleoside reverse transcriptase inhibitor; NFV, nelfinavir; NVP, nevirapine; PI, protease inhibitor; PPI, proton pump inhibitor; RTV, ritonavir; TPV, tipranavir; VPA, valproic acid.

SPECIAL CONSIDERATIONS

- **Management of HIV-Infected Patients in Critical Care Settings**
  - Among the common reasons for ICU admission among patients with HIV are respiratory failure due to bacterial pneumonias, *Pneumocystis* pneumonia, chronic obstructive pulmonary disease, and asthma exacerbation.[7] Immune reconstitution inflammatory syndrome should always be considered when HAART was recently initiated.
  - In patients already on HAART, treatment should be continued unless the HAART itself is believed to be causing harm. Common challenges in this setting are administration mode and absorption of HAART, increased chance of drug interactions, and need for renal or hepatic adjustment.
  - If the patient is diagnosed with HIV infection during the hospitalization that required ICU care, consult an HIV specialist to discuss the indication and timing of HAART.
  - If the patient has an OI with the exception of cryptococcal disease or TB, initiation of HAART should be considered, preferably within 2 weeks. HAART should be delayed 2 to 10 weeks after cryptococcal meningitis due to higher mortality with early HAART initiation. Initiation in the setting of TB infection should be individualized after consultation with an HIV specialist.
- **Antiretroviral Therapy in Specific Conditions**
  - **Chronic kidney disease.** Renal dose adjustment is required for most of the NRTIs (except ABC). TDF is associated with proximal renal tubular injury and should be used with caution in patients with chronic kidney disease (CKD). PIs, NNRTIs and INSTIs in general do not require dose adjustment and can be used in CKD.
  - **Chronic HBV infection.** A fully active HAART regimen should be constructed to include at least two drugs with HBV activity. This usually included TDF or TAF and FTC or 3TC. Of note, patients on HAART with HBV activity can experience HBV flares if HAART is stopped or change to a regimen without HBV activity.
  - **Chronic HCV infection.** HAART should be initiated in all HCV coinfected patients, regardless of CD4 cell count. If HCV is being treated, careful assessment for interaction between HAART and HCV direct acting antiviral therapy should be performed as multiple potential interactions exist.
- **Management of pregnant women**
  - **To prevent mother to child transmission, all HIV-infected pregnant women should receive HAART during pregnancy regardless of HIV RNA and CD4 cell count.** HAART should be initiated as soon as possible. Close follow-up is imperative. The goal is to achieve an undetectable viral load before delivery.[8]

○ Most currently used HAART regimens are safe in pregnancy. In the past the drug EFV was avoided in pregnancy because of concerns for potential teratogenicity arising from animal studies; however, currently available data have not demonstrated increased rates of neural tube defects in infants born to women on EFV in the first trimester.

○ Women who present for prenatal care on a well-tolerated, fully suppressive HAART regimen should continue on their existing regimen.

○ In pregnant HAART-naïve patients, preferred regimens include an NRTI backbone of TDF/FTC or ABC/3TC combined with ATVr, DRVr, or RAL.

○ Intrapartum intravenous (IV) AZT is recommended for HIV-infected pregnant women with HIV RNA >1000 copies/ml or unknown HIV RNA around delivery. AZT continuous IV infusion is administered with loading dose of 2 mg/kg over 1 hour, followed by 1 mg/kg/h until delivery.

○ Elective cesarean delivery should be scheduled at 38 weeks gestation if plasma HIV-1 RNA remains >1000 copies/mL near the time of delivery. For scheduled cesarean delivery, IV AZT should be started at least 3 hours prior.

○ Infants should be started on AZT as soon as possible after birth. AZT dosing for infants ≥35 weeks gestation at birth is 2 mg/kg orally within 6 to 12 hours of delivery, then every 6 hours for 6 weeks.

○ Breast-feeding should be avoided in developed countries with access to clean water and formula.

• **Immunization in HIV-Infected Patients:** Table 12-12 summarizes the recommendations for immunization of HIV-infected patients. **Inactivated vaccines are generally acceptable, and live vaccines are contraindicated in severely immunocompromised** (CD4 cell count <200 cells/µL).

COMPLICATIONS

Antiretroviral Adverse Drug Reactions

• **Lactic acidosis.** The clinical picture can range from asymptomatic hyperlactatemia to severe lactic acidosis with hepatomegaly and steatosis. Higher rates of lactic acidosis have been reported with the use of stavudine and didanosine. Suspected drugs should be discontinued and supportive care provided. Incidence of lactic acidosis has declined with the use of current NRTIs.

• **ABC hypersensitivity reaction.** Symptoms of hypersensitivity include fever, skin rash, fatigue; gastrointestinal symptoms such as nausea, vomiting, diarrhea, or abdominal pain; and respiratory symptoms such as pharyngitis, dyspnea, or cough. ABC may cause a fatal hypersensitivity reaction at rechallenge. To avoid these reactions, routine screening for the presence of HLA-B*5701 allele is recommended; the presence of the allele indicates high risk of ABC reactions, and ABC should be avoided

• **Hepatotoxicity caused by NVP.** NVP can cause severe hepatotoxicity, which may be fatal. Females with CD4 cell count >250 cells/µL or males with CD4 cell count >400 cells/µL are at increased risk for developing hepatotoxicity. If used, NVP should be initiated at a lower dose with close monitoring of the liver function.

• **Nephrotoxicity caused by TDF.** TDF is associated with nephrotoxicity, particularly rare cases of proximal tubular toxicity (Fanconi syndrome), and requires monitoring of kidney function.

• **Fat redistribution.** Lipodystrophy and lipohypertrophy are alterations in body fat distribution, such as accumulation of visceral fat in the abdomen, neck (buffalo hump), and pelvic areas and/or depletion of subcutaneous fat causing facial or peripheral wasting. PIs and NRTIs (stavudine, didanosine, and to a lesser extent AZT) are associated with these changes but other factors may also play a role.

TABLE 12-12   IMMUNIZATION IN HIV-INFECTED PATIENTS

Immunization	Special Considerations
Inactivated Vaccines	
Pneumococcal vaccine: 13-valent pneumococcal conjugate vaccine (PCV13) and 23 polyvalent polysaccharide pneumococcal vaccine (PPV23). Some experts recommend deferring the vaccine until the CD4 cell counts are >200 cells/µL for a better response	HIV-infected patients who have not received pneumococcal vaccine should receive a single dose of PCV13 regardless of CD4 count. PPV23 should be given at least 8 wk later if CD4 T cell counts are ≥200 cells/µL. A single PPV23 dose should be repeated 5 y later.
Hepatitis A vaccine: Recommended for MSM, IVDU, persons with chronic liver disease, and those coinfected with HBV and/or HCV. Patients with CD4 cell count >200 cells/µL or undetectable HIV RNA are more likely to achieve vaccine response.	Two doses given at 0 and 6–12 mo for HAVRIX and 0 and 6–18 mo for VAQTA
Hepatitis B vaccine: Recommended for those without evidence of past or present HBV infection. Standard dose of 20 µg may be used; however, we recommend routine use of higher dose (40 µg) as standard dose was inferior to higher dose to elicit vaccine response. Patients with CD4 cell counts of >200 cells/µL and suppressed virus have a higher chance of adequate vaccine response.	Three doses given at 0, 1, and 6 mo. Dose 40 µg. Vaccinated patients should be tested for anti-HBs antibody response after the third dose. Consider repeating the series if no response and giving a booster if low response
Influenza vaccine: Inactivated influenza vaccine is recommended for all HIV-infected patients. Use of the intranasally administered, live, attenuated vaccine is not recommended.	Vaccinate annually
Tetanus toxoid: Principles are the same as HIV-negative persons. Substitute one-time dose of Tdap vaccine at time of next booster.	Every 10 y
Human papillomavirus vaccine: Vaccine should be given to patients aged 9–26 y, but may also be considered in other groups.	Three doses given at 0, 2, and 6 mo
Meningococcal vaccine: Optional. Conjugated meningococcal vaccine should be administered to persons with asplenia, with travel exposure, of college age, or living in dormitories	Single dose, repeat every 5 y if high risk
Polio vaccine: Optional. Live OPV is contraindicated. Immunize with IPV in selected patients at high risk.	IPV consists of three doses at 0, 4–8 wk, and 6–12 mo

(Continued)

TABLE 12-12	IMMUNIZATION IN HIV-INFECTED PATIENTS (CONTINUED)
Immunization	**Special Considerations**
Haemophilus influenzae type B vaccine: Optional. The incidence of Hib infection among HIV-infected adults is low. However, asplenic patients and those with a history of recurrent *Haemophilus* infections should be considered for immunization.	Single dose
Live vaccines	
Varicella vaccine (Varivax): Varicella vaccine should be administered to HIV-infected patients with CD4 cell count >200 cells/μL if no evidence of immunity to varicella.	Two doses at 0 and 4–8 wk
Zoster vaccine (Zostavax): Zostavax consists of attenuated varicella virus at a concentration at least 14 times that found in Varivax.	Single dose for persons with history of varicella
MMR vaccine: MMR vaccine should be administered to HIV-infected patients with CD4 cell counts >200 cells/μL.	One or two doses (if two doses, minimum interval of 28 d)

HBV, hepatitis B virus; HCV, hepatitis C virus; Hib, *H. influenzae* type b; IPV, inactivated polio vaccine; IVDU, intravenous drug user; MSM, men who have sex with men; OPV, oral polio vaccine.

- **Peripheral neuropathy**
  - HIV-associated neuropathy is a common neurologic complication of HIV infection and its treatment. Diagnosis is made clinically and by excluding other possibilities for peripheral neuropathy.
  - HIV-associated neuropathy is common in advanced infection when CD4 cell count is low and HIV RNA is high. NRTIs such as d4T, ddI, and AZT are associated with this condition.
  - If onset of neuropathy is recent, optimizing HAART can improve the symptoms to some extent.
  - Treatment is largely symptomatic and includes lamotrigine, gabapentin, and antidepressants (amitriptyline, duloxetine, and venlafaxine).
- **Cardiovascular disease** associated with HIV infection and HAART
  - A number of observational studies have demonstrated higher rates of cardiovascular disease in HIV-infected patients.
  - Certain antiretroviral agents including PIs and the NRTI ABC are linked to increased cardiovascular risk in observational studies.
- **Dyslipidemia** is associated with HIV infection and HAART. Lipid abnormalities are frequently observed in persons with HIV independent of HAART. Older NRTIs and PIs are associated with dyslipidemia; however, many of the newer agents in these classes as well as the INSTI have more favorable lipid profiles.

HIV-Associated Complications

- **HIV-associated nephropathy** (HIVAN)
  - HIVAN is characterized by rapidly progressive renal dysfunction and massive proteinuria (1–3 g/d or more). Renal biopsy shows focal segmental glomerulosclerosis. Risk factors include African descent; diabetes; hypertension; hepatitis C infection; and CD4 cell count <200 cells/μL, HIV RNA level of >4000 copies/mL.
  - HAART can halt the progression when started early; angiotensin converting enzyme inhibitors may be effective, although no prospective randomized controlled trials have been performed.
- **HIV-associated neurocognitive disorders** (HANDs):
  - With wide use of HAART, the prevalence of HIV-associated dementia has diminished while less severe neurocognitive disorders have increased as individuals live longer.
  - Patients with mild forms of HAND may complain of mild difficulties in concentration, attention, and memory while the neurologic examination is unremarkable. Whether HAND improves with better central nervous system penetrating HAART is unclear.
- **HIV-associated thrombocytopenia:** Primary HIV-associated thrombocytopenia can present as the initial manifestation of HIV in 10% of cases. It is similar to idiopathic thrombocytopenic purpura. Timely initiation of HAART will reverse HIV-associated thrombocytopenia.

MONITORING/FOLLOW-UP

- HIV RNA should be monitored closely, preferably 4 weeks after initiation of HAART, and routinely monitored 3 to 4 times a year. Long-term treatment goal is to suppress HIV below the levels of detection and reconstitute CD4 T cell count.
- When patients are on HAART, CD4 T cell count can be monitored every 6 months; however, it should be monitored more frequently if the patients are not virally suppressed or their last measured count was <200 cells/μL.
- Treatment failure. Treatment failure is defined as a suboptimal response to HAART. Reasons for treatment failure include poor adherence, medication tolerability, and drug interactions.
- **Virologic failure.** Virologic failure is defined as inability to achieve or maintain HIV RNA levels below the limit of detection (<20 copies/mL).
  - Incomplete virologic response. Two consecutive plasma HIV RNA >200 copies/mL after 24 weeks of HAART.
  - Virologic rebound. Detection of HIV RNA after complete virologic suppression.
  - Antiretroviral regimens should be reviewed and genotype resistance testing should be obtained while the patient is still taking the failing regimen.
- **Inadequate immune recovery** can be defined as failure to achieve and maintain an adequate CD4 T-cell response despite virologic suppression, but a specific cutoff is difficult to establish. There is no consensus on how to manage persistent immunodeficiency; however, studies have shown that adjustment or intensification of an existing suppressive HAART regimen does not make a difference. Risk of OIs appears to be low if viral suppression is achieved.

OUTCOME/PROGNOSIS

- Mortality continues to decline with wide use of potent HAART that provides durable virologic suppression and reconstitution of the immune system. **Life expectancy in HIV infection when appropriately treated with HAART is now comparable to similar uninfected persons.**

- An increasing proportion of deaths in HIV-infected patients are attributed to non-AIDS events, in particular malignancies, liver failure secondary to viral hepatitis, and cardiovascular disease.

ADDITIONAL RESOURCES

- HIV management guideline available at http://aidsinfo.nih.gov/
- HIV knowledge base and drug interaction database: http://hivinsite.ucsf.edu/HIV resistance interpretation algorithms: http://hivdb.stanford.edu/
- Genotype interpretation algorithms and treatment guidelines at IAS-USA: http://www.iasusa.org/
- Drug interaction charts: http://www.hiv-druginteractions.org/
- HIV primary care guidelines: http://www.hivma.org/
- Useful resource for patients: www.thebody.com, www.aidsmed.com, www.avert.org/

REFERENCES

1. May MT, Gompels M, Delpech V, et al. Impact on life expectancy of HIV-1 positive individuals of CD4+ cell count and viral load response to antiretroviral therapy. *AIDS.* 2014;28(8):1193-1202.
2. Cohen MS, Chen YQ, McCauley M, et al. Antiretroviral therapy for the prevention of HIV-1 transmission. *N Engl J Med.* 2016;375(9):830-839.
3. Centers for Disease Control. HIV Risk Behaviors. Available at https://www.cdc.gov/hiv/risk/estimates/riskbehaviors.html. (last accessed 6/8/2018).
4. Group ISS, Lundgren JD, Babiker AG, et al. Initiation of antiretroviral therapy in early asymptomatic HIV infection. *N Engl J Med.* 2015;373(9):795-807.
5. Strategies for Management of Antiretroviral Therapy Study Group, El-Sadr WM, Lundgren J, Neaton JD, et al. CD4+ count-guided interruption of antiretroviral treatment. *N Engl J Med.* 2006;355(22):2283-2296.
6. Panel on Antiretroviral Guidelines for Adults and Adolescents. *Guidelines for the Use of Antiretroviral Agents in HIV-1-Infected Adults and Adolescents.* Department of Health and Human Services; 2017. http://www.aidsinfo.nih.gov/ContentFiles/AdultandAdolescentGL.pdf.
7. Huang L, Quartin A, Jones D, Havlir DV. Intensive care of patients with HIV infection. *N Engl J Med.* 2006;355(2):173-181.
8. Panel on Treatment of HIV-Infected Pregnant Women and Prevention of Perinatal Transmission. *Recommendations for Use of Antiretroviral Drugs in Pregnant HIV-1-Infected Women for Maternal Health and Interventions to Reduce Perinatal HIV Transmission in the United States;* 2017. Available at http://aidsinfo.nih.gov/contentfiles/lvguidelines/PerinatalGL.pdf.

Opportunistic Infections Associated With HIV

Jane O'Halloran and Gerome Escota

13

INTRODUCTION

- Immunosuppression occurs with progressive untreated HIV disease and manifests as declining CD4+ T-lymphocyte counts and an increased risk of opportunistic infections (OIs).
- With increased use of potent combined antiretroviral therapy (cART), the incidence of OIs has declined, resulting in a marked improvement in survival.
- OIs still occur in individuals with undiagnosed advanced HIV infection at presentation and in patients who are nonadherent to cART.
- Prophylaxis for OIs includes:
  - Primary prophylaxis instituted before an OI occurs. Initiation mainly depends on the level of immunosuppression (Table 13-1).
  - Secondary prophylaxis instituted after treatment of an episode of infection.
- **Immune reconstitution inflammatory syndrome** (IRIS) describes the clinical findings associated with immune reconstitution. This occurs in patients with advanced HIV disease who experience paradoxical worsening of a known OI or unmasking of an occult OI after initiation of cART. If IRIS occurs, ART should be continued except in rare

TABLE 13-1	COMMON OPPORTUNISTIC INFECTION PRIMARY PROPHYLAXIS		
Opportunistic Infection	Indication for Prophylaxis	Medications	Discontinue Prophylaxis
Pneumocystis pneumonia	CD4+ <200 cells/μL or oropharyngeal candidiasis or CD4+ <14%	TMP/SMX DS PO once daily or three times weekly Alternatives: Dapsone 100 mg PO once daily Atovaquone 1500 mg PO once daily	CD4+ >200 cells/ μL for >3 mo
Toxoplasmosis	CD4+ <100 cells/μL and anti-*Toxoplasma* IgG positive	TMP/SMX DS PO once daily Alternatives: Dapsone 200 mg PO once weekly + pyrimethamine 50 mg PO once weekly + leucovorin 25 mg PO once weekly. Atovaquone 1500 mg PO once daily +/− (pyrimethamine 25 mg PO once daily + leucovorin 10 mg PO once daily)	CD4+ >200 cells/ μL for >3 mo

(Continued)

TABLE 13-1	COMMON OPPORTUNISTIC INFECTION PRIMARY PROPHYLAXIS (CONTINUED)		
Opportunistic Infection	Indication for Prophylaxis	Medications	Discontinue Prophylaxis
MAC	CD4+ <50 cells/ μL after ruling out active MAC infection	Azithromycin 1200 mg PO once weekly Alternatives: clarithromycin, rifabutin (rule out active TB)	CD4+ >100 cells/ μL for >3 mo

MAC, *Mycobacterium avium* complex; TMP/SMX, trimethoprim–sulfamethoxazole.

situations (e.g., raised intracranial pressure). Symptoms can be managed supportively (i.e., use of nonsteroidal anti-inflammatory drugs and antipyretics). Addition of low-dose steroids can be considered although there are limited data to support this.

- **cART can be initiated in the setting of active OIs in most cases.** In a randomized controlled trial of patients with OIs other than TB, a significantly lower incidence of AIDS progression or death was demonstrated in subjects who initiated cART early (median of 12 d) compared with those who commenced late (median of 45 d).[1] Survival benefits have also been demonstrated when patients are treated earlier versus later for TB.[2,3] It is therefore recommended that in most cases, patients with OIs should be initiated on cART as soon as is feasible (within 2 wk). An exception to this is in cryptococcal meningitis where early cART initiation has been associated with increased mortality and therefore guidelines currently recommend cART initiation between 2 and 10 weeks after initiation of cryptococcal therapy.

Fungal Infections

Pneumocystis Pneumonia

GENERAL PRINCIPLES

- *Pneumocystis* pneumonia (PCP) is a fungal infection caused by *Pneumocystis jirovecii* (previously *Pneumocystis carinii*).
- Before the use of cART and primary PCP prophylaxis, PCP occurred in 70% to 80% of patients with AIDS. The incidence of PCP has declined dramatically, although it is still one of the most common OIs in advanced HIV disease.
- Risk factors are CD4+ cell count <200 cells/μL, history of oropharyngeal candidiasis, or prior PCP.

DIAGNOSIS

Clinical Presentation

- Presentation is subacute. Symptoms are often present for weeks and may include progressive fatigue, exertional dyspnea, nonproductive cough, fever, pleuritic chest pain, and hypoxemia.
- Lung examination is usually normal, although fine bibasilar rales may be heard. There may be a decline in oxygen saturation with exertion.

Diagnostic Testing

- **Chest radiographs** are initially normal in up to 25% of the patients. The most common findings are diffuse, bilateral, interstitial, or alveolar infiltrates progressing from peri-hilar to peripheral regions. Pneumatoceles are associated with prolonged, indolent disease and predispose to pneumothoraces. If there is a high index of suspicion for PCP but the patient has a normal chest radiograph, a **high-resolution chest CT scan** may reveal ground glass opacities.
- Although clinical examination and chest imaging can be helpful in the diagnosis of PCP, they are not pathognomonic. Definitive diagnosis depends on histopathologic or cytopathologic identification of organisms in induced sputum, bronchoalveolar lavage (BAL) fluid or in tissue.
  - Sputum induction is usually attempted, followed by bronchoscopy with BAL with or without transbronchial biopsies.
  - Sensitivity of induced sputum varies depending on the quality of the sample and experience of the laboratory, making **BAL the diagnostic procedure of choice** for obtaining adequate specimens.
  - Specimens can be stained with methenamine silver, toluidine blue, or Giemsa, but **direct fluorescent antibody staining** is the most common technique used.

TREATMENT

- Treatment duration is 21 days. Clinical response is gradual and usually occurs between day 4 to 8 of treatment.
- Trimethoprim–sulfamethoxazole (TMP-SMX) is recommended as first-line treatment for PCP (Table 13-2)
- Glucose-6-phosphate dehydrogenase deficiency should be assessed before the use of dapsone or primaquine to avoid severe hemolytic anemia.
- TMP-SMX is still the drug of choice for the pregnant patient.
- Prednisone is administered when PaO_2 <70 mm Hg or alveolar–arterial oxygen gradient >35 mm Hg (Table 13-2).

Mucocutaneous Candidiasis

GENERAL PRINCIPLES

- **Oropharyngeal candidiasis is the most common OI in HIV-infected patients.** It is most often observed in patients with CD4+ T cell count <200 cells/μL.
- *Candida albicans* is the most commonly isolated pathogen; however, *Candida tropicalis*, *Candida krusei*, and *Candida dubliniensis* have been reported.
- Infections by *Candida glabrata* and *Candida parapsilosis* tend to occur in patients with prior antifungal exposure.

DIAGNOSIS

- **Oropharyngeal candidiasis (thrush).** Patients experience burning pain in the mouth and altered taste sensation. Oropharyngeal candidiasis presents as a removable white creamy plaque on any oral mucosal surfaces. These plaques have an erythematous base when scraped.
- **Esophageal candidiasis.** Patients may present with dysphagia or odynophagia, with or without oropharyngeal lesions. Diagnosis is made by direct visualization of the esophagus by endoscopy. **This is an AIDS-defining condition.**
- **Vulvovaginal candidiasis.** Patients present with itching, white "cottage-cheese like" vaginal discharge, dyspareunia, dysuria, and erythema of the vagina and vulva.

TABLE 13-2	TREATMENT OF PNEUMOCYSTIS PNEUMONIA

Not Acutely Ill (Able to Take Oral Medication, PaO$_2$ >70 mm Hg)

- TMP-SMX two DS tabs PO every 8 h.

Acutely Ill (Not Able to Take Oral Medication, PaO$_2$ <70 mm Hg)

- TMP-SMX (5 mg/kg of TMP component per day) intravenously every 6–8 h.
- Prednisone taper is administered when PaO$_2$ <70 mm Hg or alveolar–arterial oxygen gradient >35 mm Hg. Prednisone is given 40 mg PO twice daily for 5 d, then 40 mg PO once daily for 5 d and 20 mg PO once daily for 11 d. (If oral medication is not feasible, IV methylprednisolone can be administered as 75% of prednisone dose.)

Alternative Regimens

- Clindamycin 600 mg IV every 8 h (or 300–450 mg PO four times daily) plus primaquine 30 mg PO once daily.
- Atovaquone 750 mg PO twice daily. Only for PCP of mild-to-moderate severity.
- Pentamidine 4 mg/kg/d IV once daily. Adverse reaction can be life-threatening and may include pancreatitis, hypotension, hypoglycemia, renal insufficiency, cardiac arrhythmias (including torsade de pointes).

Secondary Prophylaxis

- Should be initiated on completion of the PCP treatment. Regimen is the same as the primary prophylaxis.
- Secondary prophylaxis may be discontinued with CD4+ cell count >200 cells/μL for more than 3 mo.

PCP, pneumocystis pneumonia; TMP/SMX, trimethoprim–sulfamethoxazole.

TREATMENT

- **Oropharyngeal candidiasis.** Oral fluconazole 100 mg is the treatment of choice for management of oropharyngeal candidiasis except in pregnancy. Alternative treatments include **topical antifungal therapies** such as clotrimazole oral troches (10 mg five times daily) or nystatin oral suspension (500,000 units/5 mL four times daily).
- **Esophageal candidiasis.** Fluconazole (400 mg loading dose, followed by 200–400 mg PO or IV once daily for 14–21 d) is recommended for esophageal candidiasis. Those refractory to fluconazole after 1 week may be switched to voriconazole or posaconazole (oral therapy) or echinocandins (e.g., caspofungin) if IV is required. Amphotericin B is an alternative option, but toxicity limits its use. Pregnant patients should be treated with amphotericin B as azoles are teratogenic and safety data are not available for echinocandins. Other pathogens such as cytomegalovirus (CMV) and herpes simplex virus can cause esophagitis so endoscopic diagnosis may be required if the patient fails to respond to a trial of therapy.
- **Vulvovaginal candidiasis.** **Topical antifungal therapy** such as clotrimazole, miconazole, butoconazole, or tioconazole cream is used. **Oral fluconazole** 150 mg as a single dose is also effective. Complicated cases may require prolonged therapy, either with topical treatment >7 days or two doses of fluconazole 150 mg given 72 hours apart.

Cryptococcosis

GENERAL PRINCIPLES

- Cryptococcal infection is the most common systemic fungal infection in HIV-infected patients.
- While cryptococcal disease may occur at any CD4+ T cell count, over 75% of meningitis occurs in patients with CD4+ T cell count <50 cells/μL.

DIAGNOSIS

Clinical Presentation

- *Cryptococcus* can involve virtually any body site including central nervous system (CNS), lungs, prostate, skin, bone and joint, and ocular infections given its propensity to disseminate.
- **Cryptococcal meningitis** has an indolent course and is generally a manifestation of disseminated disease. Symptoms include headache, malaise, and prolonged fever. Meningeal irritation is uncommon. The headache often worsens with sneezing or coughing in keeping with increased intracranial pressure.
- **Cryptococcal pulmonary infection** can present with a variety of clinical manifestations including subclinical granulomatous infections of the respiratory tract with an isolated pulmonary nodule on imaging to acute respiratory.

Diagnostic Testing

- A positive cerebrospinal fluid (CSF) culture for *Cryptococcus neoformans* is the gold standard.
- CSF glucose concentration may be decreased and CSF protein increased with a raised white cell count with leukocyte predominance. Of note, the CSF may appear normal. In particular, a normal CSF white blood cell count does not rule out cryptococcal meningitis and, in fact, may be associated with poorer prognosis.
- Latex agglutination test for **cryptococcal polysaccharide antigen** is highly sensitive and specific in both serum and CSF.
- If serum cryptococcal antigen is positive in a suspected case, lumbar puncture should still be performed. **Opening pressure** should always be documented and is of prognostic significance. Elevation of intracranial pressure may require repeated CSF drainage.

TREATMENT

- Standard treatment is **amphotericin B** 0.7 to 1.0 mg/kg/d IV plus **flucytosine** (5-FC) 100 mg/kg/d PO divided over 4 doses for 2 weeks (induction therapy) followed by **fluconazole** 400 mg PO once daily for 8 weeks (consolidation therapy). **However, liposomal amphotericin dosed at 4 to 6 mg/kg/g IV is preferred as amphotericin B deoxycholate is very toxic.**
- Flucytosine blood level should be monitored to avoid toxicity; peak level drawn 2 hours after dose should not exceed 75 μg/mL.
- Close monitoring is required for any clinical signs of increased pressure or with intracranial pressure of >25 cm H_2O. Opening pressure should be reduced by 50% if it is very high or otherwise to a normal pressure of <20 cm H_2O.
- For patients intolerant of amphotericin, fluconazole 800 to 1200 mg once daily (PO or IV) plus flucytosine 100 mg/kg/d PO divided over four doses for 6 weeks can be used.
- **Secondary prophylaxis** with fluconazole 200 mg PO once daily should be given upon completion of treatment. It can be discontinued when the CD4+ T cell count is

≥100 cells/µL with an undetectable HIV RNA level for ≥3 months and receipt of cART for a minimum of 12 months. Consider reinstitution of prophylactic therapy if the CD4+ T cell count decreases to <100 cells/µL.

SPECIAL CONSIDERATIONS

- The optimal timing of cART in HIV-infected patients presenting with cryptococcal meningitis has changed in recent times. ACTG A5164 showed survival benefit of early initiation of cART (within 2 wk). However, more recently the Cryptococcal Optimal ART Timing (COAT) trial reported increased survival in patients whose ART initiation was deferred for 5 weeks after the initiation of treatment for cryptococcal meningitis.[4]
- In asymptomatic patients with positive serum cryptococcal antigen, blood cultures should be obtained and lumbar puncture be performed. If the CSF is positive, the patient should be treated for meningitis. If CSF is negative, the patient should receive fluconazole 400 mg PO once daily until CD4+ cell count >100 cells/µL for 3 months.

Histoplasmosis

GENERAL PRINCIPLES

- Histoplasmosis is caused by *Histoplasma capsulatum*, a dimorphic fungus endemic to the Ohio and Mississippi River Valleys as well as to Latin America.
- In the pre-cART era, histoplasmosis occurred in about 5% of HIV-infected patients in endemic regions with nearly all cases disseminated at the time of diagnosis.
- The incidence has declined dramatically with the use of cART, but patients in endemic regions with CD4+ T cell counts <150 cells/µL are at increased risk for histoplasmosis.

DIAGNOSIS

Clinical Presentation

- Clinical manifestations of progressive disseminated histoplasmosis in HIV-infected patients include fever, fatigue, weight loss, and hepatosplenomegaly. Oral ulcers and skin lesions may be present.
- Cough, chest pain, and dyspnea occur in half of patients.
- Neurological disease is seen in 10% of disseminated histoplasmosis, presenting as subacute meningitis or focal brain lesions.
- Disseminated disease can cause sepsis-like syndrome and acute respiratory distress syndrome. It may also cause adrenal insufficiency.

Diagnostic Testing

- Chest radiograph on presentation may show infiltrates but may be normal 50% of the time.
- Diagnosis is made by isolation of *H. capsulatum* from blood, bone marrow, lung tissue, or lymph nodes.
- Sensitivity of serologic tests may decrease with profound immunosuppression. Rapid diagnosis of disseminated histoplasmosis can be made by detection of polysaccharide antigen in the urine (sensitivity 90%) and blood (sensitivity 75%); however, there is cross-reactivity with *Blastomyces dermatitidis, Talaromyces marneffei (Penicillium marneffei)*, and *Paracoccidioides brasiliensis* antigens. Monitoring antigen levels may detect early relapse.

TREATMENT

- Liposomal amphotericin B (3 mg/kg daily) for at least 2 weeks or until clinical improvement occurs is the treatment of choice for patients with moderate to severe disseminated histoplasmosis. This should be followed by oral itraconazole for a total treatment duration of at least 1 year.
- In mild disease, oral therapy with itraconazole may be sufficient.
- Itraconazole levels should be monitored for optimal treatment. Serum concentrations of itraconazole + hydroxyitraconazole should be >1 μg/mL.
- Secondary prophylaxis can be discontinued in patients who have received >12 months of itraconazole therapy, have been on cART for 6 months or more, and have a CD4+ T cell count >150 cells/μL. Patients should also have negative blood cultures and *Histoplasma* serum antigen levels <2 units. Secondary prophylaxis should be resumed if CD4+ T count drop to <150 cells/μL.

Coccidioidomycosis

GENERAL PRINCIPLES

- *Coccidioides immitis* and *Coccidioides posadasii* are soil-dwelling dimorphic fungi.
- Most cases in HIV-infected patients occur in endemic areas (Southwestern United States, Northern Mexico, and portions of Central and South America).

DIAGNOSIS

Clinical Presentation

- The main clinical syndromes are pneumonia, skin manifestations, meningitis, bone, liver and lymph node involvement.
- Patients can be asymptomatic and have positive coccidioidal serology tests.
- Focal pneumonia can occur in patients with CD4+ T cell count >250 cells/μL, whereas other manifestations tend to occur with lower CD4+ T cell counts.

Diagnostic Testing

- Diagnosis is confirmed by culture of the organism or by demonstration of the typical spherule on histopathologic examination of involved tissue. CSF cultures in coccidioidal meningitis are positive in fewer than one third of patients.
- Serologic tests are specific and tend to reflect active disease, although they are less frequently positive in patients with low CD4+ T cell counts.
- Complement fixation IgG antibody is frequently detected in CSF in coccidioidal meningitis.

TREATMENT

- Amphotericin B (liposomal) is the treatment of choice for severely ill patients with disseminated extrapulmonary disease or those with diffuse pulmonary disease. This can be switched to fluconazole after clinical improvement.
- Fluconazole is used for treatment of mild disease such as focal pneumonia.
- Oral or IV fluconazole is the recommended treatment for coccidioidal meningitis.
- HIV-positive patients who have positive coccidioidal serologies but who are asymptomatic should be treated with fluconazole.
- Secondary prophylaxis in mild infection may be discontinued if treated for >12 months and CD4+ T cell counts are >250 cells/μL and the patient is receiving cART.
- Unlike histoplasmosis or cryptococcosis, secondary prophylaxis of severe infection and meningitis should be continued indefinitely regardless of the CD4+ T cell count.

Bacterial Infections

Mycobacterium avium Complex

GENERAL PRINCIPLES

- *Mycobacterium avium* complex (MAC) organisms are ubiquitous in the environment, and transmission is thought to be through inhalation, ingestion, or inoculation.
- Disseminated MAC infection is an important OI in patients with advanced HIV infection (CD4+ T cell counts <50 cells/μL).
- Localized MAC infection may occur with higher CD4+ T cell counts and in particular in patient with IRIS.

DIAGNOSIS

Clinical Presentation

- Symptoms of disseminated MAC are nonspecific with fever and malaise most frequent. Night sweats, abdominal pain, diarrhea, and weight loss are also seen. On examination the patient may have lymphadenopathy and hepatosplenomegaly.
- Focal inflammatory lymphadenitis may develop shortly after initiation of cART.

Diagnostic Testing

- Common laboratory abnormalities include anemia, neutropenia, and elevated alkaline phosphatase.
- Diagnosis is established by culturing the organism from blood, bone marrow, or tissue from other sterile body sites, although it often takes weeks for the organism to grow.
- Specific DNA probes for MAC are available, differentiating MAC from other mycobacteria within hours when there is sufficient mycobacterial growth in broth or agar.
- With high suspicion of disseminated MAC infection but negative blood cultures, bone marrow, liver, or lymph node biopsy may yield acid-fast bacteria or granulomas.

TREATMENT

- Combination therapy is necessary to decrease the risk of drug resistance (see Table 13-3).
- Improvement in symptoms occurs gradually, usually 2 to 4 weeks after treatment initiation.
- **Clarithromycin** 500 mg PO twice daily (or clarithromycin extended release formulation 1000 mg PO once daily) and **ethambutol** 15 mg/kg PO once daily are recommended agents.
- Adding **rifabutin** 300 mg PO once daily may be beneficial, but clinicians should evaluate potential interactions with other agents. Increased levels of rifabutin and decreased levels of clarithromycin may occur when given together. Uveitis may occur with this combination.
- Azithromycin 500 to 600 mg PO once daily may be substituted if the patient is intolerant to clarithromycin. However, some studies suggest inferiority of azithromycin to clarithromycin.[5] Adding a third or fourth agent may be considered in severe cases; however, in the setting of cART, initiation of this may not be required.
- Without immune reconstitution, treatment is lifelong. After immune reconstitution, at least 12 months of MAC treatment and 6 months of immune reconstitution (CD4+ T cell count >100 cells/μL) are suggested.

TABLE 13-3	TREATMENT OF TUBERCULOSIS	
Treatment for Drug-Susceptible Active TB		
Initial phase (2 mo)	Pulmonary TB	6 mo
INH + (RIF or RFB) + PZA + EMB (If drug susceptibility shows sensitivity to INH and RIF and PZA, then EMB may be discontinued before 2 mo of treatment is completed.)	Pulmonary TB with cavitary lung lesions and positive culture after 2 mo of TB treatment	9 mo
Continuation phase (4 plus months) INH + (RIF or RFB) once daily or three times weekly or twice weekly (if CD4+ count >100 cells/µL)	Extrapulmonary TB with CNS, bone, or joint infections	9–12 mo
	Other extrapulmonary sites	6–9 mo
MDR or XDR TB		
Therapy should be individualized based on resistance pattern		

CNS, central nervous system; EMB, ethambutol; FQ, fluoroquinolones; INH, isoniazid; MDR, multidrug resistant; PZA, pyrazinamide; RIF, rifampin; RFB, rifabutin; TB, tuberculosis; XDR, extensively drug resistant.

Mycobacterium tuberculosis

GENERAL PRINCIPLES

- HIV-infected patients are at substantially increased risk for developing TB regardless of CD4+ T cell count.
- After HIV seroconversion, rapid depletion of TB-specific T helper cells is seen.
- The annual risk of reactivation with TB disease in untreated HIV infection is at 3% to 16% per year, an annual rate that is similar to the lifetime risk of HIV-negative persons with latent TB infection (LTBI).
- **TB is the leading cause of AIDS-related death worldwide,** especially in sub-Saharan Africa. The emergence of drug-resistant TB has further increased mortality.

DIAGNOSIS

Clinical Presentation

- The clinical presentation can depend on the level of immunosuppression. Patients with higher CD4+ T cell counts (>200–300 cells/µL) tend to present with classic TB with apical cavitary lung disease, respiratory symptoms, fever, night sweats, and weight loss.
- As immunity wanes, atypical chest radiographic features and extrapulmonary TB are more common.
- The most common sites of extrapulmonary involvement are blood and extrathoracic lymph nodes, followed by bone marrow, genitourinary tract, and the CNS.

Diagnostic Testing

- Acid fast bacillus (AFB) smear can be performed on sputum; however, it may be negative in HIV infection.
- Cultures of *Mycobacterium tuberculosis* (MTB) from appropriate specimens remains the gold standard for diagnosis.
- Rapid growth detection is enabled by newer liquid culture methods; however, as MTB is a slow growing organism, this process can take weeks to months.

- Nucleic acid–based amplification (NAA) assays are used for rapid detection of TB. NAA testing is more sensitive than AFB smear and in smear-negative, culture-positive samples it is positive 50% to 80% of the time. This increases to 90% when NAA is performed on three separate specimens.
- Drug-susceptibility testing helps guide treatment and decreases the transmission of drug-resistant TB. NAA assays are available to detect resistance genes. Currently the most widely used NAA is a combined assay that detects both MTB and mutations associated with rifampicin resistance.
- Chest radiographs should be obtained; upper lung field involvement and pulmonary cavitation are both suggestive of TB.
- Appropriate AFB precautions should be initiated in all patients until TB can be ruled out.

TREATMENT

- **Primary Tuberculosis**
  - For details regarding TB treatment, see the Tuberculosis section in Chapter 5. Optimal timing of cART in patient with active TB infection remains controversial, although data suggest survival benefit in early initiation of cART after starting TB therapy and current guidelines recommend cART in all HIV-infected persons with TB. In patients with CD4+ T cell counts <50 who are cART-naive, cART should be initiated within 2 weeks of TB treatment initiation. In those with higher CD4+ T cell counts ART should be initiated within 8 weeks of starting TB treatment.[6]
  - There are important drug interactions to consider between cART and TB treatment. In particular, rifampin is a potent inducer of cytochrome P450 CYP3A, lowering the concentration of protease inhibitors, nonnucleoside reverse transcriptase inhibitors, and integrase strand transfer inhibitors.
  - Directly observed therapy is recommended for all HIV patients undergoing treatment for TB.
- **Latent Tuberculosis**
  - All HIV-infected patients should be tested for LTBI at the time of HIV diagnosis and once every year.
  - Diagnosis of LTBI can be made by tuberculin skin test (TST); **induration >5 mm is considered positive**.
  - Interferon-γ release assays are an alternative to TST with better specificity reported.[7]
  - In any HIV-infected patient, LTBI should be treated once active TB has been ruled out.
  - Isoniazid (INH) 300 mg PO once daily along with pyridoxine for 9 months is the preferred treatment of LTBI in the setting of HIV infection.
  - If INH is not tolerated, rifampin 600 mg PO once daily or rifabutin (dose adjusted based on the concomitant ART, see Table 13-4) for 4 months may be used.
  - For known exposure to drug-resistant TB, consultation with public health authorities is recommended.

Bartonellosis

GENERAL PRINCIPLES

- *Bartonella* spp. can cause a wide variety of infections including cat-scratch disease, endocarditis, bacillary angiomatosis (BA), and bacillary peliosis hepatis (BP). The latter two occur only in immunosuppressed persons.

TABLE 13-4	DOSE ADJUSTMENT WITH RIFABUTIN/RIFAMPIN AND CONCURRENT ART
ART	**Rifabutin-Related Dose Adjustment**
Boosted protease inhibitors	Decrease rifabutin to 150 mg PO three times weekly or 150 mg PO every other day
EFV	Increase rifabutin to 450–600 mg PO once daily
NVP and ETR	No need for rifabutin dose adjustment
ETR coadministered with boosted protease inhibitors	Do not use rifabutin
RAL and MVC	Under investigation
ART	**Rifampin-Related Dose Adjustment**
Boosted protease inhibitors	Do not use rifampin
EFV	Increase EFV to 800 mg PO once daily

ART, antiretroviral therapy; EFV, efavirenz; ETR, etravirine; MVC, maraviroc; NPV, nevirapine; RAL, raltegravir.

- BA is a unique vascular proliferative lesion caused by *Bartonella quintana* or *Bartonella henselae* and usually occurs in advanced HIV infection with CD4+ T cell counts <50 cells/μL. These lesions can form in different organs, including skin, bone, brain, lymph nodes, bone marrow, and gastrointestinal and respiratory tracts.
- BP is a histopathologically different vascular proliferative response that can be seen in the liver and spleen.

DIAGNOSIS

- Diagnosis can be confirmed by histopathological examination of biopsied tissue.
- **On visual inspection, BA may be indistinguishable from Kaposi sarcoma** (KS), therefore any new vascular lesion should be biopsied.
- BA lesions show characteristic vascular proliferation, and a modified silver stain (e.g., Warthin–Starry stain) usually reveals numerous bacilli. Gram stain and acid-fast stains are negative.
- Antibodies to *B. henselae* can be measured using indirect immunofluorescence. A new enzyme immunoassay is more sensitive.
- PCR for Bartonella DNA is sensitive but is not widely available.

TREATMENT

- **Erythromycin** 500 mg PO four times daily or **doxycycline** 100 mg PO twice daily is recommended. Clarithromycin and azithromycin are alternatives as erythromycin is not well tolerated. Some experts recommend doxycycline over erythromycin.
- If CNS involvement is suspected, doxycycline should be given with a rifamycin. Duration of therapy should be at least 3 months.
- Relapse can occur after the primary treatment; long-term suppression with doxycycline or a macrolide should be given if relapse occurs.
- Long-term suppression can be discontinued after the patient has received 3 to 4 months of treatment and when the CD4+ T cell count is >200 cells/μL for more than 6 months.

Protozoal Infections

Toxoplasma gondii

GENERAL PRINCIPLES

- In general, toxoplasmosis occurs because of reactivation of the intracellular protozoan parasite *Toxoplasma gondii*, generally when the CD4+ T cell count is <100 cells/μL.
- All patients with HIV infection should be screened for *T. gondii* antibodies around the time of diagnosis
- People living with HIV/AIDS who are seronegative for *T. gondii* should be counseled to avoid ingestion of undercooked or raw meat, to wash their hands after handling of raw meat or soil, to wash vegetables thoroughly, and to avoid changing cat litter. Pet cats do not need to be removed from the home.

DIAGNOSIS

Clinical Presentation

- Toxoplasmic encephalitis (TE) is the most common presentation. Patients present with headache, weakness, confusion, seizures, and coma depending on the location of the lesion.
- Disseminated toxoplasmosis, which involves the heart, lung, colon, skeletal muscles, and other organs, is rare.

Differential Diagnosis

- Both CNS lymphoma and TE can present with ring-enhancing brain lesions. It is difficult to distinguish between the two based on imaging alone.
- After obtaining appropriate diagnostic testing, empiric therapy for TE may be started and response assessed.
- TB, fungal infections, nocardiosis, syphilis, KS, chagoma, and other brain tumors are other possibilities.

Diagnostic Testing

- The presence of **IgG *T. gondii*–specific antibodies** is a marker for potential development of toxoplasmosis as most infections are because of reactivation. A patient presenting with symptoms compatible with TE but with negative *T. gondii* IgG is less likely to have toxoplasmosis (although a negative serology does not completely exclude the diagnosis).
- The level of antibody does not predict reactivation or severity of disease.
- **Multiple ring-enhancing brain lesions** often associated with edema are characteristic. MRI is more sensitive than CT scan for detection of brain lesions. Primary CNS lymphoma cannot be distinguished from TE solely on the basis of imaging. Thallium single-photon emission computed tomography and fluorodeoxyglucose positron emission tomography may be useful in distinguishing between TE and CNS lymphoma, but their value has not been established in HIV-infected patients.
- Definitive diagnosis is made by demonstrating numerous *T. gondii* tachyzoites or cysts in a **brain biopsy**. Brain tissue should also be checked by PCR for *T. gondii* DNA. Response to empiric therapy can be helpful when biopsy is not possible and is the approach taken by many clinicians in the setting of a clinical presentation consistent with TE.
- CSF may show mild mononuclear pleocytosis and elevated protein. Wright–Giemsa stain of centrifuged preparation of CSF may reveal tachyzoites. *T. gondii* DNA should also be assessed by PCR. The sensitivity of CSF PCR for *T. gondii* is between 50% and 98%, and the specificity is almost 100%.[8]

TABLE 13-5	TREATMENT OF TOXOPLASMOSIS

Standard Regimens

- Pyrimethamine 200 mg PO loading dose followed by 50 mg (<60 kg) or 75 mg (>60 kg) once daily *plus* leucovorin (folinic acid) 10–25 mg PO once daily *plus* sulfadiazine 1000 mg (<60 kg) or 1500 mg (>60 kg) PO every 6 h.
  - If the patient cannot tolerate sulfadiazine, use clindamycin 600 mg IV or PO every 6 h.

Alternative Regimens

- Pyrimethamine *plus* leucovorin *plus* one of the following:
  - Atovaquone 750 mg PO every 6 h or 1500 mg PO twice daily
  - Azithromycin 1200–1500 mg once daily
- TMP-SMX (5 mg/kg TMP and 25 mg/kg SMX) IV or PO twice daily

Other Consideration

Corticosteroids are used for significant edema and/or mass effect

Duration of Therapy

At least 6 wk of treatment regimen followed by chronic maintenance therapy (secondary prophylaxis)

Secondary Prophylaxis

- Pyrimethamine 25–50 mg PO once daily *plus* sulfadiazine 2000–4000 mg PO daily (in two to four divided dose) *plus* leucovorin 10–25 mg PO once daily
- Alternatives:
  - Clindamycin 600 mg PO every 8 h *plus* pyrimethamine 25–50 mg PO once daily *plus* leucovorin 10–25 mg PO once daily
  - Atovaquone 750 mg PO every 6–12 h and/or ([pyrimethamine 25 mg PO once daily *plus* leucovorin 10 mg PO once daily] *or* sulfadiazine 2000–4000 mg PO daily)

TMP-SMX, trimethoprim–sulfamethoxazole.

TREATMENT

Treatment of toxoplasmosis is summarized in Table 13-5.

- **Alternative regimens are clearly inferior** and should be reserved for patients who cannot tolerate the standard regimens.

Diarrhea Caused by Protozoal Infections

- Diarrhea is one of the most common symptoms in HIV-infected patients.
- Acute diarrhea may be caused by bacteria (*Campylobacter jejuni, Clostridium difficile, Salmonella, Shigella,* etc.) or enteric viruses.
- Patients with CD4+ T cell counts <200 cells/µL may have chronic diarrhea with *Cryptosporidium, Cyclospora, Cystoisospora, Microspora,* CMV, or MAC. *Giardia* and *Entamoeba histolytica* can cause persistent diarrhea regardless of CD4+ T cell counts.
- TMP-SMX prophylaxis has reduced the incidence of diarrheal illness in HIV-infected patients.

Cryptosporidiosis

GENERAL PRINCIPLES

- This is a highly infectious parasite (size 4–6 µm) that may be fatal in HIV-infected individuals.
- Transmission is primarily via fecal–oral route.
- Numerous US waterborne outbreaks have affected non–HIV-infected persons.

DIAGNOSIS

- Symptoms include diarrhea, nausea and vomiting, abdominal pain, and weight loss.
- Fulminant and extraintestinal disease can be seen in patients with CD4+ T cell counts <50 cells/µL. Infection of the biliary tree causes sclerosing cholangitis and acalculous cholecystitis.
- Laboratory studies reveal an elevated alkaline phosphatase.
- Ultrasonography may demonstrate gallbladder wall thickening and dilated bile ducts.
- Modified acid-fast stain and enzyme immunoassays of the stool or other tissue specimens are used.

TREATMENT

- **There is no reliable therapy for cryptosporidiosis.** Reconstitution of immune system with cART is key to treatment.
- Nitazoxanide has been approved for children of age <11 years, but its effectiveness in immunosuppressed adults is questionable. Paromomycin has transient or no benefit.

Microsporidiosis

GENERAL PRINCIPLES

- Microsporidia was once considered a protozoan or protist but is now known to be a fungus.
- Two species are important to be aware of in HIV-infected patients.
  - *Enterocytozoon*: Causes 90% of intestinal microsporidiosis. *Enterocytozoon bieneusi* is also associated with cholangitis and cholecystitis.
  - *Encephalitozoon*: *Encephalitozoon hellem* and *Encephalitozoon cuniculi* can disseminate to lungs and kidneys and often spare the intestine. *E. hellem* causes punctuate keratoconjunctivitis. *Encephalitozoon intestinalis* causes diarrhea, accounting for 10% of microsporidial diarrhea.

DIAGNOSIS

- Microscopic examination of stool, tissue, or corneal scraping using modified trichrome stains can establish the diagnosis.
- Transmission electron microscopy is the gold standard but is time consuming.

TREATMENT

The cornerstone of treatment is immune reconstitution with use of cART. Albendazole and fumagillin may have some activity.

CYSTOISOSPORIASIS

- *Cystoisopora belli* (previously *Isospora belli*) is an acid-fast coccidian protozoan (20–30 μm) that causes a **diarrheal illness indistinguishable from cryptosporidiosis**.
- Disseminated disease can also occur.
- There is a higher prevalence in developing countries.
- Treatment consists of **TMP-SMX** DS 1 tablet PO four times daily for 10 days followed by every 12 hours for 3 weeks. Relapse rates are high; therefore, long-term maintenance therapy (TMP-SMX 1 DS tablet three times weekly) is recommended until immune reconstitution (CD4+ T cell count >200 cells/μL for >6 mo).
- Alternatively, pyrimethamine 75 mg PO once daily plus leucovorin 10 mg PO once daily may be used if patients cannot tolerate TMP-SMX. Chronic maintenance therapy with pyrimethamine 25 mg PO once daily plus leucovorin 5 mg PO once daily.

CYCLOSPORIASIS

- *Cyclospora cayetanensis* is an acid-fast coccidian (8–10 μm) transmitted by the fecal–oral route and by contaminated water or food. It causes a diarrheal illness in advanced HIV-infected patients.
- Treatment is **TMP-SMX** DS 1 tablet four times daily for 10 days followed by 1 DS tablet three times weekly indefinitely.
- Ciprofloxacin can be tried in patients intolerant to TMP-SMX but is inferior.

Viral Infections

Cytomegalovirus

GENERAL PRINCIPLES

- With widespread use of cART, there has been a marked decline in CMV disease, although patients with CD4+ T cell counts <50 cells/μL are still at risk.
- The risk of developing disease and death in advanced HIV-infected patients is correlated with the quantity of CMV DNA measured by PCR.

DIAGNOSIS

- **Chorioretinitis**
  - Ocular disease occurs in patients with advanced HIV infection.
  - CMV chorioretinitis is because of reactivation and may not be associated with viremia.
  - Symptoms include decreased visual acuity, presence of "floaters," or unilateral visual field loss.
  - Diagnosis is made by ophthalmologic examination, revealing large creamy to yellowish white granular areas with perivascular exudates and hemorrhages. Lesions occur in the periphery but can progress to involve the macula and optic disk.
- **CMV Neurological Disease**
  - Polyradiculopathy, encephalitis, mononeuritis multiplex, and painful neuropathy can all be caused by CMV infection.
  - **Polyradiculopathy** presents with low back pain radiating to the perianal area and progressive lower extremity weakness, hypo- or areflexia and variable sensory deficit with preserved proprioception and vibratory sensation, or bladder/anal sphincter dysfunction causing urinary retention/fecal incontinence.
  - **Encephalitis** presents with rapidly progressive cognitive impairment and mental status changes. MRI may reveal meningeal or periventricular enhancement.

- ○ **Mononeuritis multiplex** causes multifocal, patchy, asymmetrical sensory, and motor deficits. Biopsy of the involved peripheral nerve can confirm the diagnosis.
- **CMV colitis and esophagitis**
  - ○ CMV colitis occurred in 5% to 10% of AIDS patients in the pre-cART era but is now uncommon.
  - ○ Diarrhea, weight loss, anorexia, abdominal pain, and fever are present.
  - ○ Diagnosis is made by colonoscopy or endoscopy with biopsy. Mucosal ulceration and submucosal hemorrhage are seen, although 10% of those with histologic evidence of CMV colitis may have normal-appearing mucosa. Biopsy shows characteristic CMV inclusions (owl eye), CMV antigen, or nucleic acid.
- **CMV pneumonitis** is less common than in transplant recipients. Isolation of CMV from pulmonary secretions is common, but the true pathogenic role of CMV in pneumonia is not well established. Diagnosis is established by finding pathognomonic intranuclear inclusion bodies in biopsy.

TREATMENT

- Treatment of CMV neurologic disease should be initiated promptly. Combination of **ganciclovir** IV plus **foscarnet** IV.
- Treatment of CMV chorioretinitis is presented in Table 13-6.

TABLE 13-6	TREATMENT OF CYTOMEGALOVIRUS CHORIORETINITIS

For Small Peripheral Lesions

- Valganciclovir 900 mg PO twice daily for 14–21 d, then 900 mg PO once daily

For Immediate Sight-Threatening Lesions

- Ganciclovir intraocular implants are no longer available
- Intravitreal injections of ganciclovir (2 mg) or foscarnet (2.4 mg) for 1–4 doses over a period of 7–10 days *plus* valganciclovir 900 mg PO (twice daily for 14–21 d, then once daily)
- Alternatives
  - ○ Ganciclovir 5 mg/kg IV every 12 h for 14–21 d, then 5 mg/kg IV once daily
  - ○ Ganciclovir 5 mg/kg IV every 12 h for 14–21 d, then valganciclovir 900 mg PO once daily
  - ○ Foscarnet 60 mg/kg IV every 8 h or 90 mg/kg IV every 12 h for 14–21 d, then 90–120 mg/kg IV once daily
  - ○ Cidofovir 5 mg/kg/wk IV for 2 wk, then 5 mg/kg every other week with saline hydration before and after therapy and probenecid 2 g PO 3 h before the dose followed by 1 g PO 2 h after the dose and 1 g PO 8 h after the dose (total of 4 g)

Secondary Prophylaxis (Until Immune Reconstitution)

- Valganciclovir 900 mg PO once daily
- Alternatives for secondary prophylaxis
  - ○ Ganciclovir 5 mg/kg IV five to seven times weekly
  - ○ Foscarnet 90–120 mg/kg IV once daily
  - ○ Cidofovir 5 mg/kg IV every other week with saline hydration and probenecid

- Treatment of CMV colitis and esophagitis consists of ganciclovir IV or foscarnet IV for at least 21 days or until resolution of signs and symptoms. Oral valganciclovir may be used when symptoms (and oral absorption) improve.
- Maintenance therapy with an oral anti-CMV agent is only necessary for CMV retinitis. It is not recommended in other CMV end-organ disease except with documented relapse or with concurrent retinitis.
- Treatment for CMV pneumonitis should be considered in patients with histologic evidence or when CMV is the only pathogen identified in a progressive, deteriorating pneumonia not responding to other treatments. Ganciclovir IV can be used.

Varicella-Zoster Virus

GENERAL PRINCIPLES

- Reactivation of varicella-zoster virus (VZV) infection is more frequent among HIV-infected persons than among age-matched non–HIV-infected controls.
- Most herpes zoster–related complications, including disseminated disease, occur in patients with CD4+ T cell count <200 cells/µL.

DIAGNOSIS

- Patients may present with typical, single-dermatome zoster. Disseminated skin involvement and organ involvement are more common in immunocompromised hosts.
- VZV-related neurologic disease includes CNS vasculitis, multifocal leukoencephalitis, ventriculitis, myelitis and myeloradiculitis, optic neuritis, cranial nerve palsies, focal brain stem lesions, and aseptic meningitis.
  ○ **HIV-associated zoster ophthalmicus** occurs with reactivated infection involving the ophthalmic division of the trigeminal nerve, which may cause keratitis and retinitis.
  ○ **Acute retinal necrosis** (ARN) is a necrotizing herpetic retinopathy characterized by marked anterior and intermediate uveitis, retinal arteritis, papillitis of the optic disk, and retinal and choroidal occlusive vasculitis. Retinal detachment is common. ARN can occur regardless of CD4+ T cell count. It is also seen with CMV or HSV infections.
  ○ **Progressive outer retinal necrosis (PORN)** is caused almost exclusively by VZV and occurs in severely immunosuppressed patients with CD4+ T cell count <50 to 100 cells/µL. PORN presents with pain in the eye with movement as a result of optic nerve involvement. Retinal findings are multifocal necrotic lesions that rapidly coalesce. There is no or minimal vitreous inflammation. Most patients with PORN will become blind within 1 month due to retinal detachment, optic neuropathy, or widespread retinal necrosis.

TREATMENT

- For uncomplicated varicella (primary infection), oral **acyclovir** 20 mg/kg/d (commonly 800 mg PO five times daily), **valacyclovir** 1 g PO three times daily, or **famciclovir** 500 mg PO three times daily for 5 to 7 days are used.
- For recurrent infection, oral valacyclovir, famciclovir, or acyclovir for 5 to 7 days is recommended.
- If cutaneous lesions are extensive or with concerns for visceral involvement, IV acyclovir should be initiated.

- ARN requires aggressive treatment with high-dose IV acyclovir (10 mg/kg every 8 h) for 10 to 14 days followed by prolonged oral valacyclovir (1 g PO three times daily for 6 wk); early laser retinopexy to prevent extension of peripheral detachments may result in good vision.
- Optimal treatment for PORN is unknown. Some success has been observed with a combination IV ganciclovir and foscarnet, plus intravitreal ganciclovir and/or foscarnet. Optimization of cART is recommended.

SPECIAL CONSIDERATIONS

- **Postexposure prophylaxis.** HIV-infected patients who are susceptible to VZV should receive varicella-zoster immune globulin within 96 hours of close contact with a person who has active varicella or herpes zoster.
- **Vaccination.** The live attenuated varicella vaccine can be safely given to HIV-infected patients with CD4+ T cell count >200 cells/μL.

Progressive Multifocal Leukoencephalopathy

GENERAL PRINCIPLES

- Progressive multifocal leukoencephalopathy (PML) is characterized by deep white matter changes due to focal demyelination caused by infection of oligodendrocytes by the JC polyoma virus.
- In the pre-cART era, PML occurred in approximately 4% of AIDS patients and progressed to death within months from diagnosis.
- Despite the fact that the incidence of PML has declined with cART, morbidity and mortality associated with PML remain high.
- PML may occur in patients with high CD4+ T cell counts and even on cART.

DIAGNOSIS

Clinical Presentation

- Clinical presentation varies from diffuse encephalopathy to focal deficits.
- Initial symptoms may begin as partial neurologic deficits and evolve to hemiparesis. Symptoms tend to progress over several weeks to months.
- Seizures may develop in up to 20% of affected patients.

Diagnostic Testing

- Definitive diagnosis is made by a **brain biopsy**. However, PML is usually diagnosed with a combination of clinical and neuroimaging findings.
- **MRI** lesions are hyperintense on T2-weighted and fluid-attenuated inversion recovery sequences and hypointense on T1-weighted sequence. PML is most commonly noncontrast enhancing.
- PCR detection of JC virus from CSF has sensitivity of 72% to 92% and specificity of 92% to 100% in patients not on cART.[9] Immune recovery decreases the sensitivity of the test.

TREATMENT

- **No established treatment exists for PML.**
- Patients should be started on cART immediately. Immune reconstitution (IRIS) can cause a paradoxical response.
- Corticosteroids have been used in this setting to control the local inflammation and reduce cerebral edema although data are limited.

HUMAN PAPILLOMAVIRUS INFECTION

- Human papillomavirus (HPV) is a common sexually transmitted virus and the cause of cervical cancer. Other types of lesions caused by HPV infection include genital, anal, and oral warts. Anal and some oropharyngeal cancers are caused by HPV.
- **Women with HIV infection have a sevenfold higher rate of cervical cancer.**
- Most infections resolve or become latent and undetectable; persistent infection with oncogenic types is required to develop cancerous lesions.
- There are more than 100 HPV serotypes.
  - The most important serotypes are types 16 and 18, which account for approximately 50% and 10% to 15% of cervical cancer, respectively.
  - HPV types 6 and 11 cause 90% of genital warts.
- There are several HPV **vaccines** currently available:
  - A quadrivalent HPV vaccine targets types 6, 11, 16, and 18.
  - A bivalent vaccine targets types 16 and 18.
  - A 9-valent HPV vaccine is designed to target types 6, 11, 16, 18, 31, 33, 45, 52, and 58.
- HPV vaccine is indicated for all women and men under the age of 26 years.

Human Herpesvirus 8 Disease

GENERAL PRINCIPLES

- Human herpesvirus (HHV)-8 is associated with KS as well as **primary effusion lymphoma** (PEL) and **multicentric Castleman disease** (MCD) and can occur at any CD4+ T count, although KS and PEL usually occur in those with CD4+ T cell counts <200 cells/μL.
- HHV-8 seroprevalence in the general population of the United States is 1% to 5%; men who have sex with men have a seroprevalence of 20% to 70%.
- The incidence of KS in the pre-cART era was about 20%, which has since dramatically declined.
- PEL is an uncommon AIDS-related lymphoma, associated with HHV-8 and presents as a body cavity effusion.
- MCD is a lymphoproliferative disorder associated with HHV-8. The incidence of MCD has been increasing with the use of cART. MCD has been linked with overexpression of interleukin-6.

DIAGNOSIS

- KS is a multicentric tumor that initially presents as purplish nodules on the skin or mucous membranes.
  - Patients with CD4+ T cell count >300 cells/μL may develop limited cutaneous lesions.
  - Oral lesions are common on the hard palate and gingival margins and are often asymptomatic.
  - Lymphatic and visceral sites of disease are common, with 40% having gastrointestinal involvement at diagnosis. Lymph node involvement may result in edema of the legs and scrotum.
  - Biopsy should be performed to distinguish from BA.
- PEL originates on serosal surfaces such as pleura, pericardium, peritoneum, joint spaces, and meninges and produces a symptomatic serous effusion with high-grade malignant lymphocytes, but without detectable mass. Diagnosis is made by fluid cytology; the presence of HHV-8 in the nuclei of the malignant cell is diagnostic. Immunohistochemical staining for latent viral gene product (latency-associated nuclear antigen LANA-1) is used.

- MCD is characterized by polyclonal hypergammaglobulinemia, generalized lymphadenopathy, hepatosplenomegaly, constitutional symptoms (e.g., fever, weakness, and weight loss), and autoimmune hemolytic anemia. KS is also commonly found.

TREATMENT

- All HIV-infected patients presenting with KS should be started on cART as the lesions may regress in response to HIV treatment. Management of KS is largely palliative. In advanced KS or with lesions associated with pain, extremity edema, soft tissue infection, and GI and respiratory symptoms, therapy is recommended.
  - Local therapies include radiotherapy, intralesional chemotherapy with vinblastine, cryotherapy, and alitretinoin gel.
  - Systematic therapies include chemotherapy and interferon α. First-line chemotherapy is liposomal doxorubicin. For poor response or relapse, paclitaxel has been shown to have a high response rate.[10] Other agents are etoposide and vinorelbine.
- The overall prognosis of PEL is poor. All patients should receive cART. There are only limited data regarding chemotherapy in patients who fail cART alone. Patients may be treated with liposomal doxorubicin with or without bortezomib and prednisone.
- Treatment for MCD has not been well established, although there are anecdotal reports of use of steroids, chemotherapy (e.g., rituximab, tocilizumab, vinblastine, etoposide, cyclophosphamide/hydroxydaunorubicin/vincristine/prednisone [CHOP]), and antiviral therapy such as ganciclovir, foscarnet, and cidofovir.

REFERENCES

1. Zolopa A, Andersen J, Powderly W, et al. Early antiretroviral therapy reduces AIDS progression/ death in individuals with acute opportunistic infections: a multicenter randomized strategy trial. *PLoS One.* 2009;4(5):e5575.
2. Blanc FX, Sok T, Laureillard D, et al. Earlier versus later start of antiretroviral therapy in HIV-infected adults with tuberculosis. *N Engl J Med.* 2011;365(16):1471-1481.
3. Abdool Karim SS, Naidoo K, Grobler A, et al. Timing of initiation of antiretroviral drugs during tuberculosis therapy. *N Engl J Med.* 2010;362(8):697-706.
4. Boulware DR, Meya DB, Muzoora C, et al. Timing of antiretroviral therapy after diagnosis of cryptococcal meningitis. *N Engl J Med.* 2014;370(26):2487-2498.
5. Ward TT, Rimland D, Kauffman C, Huycke M, Evans TG, Heifets L. Randomized, open-label trial of azithromycin plus ethambutol vs. clarithromycin plus ethambutol as therapy for *Mycobacterium avium* complex bacteremia in patients with human immunodeficiency virus infection. Veterans Affairs HIV Research Consortium. *Clin Infect Dis.* 1998;27(5):1278-1285.
6. Panel on Opportunistic Infections in HIV-Infected Adults and Adolescents. *Guidelines for the Prevention and Treatment of Opportunistic Infections in HIV-infected Adults and Adolescents: Recommendations from the Centers for Disease Control and Prevention, the National Institutes of Health, and the HIV Medicine Association of the Infectious Diseases Society of America*; 2017. Available at http:// aidsinfo.nih.gov/contentfiles/lvguidelines/adult_oi.pdf.
7. Menzies D, Pai M, Comstock G. Meta-analysis: new tests for the diagnosis of latent tuberculosis infection: areas of uncertainty and recommendations for research. *Ann Intern Med.* 2007;146(5):340-354.
8. Mesquita RT, Ziegler AP, Hiramoto RM, Vidal JE, Pereira-Chioccola VL. Real-time quantitative PCR in cerebral toxoplasmosis diagnosis of Brazilian human immunodeficiency virus-infected patients. *J Med Microbiol.* 2010;59(Pt 6):641-647.
9. Cinque P, Scarpellini P, Vago L, Linde A, Lazzarin A. Diagnosis of central nervous system complications in HIV-infected patients: cerebrospinal fluid analysis by the polymerase chain reaction. *AIDS.* 1997;11(1):1-17.
10. Cianfrocca M, Lee S, Von Roenn J, et al. Randomized trial of paclitaxel versus pegylated liposomal doxorubicin for advanced human immunodeficiency virus-associated Kaposi sarcoma: evidence of symptom palliation from chemotherapy. *Cancer.* 2010;116(16):3969-3977.

Infection in Non-HIV Immunocompromised Hosts

Anupam Pande and Ige George

14

Hematopoietic Stem Cell Transplantation

GENERAL PRINCIPLES

- There are two **major types** of hematopoietic stem cell transplant (HSCT).
  - **Autologous:** the patient serves as his or her own source of stem cells. This is commonly used for the treatment of lymphoid malignancies and myeloma to facilitate cytotoxic chemotherapy.
  - **Allogeneic:** the stem cell source is a human leukocyte antigen (HLA)–matched donor (e.g., family member or unrelated volunteer donor) or banked cord blood cells. This is commonly used for the treatment of myeloid malignant diseases (e.g., acute and chronic leukemia). Haploidentical HSCT is where one HLA haplotype-matched family member donor is used.
- The three **major steps** of HSCT are as follows:
  - **Stem cell harvest and manipulation.** Stem cells are obtained either directly from the bone marrow, growth factor–stimulated peripheral blood, or umbilical cord blood. The stem cell graft is sometimes manipulated before transplantation. Most commonly, T-cell depletion is performed to reduce the risk of graft versus host disease (GVHD).
  - **Conditioning.** Before the infusion of the stem cell graft, a conditioning regimen is chosen based on the type of stem cell graft and reason for HSCT. Most commonly, prospective allogeneic HSCT recipients are given an intensive myeloablative regimen consisting of cyclophosphamide, total body irradiation, and antithymocyte globulin (ATG). Nonmyeloablative regimens are increasingly being used for patients who may not tolerate intensive conditioning regimens.
  - **Stem cell graft infusion, engraftment, and posttransplant care.** The duration of neutropenia after stem cell graft infusion varies according to the type of HSCT performed (10–14 d for autologous, 15–30 d for allogeneic with an ablative regimen, 5–7 d for allogeneic with a nonmyeloablative regimen). Primary graft failure is the absence of engraftment (absolute neutrophil count [ANC] < 500 cells/μL) by day 42 after transplant. An immunosuppressive regimen commonly consisting of a calcineurin inhibitor (cyclosporine or tacrolimus) plus mycophenolate mofetil or a short course of methotrexate is given to allogeneic HSCT recipients to prevent both stem cell graft rejection and GVHD. The immunosuppressive regimen is typically tapered over 4 to 6 months and discontinued unless GVHD occurs. **Immune reconstitution after allogeneic HSCT may take a year or more.** Autologous HSCT does not require posttransplant immunosuppression and therefore takes only 3 to 9 months for immune recovery. While there is currently no definitive laboratory marker for immune reconstitution, several studies have shown that CD4+ cell counts are the most accessible and predictive marker for restoration of immune competence after HSCT.

INFECTION RISK

- The risk and type of infection with HSCT differ depending on the type of transplant, type of stem cell graft, conditioning regimen, immunosuppressive regimen, and development of posttransplant complications such as GVHD.
- **Allogeneic HSCT**, especially transplants from **unrelated** or **mismatched donors**, results in slower immune reconstitution and elevated infection risk.
- **Myeloablative conditioning regimens** result in rapid-onset and prolonged neutropenia and more mucosal injury compared with nonmyeloablative regimens and therefore have a higher risk of neutropenic infections, especially typhlitis.
- **ATG** results in profound T-cell immunodeficiency; **methotrexate** results in delayed neutrophil recovery and more mucosal injury; these drugs elevate the risk of invasive fungal infections (IFIs) and herpesvirus infections.
- **Central venous catheters** breach the skin barrier and predispose patients to bacterial and yeast infections. Catheter-associated infections are the leading cause of bloodstream infections in HSCT recipients, particularly during the pre-engraftment period and in patients with GVHD.
- **Mucositis** serves as a portal of entry for oral or intestinal infections and is common with methotrexate-containing regimens.
- **GVHD** results in markedly elevated infection risk because of prolonged and intensive administration of immunosuppressive medications and splenic dysfunction.
- The types of infections at various times after HSCT are outlined in Table 14-1.

TABLE 14-1	RISK FACTORS AND TYPES OF INFECTIONS IN HSCT RECIPIENTS[a]		
Type of Pathogen	Early Pre-engraftment (<2–4 wk): Neutropenia, barrier breakdown from mucositis, and central venous catheters.	Early Postengraftment (<3 mo): Impaired cellular and humoral immunity, with restricted T-cell repertoire.	Late Postengraftment (>2–3 mo)[b]: Impaired cellular and humoral immunity (B-cell and CD4+ T-cell recovery, diversified repertoire).
Bacteria	**Gram positive:** Including CONS, *Staphylococcus aureus*, viridans *Streptococcus*. Risk factors: mucositis and central venous catheter use. **Gram negative:** Including *Legionella*, *Pseudomonas aeruginosa*, *Enterobacter*, and *Stenotrophomonas maltophilia*. Risk factors: mucositis/cutaneous injury and neutropenia. ***Clostridium difficile:*** Risk factors: antibiotic use, neutropenia.	**Gram positive:** Including *Listeria*. Risk factors: central venous catheter use. **Gram negative:** Including *Legionella*. Risk factors: enteric involvement of GVHD and use of central venous catheters. ***Mycobacterium:*** Rare. Because of reactivation of TB or MAC; new exposure with atypical mycobacterium.	**Encapsulated bacteria:** Including *Streptococcus pneumoniae*, *Haemophilus influenzae*, *Neisseria meningitidis*. Risk factors: immunoglobulin deficiency, hyposplenism, severe chronic GVHD (poor opsonization). **Gram positive:** Including *Staphylococcus*, *Nocardia*. **Gram negative:** Including *Pseudomonas*. Risk factor: chronic GVHD.

TABLE 14-1	RISK FACTORS AND TYPES OF INFECTIONS IN HSCT RECIPIENTS[a] (CONTINUED)

| Viruses | **HSV:** Because of viral reactivation. **Respiratory viruses:** Including RSV, parainfluenza, rhinovirus, influenza, human metapneumovirus. Follows community outbreak patterns. | **CMV:** Risk factors: acute GVHD, older age, total body irradiation conditioning, matched unrelated donor, and impaired CMI. Decreased incidence with prophylaxis. **EBV:** Risk factors: mismatched donors and T-cell-depleted grafts. **BK virus:** Risk factors: GVHD, cyclophosphamide conditioning regimens. **Respiratory viruses:** Including RSV, influenza, parainfluenza, rhinovirus, human metapneumovirus. Follows community outbreak patterns. **Adenovirus:** Because of reactivation. Risk factor: acute GVHD. **HHV-6:** Related to anti-CD3 mAb use, GVHD. **Enteric viruses:** Including coxsackie, echovirus, rotavirus, norovirus. Usually summer/fall months. | **CMV:** Risk factors: GVHD, impaired CMI, and viral latency pretransplant. **EBV:** Including PTLD. Risk factors: mismatched donors, and T-cell-depleted grafts. **VZV:** Decreased incidence with acyclovir prophylaxis. Risk factors: viral latency or infection pretransplant, total body irradiation, antithymocyte globulin therapy, GVHD, and lymphopenia. **Respiratory viruses, Adenovirus:** Because of reactivation. Risk factor: GVHD. **HBV, HCV:** Because of reactivation. **Other viruses:** Measles, mumps, rubella, parvovirus B19, BK/JC virus, HHV-8. Because of loss of specific B-cell immunity. |

(Continued)

TABLE 14-1	RISK FACTORS AND TYPES OF INFECTIONS IN HSCT RECIPIENTSᵃ (CONTINUED)		
Fungi	***Candida:*** Because of mucositis, antibiotic use, and neutropenia. Decreased incidence with antifungal prophylaxis, except triazole-resistant species (*Candida krusei, Candida glabrata*). **Molds:** Including *Aspergillus, Fusarium, Zygomycetes*, others. Risk factors with allogeneic HSCT: prolonged neutropenia, older age, HLA match, delayed engraftment.	***Aspergillus:*** Risk factors: GVHD, diminished CMI, older age, corticosteroid therapy, graft failure, cytopenia, iron overload. **Other molds:** Including *Fusarium, Mucorales.* Risk factors with allogeneic HSCT: GVHD, CMV infection pretransplantation. ***Candida:*** Decreased incidence with antifungal prophylaxis. ***Pneumocystis jirovecii:*** Related to GVHD. Decreased incidence with prophylaxis use.	***Aspergillus,* other molds:** Risk factors: GVHD, older age, corticosteroid therapy, graft failure, cytopenia, iron overload. ***Pneumocystis jirovecii:*** Related to GVHD. Decreased incidence with prophylaxis.
Parasites		***Toxoplasma:*** Because of reactivation. Risk factors: T-cell depletion, severe immunosuppressed allogeneic HSCT.	

ᵃBased primarily on studies with myeloablative regimens. Paradigm for the early pre-engraftment period differs significantly for nonmyeloablative regimens but is similar in the postengraftment period.

ᵇLate postengraftment infections are usually only seen in allogeneic HSCT and not autologous HSCT due to posttransplant immunosuppressive regimens and chronic GVHD.

CONS, coagulase-negative staphylococci; CMI, cell-mediated immunity; CMV, cytomegalovirus; EBV, Epstein–Barr virus; GVHD, graft versus host disease; HBV, hepatitis B virus; HCV, hepatitis C virus; HHV, human herpes virus; HSCT, hematopoietic stem cell transplantation; HSV, herpes simplex virus; mAb, monoclonal antibody; MAC, *Mycobacterium avium* complex; NK, natural killer; PTLD, posttransplant lymphoproliferative disorder; RSV, respiratory syncytial virus; TB, *Mycobacterium tuberculosis*; VZV, varicella zoster virus.

Common Infectious Complications After HSCT

Neutropenic Fever

GENERAL PRINCIPLES

- Fever frequently occurs in patients with neutropenia (ANC < 500 cells/μL) and may be a sign of infection. Likely **sites of infection include the lungs, central venous catheters, genitourinary tract, bloodstream, skin, and intestine.** Overt inflammation is usually not present, and a high index of suspicion must be maintained while searching for foci of infection.
- Frequently identified causative organisms include staphylococci, enterococci, streptococci, several gram-negative bacilli, and anaerobes. Infections caused by *Candida*, *Aspergillus*, and other molds are less common but may occur[1] (see Table 14-2).

DIAGNOSIS

- A thorough workup must include two separately drawn blood cultures, urinalysis and urine culture, chest radiograph, and abdominal imaging as indicated.
- Patients with profound (ANC < 100 cells/μL) or prolonged (anticipated to last >7 d) neutropenia or those with significant medical comorbidities including hypotension, neurologic changes, pneumonia, or new-onset abdominal pain are considered high-risk for IFIs and should have CT-imaging of the chest and abdomen with a careful examination of skin for lesions that can be biopsied.
- Select cases may require CT of the sinuses, testing for cytomegalovirus (CMV) PCR, and fungal or mycobacterial blood cultures.

TREATMENT

- Timely and appropriate administration of broad-spectrum antibiotics is essential, with the choice of therapy determined by the most likely site of infection, causative organisms, and institutional bacterial susceptibility patterns.
- For high-risk patients, this typically involves the use of a third- or fourth-generation antipseudomonal β-lactam agent, with vancomycin added only if indicated (skin or soft tissue infection, suspected catheter-related infection, pneumonia, hemodynamic instability, known colonization with resistant gram-positive organisms, severe mucositis, or fluoroquinolone prophylaxis).
- Modification to the initial empiric regimen should be guided by clinical and microbiologic data. Empiric antifungal coverage should be considered in high-risk patients who have persistent fever after 4 to 7 days of broad-spectrum antibacterials and no identified source of fever.
- Treatment duration is dictated by organism and site, and appropriate antibiotics should be continued for at least the duration of neutropenia.
- **In adult patients expected to be profoundly neutropenic (ANC ≤ 100 cells/μL) for more than 7 days, it is recommended that antibacterial prophylaxis with a fluoroquinolone be initiated.** Antibacterial prophylaxis is usually started at the time of HSCT and continued until WBC recovery or initiation of empiric antibacterial therapy for neutropenic fever.
- Growth factors such as granulocyte macrophage colony-stimulating factor (GM-CSF) and granulocyte colony-stimulating factor (G-CSF) have been shown to reduce the duration of neutropenia after HSCT but have not been shown to reduce mortality.

TABLE 14-2	DIFFERENTIAL DIAGNOSIS OF CLINICAL MANIFESTATIONS OF DISEASE AFTER HSCT BY TIME PERIOD			
Illness	Early Pre-engraftment (<2–4 wk)	Early Postengraftment (1–3 mo)	Late Postengraftment (>2–3 mo)
Bloodstream infections	Bacteria (CONS, Viridans Streptococci, *Candida* (especially associated with central venous catheters and those receiving TPN)	Bacteria (especially CONS), *Candida*	Encapsulated organisms including *Streptococcus pneumoniae, Neisseria meningitidis*
Bone marrow suppression	Drug toxicity, CMV, HHV-6, acute GVHD, graft failure	CMV, HHV-6, acute GVHD, graft failure, drug toxicity	Parvovirus, CMV, graft failure, HHV-6, drug toxicity, chronic GVHD
CNS disease	**Focal:** Bacteria, molds, *Candida*, stroke, drug toxicity **Diffuse:** Bacteria, HSV, *Candida*, drug toxicity	**Focal:** bacteria including Listeria, toxoplasmosis, molds, tumor relapse **Diffuse:** HHV-6, CMV, *Cryptococcus*, drug toxicity	**Focal:** bacteria, molds, PML, tumor relapse, drug toxicity **Diffuse:** VZV, drug toxicity
Diarrhea/colitis	*Clostridium difficile, Candida*, enteric viruses, neutropenic enterocolitis (typhlitis), noninfectious (mucosal injury from conditioning regimen, GI bleed, infarct)	*C. difficile*, CMV, enteric viruses, adenovirus, acute GVHD, GI bleed, infarct, drug toxicity	CMV, EBV, adenovirus, *C. difficile*, enteric viruses, drug toxicity, chronic GVHD, GI bleed, infarct
Esophagitis	Drug toxicity, *Candida*, HSV	Drug toxicity, CMV	Drug toxicity

Neutropenic fever: severity risk related to duration and degree of neutropenia, degree of mucosal damage	Usually bacteria including *Staphylococcus epidermidis*, viridans streptococci, *Staphylococcus aureus, Enterobacter, Escherichia coli, Klebsiella, Pseudomonas, Stenotrophomonas; Candida, Aspergillus;* HSV; respiratory viruses; tumor fever; drug fever; acute GVHD; PE	Bacteria, CMV, adenovirus, PCP, *Aspergillus* and other molds, chronic disseminated candidiasis, respiratory viruses, acute GVHD, drug fever	CMV, VZV, EBV, PCP, molds, encapsulated bacteria, chronic GVHD, drug fever
Non-neutropenic fever	Engraftment syndrome, acute GVHD, drug fever, bacteria, respiratory viruses	CMV, sinusitis, central line infection, fungal infection, drug fever	CMV, sinusitis, central line infection, fungal infection, drug fever
Hemorrhagic cystitis	Cyclophosphamide toxicity, adenovirus (rare)	CMV, cyclophosphamide toxicity, adenovirus	BK virus
Hepatitis	Bacteria, HSV, chronic disseminated candidiasis, veno-occlusive disease (sinusoidal obstructive syndrome) from conditioning regimen, drug toxicity, iron overload	Acute GVHD, HSV, CMV, HHV-6, PCP, chronic disseminated candidiasis, drug toxicity, iron overload	HBV, HCV, EBV, VZV (fulminant hepatitis, even in absence of rash), veno-occlusive disease, drug toxicity, chronic GVHD, iron overload
Mucositis	HSV, *Candida*, drug toxicity (conditioning regimen), acute GVHD, viridans *Streptococci*	HSV, *Candida*, acute GVHD	*Candida*, HSV, chronic GVHD
Nephritis	Bacteria	CMV, adenovirus	BK/JC viruses
Ocular disease	Candida, molds	CMV, PCP, toxoplasmosis	VZV

(Continued)

TABLE 14-2	DIFFERENTIAL DIAGNOSIS OF CLINICAL MANIFESTATIONS OF DISEASE AFTER HSCT BY TIME PERIOD (CONTINUED)			
Illness	Early Pre-engraftment (<2–4 wk)	Early Postengraftment (1–3 mo)	Late Postengraftment (>2–3 mo)
Pneumonia: Focal infiltrate	Bacteria, *Aspergillus*, or other molds (halo sign or cavitary lesions), chemotherapy, PE, aspiration pneumonitis	Bacteria, *Aspergillus* or other molds, *Legionella*, PCP, TB, *Nocardia*, MAC, tumor relapse	Bacteria, *Aspergillus*, or other molds, PCP, *Legionella, Nocardia*, VZV, EBV-associated lymphoma
Diffuse	ARDS from conditioning regimen, pulmonary edema from CHF (cardiotoxic drugs) or volume overload, acute GVHD, radiation pneumonitis, hemorrhagic alveolitis, hypersensitivity drug reaction, respiratory viruses, HSV	Respiratory viruses, CMV, PCP, adenovirus, *Legionella*, Mycoplasma, TB, MAC, Cryptococcus, acute GVHD, idiopathic interstitial pneumonitis, radiation pneumonitis, hemorrhagic alveolitis, pulmonary veno-occlusive disease	CMV, respiratory viruses, PCP, adenovirus, chronic GVHD, bronchiolitis obliterans with organizing pneumonia, alveolar proteinosis
Rash	HSV, *Candida*, bacteria, molds, drug toxicity, acute GVHD	Acute GVHD, bacteria, *Candida*, molds, CMV, HHV-6, atypical mycobacteria, drug toxicity	VZV, molds, drug toxicity, chronic GVHD

ARDS, acute respiratory distress syndrome; CONS, coagulase-negative staphylococci; CMV, cytomegalovirus; CNS, central nervous system; CV, cardiovascular; EBV, Epstein–Barr virus; GI, gastrointestinal; GVHD, graft versus host disease; HBV, hepatitis B virus; HCV, hepatitis C virus; HHV, human herpes virus; HSCT, hematopoietic stem cell transplant; HSV, herpes simplex virus; MAC, *Mycobacterium avium* complex; PCP, *Pneumocystis jirovecii* pneumonia; PE, pulmonary embolism; PML, progressive multifocal leukoencephalopathy; TB, *Mycobacterium tuberculosis*; TPN, total parenteral nutrition; VZV, varicella zoster virus.

NON-NEUTROPENIC FEVER

- Fever without localizing signs occurring after engraftment is typically from an infectious cause (see Table 14-2). Diagnostic workup is similar to that of neutropenic fever.
- **Fever occurring at the time of engraftment is usually secondary to engraftment syndrome.**
  - Engraftment syndrome consists of fever occasionally accompanied by rash, pneumonitis, hyperbilirubinemia, or diarrhea.
  - Infections must be excluded with a full septic workup.
  - If no infections are identified, a trial of short-course high-dose corticosteroids should be considered.

Pneumonia

GENERAL PRINCIPLES

- Pneumonia commonly occurs in HSCT recipients. There are many infectious causes of pneumonia, and these vary by the time after transplantation and type of infiltrate (Table 14-2). Multiple pathogens are frequently present.
- **Focal infiltrates** are typically due to bacteria (e.g., *Streptococcus pneumoniae, Pseudomonas aeruginosa*), *Nocardia, Aspergillus*, and other molds. Noninfectious causes include aspiration, wedge infarction from pulmonary embolism, and chemotherapy-induced micronodules.
- **Diffuse infiltrates** are typically due to respiratory viruses (e.g., influenza, parainfluenza, adenovirus, and respiratory syncytial virus [RSV]), CMV, *Pneumocystis jirovecii* pneumonia (PCP), and *Legionella*. Noninfectious causes include adult respiratory distress syndrome, pulmonary edema, diffuse alveolar hemorrhage, and chronic GVHD.

DIAGNOSIS

- A chest radiograph or CT scan of the chest should be performed for patients with suspected pneumonia.
- Blood and sputum cultures, nasopharyngeal swab for viral immunofluorescence assay and culture, blood CMV quantitation, urine *Legionella* antigen, and serum galactomannan determination should be performed as indicated.
- Bronchoscopy with bronchoalveolar lavage (BAL) is often useful and should be considered especially for patients who fail standard therapy.
- Nodules may be biopsied with CT guidance in the absence of severe thrombocytopenia.

TREATMENT

- Empiric treatment should be targeted toward the most likely pathogens.
- Antibiotic choice is guided by the institutional bacterial susceptibility patterns and the patient's own microbiome.
- If bacterial pneumonia is suspected, a **third- or fourth-generation cephalosporin with or without vancomycin is typically started**. If *Legionella* is suspected, azithromycin or a quinolone may be added.
- If fungal pneumonia is suspected, a mold-active antifungal agent is typically started.
- Treatment for viruses, PCP, mycobacteria, or *Nocardia* is typically withheld until such infections are identified because of potential harm from polypharmacy.

Diarrhea

GENERAL PRINCIPLES

- Diarrhea commonly ensues after HSCT and has myriad causes (Table 14-2); it is associated with infection in fewer than 20% of cases.[2]
- In the **pre-engraftment period**, typical causes are mucosal injury from conditioning chemotherapy, *Clostridium difficile* enterocolitis, viral enteritis, and neutropenic enterocolitis (typhlitis).
- In the **postengraftment period**, usual causes are GVHD, CMV, adenovirus, norovirus, and *C. difficile* enterocolitis. Rarely, pathogenic bacteria (e.g., *Salmonella*, *Shigella*, *Yersinia*, and *Campylobacter*) and parasites (e.g., *Cryptosporidium* and *Giardia*) are encountered.

DIAGNOSIS

- A CT scan of the abdomen and pelvis should be performed for patients with moderate to severe diarrhea.
- Stool cultures, stool *C. difficile* toxin testing, and stool examination for ova and parasites should be performed as indicated.
- Transaminases and blood CMV quantitation should be carried out. However, CMV enteritis is a predominantly local disease and could present without detectable viremia.
- Persistent diarrhea in the postengraftment period should prompt consideration of an endoscopy as GVHD and infectious agents such as CMV exist with equal probability and may at times coexist.

TREATMENT

- Empiric treatment for *C. difficile* should be considered.
- If proven, neutropenic enterocolitis warrants broad-spectrum antibiotic therapy including anaerobic coverage.
- Treatment for other conditions such as CMV enterocolitis and GVHD are typically withheld until a definite diagnosis is made.

Herpes Simplex Virus

GENERAL PRINCIPLES

- The incidence of herpes simplex virus (HSV) disease has decreased with antiviral prophylaxis. Before routine administration of antiviral prophylaxis, up to 80% of HSCT recipients developed HSV reactivation.
- HSV disease usually occurs in HSCT recipients with chronic GVHD.
- **All HSV-seropositive HSCT recipients should receive acyclovir or valacyclovir during the pre-engraftment and early postengraftment period.**[3]
- Use of HSV prophylaxis is not indicated for HSV-seronegative recipients, even if the donor is HSV seropositive.
- Use of valganciclovir or ganciclovir for CMV prophylaxis protects against HSV reactivation as well.

DIAGNOSIS

- Patients generally present with oral ulcers; however, this can progress to severe mucositis and esophagitis.

- Disseminated disease is rare, with viral replication in the lungs, liver, gastrointestinal tract, and central nervous system (CNS).
- Genital HSV accounts for only a small percentage of HSV reactivation cases.
- Testing is similar to that in solid organ transplant (SOT) recipients and is discussed below.

TREATMENT

Treatment is similar to SOT recipients and is discussed in the following section.

Varicella Zoster Virus

GENERAL PRINCIPLES

- The incidence of varicella zoster virus (VZV) disease has decreased with antiviral prophylaxis. However, it remains common and occurs in up to 40% of HSCT recipients, usually starting after prophylactic antivirals have been discontinued.
- VZV disease usually occurs within the first 12 months postengraftment or in HSCT recipients with chronic GVHD.
- **All VZV-seropositive HSCT recipients should receive acyclovir or valacyclovir for at least 12 months after engraftment.**[3] Prophylactic antivirals should be continued in the presence of chronic GVHD.
- Use of valganciclovir or ganciclovir for CMV prophylaxis protects against VZV reactivation as well.
- VZV-seronegative HSCT recipients who are exposed to persons with active VZV disease should receive a course of acyclovir with or without human varicella zoster immunoglobulin (VariZIG) within the first 96 hours postexposure.

DIAGNOSIS

- VZV reactivation usually presents as a cutaneous infection, with involvement of single dermatome. Occasionally, multiple dermatomes are affected.
- Rarely, disseminated VZV infection, with involvement of the lungs, liver, gastrointestinal tract, and skin, and meningoencephalitis or myelitis can occur.
- Cutaneous lesions consistent with herpes zoster usually do not need confirmatory testing for a definitive diagnosis.
- Suspected cases of VZV dissemination or CNS disease should have blood and CSF sent for VZV detection using nucleic acid detection.

TREATMENT

Treatment is similar to SOT recipients and is discussed in the following section.

Cytomegalovirus

GENERAL PRINCIPLES

- The incidence of CMV disease among HSCT recipients has decreased with the advent of **preemptive treatment**[3] for asymptomatic CMV infection. Without prophylaxis, up to 35% of patients develop CMV disease.

- All allogeneic and autologous HSCT recipients who are CMV seropositive and at high risk should undergo screening for CMV viremia using a nucleic acid test or pp65 antigen on a weekly basis. **Two consecutive positive tests should prompt preemptive therapy.**
  - Ganciclovir is the preferred antiviral choice; alternatives are valganciclovir, foscarnet, and cidofovir. Letermovir has recently been approved for prophylaxis in seropositive allogeneic HSCT recipients.
  - A minimum of 2 weeks of treatment and a negative indicator test are required before the antiviral drug can be discontinued.
- **Risk factors** for CMV disease include the following:
  - In **allogeneic** HSCT recipients, CMV seropositivity in either the donor or the recipient, high-dose corticosteroid use, T-cell depletion, acute and chronic GVHD, and the use of mismatched or unrelated donors.
  - In **autologous** HSCT recipients, CD34+ selection, high-dose corticosteroid use, and the use of total body irradiation or fludarabine as part of the conditioning regimen.
- **CMV disease** usually occurs within the first 100 days postengraftment. However, widespread use of preemptive therapy has led to increased incidence of late-onset (>100 d postengraftment) CMV disease.
- CMV disease may coexist with other conditions, such as GVHD, coinfections with bacteria, *P. jirovecii*, and *Aspergillus.*

DIAGNOSIS

- HSCT recipients commonly develop pneumonitis.
- Patients may also develop esophagitis, gastritis, enterocolitis, and hepatitis.
- Rarely, meningoencephalitis and retinitis may ensue.
- Diagnosis depends on demonstrating viral replication in the presence of a clinical syndrome consistent with invasive CMV disease.
- Suspected cases of CMV pneumonia should have BAL specimens sent for **nucleic acid testing**. However, caution must be taken in interpreting the results, as CMV shedding into the respiratory tract is common and does not necessarily correlate with disease. A negative nucleic acid test, however, makes a diagnosis of CMV pneumonia highly unlikely.
- An assay to detect CMV in blood, using **nucleic acid testing or pp65 antigen**, should be performed as it is sensitive and specific. Higher viral loads by PCR are associated with tissue-invasive disease, with lower loads usually indicating asymptomatic infection. Pneumonitis, hepatitis, and disseminated disease generally have detectable viremia; gastrointestinal disease, however, is usually local and can have no detectable viremia. Levels can be followed to guide management and monitor treatment response, although standardization varies among institutions.
- Histopathologic evidence for CMV disease, such as characteristic "owls eye" nuclear inclusions, is useful in the diagnosis of invasive disease. Gastrointestinal disease usually requires a biopsy for proof of CMV disease.

TREATMENT

- Treatment with intravenous **ganciclovir** is first-line therapy. Valganciclovir is often substituted for mild to moderate CMV disease. Foscarnet and cidofovir are alternatives but typically reserved for resistant cases due to nephrotoxicity.
- Intravenous immunoglobulin (IVIG) or pooled CMV immunoglobulin is often added for the treatment of CMV disease, but there is no significant benefit compared with antiviral monotherapy.
- Failure to decrease viral replication after around 2 weeks should prompt resistance testing with UL97 and UL54 mutational analysis to determine appropriate treatment.

HUMAN HERPES VIRUS 6

- Human herpes virus (HHV) 6 is the cause of **roseola**, a febrile childhood rash which affects nearly all children by age 3. Like all herpesviruses, **it can establish latency**.
- HHV-6 reactivation is common among allogeneic HSCT recipients in the early post-transplant period. The clinical significance of HHV-6 viremia is unknown but has been associated with fever, rash, hepatitis, idiopathic pneumonia syndrome, bone marrow suppression, and delayed platelet and monocyte engraftment.
- Uncommonly, **acute limbic encephalitis** is associated with HHV-6 reactivation in the CNS. This usually occurs in the early postengraftment period; is more common with umbilical cord blood, use of anti-CD3 monoclonal antibodies, or HLA-mismatched grafts; and can lead to profound memory loss, seizures, mild CSF pleocytosis, and significant mesial temporal lobe abnormalities on MRI.
- Treatment with **ganciclovir and foscarnet** has been used with mixed success in case reports.

RESPIRATORY VIRUS INFECTIONS

- Respiratory virus infections occur in up to 20% of HSCT recipients; 30% to 40% of patients who initially present with upper respiratory tract infection develop lower respiratory tract disease. Risk factors for progression to lower respiratory tract disease include age greater than 65 years, use of myeloablative conditioning, severe neutropenia or lymphopenia, and an underlying diagnosis of leukemia.
- The etiology of respiratory virus infections should be determined by nasopharyngeal viral swab or BAL.
- **The most common viral etiologies of lower respiratory tract disease in HSCT recipients are influenza, parainfluenza, RSV, and adenovirus.**[4] Emerging viruses such as human metapneumovirus, coronavirus, enteroviruses, and rhinovirus are increasingly being recognized.
- Symptoms for viral respiratory infections are similar; dyspnea may indicate progression to lower tract disease or bacterial superinfection.
- HSCT recipients typically have prolonged shedding of virus and require extended isolation precautions.

Influenza

GENERAL PRINCIPLES

- **All HSCT candidates, recipients, household contacts, and health care workers should receive the annual inactivated influenza vaccine.** Among HSCT recipients, the vaccine should be administered 6 months posttransplantation, given an absent immune response in the early period.
- **Chemoprophylaxis** should be considered for unvaccinated HSCT candidates, recipients, household contacts, and health care workers who are exposed to influenza.
- Complications of influenza virus infection are common in HSCT recipients and include a high rate of progression to pneumonia, bacterial or fungal superinfection, and death. Risk factors for complications include absolute lymphopenia, steroids, and influenza infection early after transplantation.[4]

DIAGNOSIS

Diagnosis can be made by nucleic acid testing or direct fluorescent antibody (DFA) of nasopharyngeal swab or lower respiratory samples. The rapid antigen detection assays have lower sensitivity compared with molecular assays and hence false-negative results are common during peak influenza activity.

TREATMENT

- Treatment options include neuraminidase inhibitors **oseltamivir and zanamivir**. Only patients who cannot receive or tolerate these agents should receive **peramivir**.
- There is increasing resistance to M2 inhibitors amantadine and rimantadine.
- Antiviral choice depends on annual viral strain susceptibility and guidelines from the Centers for Disease Control and Prevention.
- Immunosuppressed hosts still benefit from treatment **even if begun after 48 hours of the onset** of symptoms.
- Some experts recommend prolonging therapy to 10 days if patients are still symptomatic after 5 days of treatment.

PARAINFLUENZA

- Parainfluenza virus occurs year-round and can range from asymptomatic infections to severe pneumonia and respiratory failure among HSCT recipients. Other manifestations include Guillain–Barré syndrome, acute disseminated encephalomyelitis, and parotitis.
- Coinfections with bacterial and fungal organisms are common; lower respiratory tract disease has a very poor prognosis.
- Diagnosis is typically made by nucleic acid testing, DFA or viral culture of nasopharyngeal swab or BAL fluid.
- Treatment options are limited; intravenous and oral **ribavirin** has been used with mixed results.

Respiratory Syncytial Virus

GENERAL PRINCIPLES

- RSV infections in HSCT recipients usually manifest as upper respiratory tract symptoms but can lead to severe lower respiratory tract infections.
- Lower tract infections are associated with high morbidity and mortality and are frequently associated with significant copathogens.
- **Risk factors** for severe disease include older age, myeloablative regimen, GVHD, pre-engraftment, lymphopenia, and preexistent obstructive airway disease.[4]

DIAGNOSIS

Diagnosis can be made by nucleic acid testing, DFA or viral culture of nasopharyngeal swab or BAL fluid.

TREATMENT

- Treatment options include aerosolized ribavirin, IVIG, and RSV monoclonal antibody palivizumab. No randomized controlled trials have been performed to define the best treatment option.
- **Aerosolized ribavirin** has been most frequently used; however, it needs to be administered in a negative pressure room because of its potential for teratogenicity. It is likely most useful in preventing progression of upper airway infection to lower tract disease.
- Intravenous or oral ribavirin has been proposed as an alternative; systemic ribavirin use has potential risk and unknown efficacy.
- Palivizumab is typically reserved for RSV treatment or prophylaxis in pediatric patients.

Adenovirus

GENERAL PRINCIPLES

- Adenovirus commonly causes upper or lower respiratory tract infection but can also cause conjunctivitis, hepatitis, enteritis, and hemorrhagic cystitis.
- Adenovirus reactivation in HSCT recipients is relatively common, with high mortality rates in fulminant hepatitis and disseminated disease.
- Risk factors for severe disease include T-cell-depleted grafts, HLA-mismatched transplants, GVHD, total body irradiation, and use of anti-T-cell agents including ATG and alemtuzumab.[4]

DIAGNOSIS

- Diagnosis is typically made by PCR testing with quantitative viral loads shown to predict clinical response and prognosis, with high titers correlating with increased risk of death.
- Detection of adenovirus at two or more sites is predictive of invasive disease in HSCT recipients.

TREATMENT

- Treatment options include cidofovir, or the newer lipid conjugated derivative brincidofovir (CMX001) and IVIG.
- **Cidofovir** has mixed results, and care must be taken to avoid irreversible nephrotoxicity.
- Decreasing immunosuppression, if possible, should be attempted.

Invasive Fungal Infections

- IFIs may be caused by endemic or opportunistic fungi with a wide variety of clinical presentations from nonspecific respiratory illness to fulminant pneumonia.[5]
- HSCT patients are more susceptible to ubiquitous opportunistic fungi due to immunosuppressive regimens.
- **The most common IFIs encountered in HSCT recipients are *Aspergillus* (43%), *Candida* (28%), other molds such as *Fusarium* and *Scedosporium* (16%), and zygomycetes (8%).**[5]
- Risk factors include antibiotic use, central line placement, neutropenia, GVHD, and prolonged corticosteroid use.
- Topical agents may reduce colonization of mouth and skin but do not prevent locally invasive or disseminated fungal infections.
- Patients at high risk for IFIs (i.e., patients with prolonged neutropenia and patients with GVHD necessitating corticosteroid use) should receive triazole prophylaxis, preferably posaconazole.[6]

Aspergillosis

GENERAL PRINCIPLES

- Invasive aspergillosis is the most common fungal infection in HSCT patients.
- Risk factors for invasive aspergillosis include HSCT recipients (highest risk), prolonged neutropenia, corticosteroid use, GVHD, CMV disease, and older age. Patients with chronic lung diseases such as chronic obstructive pulmonary disease and those on corticosteroids are at higher risk for chronic necrotizing aspergillosis and invasive pulmonary aspergillosis.

- In patients with prior invasive aspergillosis despite fluconazole prophylaxis, voriconazole may be used as secondary prophylaxis.
- The use of laminar airflow or high-efficiency particulate air filtration for patients who receive bone marrow transplants and other high-risk patients prevents invasive aspergillosis.

DIAGNOSIS

- *Aspergillus* infection mainly manifests as pulmonary diseases, from hypersensitivity to angioinvasion, causing four main syndromes: allergic bronchopulmonary aspergillosis, chronic necrotizing *Aspergillus* pneumonia, aspergilloma, and invasive pulmonary aspergillosis.
- In severely immunocompromised patients, *Aspergillus* can hematogenously disseminate and can lead to endophthalmitis, endocarditis, and abscesses in the heart, kidney, liver, spleen, soft tissue, brain, and bone.
- Diagnosis of infection can be accomplished by culture and galactomannan assay in serum or BAL fluid and is suggested by certain radiographic features.
- The **galactomannan assay** is specific and shows higher sensitivity in the detection of *Aspergillus* in HSCT patients than in SOT recipients.
  - Serum galactomannan sensitivity is 70% but can be lower in non-neutropenic patients and with concurrent use of antifungals.[7]
  - Galactomannan assay on BAL fluid has greater sensitivity. Confounding factors include timing of bronchoscopy with regard to infection and processing of BAL samples.
- Typical appearance of invasive aspergillosis on CT scan involves nodular lesions with a halo sign or cavity. However, neutrophil count, GVHD, and immunosuppression can affect the appearance on CT with tree-in-bud opacities and other lesions reported.

TREATMENT

- The drug of choice for the treatment of invasive aspergillosis is **voriconazole** because of higher tolerance and improved survival with its use when compared with amphotericin B.[7]
  - Serum levels must be monitored.
  - Side effects include visual disturbances, rash, and liver function test abnormalities.
- **Liposomal amphotericin B** is an alternative in patients unable to tolerate voriconazole, with improved outcomes with earlier initiation of treatment.
- **Isavuconazole** does not require drug level monitoring, has less drug interactions, and is noninferior to voriconazole in treating aspergillosis.
- **Posaconazole** can also be used for salvage when patients who cannot tolerate voriconazole as primary or salvage therapy. Absorption requires adequate caloric intake; serum levels must also be monitored. **Caspofungin** has also been reported to be an effective primary therapy and salvage therapy in HSCT recipients.
- Dual therapy with voriconazole plus caspofungin or liposomal amphotericin B plus caspofungin can be considered in patients with refractory or progressive disease. However, there is no evidence that combination therapy is more effective for treatment.

CANDIDIASIS

- Invasive candidiasis is usually caused by dissemination of endogenous *Candida* colonizing the gastrointestinal tract.
- Risk factors include neutropenia, severe mucositis, central venous catheters, broad-spectrum antibiotics, severe gastrointestinal GVHD, and prior colonization with *Candida*.

- An erythematous, maculopapular rash can sometimes be the first sign of disseminated infection.
- Hepatosplenic candidiasis often manifests with fever, abdominal complaints, transaminitis and typical radiologic findings with multiple microabscesses in the liver and spleen. This occurs during the phase of recovery from neutropenia.
- **Antifungal prophylaxis with triazole antifungals** has significantly decreased the morbidity and mortality from invasive *Candida*; current cumulative incidence during the first year after HSCT is < 5%.
  - However, an increased incidence of infection with **fluconazole-resistant *Candida***, including *Candida krusei* and some *Candida glabrata* strains, has been noted.
  - Autologous HSCT recipients are at lower risk for invasive candidiasis and generally do not require routine prophylaxis for *Candida*.
  - **Fluconazole** is the drug of choice for *Candida* prophylaxis and is usually initiated when starting conditioning regimens.[8] High-dose fluconazole treatment has not shown increased benefit over regular doses of 200 mg/d, but dosages less than 200 mg/d have variable efficacy and are not recommended.
  - Treatment is guided by site of infection, susceptibility pattern of *Candida* species, and immunosuppression. The **echinocandins** (i.e., caspofungin, micafungin, and anidulafungin) are first-line treatments for candidemia in HSCT recipients.[9] *C. glabrata* may be resistant to fluconazole and voriconazole, and *C. krusei* may also be relatively resistant to fluconazole but is susceptible to voriconazole. *Candida parapsilosis* may be less responsive to the echinocandins. Refractory cases, or cases with endocarditis or CNS disease, require treatment with amphotericin B with or without oral flucytosine.[9]
  - Duration of treatment depends on site of infection, resolution of infection, and state of immunosuppression.

Mucormycosis

GENERAL PRINCIPLES

- **Mucormycosis** refers to infections with fungi in the order of Mucorales, of which *Rhizopus* species are most common. The usual route of exposure is inhalation of spores.
- Mucormycosis is a fungal emergency, with an incidence of 0.1% to 2% of HSCT recipients and a high fatality rate (24%–49%).[10] Even if successfully treated, infection can result in serious disfigurement among survivors.
- **Types of infection** include pulmonary, rhinocerebral disease, cutaneous, gastrointestinal, and CNS.
  - Disseminated infections usually follow pulmonary or rhinocerebral disease.
  - **Pulmonary infection** usually occurs in diabetic patients or immunocompromised hosts, especially those with neutropenia. **This is the most common form of infection in HSCT recipients**, followed by disseminated disease. In HSCT recipients, pulmonary mucormycosis often occurs after resolution of neutropenia and after engraftment and is associated with corticosteroid therapy for GHVD.
  - Rhinocerebral disease usually occurs in diabetic patients; this is rare among HSCT patients.
  - Cutaneous involvement has been reported in HSCT recipients and those with hematologic malignancies. It can also be found at the site of central catheter placement.
  - CNS mucormycosis usually results from dissemination from pulmonary or rhinocerebral sources.

DIAGNOSIS

Clinical Presentation

- Clinical features vary depending on the type of infection.
- Symptoms of pulmonary infection include fever unresponsive to antibiotics, dyspnea, cough, and pleuritic chest pain. Angioinvasion and resultant tissue necrosis can lead to hemoptysis and may be fatal with major blood vessel involvement.
- Rhinocerebral mucormycosis may present with facial pain, black necrotic lesions, discharge from the nasal and palatal mucosa, fever, periorbital cellulitis, proptosis, and visual deficits.

Diagnostic Testing

- Establishing **diagnosis** can be difficult as clinical presentation may mimic other IFIs and *Mucorales* are environmental isolates and frequent contaminants/colonizers.
- **The gold standard for diagnosis requires a positive culture or histopathology from a sterile site** such as needle aspirate, tissue biopsy, or pleural fluid.[10] Culture is unreliable: tissue processing that includes grinding kills the organism; biopsy with histopathology is the most sensitive and specific test.
- Probable infection is indicated with positive culture from nonsterile site (for example, BAL fluid) in a patient with appropriate risk factors and clinical/CT evidence consistent with mucormycosis.
- Chest CT is the best test for determining the extent of pulmonary disease. Radiographic findings include cavitations, lobar consolidation, isolated masses, nodular disease, or wedge-shaped infarcts. More than 10 pulmonary nodules, pleural effusion, or concurrent invasive sinusitis can help distinguish *Mucorales* from *Aspergillus*.[10]

TREATMENT

- **Rapid diagnosis is crucial as delay in initiation of appropriate antifungal therapy is associated with increased mortality.**
- Tight diabetic control and rapid correction of underlying ketoacidosis, dose reduction or discontinuation of corticosteroids or other immunosuppressants, and consideration of G-CSF in neutropenic patients are important measures.
- **Surgical debridement** of infected and necrotic tissue is critical and should be performed for rhinocerebral disease and considered in other types of infection including pulmonary infection, if possible. Owing to the superficial nature of cutaneous disease, early diagnosis and surgical debridement with skin grafting yield favorable outcomes.
- The optimal duration of any antifungal for treating these infections has not been established, although treatment length is at least 3 to 6 weeks.
- High doses of **lipid formulations of amphotericin B** (liposomal amphotericin B or amphotericin B lipid complex at 5–7.5 mg/kg per day) are the drug of choice for treatment of *Mucorales* infections. They also have better lung penetration, lower side-effect profiles, with improved survival demonstrated as compared with amphotericin B deoxycholate.[10]
- Posaconazole has in vitro activity, but the suspension usually achieves serum concentrations typically below MIC_{90}. However, delayed release formulation of posaconazole more reliably achieves therapeutic levels and is an alternative for those who cannot tolerate amphotericin B or as salvage therapy. Recently, isavuconazole has also been approved and has the advantage of lower risk of prolonging QTc interval and obviates the need for drug-level monitoring.

Fusariosis

GENERAL PRINCIPLES

- *Fusarium* species are found commonly in the soil and on plants. Pathogenesis relies on three factors: colonization, tissue damage, and immunosuppression.
- Risk factors in HSCT patients include severity and duration of neutropenia (especially in the early pre-engraftment period), corticosteroid therapy (especially in the postengraftment period in the setting of chronic GVHD), colonization, tissue damage, or receipt of a graft from an HLA-mismatched or unrelated donor.

Diagnosis

- The clinical presentation includes refractory fever, skin lesions, sinopulmonary infections, and onychomycosis.
- Skin lesions include purpura, macules, target lesions, and multiple tender subcutaneous nodules, but the characteristic skin lesion in disseminated fusariosis is "ecthyma gangrenosum": red or gray macules with central ulceration or black eschar.
- Diagnosis can be made by biopsy of skin lesions during disseminated fusariosis.
- The clinical and radiographic features of invasive mucormycosis and fusariosis are similar and nonspecific and impossible to distinguish.
- In contrast to other types of invasive molds, *Fusarium* can frequently be recovered from blood cultures in the setting of disseminated disease probably as it can sporulate in vivo.[11]

TREATMENT

- Fusarium demonstrates inherent resistance to echinocandins and mediocre susceptibility to amphotericin B. **Voriconazole appears to be more effective than liposomal amphotericin B both in vitro and in vivo for primary therapy and salvage therapy in most species** and has a better side-effect profile.[12]
- Surgical resection of infected necrotic tissue is a significant component of therapy, along with prompt removal of central venous catheters and reversal of underlying immunosuppression.

Infectious Complications Associated With Solid Organ Transplantation

- Improved immunosuppressive regimens and surgical techniques have reduced the incidence of graft rejection and patient survival after organ transplantation. There has also been a parallel decline in infectious mortality with pretransplant screening, antimicrobial prophylaxis, and treatment of infections. However, infections continue to be among the leading causes of morbidity and mortality in solid organ transplant recipients along with vascular events and graft failure. Early and specific diagnosis of invasive infection along with rapid, aggressive treatment is essential. Etiology of infection includes complications related to surgery, health care–associated infections, opportunistic infections, reactivation of latent organisms, and donor-derived infections.
- Clinical diagnosis is complicated by lack of the usual signs and symptoms of inflammation or infection, resulting in advanced or disseminated infection at the time of clinical presentation.
  - Additionally, alterations in anatomy due to organ transplantation can impair diagnosis; noninfectious causes of fever including graft rejection, drug toxicities, and autoimmune reactions can mimic infectious processes.

○ Serologic testing is usually not useful in diagnosis due to delayed seroconversion in these immunosuppressed individuals. Fortunately, the recent availability of quantitative antigen or nucleic acid–based assays facilitates early diagnosis; however, invasive diagnostic procedures including tissue biopsies and advanced imaging procedures are often necessary for diagnosis.

• Once diagnosis is established, choice of antimicrobials is complicated by drug interactions with immunosuppressive medications.

• The risk of infection is mainly determined by two factors: the epidemiologic exposures and the net state of immunosuppression.

○ To assess **epidemiologic exposures**, a detailed history of potential pathogen encounters and risk factors for both the recipient and the donor, including contact with common community-acquired pathogens for their specific region, is necessary.

○ The **net state of immunosuppression** takes into account the type, dose, duration, and sequence of immunosuppressive therapies; underlying diseases or comorbid conditions; the presence of devitalized tissues or fluid collections in the transplanted organ; invasive devices (central venous catheters, urinary catheters, drains, etc.); neutropenia and hypogammaglobulinemia; metabolic problems (uremia and malnutrition); and infection with immunomodulating viruses such as CMV, Epstein–Barr virus (EBV), HHV-6, hepatitis B virus (HBV), and hepatitis C virus (HCV).

• Additionally, some asymptomatic infections can be unveiled or their course accelerated with the use of immunosuppressive medications, including West Nile virus, HSV, HCV, and lymphocytic choriomeningitis virus.

• The risk and etiologies of infection posttransplantation can be divided into three time periods: **early posttransplantation** (first month), **intermediate period** (1–6 mo), and **late period** (greater than 6 mo) (see Table 14-3). This time line may vary between transplant centers using different immunosuppressive regimens, between different types of transplantation, and with different patient populations but can serve as a general guide.

Herpes Simplex Virus

GENERAL PRINCIPLES

• Disease in SOT recipients differs in that they **shed virus more frequently, have more frequent and severe manifestations of disease, may present atypically**, delaying diagnosis with slower response to therapy.

• Disease usually results from **reactivation of the virus**, although disease has been documented from allograft or primary infection. It typically occurs within the first month posttransplant in the absence of prophylaxis.

• Risk factors include HSV-seropositive recipients with an incidence around 35% to 68% without prophylaxis; therefore, the serostatus of all SOT recipients should be checked before transplant.[13]

• Prevention by use of **acyclovir or valacyclovir** should be considered for all seropositive organ recipients not receiving CMV prophylaxis.

○ Prophylaxis should be continued at least 1 month. If they continue to experience frequent symptomatic reactivation, suppressive therapy should be continued.

○ **Suppressive therapy** can be given safely for several years and is associated with less acyclovir resistance than intermittent therapy.

Early Posttransplant Period (<1 mo)	Intermediate Period (1–6 mo)	Late Posttransplant Period (>6 mo)
Caused by donor- or recipient-derived infections; infectious complications of transplant surgery and hospitalization	Caused by activation of latent infections. Highest risk of opportunistic infections	Usually caused by community-acquired infections as decreased immunosuppression; rare infections from transplanted organ
Antimicrobial-resistant infections acquired during hospitalization, including gram-negative enteric bacilli, MRSA, VRE, non-*albicans* *Candida*, resistant *Aspergillus*	**With prophylaxis (i.e., PCP, CMV, HSV, HCV):** Polyomavirus infections (BK), nephropathy	**Reduced immunosuppression:** CMV (colitis, retinitis)
Aspiration	Infectious diarrhea: *C. difficile* colitis; *Cryptosporidium*, *Microsporidia*, CMV, rotavirus	Hepatitis (HBV, HCV)
Catheter infection	HCV infection	HSV encephalitis
Wound infection	Respiratory viruses including adenovirus, influenza, RSV, parainfluenza	Community-acquired (West Nile)
Anastomotic leaks and ischemia	*Cryptococcus neoformans*	BK virus (PML)
Clostridium difficile colitis	Latent infection with protozoal diseases, i.e., toxoplasmosis, *Leishmania*, Chagas disease	Skin cancer
	Mycobacterium tuberculosis and nontubercular mycobacteria	EBV-associated lymphoma, PTLD
		Community-acquired pneumonia: respiratory viruses, pneumococcus, Legionella, etc.
		Urinary tract infection
		Aspergillus, atypical molds, *Mucor*, *Nocardia*, *Rhodococcus*
Donor-derived infections: bacterial and fungal disease	**Without prophylaxis:** PCP	**Higher immunosuppression due to inadequate graft function:**
Endemic infections (e.g., histoplasmosis, tuberculosis) (uncommon)	Herpesviruses (EBV, HSV, VZV, CMV)	Opportunistic infections: PCP, *Cryptococcus*, nocardiosis, etc.
Graft-associated infections including HSV, LCMV, rhabdovirus, West Nile virus, HIV, *Trypanosoma cruzi*, toxoplasmosis	HBV infection	Severe community-acquired infections, especially influenza, *Listeria*
	Endemic fungal infections including histoplasmosis, coccidioidomycosis, blastomycosis	
Recipient-derived infections (colonization): Aspergillus, *Pseudomonas*, *Burkholderia*	*Listeria, Nocardia, Toxoplasma, Strongyloides, Leishmania, T. cruzi*	

CMV, cytomegalovirus; EBV, Epstein–Barr virus; HBV, hepatitis B virus; HCV, hepatitis C virus; HSV, herpes simplex virus; LCMV, lymphocytic choriomeningitis virus; MRSA, methicillin-resistant *Staphylococcus aureus*; PCP, *Pneumocystis jirovecii* pneumonia; PML, progressive multifocal leukoencephalopathy; PTLD, posttransplantation lymphoproliferative disorder; RSV, respiratory syncytial virus; VRE, vancomycin-resistant *Enterococcus*; VZV, varicella zoster virus.

DIAGNOSIS

- The clinical presentation is usually **vesicles or ulcerative disease in the orolabial, genital, or perianal region.**
- Visceral and disseminated disease (esophagitis, hepatitis, and pneumonitis) can also occur. Usual presentation with dissemination is fever, leukopenia, and hepatitis. Pneumonitis is more common in lung–heart transplants. Keratitis and other ocular complications may occur.
- **Diagnosis is made by PCR** (more sensitive than tissue culture) which is the test of choice, DFA testing of lesions and other samples, and culture.

TREATMENT

- Treatment regimen depends on the severity and location of disease and should be continued until complete resolution of all lesions.
  - Limited mucocutaneous disease can be treated with oral **acyclovir, valacyclovir, or ganciclovir.**
  - **IV acyclovir** should be rapidly initiated with disseminated or visceral disease or extensive cutaneous or mucosal disease.[13]
  - Consideration should be given to decreasing immunosuppressive regimen.
- **With patients not responding to appropriate therapy with acyclovir, resistance should be considered.** Workup in these cases should include laboratory confirmation of HSV with acyclovir resistance testing. If resistance is found, foscarnet or cidofovir can be used.

Cytomegalovirus

GENERAL PRINCIPLES

- CMV seroprevalence ranges from 30% to 97% in the general population and is one of the main causes of morbidity in SOT patients.[14] In the absence of prophylaxis, CMV occurs in the first 3 months after transplant.
- **CMV tends to invade the allograft and has been implicated in acute and chronic graft injury and increased risk of graft rejection.**
- The greatest risk factor for CMV disease is organ transplantation from seropositive donors to seronegative recipients (D+R−), followed by seropositive recipients (R+). SOT from seronegative donor to seronegative recipient (D−R−) is lowest risk and does not need prophylaxis as long as recipients receive CMV-negative blood or leukodepleted blood products to prevent primary CMV infection. Other risk factors include receipt of antilymphocyte antibodies, especially during antirejection therapy, and lung, small intestine, and pancreas transplant recipients.
- Preventive strategies include either prophylaxis or preemptive therapy. There currently is no consensus on the best method with considerable variation in practice across centers.
  - **Prophylaxis** involves giving **valganciclovir, oral ganciclovir, or IV ganciclovir** for all at-risk patients (D+R− and R+) beginning within 10 days posttransplant and continuing usually for 3 to 6 months (some centers use 12 mo or longer durations for D+R− lung and heart–lung recipients). In R+ patients, regimen can be given for 3 months (6–12 mo for lung and lung–heart recipients). Benefits include preventing reactivation of other herpesviruses and **decreased graft loss and improved survival.**[14] Unfortunately, late-onset CMV disease may occur once off prophylaxis and is associated with higher mortality. For heart or lung transplant recipients, CMV immunoglobulin can be considered as adjunct therapy. Prophylaxis should also be given to patients receiving antilymphocyte therapies or high-dose steroids.

- **Preemptive therapy** involves weekly monitoring of CMV replication in higher risk patients by PCR or pp65 antigen, with valganciclovir or IV ganciclovir initiated in those with signs of early CMV replication above established threshold for that assay. Benefits for preemptive therapy include decreased drug costs and toxicity; however, this requires close monitoring.

DIAGNOSIS

- Most common type of CMV disease is a mononucleosis syndrome of fever, malaise, leukopenia, and thrombocytopenia. Tissue-invasive disease manifests as hepatitis, pneumonitis with nonproductive cough, retinitis, colitis, adrenalitis with adrenal insufficiency, or meningoencephalitis.
- Diagnostic testing is similar to that in HSCT recipients.

TREATMENT

Treatment is similar to that in HSCT recipients.

Epstein–Barr Virus and Posttransplantation Lymphoproliferative Disorder

GENERAL PRINCIPLES

- In SOT recipients, **EBV is transmitted from a seropositive donor graft, when non-leukoreduced blood products are used or less commonly, exposure to body fluids like saliva**. Therefore, EBV serostatus should be determined before transplantation to stratify risk of EBV-related diseases.[15]
- **EBV is associated with most posttransplantation lymphoproliferative disorder (PTLD) cases**, and the incidence of PTLD is increasing among organ transplant recipients.
  - The highest rate of PTLD in SOT occurs in the first year posttransplantation. Most cases are of recipient origin (primary infection after SOT) except for very early PTLD limited to allograft.
  - EBV genome is found in the majority of B-cell PTLD diagnosed within the first year after SOT, but a quarter to one-third of late PTLD cases are EBV B-cell negative. EBV-negative PTLD is more likely to occur more than 1 year after SOT.
  - **Risk factors** for early PTLD disease include primary EBV infection, young age, CMV mismatch or CMV disease, seronegative recipients (immune naive) with seropositive donor organs, and receipt of polyclonal antilymphocyte antibodies. Risk factors for late disease include longer duration of immunosuppression and older recipient age.
  - Type of organ transplanted changes the risk stratification for both early and late PTLD, with small intestinal transplant recipients at greatest risk (up to 32%) and renal transplant patients at low risk (1%–2%).[15]
- Other than limiting immunosuppression where possible, **there is no accepted prophylaxis for PTLD**.

DIAGNOSIS

Clinical Presentation

PTLD may resemble a mononucleosis syndrome with fever, tonsillar and peripheral node involvement, or a diffuse polymorphous B-cell infiltration in visceral organs, preceded by a mononucleosis-like episode. The third type of presentation is with extra-nodal B-cell lymphomas containing EBV genome.

Diagnostic Testing

- Diagnosis of PTLD requires tissue examination for EBV-specific nucleic acids by **RNA hybridization as well as immunostaining for EBV-specific latent antigens**.
- The role of EBV viral load remains uncertain because of poor positive predictive value.
- In lung and heart–lung transplant recipients, determination of EBV load in BAL fluid may be a good predictor of PTLD in the presence of consistent clinical findings.[15]
- Total body CT scan and, of late, positron emission tomography can be considered for initial assessment of PTLD.

TREATMENT

- **Treatment usually starts with reductions in immunosuppression, which can result in regression of PTLD in 45% of patients.**[15]
- Surgical resection and local radiation therapy have been used as adjunct treatments.
- Antiviral therapy (ganciclovir/valganciclovir) is not efficacious: although these agents offer a theoretical benefit, they do not affect the proliferation of EBV-immortalized cells.
- Increasing evidence supports the use of **rituximab with or without chemotherapy**, the humanized chimeric monoclonal antibody against CD20, to treat refractory PTLD that is CD20 marker positive.[15]
- In patients with high viral load on diagnosis, response to therapy can be determined by following decline and clearance of EBV. With the exception of those on rituximab, this usually corresponds to clinical and histologic regression.

Varicella Zoster Virus

GENERAL PRINCIPLES

- Varicella is rare in SOT recipients but can be devastating, with severe skin and visceral disease and disseminated intravascular coagulation. Zoster is frequent in SOT patients with an incidence of around 10% in the first 4 years posttransplant.[11]
- All patients considered for SOT should undergo serologic testing to document prior exposure to VZV. Short-term prevention can be accomplished with oral acyclovir or other regimen for CMV or HSV prophylaxis. Insufficient data exist to recommend long-term suppression.
- **Before transplantation, VZV-naive patients should be vaccinated with the varicella virus vaccine** (if no other contraindications exist) at least 2 to 4 weeks before transplant and 4 to 6 weeks in end-stage organ disease due to decreased seroconversion rates. Zoster vaccine can be considered pretransplant if the patient meets criteria for this vaccine but is contraindicated posttransplant.
- **Postexposure prophylaxis** should be given to naive SOT recipients with significant exposure to an infected individual (i.e., household contact, significant face-to-face contact, or roommate in the hospital).[11]
  - VariZIG may be of benefit but must be given within 96 hours of exposure. It does not prevent disease but decreases severity.
  - Antiviral therapy as postexposure prophylaxis has not been evaluated in SOT patients but is an alternative when VariZIG is not available and comprises a 7- to 10-day course of valacyclovir or acyclovir.

DIAGNOSIS

- Clinical presentation of varicella and zoster is similar to that in other patients but tends to be more severe. Dissemination of zoster occurs uncommonly. Postherpetic neuralgia may be more common in SOT recipients.

- **Diagnosis can be made clinically in typical cases or by PCR** (the most sensitive test) or direct fluorescent assay in atypical cases or suspected disseminated or visceral disease.

TREATMENT

- **Treatment with IV acyclovir should be initiated early in SOT patients with primary varicella, as they are at risk for severe disease.**[15] Reduction of immunosuppression should be considered, with steroids continued or increased for stress response. IVIG or VZIG has not shown any significant benefit.
- Localized dermatomal zoster can be treated with oral valacyclovir or famciclovir on an outpatient basis with close monitoring. However, VZV reactivation in the trigeminal ganglion (herpes zoster ophthalmicus) or in the geniculate ganglion (Ramsay Hunt syndrome) requires IV acyclovir as it can lead to blindness, facial palsy, or hearing loss.
- Disseminated zoster should be treated with IV acyclovir. In cases of acyclovir resistance, foscarnet or cidofovir can be used.

Polyomavirus Infections

GENERAL PRINCIPLES

- Polyomavirus infections can be detected in almost 60% of renal transplant recipients and are **a significant cause for graft failure**. Infectious nephropathy can occur in 1% to 10% of cases.[16]
- JC virus and SV40 can cause nephropathy in this population; however, **the usual cause is BK virus**.
- BK virus infection has been associated with two **major complications in transplant recipients**: nephropathy, usually in renal transplant patients, with a rate of 1% to 10%; and hemorrhagic cystitis, usually affecting allogeneic HSCT patients at rates of 5% to 15%.[16]
  - It is less commonly associated with pneumonitis, retinitis, and encephalitis.
  - In renal allograft recipients, it can also cause hemorrhagic cystitis, asymptomatic viruria, interstitial nephritis, and ureteric obstruction.
- Primary BK virus infection is usually asymptomatic and occurs in the first decade of life. Latent infection is then usually established in the genitourinary tract.
- Asymptomatic BK viruria occurs in immunocompetent hosts intermittently at a low rate but at high levels in immunocompromised individuals, particularly after SOT or HSCT.
- One-third of renal transplant patients with high-level BK viruria progress to viremia and nephropathy.[16]
- The virus directly causes loss of renal tubular epithelial cells (decoy cells in urine cytology), and inflammation elicited by necrosis and denudation of tubular basement membrane leads to infiltration by lymphocytes, tubular atrophy, and fibrosis.
- Graft loss after nephropathy occurs in <10%.
- To prevent nephropathy, kidney transplant recipients should be screened at least every 3 months in the first 2 years and then annually for the next 3 years for BK virus replication (either by viruria/viremia or decoy cells in urine cytology) to identify at-risk individuals before significant allograft damage.

DIAGNOSIS

- The first clinical sign of BK-associated nephropathy is frequently a gradual increase in serum creatinine, which indicates extensive tubular damage and inflammation.
- Definitive diagnosis is made by histologic examination of tissue and identification of BK virus–associated cytopathic changes. A minimum of two biopsies must be taken because of the focal nature of the destruction.

TREATMENT

- Treatment of BK nephropathy in renal transplant patients without signs of acute graft rejection is to **reduce immunosuppression**.[16] The primary goal is to control BK virus replication and preserve renal allograft function, which can be monitored by serum creatinine, BK viral load, and allograft histology.
- BK virus–specific immune recovery generally takes 1 to 2 months. In patients with sustained high-level plasma BK virus load despite reduced immunosuppression, antiviral therapy with cidofovir can be considered, which improves graft survival despite no change in rate of BK virus clearance, but has significant toxicities.[16] Leflunomide, IVIG, and fluoroquinolones have also been used without consistent benefit.

Hepatitis C Virus

GENERAL PRINCIPLES

- Hepatitis C is discussed in Chapter 6. This is a rapidly evolving field with several new drugs recently available. For SOT, certain key aspects should be noted.
- Ideally, patients with chronic hepatitis C and advanced liver disease should complete treatment before liver transplant with regimens discussed in Chapter 6. However, liver transplant candidates with decompensated liver disease may be better served by liver transplant rather than direct-acting antivirals (DAAs) for two reasons: they may receive a liver from HCV+ donor which will require treatment and their morbidity is from decompensated liver disease which is not reversed by DAAs. Treatment with DAAs should be offered after transplant as it improves graft and patient survival.[17]
- In HCV-infected individuals, HCV infection of allograft occurs universally in those with viremia at the time of liver transplantation.

TREATMENT

- After liver transplant, combinations of glecaprevir and pibrentasvir or ledipasvir and sofosbuvir for 12 weeks are approved if allograft is noncirrhotic. If allograft is cirrhotic, only the latter combination is approved, and ribavirin is added if cirrhosis is decompensated.
- Glecaprevir and pibrentasvir (all HCV genotypes) or ledipasvir and sofosbuvir (only genotypes 1 and 4) for 12 weeks are regimens that can also be used in kidney transplant patients with or without compensated cirrhosis.[17]
- For individual cases that may need alternative regimens, consultation with specialists should be sought.
- Close monitoring of tacrolimus levels is required due to drug interactions with various DAAs.

Pneumocystis Pneumonia

GENERAL PRINCIPLES

- *Pneumocystis* pneumonia caused by *P. jirovecii* has been increasingly recognized as an opportunistic infection among non–HIV immunosuppressed patients.
- Similar to HIV positive patients, it usually manifests as dyspnea, hypoxemia, cough, fever, and bilateral infiltrates in the majority of infected patients. However, the clinical presentation in non-HIV patients is characterized by a more fulminant course, shorter duration of symptoms, and a higher mortality rate.[18]

DIAGNOSIS

The parasite burden of infection in non-HIV patients is lower which has important implications for diagnostic strategies. DFA performed on lung tissue biopsy has the highest yield (sensitivity >95%) compared to BAL (sensitivity 80%–95%) or induced sputum (sensitivity 30%–55%).

TREATMENT

- Trimethoprim-sulfamethoxazole, administered orally or intravenously, is the first-line agent for the treatment of any form or severity of PCP. Doses and alternative agents are listed in Chapter 13.
- There are no randomized controlled trials in non-HIV patients with PCP that clearly demonstrate that adjunctive corticosteroids in moderate-to-severe disease accelerate symptomatic and physiologic improvement and prolong survival. Small retrospective studies have shown no significant difference in mortality, respiratory failure, or pulmonary coinfection with the use of adjunctive corticosteroids.[19]
- Although widely prescribed, there are no data on secondary prophylaxis in this population.

Nocardiosis

GENERAL PRINCIPLES

- *Nocardia* species are ubiquitous saprophytic gram-positive bacteria in the "aerobic actinomycetes" group, causing infections in 0.7% to 3.5% of SOT recipients, mostly heart, kidney, and liver transplant recipients. The most common species causing infection in SOT recipients are *N. nova, N. brasiliensis, N. farcinica and N. cyriacigeorgica.*[20]
- High-dose steroids, CMV infection in the preceding 6 months, and ATG are risk factors for nocardiosis. In addition, high calcineurin inhibitor levels, rituximab, hypogammaglobulinemia, tumor necrosis factor (TNF) antagonists, and alemtuzumab are implicated.

DIAGNOSIS

- Nocardiosis usually presents as an indolent focal or nodular pneumonia that may cavitate. Local spread to contiguous structures and the chest wall has been noted.
- Skin and subcutaneous nodules may occur as primary infection from direct inoculation or from hematogenous spread. Other cutaneous forms of nocardiosis include lymphocutaneous disease (sporotrichoid lesions) and mycetoma. Disseminated nocardiosis can lead to pyomyositis, bone abscess, or infection of any number of other sites.
- Brain abscess is a dreaded and common complication. It should be ruled out even in patients without neurologic symptoms.
- Diagnosis depends on biopsy and culture of the affected site.

TREATMENT

- Antibiotic therapy depends on site and severity of disease, drug interactions, and the species of *Nocardia* and should be guided by susceptibility testing.
- Primary antimicrobials recommended include trimethoprim-sulfamethoxazole, linezolid, imipenem, amikacin, amoxicillin-clavulanate, and minocycline. Combination therapy is recommended for immunocompromised patients.
- Surgical therapy may be required to drain abscesses, especially for cerebral abscesses not responding to medical therapy.
- Duration of therapy ranges from 8 weeks to 12 months (for brain abscess).[20]

Invasive Fungal Infections

- Risk factors for invasive aspergillosis include retransplantation, requirement for renal replacement therapy in immediate posttransplant period, repeat operation (liver and heart), *Aspergillus* colonization pre- or posttransplant within a year, induction with alemtuzumab or thymoglobulin. Other factors specific to lung transplant include single lung transplant, rejection with augmented immunosuppression, hypogammaglobulinemia, early airway ischemia. For heart transplants, prior invasive aspergillosis and CMV disease have also been noted as risk factors.[21] For these high-risk patients, prophylaxis with echinocandin or intravenous liposomal amphotericin B (preferred in liver transplant recipients), inhaled amphotericin B (preferred in lung transplant recipients) and azoles (in heart transplant recipients) for variable durations from few weeks to months can be given. Therapy of invasive aspergillosis is similar to in patients with HSCT.
- SOT, especially liver and lung transplantation, is a risk factor for cryptococcosis. Clinical presentation is often less typical (skin and soft tissue infections), with delayed diagnosis and worse prognosis compared with HIV-infected patients.[22] Diagnosis and initial treatment is similar to that of cryptococcal meningitis (see Chapter 13). Maintenance treatment is often prolonged to 6 to 12 months due to continued immunosuppression.
- SOT is a risk factor for endemic mycoses, which are more common in recipients from endemic areas, and can have more severe presentations. Donor infections have been reported in all endemic mycoses except blastomycosis.[23] Diagnosis and management are similar to immunocompetent patients (Chapter 15). For coccidioidomycosis, lifelong fluconazole prophylaxis is recommended for all transplant recipients after treatment of active infection. Prophylaxis is also indicated for 12 months for patients undergoing SOT with previous coccidioidomycosis. Other endemic mycoses do not require similar measures but are treated for prolonged duration (usually 6–12 mo, but could be longer in certain cases).
- Drug interactions with azoles are an important consideration in transplant recipients with IFIs.

Candidiasis

GENERAL PRINCIPLES

- **Candida infections are the most common IFI in SOT patients**, accounting for over half of cases, and overall rates of invasive candidiasis have increased slightly over time.[24]
- Invasive candidiasis usually occurs within the first 3 months posttransplant, earlier than other invasive mycoses.
- **In liver transplant patients,** based on prospective data and meta-analyses, prophylaxis should be given for 4 weeks to those with at least two of the following risk factors: retransplantation, prolonged or repeat surgery, renal failure, high transfusion requirement (>40 units of blood products), choledocojejunostomy, and *Candida* colonization preoperatively.[24] **Fluconazole** is the treatment of choice, unless at risk for *Aspergillus*, in which case an antifungal with activity against both agents should be used. Of note, fluconazole prophylaxis has also been shown to increase the rate of non-*albicans Candida* infections.
- Among pancreatic transplant recipients, prophylactic fluconazole is used if recipients had enteric drainage, vascular thrombosis, or postperfusion pancreatitis.
- Although clinical data are lacking in small bowel transplant patients, because of the high rates (up to 28%) of *Candida* infection, antifungal prophylaxis is routinely used with either fluconazole or, if non-*albicans Candida* is suspected, lipid formulations of amphotericin B.[24] Prophylaxis is recommended for at least 4 weeks or until the anastomosis has completely healed.

- For lung transplant recipients, agents with activity against Aspergillus are used; duration varies according to risk factors and transplant center.
- Kidney and heart transplant recipients are low-risk and do not require prophylaxis.

DIAGNOSIS

- Diagnosis is made by recovery of *Candida* from a sterile body site/fluid.
- In invasive candidiasis, cultures are sensitive for isolation of *Candida* only about 50% of the time.[9]
- *Candida* isolated from the respiratory tract is rarely indicative of invasive infection and does not require treatment unless it is in a lung transplant patient and anastomotic tracheobronchitis is a concern.[24] Diagnosis of *Candida* tracheobronchitis is based on visual inspection and histologic confirmation.
- The $(1,3)$-β-D-glycan assay has a sensitivity of 75% to 80% and a specificity of 80%.[9]

TREATMENT

Treatment recommendations are similar to those in HSCT recipients.

Parasitic Infections

- Parasitic infections remain the most under-recognized of all infections in organ transplantation, with only limited studies and most treatment recommendations based on expert opinion alone.
- Parasitic disease can occur as a result of reactivation of latent infection in the recipient, new infection, or transmission from the organ donor.
- Coinfection is a common feature. CMV has been associated with increased risk of invasive parasitic disease, but disseminated bacterial infections are also common coinfections.
- The incidence of parasitic infection is expected to increase, in part because of the decreased use of cyclosporine-based immunosuppressive regimens in favor of other regimens that lack the antiparasitic effect of cyclosporine.[25]
- Toxoplasmosis has been discussed in Chapter 13 and 17 and management is similar to that in HIV-infected hosts.

Strongyloides

GENERAL PRINCIPLES

- Epidemiology, pathophysiology, clinical presentation, diagnosis, and treatment of strongyloidiasis are discussed in Chapter 18.
- Strongyloidiasis has been described in transplant recipients with activation of latent infection and from donor-derived infection.
- Risk factors for **hyperinfection syndrome and disseminated disease** include severe immunosuppression and corticosteroid use and are most likely to occur in the initial months posttransplant with the highest level of immunosuppression. Cyclosporine-sparing therapies, including the T-cell depletion regimens, have also been implicated.
- Mortality for hyperinfection syndrome is almost 50%, and around 70% in disseminated disease.[25]
- Organ donors and high-risk organ recipients from endemic areas with appropriate exposure history should be screened with serology.

DIAGNOSIS

- Clinical syndromes include acute or chronic infection, hyperinfection syndrome, and disseminated disease.
- Acute or chronic infection includes pulmonary involvement, skin rash, bacterial sepsis or bacterial meningitis from intestinal flora exposed by larval damage; or acute and severe abdominal disease with bloody diarrhea, ileus, intestinal obstruction, or hemorrhage.
- Definitive diagnosis is made by identifying larvae in clinical specimens, but ELISA and gelatin particle indirect agglutination assays are also highly sensitive and specific.
- Eosinophilia can be found during acute infection but may not be present with chronic or severe disease.

TREATMENT

- The drug of choice is **ivermectin**, with length of treatment dependent on severity.[25]
- Albendazole can be used as an alternative treatment option.

Infectious Complications Associated With Immunomodulating Biologic Agents

GENERAL PRINCIPLES

- Many novel biologics have the ability to modulate the immune system. While these agents carry fewer infectious risks than traditional nontargeted immunosuppression with corticosteroids or azathioprine, **susceptibility to infection remains elevated**, and clinicians must continue to be vigilant. Broadly, the commonly used biologic agents can be classified into two major categories.
  - **Antilymphocyte therapies,** which include the following:
    - T-lymphocyte-depleting agents, ATGs, and alemtuzumab
    - Nondepleting costimulatory blockade therapies such as the interleukin (IL)-2 receptor antagonists basiliximab and daclizumab and the cytotoxic T-lymphocyte antigen (CTLA)-4 antagonists belatacept and abatacept
    - B-cell-depleting agents such as rituximab
  - **TNF-α inhibitors** that treat chronic inflammatory conditions such as rheumatoid arthritis, Crohn disease, sarcoidosis, psoriasis, and ankylosing spondylitis. These include monoclonal antibodies such as infliximab, adalimumab, and certolizumab pegol and the soluble TNF-α receptor etanercept. Further details are discussed in the following section (see Table 14-4).[26-28]
- The profound and long-standing immunosuppression associated with ATG and alemtuzumab necessitates anti-infective prophylaxis. Trimethoprim–sulfamethoxazole, dapsone, or atovaquone should be given for *Pneumocystis* prophylaxis. Seropositivity to herpesviruses should be determined, and relevant antiviral preventive measures should be instituted.[26] Antifungal prophylaxis is controversial as universal azole administration can breed resistance; definitive studies are needed.
- Clinical data suggest that infectious complications associated with interleukin (IL)-2 receptor antagonists basiliximab and daclizumab are reduced compared with other induction therapies.
- **Hepatitis B screening** should be performed before starting **rituximab**, and either periodic monitoring for reactivation or administration of antiviral agents such as tenofovir, entecavir, or lamivudine should be performed for infected patients.

- **Screening for latent TB infection** must be carried out among **prospective anti-TNF-α recipients**, and treatment should be instituted if warranted. Concurrent TNF-α blockade does not interfere with treatment of latent TB.
- Patients who develop TB while on anti-TNF-α therapy should have TNF blocker therapy stopped until response to anti-infectives is observed. Stopping anti-TNF-α therapy, however, can lead to a paradoxical reaction wherein patients develop worsening inflammation, as a result of immune reconstitution. This usually occurs with disseminated or extrapulmonary disease and resolves with reinstitution of the TNF blockade.

TABLE 14-4	INFECTIONS IN RECIPIENTS OF BIOLOGIC AGENTS		
Drug	**Mechanism of Immunomodulation**	**Indications**	**Infection Risk, Comments**
T-Lymphocyte-Depleting Agents[26,27]			
Antithymocyte globulin	Rabbit/horse polyclonal antibodies to human thymocytes or T cells Induce T- and B-cell depletion and interfere with dendritic cells and NK cell function. Effects persist for > 1 y.	Treatment or prevention of graft rejection or GVHD	Bacteria: urinary tract infections, pneumonia, bloodstream infections, surgical site infections, mycobacterial infections Viruses: CMV, EBV (including PTLD), BK Fungi: *Pneumocystis*, *Candida*, *Aspergillus*, other molds, *Cryptococcus*, and endemic mycoses
Alemtuzumab	Humanized monoclonal antibody directed against CD52, a membrane glycoprotein of T and B cells, monocytes and macrophages, and NK cells. Effects persist for at least 9 mo.	Treatment or prevention of graft rejection; certain lymphomas	Bacteria: bloodstream infections, pneumonia, meningitis, mycobacterial infections Viruses: HSV, VZV, and CMV reactivation, respiratory viral infections (e.g., influenza, parainfluenza, RSV, and adenovirus) can progress from upper tract to lower tract disease; PML, HHV-6, BK, parvovirus Fungi: *Pneumocystis*, *Candida*, *Aspergillus*, other molds, *Cryptococcus*, and endemic mycoses Parasites: *Toxoplasma* *(Continued)*

TABLE 14-4	INFECTIONS IN RECIPIENTS OF BIOLOGIC AGENTS (CONTINUED)		
Drug	**Mechanism of Immunomodulation**	**Indications**	**Infection Risk, Comments**
Muromonab	Murine monoclonal antibody to CD3 on mature T cells, removing them from the circulation	Solid organ transplant rejection	Bacteria: including *Listeria*, *Nocardia*, non-TB mycobacteria Fungi: *Candida*, molds, dermatophytes *Pneumocystis* Viruses: All herpesviruses, adenovirus. RSV, parainfluenza virus, enterovirus
Interleukin-2 Receptor Antagonists[26,27]			
Basiliximab	Chimeric human-murine monoclonal antibody against CD25, part of the IL-2 receptor (expressed on the surface of progenitor T and B cells and activated mature T and B cells). Effects last 4–6 wk after induction; resting lymphocytes not affected.	Induction and maintenance therapy for prevention of graft rejection (higher risk of infection with HSCT over SOT)	Bacterial, nocardiosis CMV, HSV, *Candida*, *Aspergillus*, other molds
Daclizumab	Humanized monoclonal antibody against IL-2 receptor Effects last 3 mo after induction; resting lymphocytes not affected.	Induction and maintenance therapy for prevention of graft rejection (higher risk of infection with HSCT over SOT)	Bacteria: including legionellosis, nocardiosis, mycobacterial Viruses: CMV, HSV, RSV, influenza, BK Fungi: *Candida*, *Aspergillus*, other molds

TABLE 14-4	INFECTIONS IN RECIPIENTS OF BIOLOGIC AGENTS (CONTINUED)		
Drug	Mechanism of Immunomodulation	Indications	Infection Risk, Comments
Cytotoxic T-Lymphocyte Antigen-4 Antagonists[26]			
Abatacept, belatacept	Fusion proteins comprised of the Fc fragments of human IgG1 connected to the extracellular domain of CTLA-4 blocking T-cell costimulation, thereby preventing T-cell activation	RA, prevention of graft rejection	Less clear infection risk when used as monotherapy; infections reported when combined with other immunosuppression for rheumatoid arthritis PTLD reported with belatacept
B-cell-depleting agents[28]			
Rituximab	Chimeric human-murine monoclonal antibody against CD20, a transmembrane protein on pre-B and mature cells, but not plasma cells. Effects last 6–9 mo.	Various hematologic malignancies, induction therapy and treatment of GVHD, RA, immune mediated cytopenias, lupus nephritis, PTLD, GPA	With monotherapy, main concerns are reactivation of HBV and PML. Pneumocystis is a concern when used as R-CHOP. Other infections (serious bacterial infections, HSV, VZV, CMV, parvovirus, HCV) occur when used in patients with hematologic malignancy with prolonged cytopenias and/or hypogammaglobulinemia or in SOT recipients in conjunction with other immunosuppression.
90Y-Ibritumomab	Radioconjugated murine monoclonal antibody against CD20	NHL	Various bacterial and viral infections due to prolonged and severe cytopenias

(Continued)

TABLE 14-4	INFECTIONS IN RECIPIENTS OF BIOLOGIC AGENTS (CONTINUED)		

Drug	Mechanism of Immunomodulation	Indications	Infection Risk, Comments
Tumor necrosis factor (TNF)-α inhibitors[27]			
Adalimumab	Human monoclonal antibody against TNF-α; prevents differentiation of monocytes into macrophages, macrophage activation, and recruitment of neutrophils and macrophages for granuloma formation	RA, AS, IBD, plaque psoriasis, uveitis, hidradenitis suppurativa, pyoderma gangrenosum	Granulomatous infections (TB especially extrapulmonary and disseminated disease-risk 2–12 times placebo, histoplasmosis, coccidioidomycosis) Other: Bacterial pneumonia, *Candida*, *Toxoplasma*, *Nocardia*, CMV, VZV
Infliximab	Chimeric human-murine monoclonal antibody against TNF-α composed of human IgG1 constant region fused to the murine variable region	RA, AS, IBD, plaque psoriasis	Granulomatous infections (TB – especially extrapulmonary and disseminated disease - risk 2–12 times placebo, other mycobacteria, histoplasmosis, coccidioidomycosis, cryptococcosis) Viruses: CMV, VZV and HBV reactivation Other: Bacterial sepsis, *Listeria*, *Toxoplasma*, *Brucella*, *Bartonella*, *Leishmania*, *Candida*, molds
Etanercept	Soluble TNF-α receptor composed of two extracellular domains of human TNF receptor 2 fused to the Fc fragment of human IgG1 and, therefore, binds TNF as well as related cytokines	RA, AS, plaque psoriasis, acute GVHD	Lesser risk of granulomatous infections than other TNF-α inhibitors; longer time to onset of TB and lesser risk of extrapulmonary and disseminated disease Other infections occur when used in combination (e.g., with IL-1 receptor antagonist anakinra)

TABLE 14-4	INFECTIONS IN RECIPIENTS OF BIOLOGIC AGENTS (CONTINUED)		
Drug	Mechanism of Immunomodulation	Indications	Infection Risk, Comments
Certolizumab pegol	Pegylated human-ized Fab fragment against TNF-α	RA, AS, IBD, psoriatic arthritis	Tuberculosis (risk 8.5–12.2 times pla-cebo); other viral and fungal infections as for other agents in this group; other mold infections, Legionella and Pneumocystis also reported
Integrin antagonists			
Natalizumab	Monoclonal anti-body against α4 subunit of integrin; limiting adhesion and transmigration of leukocytes	Multiple sclerosis, IBD	PML HSV, VZV
Vedolizumab	Humanized mono-clonal antibody against α4β7 integrin, blocking migration of mem-ory T cells across endothelium into parenchymal tissue	IBD	Respiratory and gas-trointestinal infections; anal abscess, sepsis, TB, Listeria, Giardia, CMV; PML

AS, ankylosing spondylitis; CMV, cytomegalovirus; CTLA, cytotoxic T-lymphocyte antigen; EBV, Epstein–Barr virus; GPA, granulomatosis with polyangiitis; GVHD, graft versus host disease; HBV, hepatitis B virus; HHV-6, human herpes virus-6; HSCT, hematopoietic stem cell transplant; HSV, herpes simplex virus; IBD, inflammatory bowel disease; IL, interleukin; NHL, non-Hodgkin lymphoma; NK; natural killer; PML, progressive multifocal leukoenceph-alopathy; PTLD, posttransplantation lymphoproliferative disorder; RA, rheumatoid arthritis; R-CHOP, rituximab, cyclophosphamide, hydroxydaunorubicin, oncovin (vincristine) and prednisone; RSV, respiratory syncytial virus; SOT, solid organ transplant; TB, tuberculosis; TNF, tumor necrosis factor; VZV, varicella zoster virus.

REFERENCES

1. Freifeld AG, Bow EJ, Sepkowitz KA, et al. Clinical practice guideline for the use of antimicrobial agents in neutropenic patients with cancer : 2010 update by the Infectious Diseases Society of America. *Clin Infect Dis.* 2011;52(4):e56-e93.
2. van Kraaij MGJ, Dekker AW, Verdonck LF, et al. Infectious gastro-enteritis: an uncommon cause of diarrhoea in adult allogeneic and autologous stem cell transplant recipients. *Bone Marrow Transplant.* 2000;26(3):299-303.
3. Tomblyn M, Chiller T, Einsele H, et al. Guidelines for preventing infectious complications among hematopoietic cell transplantation recipients: a global perspective. *Biol Blood Marrow Transplant.* 2009;15(10):1143-1238.

4. Shah DP, Ghantoji SS, Mulanovich VE, Ariza-Heredia EJ, Chemaly RF. Management of respiratory viral infections in hematopoietic cell transplant recipients. *Am J Blood Res.* 2012;2(4):203-218.

5. Kontoyiannis DP, Marr KA, Park BJ, et al. Prospective surveillance for invasive fungal infections in hematopoietic stem cell transplant recipients, 2001–2006: overview of the Transplant-Associated Infection Surveillance Network (TRANSNET) Database. *Clin Infect Dis.* 2010;50(8):1091-1100.

6. Fleming S, Yannakou CK, Haeusler GM, et al. Consensus guidelines for antifungal prophylaxis in haematological malignancy and haemopoietic stem cell transplantation, 2014. *Intern Med J.* 2014;44(12):1283-1297.

7. Patterson TF, Thompson GR, Denning DW, et al. Practice guidelines for the diagnosis and management of aspergillosis: 2016 update by the Infectious Diseases Society of America. *Clin Infect Dis.* 2016;63(4):e1-e60.

8. Tacke D, Buchheidt D, Karthaus M, et al. Primary prophylaxis of invasive fungal infections in patients with haematologic malignancies. 2014 Update of the recommendations of the Infectious Diseases Working Party of the German Society for Haematology and Oncology. *Ann Hematol.* 2014;93(9):1449-1456.

9. Pappas PG, Kauffman CA, Andes DR, et al. Clinical practice guideline for the management of candidiasis: 2016 update by the Infectious Diseases Society of America. *Clin Infect Dis.* 2016;62(4):e1-e50.

10. Cornely OA, Arikan-Akdagli S, Dannaoui E, et al. ESCMID and ECMM joint clinical guidelines for the diagnosis and management of mucormycosis 2013. *Clin Microbiol Infect.* 2014;20(S3):5-26.

11. Pergam SA, Limaye AP. Varicella zoster virus in solid organ transplantation. *Am J Transplant.* 2013;13(suppl 4):138-143.

12. Tortorano AM, Richardson M, Roilides E, et al. ESCMID and ECMM joint guidelines on diagnosis and management of hyalohyphomycosis: Fusarium spp., Scedosporium spp. and others. *Clin Microbiol Infect.* 2014;20(S3):27-46.

13. Wilck MB, Zuckerman RA. Herpes simplex virus in solid organ transplantation. *Am J Transplant.* 2013;13(suppl 4):121-127.

14. Razonable RR, Humar A. Cytomegalovirus in solid organ transplantation. *Am J Transplant.* 2013;13(suppl 4):93-106.

15. Allen UD, Preiksaitis JK. Epstein-barr virus and posttransplant lymphoproliferative disorder in solid organ transplantation. *Am J Transplant.* 2013;13(suppl 4):107-120.

16. Hirsch HH, Randhawa P. BK polyomavirus in solid organ transplantation. *Am J Transplant.* 2013;13(suppl 4):179-188.

17. Chung RT, Ghany MG, Kim AY, et al. Hepatitis C guidance 2018 update: AASLD-IDSA recommendations for testing, managing, and treating hepatitis C virus infection. *Clin Infect Dis.* 2018;67(10):1477-1492.

18. Sepkowitz KA. Opportunistic infections in patients with and patients without Acquired Immunodeficiency Syndrome. *Clin Infect Dis.* 2002;34(8):1098-1107.

19. Moon SM, Kim T, Sung H, et al. Outcomes of moderate-to-severe Pneumocystis pneumonia treated with adjunctive steroid in non-HIV-infected patients. *Antimicrob Agents Chemother.* 2011;55(10):4613-4618.

20. Clark NM, Reid GE. Nocardia infections in solid organ transplantation. *Am J Transplant.* 2013;13(suppl 4):83-92.

21. Singh NM, Husain S. Aspergillosis in solid organ transplantation. *Am J Transplant.* 2013;13(suppl 4):228-241.

22. Baddley JW, Forrest GN. Cryptococcosis in solid organ transplantation. *Am J Transplant.* 2013;13(suppl 4):242-249.

23. Miller R, Assi M. Endemic fungal infections in solid organ transplantation. *Am J Transplant.* 2013;13(suppl 4):250-261.

24. Silveira FP, Kusne S. Candida infections in solid organ transplantation. *Am J Transplant.* 2013;13(suppl 4):220-227.

25. Schwartz BS, Mawhorter SD. Parasitic infections in solid organ transplantation. *Am J Transplant.* 2013;13(suppl 4):280-303.

26. Issa NC, Fishman JA. Infectious complications of antilymphocyte therapies in solid organ transplantation. *Clin Infect Dis.* 2009;48(6):772-786.

27. Salvana EMT, Salata RA. Infectious complications associated with monoclonal antibodies and related small molecules. *Clin Microbiol Rev.* 2009;22(2):274-290.

28. Gea-Banacloche JC. Rituximab-associated infections. *Semin Hematol.* 2010;47(2):187-198.

Dimorphic Mycoses

15

Krunal Raval and Andrej Spec

INTRODUCTION

- Dimorphic mycoses are a group of fungi that exist in mold form at environmental temperatures and in yeast forms (or spherules, for coccidioidomycosis) at body temperatures.
- Coccidioidomycosis is not a true dimorphic fungus as it forms spherules, not yeast, at body temperature; however, because of overwhelming similarities it is often discussed in concert with and treated as an endemic mycosis.
- The majority of dimorphic mycoses are also endemic mycoses (*Blastomyces dermatitidis, Coccidioides* spp., *Histoplasma capsulatum, Paracoccidioides brasiliensis,* and *Talaromyces marneffei*) due to a specific environmental niche that limits their distribution.
- Although the endemic mycoses may cause disease in healthy individuals, immunocompromised individuals are at greater risk of severe or disseminated disease.
- These infections are characterized by long periods of latency. Clinical disease can present up to 30 years after exposure. Therefore, disease can be identified in patients who have moved away from an endemic region.
- Definitive diagnosis of endemic mycosis infection is by growth of the organism in culture. As there is no commensal component to the life cycle of endemic mycoses, all cultures represent an infection. However, the sensitivity of cultures is low and growth rates can be slow. To improve diagnostics, several species specific-serologies and antigen tests have been developed.
- The specific pathogens covered in this chapter include *B. dermatitidis, Coccidioides* spp., *H. capsulatum, P. brasiliensis,* and *Sporothrix schenckii, Emmonsia crescens, T. marneffei.*
- Infections caused by *Candida* spp., *Aspergillus* spp., *Cryptococcus* spp., dermatophytes, and invasive molds are covered in Chapters 13 and 14.

Blastomycosis

GENERAL PRINCIPLES

- *B. dermatitidis* is a dimorphic fungus that is endemic to North America. This includes southeastern, midwestern and south-central US states bordering the Mississippi and Ohio River basins and Canadian provinces bordering the Great Lakes as well as St. Lawrence River and the Nelson River.
- The primary habitat is thought to be soil and decaying wood, although the evidence for this is weak.
- The usual route of entry is via inhalation of the conidia of the mold form. Less commonly, entry may occur through direct inoculation by skin puncture. Once inhaled, the organisms change to the yeast form and multiply by budding. Infection can then disseminate hematogenously to affect other organs or tissues.
- Infection with *B. dermatitidis* does not appear to be significantly more common in immunocompromised hosts than in immunocompetent hosts; however, infection tends to be more severe and dissemination and central nervous system (CNS) involvement are more common. The mortality also appears to be higher.
- When thinking of blastomycosis, remember the "B's": **B**lastomycosis, **B**road **B**ased **B**udding, **B**reath (pneumonia), **B**rain, **B**one, **B**ody covering (skin).

DIAGNOSIS

Clinical Presentation

- *B. dermatitidis* **most commonly causes pneumonia.** Initial infection ranges from asymptomatic infection to self-limited pneumonia (acute or chronic) to severe infection with potential for dissemination of disease or acute respiratory distress syndrome (ARDS). Chest radiography may reveal a lobar infiltrate and may frequently have a mass-like or cavitary lesion. Atypical presentations are often confused with lung cancer, tuberculosis, or other fungal infections.
- Blastomycosis may present as a community-acquired ARDS, which usually happens when a large, often asymptomatic peritracheal lymph node erodes into the airways and drains into the lungs, leading to an overwhelming immune response.
- **Skin lesions** are the second most common manifestation of blastomycosis. Skin lesions are typically well-circumscribed nonpainful papules or nodules; however, appearance may vary. Most commonly, skin manifestations follow subclinical pulmonary infection with hematogenous dissemination. Rarely, infection may occur as a result of direct inoculation from breaks in the skin.
- Osteomyelitis is the third most common manifestation of blastomycosis. Septic arthritis can develop from direct extension of osteomyelitis.
- CNS involvement including brain abscess is fourth most common manifestation and can be devastating.
- Other less common manifestations include prostatitis and epididymo-orchitis in men. Less commonly, ocular infection and oral or laryngeal infection can also be seen.

Diagnostic Testing[1]

- **Microbiologic cultures may take up to several weeks to grow.**
- Rapid diagnosis can be achieved by **visualizing the organism in a tissue sample or clinical specimen**. Organisms can be identified from sputum or pus samples using a KOH wet prep followed by Gomori methenamine silver (GMS) stain or periodic acid–Schiff (PAS) stain.
- *B. dermatitidis* is often identified by its classic morphology described as **broad-based budding yeast.**
- Blastomycosis is the most common cause of pseudoepitheliomatous hyperplasia on pathology and is often confused with squamous cell carcinoma. In those situations, GMS and PAS stains are usually positive.
- Serologic antibody assays are available but not routinely recommended due to poor sensitivity and specificity as well as cross-reactivity with other fungal organisms.
- Immunodiffusion assays that measure antibody to *B. dermatitidis* A antigen are relatively specific, but sensitivity is only 28% to 64% and lower in immunocompromised individuals.
- Antigen test is more sensitive than the available serologic tests, but cross-reactivity exists with other fungal organisms, specifically *H. capsulatum*. Because of overlapping geographic distribution and similar presentation and treatment, the *Histoplasma* urine antigen is often used to test for both *B. dermatitidis* and *H. capsulatum* infection.

TREATMENT[1]

- For moderately severe to severe pneumonia, severe disseminated disease, CNS disease, or disease in the immunocompromised host, initial treatment should be with a **liposomal formulation of amphotericin B**, 5 mg/kg IV daily (see Table 15-1).[1] Once clinically improved, oral itraconazole may be substituted.

TABLE 15-1	TREATMENT OF BLASTOMYCOSIS		
Manifestation	**Treatment**	**Duration**	**Notes**
Nonmeningeal disease; mild to moderate disease; immunocompetent	Itraconazole 200 three times daily × 3 d followed by itraconazole 200-400 mg/d PO	6-12 mo	Itraconazole levels must be followed
Meningitis; acute dissemination; severe disease; immunocompromised	Lipid formulation of amphotericin B, 3-5 mg/kg per day IV until clinically improved, then itraconazole 200 three times daily × 3 d followed by once or twice daily	6-12 mo	Lifelong suppression should be considered in the immunocompromised

Adapted from Chapman SW, Dismukes WE, Proia LA, et al. Clinical practice guidelines for the management of blastomycosis: 2008 update by the Infectious Diseases Society of America. *Clin Infect Dis.* 2008;46:1801-1812.

- Less severe infection may be treated with oral **itraconazole** suspension 200 mg three times daily for 3 days, followed by once or twice daily dosing for 6 to 12 months.
- Itraconazole tablets can be substituted for suspension; they are better tolerated as the suspension is associated with poor taste and increased rate of diarrhea, but the absorption is less reliable.
- Because of inconsistent absorption of both formulations, itraconazole levels should be monitored. Suspension is preferred for those with severe disease, history of poor absorption of oral medications, or those on acid-suppressive medications.
- Chronic lifelong suppression may be indicated for immunocompromised hosts if the immunosuppression cannot be reversed or at least reduced.
- The new azole antifungal agents, posaconazole, voriconazole, and isavuconazole, have in vitro and in vivo activity against *B. dermatitidis*, but there is less clinical experience with their use. They should be used only in cases of itraconazole intolerance; further investigation into their use is warranted.
- The echinocandins (e.g., caspofungin, anidulafungin, and micafungin) do not have good activity and should not be used for *B. dermatitidis* infection.

Coccidioidomycosis

GENERAL PRINCIPLES

Epidemiology

- *Coccidioides* spp. are dimorphic fungi that are endemic to the soil in the desert southwest of the United States, northern Mexico, and parts of Latin America. However, there is growing evidence of spread to new areas due to global warming.
- Two species have been identified, *Coccidioides immitis* and *Coccidioides posadasii*. They are the causative agents of **"San Joaquin valley fever."**

- *Coccidioides* spp. exist either in the mycelial form or as unique spherules. Infection occurs by inhalation of arthroconidia of the mycelial form. In the lungs, the arthroconidia transform into spherules, which in turn form internal endospores. On rupture, hundreds of endospores are released, each of which is capable of maturing into viable fungi.
- The time of highest incidence of infection is after the rainy season. During the wet season, *Coccidioides* spp. proliferate and increase their biomass significantly. When the soil dries out, production of arthroconidia is increased, and resulting sand and dust storms pick up the arthroconidia leading to spread.
- The incidence of infection has been rising over recent decades because of an increase in the population of cities in the southwestern United States and worsening draught cycles due to climate change. There have been reports of outbreaks associated with disruption of soil following excavations, earthquakes, and dust storms.
- Extrapulmonary disease is caused by hematogenous dissemination. Cutaneous inoculation has been reported but is exceedingly rare; cutaneous infections almost always represent disseminated disease.

DIAGNOSIS[2]

Clinical Manifestations

- The majority of *Coccidioides* exposures result in subclinical disease. Some patients develop pulmonary infection indistinguishable from community-acquired pneumonia. This may be associated with fevers, erythema nodosum, headache, and migratory polyarthralgia. This does not represent a true dissemination and is related to immune complex deposition. Diffuse pneumonia is usually seen in immunocompromised patients or due to a large infectious inoculum. Diffuse pneumonia usually indicates the presence of fungemia.
- Approximately 4% of lung infections due to *Coccidioides* result in the formation of pulmonary nodules or cavities. These frequently have no associated symptoms but may be indistinguishable from lung cancer or other infections such as tuberculosis. Cavities may rupture, resulting in hydropneumothorax. These nodules may persist even after treatment, and they do not represent treatment failure, unless they start to increase in size, are culture positive, or have increasing serology titers.
- Chronic fibrocavitary pneumonia is characterized by pulmonary cavitation and interstitial fibrosis. This is more common among diabetics and patients with underlying lung disease.
- Extrapulmonary or disseminated disease is rare but is seen more frequently in certain ethnic groups. People of Filipino or African ancestry seem to have a risk of disseminated disease that is several-fold higher than the Caucasian population. Extrapulmonary disease is often not associated with any pulmonary symptom, and chest radiograph may be normal. The most common sites of extrapulmonary involvement include the brain, skin, bones, and joints.
- The most severe manifestation of coccidioidomycosis is meningitis, which is universally fatal if not treated. Complications of *Coccidioides* meningitis include CNS vasculitis and hydrocephalus.

Diagnostic Testing

- Cultures usually grow within 5 to 7 days of incubation in anaerobic conditions. Once growth is evident, samples should only be handled in an appropriate biocontainment cabinet as the mycelial form is highly contagious.
- *Coccidioides* spp. may also be identified by direct **visualization of the organisms in clinical specimen.** Human-to-human transmission has not been reported outside of organ donation, and tissue samples can be handled without specific precautions. Sputum and respiratory secretions may be examined with KOH prep or calcofluor white smear. Organisms can be identified in tissue stained with hematoxylin and eosin (H&E), GMS, or PAS stains.

- Unlike blastomycosis, **serologic testing for *Coccidioides* spp. is sensitive and specific**. Latex agglutination tests and complement fixation are useful screening tools. Complement fixation titers higher than 1:16 may indicate disseminated disease.
- CSF findings in *Coccidioides* meningitis are similar to bacterial meningitis, but can exhibit lymphocytic predominance and highly elevated protein (>1 g). Cultures of CSF are frequently negative for *Coccidioides*, so a high index of suspicion and confirmation with serologic tests are required.

TREATMENT[2]

- Treatment of acute pulmonary infection is controversial. Some experts advocate treatment of all symptomatic patients. Others advocate watchful waiting for otherwise healthy individuals. Immunosuppressed, pregnant, severely ill patients, as well as those with underlying diabetes, heart, or lung disease should receive treatment. The initial treatment of choice is usually **amphotericin B lipid formulation** (Table 15-2). After initial improvement, therapy can be continued with an oral azole antifungal for at least 12 months. Fluconazole and itraconazole are the most commonly used azole antifungal agents for *Coccidioides* infection.
- Asymptomatic pulmonary nodules or cavities likely do not require treatment with antifungal medications. Patients with symptoms such as pain, superinfection, or hemoptysis may benefit from treatment, although recurrence may occur once medications are stopped.
- For severe symptoms or cavity rupture, surgical evaluation with thoracotomy, lobectomy, and decortication may be required.
- Chronic fibrocavitary pneumonia requires treatment with oral azole antifungal agents for duration of at least 1 year. If not improved on azoles, amphotericin B is the alternative treatment.

TABLE 15-2	TREATMENT OF COCCIDIOIDOMYCOSIS		
Manifestation	**Treatment**	**Duration**	**Notes**
Nonmeningeal disease	Itraconazole 200 mg PO twice daily or fluconazole 400 mg PO daily	12 mo Lifelong suppression if disseminated	Follow serum titers after treatment. Rising titers suggest recurrence.
Meningitis	Fluconazole 400-800 mg IV/PO daily. Intrathecal amphotericin B 0.1-1.5 mg daily to once weekly may be added for severe meningeal disease	Chronic lifelong suppression recommended	For pulmonary nodules and asymptomatic cavitary disease, no therapy indicated. Consider surgery if cavitary disease persists >2 y, progresses >1 y, or is located near pleura
Chronic fibrocavitary pneumonia	Fluconazole 400 mg PO daily or itraconazole 200 mg PO twice daily	12 mo	Amphotericin B is an alternative. Goal serum itraconazole level >1 µg/mL

- *Coccidioides* meningitis is treated with fluconazole at doses of 400 mg or higher. Some experts propose the addition of intrathecal amphotericin B for initial treatment in severe cases. Liposomal amphotericin has been successfully used for salvage therapy, despite the fact that the deoxycholate formulation is inferior to fluconazole. Fluconazole should be continued for life, if tolerated, as relapse rate is 78% after discontinuation. Hydrocephalus almost always requires shunt placement for decompression, which often requires multiple revisions.
- The newer antifungals, isavuconazole, voriconazole, posaconazole, and the echinocandins, show some promise in the treatment of *Coccidioides* infection, although more studies are needed.

Histoplasmosis

GENERAL PRINCIPLES

- *H. capsulatum* is a dimorphic fungus that grows in soil. The fungus is endemic to several regions of North and South America, as well as areas in Asia and Africa. In the United States, it is most commonly found in the Mississippi and Ohio River valleys. *Histoplasma* is most abundant in nitrogen-rich soil, such as those contaminated with pigeon or bat excretions, as this accelerates sporulation.
- Entry into the body is by inhalation of microconidia. In the alveoli, these microconidia are phagocytosed by macrophages and neutrophils where they may disseminate, first to the hilar and mediastinal lymph nodes, followed by the reticuloendothelial system.
- **Infection is extremely common in endemic areas, and most residents of these areas have been exposed by the time they reach adulthood.** Disease can occur in anyone, but immunosuppressed individuals are far more likely to experience severe or disseminated forms of disease.

DIAGNOSIS[3]

Clinical Manifestations

- **Pneumonia is the most common manifestation** of infection with *H. capsulatum*. Most patients are asymptomatic or experience mild, subclinical infection. Patients exposed to a massive inoculum of *H. capsulatum* or the immunosuppressed may experience severe or life-threatening pneumonia.
- Complications of pulmonary histoplasmosis include pericarditis, mediastinal lymphadenitis, mediastinal granuloma, mediastinal fibrosis, arthralgias, erythema nodosum, and erythema multiforme.
- Chronic pulmonary histoplasmosis and cavitary histoplasmosis are more commonly seen in older patients with underlying chronic lung disease such as emphysema.
- **Progressive disseminated histoplasmosis** (PDH) can affect any individual but most commonly occurs in the setting of immunosuppression, such as those with AIDS and hematologic malignancy, recipients of organ transplantation, and patients receiving antitumor necrosis factor α agents.
- Disseminated disease results from hematogenous spread of the organism and can affect almost any organ, but most commonly the GI system, skin, brain, adrenal glands, and bone.
- Signs and symptoms may include fevers, chills, weight loss, dyspnea, abdominal pain, diarrhea, hypotension, ARDS, anemia, thrombocytopenia, hepatosplenomegaly, elevated liver enzymes, disseminated intravascular coagulation, Addisonian crisis, or meningitis.
- There are acute, subacute, and chronic forms of PDH, which are distinguished by decreasing severity and increasing duration of symptoms.
- Laboratory tests that may suggest disseminated histoplasmosis include elevated LDH, ferritin, alkaline phosphatase, and a high AST to ALT ratio.

Diagnostic Testing

- Cultures can take up to several weeks to grow. In disseminated disease, the organism is frequently cultured from blood or bone marrow samples. *H. capsulatum* is the slowest growing of all endemic mycoses.
- Rapid diagnosis can be achieved by **visualizing the organism in a tissue sample or clinical specimen**. Organisms can be identified from tissue samples using GMS or PAS fungal stains. Unlike *Blastomyces*, the organisms are not generally identified by direct examination of sputum or bronchiolar alveolar lavage fluid. The organism can be detected on Wright–Giemsa stain of peripheral blood in up to 40% of acute PDH cases.
- Antigen detection is a useful tool in the diagnosis of histoplasmosis. Antigen concentrations in the urine are higher, and **detection of antigen in the urine** is more sensitive than in the serum. Urinary antigen is detected in over 90% of cases of PDH but is not as sensitive for isolated pulmonary disease. Titers of urine *Histoplasma* antigen can be used to monitor treatment.
- Serology testing is available for the detection of antibodies against *H. capsulatum*. A fourfold rise in acute and convalescent antibody titers by complement fixation is useful for the retrospective diagnosis of acute pulmonary histoplasmosis. Serology testing is not as useful for the diagnosis of chronic or disseminated disease.

TREATMENT[4]

- Treatment is not required for the vast majority of patients with mild to moderate **acute pulmonary histoplasmosis**. For persistent infection (symptoms >1 mo duration), oral **itraconazole** 200 mg three times daily for 3 days followed by twice daily dosing for 6 to 12 weeks may be used. Alternatively, intravenous **lipid formulation of amphotericin B** should be used for more severe infections, such as those with hypoxia. Treatment recommendations are summarized in Table 15-3.
- Antifungal treatment is usually not indicated for asymptomatic hilar or mediastinal lymphadenitis, granuloma, histoplasmoma, pericarditis, or arthralgias associated with acute infection. If symptoms are present, treatment is the same as acute pulmonary histoplasmosis. Surgery may be indicated if lymphadenopathy, granuloma, or histoplasmoma causes compressive symptoms in contiguous structures.
- Mediastinal fibrosis is an immune response to past infection and is thus unlikely to respond to antifungal treatment. Intravascular stenting may be required if the pulmonary vessels are compressed. Surgery should be approached with great caution as there is high perioperative mortality. Overall prognosis is poor.
- Chronic or cavitary pulmonary histoplasmosis should be treated with itraconazole 200 mg three times daily for 3 days followed by once or twice daily dosing for at least 1 year.
- **PDH** should be treated initially with intravenous **lipid formulation of amphotericin B** 3 to 5 mg/kg per day for 2 weeks or until clinically improved, followed by itraconazole 200 mg three times daily for 3 days then twice daily for 12 months. Itraconazole should be continued in patients with HIV/AIDS until CD4 count is > 200 cells/μL for at least 6 months. Longer treatment or lifelong suppression should be considered in immunosuppressed patients where the immunosuppression cannot be reversed or reduced.
- **CNS histoplasmosis** should be treated with **lipid amphotericin B** 5 mg/kg per day for 4 to 6 weeks followed by itraconazole 200 mg PO twice daily for a minimum of 6 months. However, the mortality is high.
- When itraconazole is used, it is important to check serum itraconazole levels with a goal of >1 μg/mL to ensure absorption.
- Arthralgias, pericarditis, and erythema nodosum should be treated with anti-inflammatory agents such as nonsteroidal anti-inflammatory drugs or corticosteroids.

TABLE 15-3	TREATMENT OF HISTOPLASMOSIS		
Manifestation	**Primary Therapy**	**Duration**	**Notes**
Acute pulmonary disease	If symptoms <4 wk – No treatment.		
	If symptoms persist >1 mo treat with itraconazole 200 mg three times daily for 3 d followed by twice daily.	6-12 wk	Goal serum itraconazole level >1 µg/mL
	In severe disease, lipid amphotericin B 3-5 mg/kg per day for 2 wk followed by itraconazole.	12-24 wk	
Acute dissemination; severe disease; immunocompromised	Lipid amphotericin B, 3-5 mg/kg per day IV for 2 wk or until clinically improved, then itraconazole 200 mg PO twice daily	12 mo followed by long-term suppression for immunosuppressed; if HIV/AIDS, until CD4 count >200 cells/µL for 6 mo	Goal serum itraconazole level >1 µg/mL
CNS histoplasmosis	Lipid amphotericin B 5 mg/kg per day for 4-6 wk followed by itraconazole 200 mg PO 2-3 × daily	Minimum 6 mo followed by lifelong suppression in the immunocompromised	Goal serum itraconazole level >1 µg/mL
Chronic or cavitary pulmonary histoplasmosis	Itraconazole 200 mg PO once or twice daily	Minimum 12 mo	Goal serum itraconazole level >1 µg/mL
Mediastinal fibrosis	Antifungal therapy likely of no benefit		

Adapted from Wheat LJ, Freifeld AG, Kleiman MB, et al. Clinical practice guidelines for the management of patients with histoplasmosis: 2007 update by the Infectious Diseases Society of America. *Clin Infect Dis.* 2007;45:807-825.
CNS, central nervous system.

Paracoccidioidomycosis

GENERAL PRINCIPLES

- *P. brasiliensis* is a thermally dimorphic fungus that is limited to Latin America, from Mexico to Central and South America. The highest incidence of disease is in Brazil, Venezuela, and Colombia.

- *P. brasiliensis* **disproportionately affects men over the age of 30 years** with a ratio of men to women of 15:1. It is more prevalent among rural workers engaged in agriculture. There has been a decrease in incidence of the disease as farming techniques have become more industrialized.

DIAGNOSIS

Clinical Presentation

- Disease occurs by inhalation of microconidia into the lungs. Only a minority of patients (<5%) eventually develop clinical disease.
- Acute/subacute paracoccidioidomycosis (juvenile paracoccidioidomycosis) is almost always observed in children, adolescents, and adults under 30 years of age, and it represents less than 10% of cases. After a period of latency, it presents with dissemination of infection to the reticuloendothelial system resulting in lymphadenopathy, hepatosplenomegaly, and/or bone marrow dysfunction.
- Chronic paracoccidioidomycosis represents reactivation of the primary infection and is much more frequent in adult men. It predominantly involves the lungs.
- Pneumonia from paracoccidioidomycosis is commonly diagnosed only after disease has progressed to severe, chronic lung disease with fibrosis and emphysematous changes.

Diagnostic Testing

- Cultures have low sensitivity and can take up to 1 month to grow.
- Rapid identification can be achieved by **visualizing the organism in clinical specimens** such as sputum, pus, or tissue. A simple KOH prep has a relatively high yield. Tissues can be stained with GMS to identify the organisms. In clinical specimens, the yeast are described as small, with thick walls and multiple buds, resembling a captain's wheel.
- Serologic testing is the most reliable and widely used assay. It is 97% sensitive and 100% specific. Skin testing is not useful due to low sensitivity.

TREATMENT[5,6]

- For mild to moderate paracoccidioidomycosis, itraconazole is the drug of choice. Alternatively, trimethoprim/sulfamethoxazole (TMP/SMX) can also be used. Duration of therapy is usually 6 to 12 months.
- For severe disease (shock or respiratory failure) or CNS infection, initial therapy with amphotericin B (preferably lipid formulation if available) is recommended followed by itraconazole or TMP/SMX for extended duration.
- Serologic testing should be performed before the initiation of therapy, after 3 months of therapy, and every 6 months thereafter until the completion of therapy.

Talaromycosis (Previously Referred to as Penicilliosis)

GENERAL PRINCIPLES

- *T. marneffei* is a thermally dimorphic fungus found in Southeast Asia, often associated with exposure to the bamboo rat. Disease from *T. marneffei* was exceedingly rare before the HIV/AIDS epidemic.
- Disease from *T. marneffei* **should be considered in immunocompromised individuals residing in, or in visitors to, the endemic region of Southeast Asia.**

- Talaromycosis typically develops in immunocompromised individuals, especially those with HIV infection (CD4 <100 cells/µL) and other acquired cellular immune deficits.
- *T. marneffei* infection occurs after inhalation of the microconidia into the lungs.

DIAGNOSIS

Clinical Presentation

- Clinical manifestations of talaromycosis are secondary to hematogenous dissemination. Presentation ranges from isolated skin/mucosal lesions to respiratory failure and circulatory collapse.
- GI involvement, arthritis, osteomyelitis and neurologic manifestations, presenting as fevers and altered mental status, have been associated with talaromycosis.
- In HIV-infected individuals, the skin lesions may be umbilicated and confused with molluscum contagiosum.

Diagnostic Testing

- *T. marneffei* has a very characteristic appearance in culture due to a striking red pigment.
- The organism can also be identified on smear or histopathologic studies.
- Serologic assays are not widely used because of limited data regarding diagnostic accuracy and restricted availability.
- Galactomannan testing, which is primarily used for detection of aspergillosis, has significant cross-reactivity with *T. marneffei*.

TREATMENT[7]

- Owing to high mortality (97%) associated with untreated talaromycosis, prompt treatment is strongly recommended.
- For CNS infections, initial treatment should consist of liposomal amphotericin B for 4 to 6 weeks followed by itraconazole for 10 weeks.
- For moderate to severe non-CNS infections, length of induction with liposomal amphotericin B is 2 weeks followed by itraconazole.
- For mild cases, 10 weeks of itraconazole is recommended. Voriconazole can also be considered.
- Maintenance therapy with daily itraconazole is recommended in the immunocompromised host until restoration of cellular immunity. In HIV patients, maintenance therapy should be continued until CD4 >100 cells/µL for at least 6 months.

Sporotrichosis

GENERAL PRINCIPLES

- *S. schenckii* is a dimorphic fungus that exists in its hyphal form in the environment and as an oval- or cigar-shaped yeast at body temperature. *S. schenckii* lives in decaying wood and other vegetation, hay, and soil. It has been isolated throughout the world, but it is most common in tropical or subtropical regions of the Americas.
- Unlike the other dimorphic mycoses, sporotrichosis infection is usually introduced by **direct inoculation into the skin or soft tissue**. This usually occurs after minor trauma and contact with soil or decaying plant matter.
- Pulmonary sporotrichosis is rare but can occur after inhalation of microconidia. Pulmonary infection is more common among individuals with underlying lung disease and alcoholics.

DIAGNOSIS

Clinical Presentation

- Lymphocutaneous sporotrichosis is predominately a cutaneous disease. Following inoculation, the organism spreads via lymphatic channels.
- The primary lesion develops at the site of inoculation. A papule initially develops, which later ulcerates. The ulcer may or may not be painful. After lymphatic spread, nodules may form and then ulcerate along the distribution of the lymphatics.
- **Pneumonia** due to *S. schenckii* presents with fever, night sweats, weight loss, fatigue, and cough. Nodular and cavitary lesions may be seen on chest radiograph. Presentation may mimic that of reactivation tuberculosis.
- **Osteomyelitis and septic arthritis are uncommon manifestations usually due to hematogenous spread and occur most often in alcoholics.**
- Multifocal extracutaneous disease and meningitis have been described but are exceedingly rare. Disseminated disease may be more common among the severely immunocompromised, such as patients with advanced AIDS.

Diagnostic Testing

- Culture material may be obtained from aspiration of a lesion or tissue biopsy. The organism usually grows within a week at room temperature.
- Histopathologic examination is less reliable and has a lower yield. The organism may be seen as tiny oval- or cigar-shaped yeasts with multiple buds.
- Serologic testing for sporotrichosis is not available.

TREATMENT[8]

- Treatment of cutaneous or lymphocutaneous sporotrichosis is with **itraconazole** 200 mg daily for 2 to 4 weeks after all lesions have resolved, usually a total of 3 to 6 months.
- Treatment of osteoarticular sporotrichosis is with itraconazole 200 mg twice daily for 12 months. Alternatively, amphotericin B may be used for initial therapy, followed by oral itraconazole.
- For pulmonary, meningeal, and disseminated sporotrichosis, initial therapy should be with IV **amphotericin B** followed by itraconazole for at least 12 months. Patients with AIDS or other severely immunocompromised individuals should continue prophylactic itraconazole until immune recovery.

Emansiosis

GENERAL PRINCIPLES

- Emansiosis is due to infections caused by genus *Emmonsia*, a thermally dimorphic opportunistic fungal pathogen. It consists of three species that are associated with human diseases – *E.pasteuriana, E.crescens,* and *E.parva*.
- In South Africa, *Emmonsia* been reported to cause disseminated infection in HIV-infected patients with low CD4 counts (usually <100 cells/μL).

DIAGNOSIS

Clinical Manifestations[9]

- Emansiosis typically presents with fever, night sweats, weight loss, and lymphadenopathy. Chest radiography findings can mimic tuberculosis.

- Dermatologic manifestations are seen in almost every case in immunocompromised individuals. Presentation ranges from erythematous papules to plaques to ulcers.
- In patients with HIV, lesions can be misdiagnosed as Kaposi sarcoma.

Diagnostic Testing

- Culture material may be obtained from aspiration of a lesion or tissue biopsy. The organism usually grows within a week at room temperature.
- Histopathologic examination is reliable and has good yield. The organism may be seen as septate, hyaline hyphae, 1 to 1.2 μm in diameter, with numerous smooth-walled conidia that are oval to subglobose.
- Serologic testing is not available.

TREATMENT

- In a recent study, most patients had dramatic and rapid responses to amphotericin B deoxycholate at a dose of 1 mg/kg of body weight per day for 14 days, followed by itraconazole maintenance therapy.
- Antiretroviral therapy should be initiated in patients with AIDS.

REFERENCES

1. Chapman SW, Dismukes WE, Proia LA, et al. Clinical practice guidelines for the management of blastomycosis: 2008 update by the Infectious Diseases Society of America. *Clin Infect Dis.* 2008;46:1801-1812.
2. Galgiani JN, Ampel NM, Blair JE, et al. Coccidioidomycosis. *Clin Infect Dis.* 2005;41:1217-1223.
3. Hage CA, Ribes JA, Wengenack NL, et al. A multicenter evaluation of tests for diagnosis of histoplasmosis. *Clin Infect Dis.* 2011;53:448-454.
4. Wheat LJ, Freifeld AG, Kleiman MB, et al. Clinical practice guidelines for the management of patients with histoplasmosis: 2007 update by the Infectious Diseases Society of America. *Clin Infect Dis.* 2007;45:807-825.
5. Queiroz-Telles F, Goldani LZ, Schlamm HT, et al. An open-label comparative pilot study of oral voriconazole and itraconazole for long-term treatment of paracoccidioidomycosis. *Clin Infect Dis.* 2007;45:1462-1469.
6. Shikanai-Yasuda MA, Benard G, Higaki Y, et al. Randomized trial with itraconazole, ketoconazole and sulfadiazine in paracoccidioidomycosis. *Med Mycol.* 2002;40:411-417.
7. Kaplan JE, Benson C, Holmes KH, et al. Guidelines for prevention and treatment of opportunistic infections in HIV-infected adults and adolescents: recommendations from CDC, the National Institutes of Health, and the HIV Medicine Association of the Infectious Diseases Society of America. *MMWR Recomm Rep.* 2009;58(RR-4):1-207.
8. Kauffman CA, Bustamante B, Chapman SW, Pappas PG. Clinical practice guidelines for the management of sporotrichosis: 2007 update by the Infectious Diseases Society of America. *Clin Infect Dis.* 2007;45:1255-1265.
9. Kenyon C, Bonorchis K, Corcoran C, et al. A dimorphic fungus causing disseminated infection in South Africa. *New Engl J Med.* 2013;369(15):1416-1424.

Zoonotic Infections and Ectoparasites

16

Abigail L. Carlson and Steven J. Lawrence

INTRODUCTION

- Zoonoses are a broad group of over 200 diseases that are acquired from nonhuman animal reservoirs; human disease can form an occasional part of the life cycle of the pathogen or may represent a "dead-end" event.
- Ectoparasites are arthropods that infest the exterior surface of the host (e.g., skin and hair). They feed on host blood and/or tissue; disease is the result of tissue necrosis or hypersensitivity to substances injected as part of the feeding process.
- Zoonotic diseases make up the majority of emerging infections caused by the intersection of human and animal habitats and arthropod vectors. This can be due to natural phenomena, climate change, and/or human behavior such as migration, rapid urbanization, and recreational or occupational activities. This interaction between humans, animals, and the environment forms the basis of the One Health model of disease that is essential for understanding these infections.
- Infection in humans occurs by a variety of routes: direct contact via broken skin or animal bites, ingestion of contaminated food or water, inhalation, or via an arthropod vector. Human-to-human transmission is possible with some infections in unusual circumstances, such as blood transfusion.
- A high index of suspicion and awareness of risk factors are important in diagnosis, as laboratory diagnosis is often difficult, requiring paired sera in many cases. An appropriate history should include attention to travel and location of residence, occupation and hobbies, pets and other animal exposures, arthropod exposure, and food history. High-risk occupations and hobbies include abattoir workers, farmers, veterinarians, pet store employees, and hunters.
- Included in this category are several highly fatal and easily produced microorganisms that have the potential to be used as agents of bioterrorism and produce substantial illness in large populations via an aerosol route of exposure.
- A bioterrorism-related outbreak should be considered if an unusually large number of patients present simultaneously with a respiratory, gastrointestinal (GI), or febrile rash syndrome; if several otherwise healthy patients present with unusually severe disease; or if an unusual pathogen for the region is isolated.

Animal and Human Bite Wounds

GENERAL PRINCIPLES

- Bite wounds are common, but most do not require treatment. Those who do receive treatment account for 300,000 emergency department (ED) visits, 10,000 hospitalizations (1% of all admissions originating within the ED), and approximately 20 deaths annually in the United States.[1]
- Infection is the most common complication of bites.
- **Dog bites** are the most common of animal bites, accounting for 80% to 90% of cases. Half of the patients are bitten on the hand. **Cat bites** are 5% to 15% of bite wound injuries, which occur on the upper extremity in approximately two-thirds of cases.

- Cellulitis occurring within 24 hours after a dog or cat bite is **likely to be secondary to *Pasteurella multocida*,** a facultative anaerobic gram-negative bacillus. This organism can cause severe infections of soft tissues, bones, and joints.[1]
- The next most common bacteria causing infection associated with both cat and dog bites are *Streptococcus, Staphylococcus* (including MRSA), *Moraxella, Corynebacterium,* and *Neisseria. Capnocytophaga* species are facultative anaerobes that are normal flora of cat and dog saliva and may cause fulminant sepsis in immunocompromised or asplenic patients.[1,2] Numerous other organisms have been found to cause infection following animal bites, and polymicrobial infection is common.
- **Humans are the third most common cause of bite wounds.** The microbiology of human bite infections is complex. **Human bites develop infection more frequently than animal bites.** Most infections are polymicrobial and involve anaerobes that are commonly β-lactamase producers and penicillin resistant. *Streptococcus viridans* is the most frequent organism reported. *Staphylococcus aureus* is reported in up to 40% of wounds and may have a particular association with a patient's attempts at self-debridement.
- Most infections after venomous **snake bites** are caused by organisms that colonize the devitalized tissue that results from local envenomation. Enteric gram-negatives must also be considered when evaluating the patient with an infection secondary to snake bite, as the prey of snakes often defecate in their mouths during ingestion.

DIAGNOSIS

Clinical Presentation

- When evaluating a bite wound, a careful history should include an assessment of the source of the bite, rabies vaccination status of the animal, and any evidence of rabid behavior, as well as the patient's vaccination history, with attention to rabies vaccination and tetanus immune status. The possibility of a human bite wound or closed fist injury should be considered when examining any injury over the MCPs, as these wounds are often minimized by patients.
- Immediately after a bite, the wound area should be examined for hemorrhage, trauma to vital structures, and crush injury. In certain wounds, careful examination under local anesthesia should evaluate for damage to tendon sheath, fascia, joint capsule, or bone. Once the wound is stabilized, concern for infectious complications can be addressed.
- Complications include **cellulitis, tenosynovitis, local abscess formation, septic arthritis, osteomyelitis, and occasionally sepsis, endocarditis, meningitis, and brain abscess**. Concerning symptoms include fever, lymphangitis, lymphadenopathy, and decreased range of motion in or tenderness over a joint, tendon, or muscle in the proximity of the bite.
- Deep puncture wounds such as those caused by cat bites are more likely to cause anaerobic abscesses. Additionally, occult inoculation of deep structures such as tendon and bone is possible, as bites can be significantly deeper than is apparent from the surface injury.
- **Human bites** are best divided into two categories:
  - **Occlusive bite wounds** are those that occur when the teeth are closed forcibly and break the skin. The affected anatomic site varies by gender: In men, human bites typically occur on the hand, arm, and shoulder, whereas women are more often bitten on the breast, genitals, leg, and arm. Complications arise more frequently after occlusive bites to the hand than to any other site.
  - **Clenched-fist injuries** account for the remainder of human bite wounds. These result when one person punches another person in the mouth, typically causing a break in the skin overlying the third metacarpophalangeal (MCP) joint. This is the most serious type of human bite infection, as the metacarpal joint capsule is frequently perforated and often develops into septic arthritis. Cellulitis, tendonitis, and, rarely, nerve laceration or bone fracture are other possible complications of clenched-fist injuries.

Diagnostic Testing

- When patients present with an infected bite wound or any associated infectious complication, data obtained from blood and wound cultures should be used to guide the choice of antimicrobial agents.
- Plain radiographs should be obtained to evaluate for foreign body retention or bone/joint involvement, especially in the case of cat bites and other deep puncture wounds.

TREATMENT

- The treatment of bite wounds centers on aggressive local wound cleaning, pressure irrigation with sterile saline solution, debridement of devitalized tissue, and antibiotic therapy, if appropriate. Local anesthesia may help in achieving deeper cleaning of affected tissue.
- **Closure of open wounds should be considered carefully.** In general, bite wounds, especially cat or human bites, should be closed by secondary intention unless there is significant concern for cosmetic outcome. Bite wounds should not be closed unless they are clinically uninfected, are less than 12 hours old (24 h on the face), and are located in a cosmetically sensitive area. Wounds on the hands or feet should not be closed by primary intention.
- Prophylactic antibiotics should be given to all patients who present with a bite that penetrates the skin of the hand, face, or genitals or is in close proximity to bone, tendon, or muscle. **All clenched-fist injuries should receive prophylaxis. Cat bites generally require prophylaxis** because of the higher risk of infection due to the puncture wounds. Length of prophylactic therapy is generally 7 days. Patients should be evaluated for need for tetanus or rabies postexposure prophylaxis.[1]
- **Empiric treatment with oral amoxicillin plus clavulanate** or IV ampicillin plus sulbactam is usually indicated for infected bite wounds. These are also the medications of choice for prophylaxis. Moxifloxacin or doxycycline are alternatives for penicillin-allergic patients.
- Definitive treatment should be directed by microbiologic data.
- Tetanus prophylaxis should also be provided.
  - If vaccination history is unknown or the patient has received < 3 lifetime doses of tetanus toxoid-containing vaccine, Tdap and complete catch-up vaccination series should be given. If the wound is a major wound or dirty wound, tetanus immune globulin should also be given.
  - If the patient has received 3 or more lifetime doses of tetanus toxoid-containing vaccine and it has been > 5 years since the last dose (or >10 years for clean, minor wounds), a Td or Tdap booster should be given.
- **Rabies** postexposure prophylaxis is detailed below.

Rabies

GENERAL PRINCIPLES

- Rabies viruses are of the family *Rhabdoviridae*, genus *Lyssavirus*, all of which may cause rabies disease.[3]
- Rabies is rare in the United States, and in the majority of recently reported cases, there was no clear history of animal bite or high-risk exposure.
- **Undetected bites from bats may be the most common source of infection in the United States.**[3,4]
- **Rabies is more common in the developing world, where dog bites are the primary source.**

DIAGNOSIS

- After a widely variable incubation period of days to months (or even years), patients may present with a prodrome of fever, headache, malaise, and personality changes lasting approximately 1 week. This is followed by agitated delirium, hydrophobia, and seizure ("furious rabies," 80%) or a meningitis syndrome with ascending paralysis ("paralytic rabies," 20%). Progression to coma and death is rapid.
- Cerebrospinal fluid (CSF) may show a lymphocytic pleocytosis.
- Diagnosis is best made by direct fluorescent antibody of a skin biopsy specimen taken from the nape of the neck above the hairline, polymerase chain reaction (PCR) of tissue or saliva, or serology. Sensitivity of all tests increases with time after symptom onset.

TREATMENT

- **Preexposure rabies prophylaxis** is indicated for persons at high risk, such as veterinarians, animal handlers, and certain travelers to areas where rabies is enzootic.[3] Vaccination should include three doses administered IM or intradermally on days 0, 7, and 21, or 28. Booster doses based on antibody titers are recommended for persons in certain high-risk categories.
- **Postexposure rabies prophylaxis** should be immediately given to any person who reports a nondomestic dog bite, or a scratch, bite, or contact with mucous membranes of skunks or raccoons. Additionally, prophylaxis is warranted for any person who is bitten by a bat or comes in contact with a bat and cannot rule out a bite. This includes situations in which a bat is found in the room of an infant or a person sleeping or incapacitated. Prophylaxis is not indicated if the bat is captured and tests negative for rabies. Further consultation with local public health officials may be required to determine the risk of exposure.
  - Bites of foxes and most other wild carnivores also warrant prophylaxis. Bites from rodents, hares, and livestock should be considered on a case-by-case basis, consulting with public health officials if there is concern that prophylaxis may be needed.
  - **Routine domestic dog and cat bites in the United States do not warrant immediate rabies prophylaxis unless the animal was displaying unusual behavior or signs of hydrophobia.** Instead, it is recommended that the local health department be contacted immediately; the pet is observed for 10 days for the development of signs of rabies.[3,5]
  - Soap solution and povidone iodine wound irrigation reduces the risk of rabies by 90%. Early suturing may increase the risk of rabies.
  - If the patient **has not had a rabies vaccination within the last 3 years**, rabies immune globulin (RIG) 20 IU/kg should be administered, injected as much as possible around the wound site, with the rest given IM. Rabies vaccine should be administered in the deltoid or thigh (away from the site of RIG injection) at days 0, 3, 7, and 14. Immunocompromised patients should receive an additional dose at day 28.
  - If the patient has been previously vaccinated against rabies, booster should be administered at days 0 and 3 only, without administration of RIG.
  - Survival after the development of disease is exceedingly rare, with only 15 cases published in the literature.[6,7] Nearly all had severe neurologic sequelae.

TICK-BORNE ILLNESSES

- Several human diseases are transmitted or caused by ticks. Two families of tick species can transmit human disease: *Ixodidae* (hard ticks) and *Argasidae* (soft ticks). All tick species have complex life cycles that involve progression from eggs to larvae (commonly known as seed ticks) to nymphs to adults. Blood meals are required for progression from stage to stage. Larvae, nymphs, and adults can all serve as vectors of infection while feeding on mammals, including humans. The soft ticks can survive for years in the adult form without taking blood meals.

- Diagnosis can be challenging, as <50% of the patients who are diagnosed with tick-borne illnesses recall having been bitten by a tick. A high level of clinical suspicion is thus necessary for patients living in or traveling to tick-endemic areas who present with compatible symptoms during warmer months. In most cases, serologic tests must be carefully used in the correct context of clinical presentation and epidemiologic information. **Coinfection with more than one tick-borne illness can occur** and can confuse the clinical presentation.
- **Prevention of tick bites is the most important preventative intervention.** This includes wearing light-colored, long-sleeved clothing, tucking pant legs into socks, application of DEET to skin and permethrin to clothing, and performing full-body tick checks after exposure to tick-infested areas.

Lyme Disease

GENERAL PRINCIPLES

- Lyme disease is the most frequently reported vector-borne disease in the United States, with 20,000 cases yearly. Most cases are reported between May and October.
- It is caused by the spirochete **Borrelia burgdorferi**, which is endemic in >15 US states but mostly occurs in three foci: the Northeast, the upper Midwest (Wisconsin and Minnesota), and the West (California and Oregon). It is also endemic in Eurasia.
- The principal vector in the Northeast and Upper Midwest is the deer tick *Ixodes scapularis*; in Western regions, it is the black-legged tick *Ixodes pacificus*. The infection is usually transmitted by the nymph stage, which is very small and consequently often unnoticed. In most cases, prolonged attachment (>36 h) is required for transmission of the infection. The overall risk of Lyme disease after a deer tick bite is 3.2% in areas of highest prevalence.[8,9]

Diagnosis

CLINICAL PRESENTATION

- Lyme disease has three distinct stages:
  - In the **early localized stage**, Lyme disease manifests with a rash (erythema migrans, EM) at the site of the tick bite in 70% to 80% of patients.[10] The most common sites are the thighs, groin, and axilla. There is significant variation in the final size and shape, but classically this begins as a nontender, red macule or papule that slowly expands to a final median diameter of about 15 cm. Central clearing occurs in larger lesions, causing the stereotypic "bull's-eye" appearance. This is frequently accompanied by influenza-like symptoms and regional lymphadenopathy. Headache and meningismus can sometimes be seen. Within 3 to 4 weeks, EM spontaneously resolves (range, 1-14 mo).
  - Within weeks to months after inoculation, multiple annular EM-like skin lesions may herald **early disseminated infection**, associated with more prominent fever and systemic symptoms. Malar rash, conjunctivitis, mild hepatitis, and migratory arthralgia without arthritis may also be seen. The most commonly involved end organs include the central nervous system (CNS) and the cardiovascular system.

- **Neuroborreliosis** occurs in 10% to 15% of untreated patients with early disseminated disease.[11] This can include cranial neuritis (most commonly unilateral or bilateral facial nerve palsy), lymphocytic meningitis, mononeuritis multiplex, motor and sensory radiculopathy, myositis, and cerebellar ataxia. These symptoms can occur in various combinations, are usually fluctuating, and may be accompanied by CSF abnormalities (lymphocytic pleocytosis and increased protein). Symptoms commonly improve within weeks to months, even in untreated patients.
  - **Cardiac involvement** occurs in 4% to 10% of untreated patients with early disseminated disease.[12] The most common abnormality is atrioventricular block (first-degree, Wenckebach, or transient complete heart block); rarely, diffuse myocardial involvement consistent with myopericarditis can occur.
- **Late persistent infection** most prominently affects the joints and CNS. Chronic skin manifestations of late Lyme disease are seen in Europe but not in the United States, except in immigrants. Late persistent symptoms develop months to years after untreated primary disease and are largely related to the immune response to borrelial surface proteins. As a result, the response to antibiotics is varied, and symptoms occasionally persist after successful eradication of the organism with antibiotic therapy.
  - **Lyme arthritis** occurs in approximately 60% of untreated patients, months after the onset of illness in the context of strong cellular and humoral immune responses to *B. burgdorferi*.[13] Patients may experience intermittent episodes of oligoarticular joint swelling, especially involving the knee. These episodes last from a few weeks to months, with periods of remission between episodes. Synovial fluid white blood cell counts (WBCs) range from 50,000 to 110,000 and are predominantly polymorphonuclear. *B. burgdorferi* PCR is positive in the synovial fluid or tissue. Chronic Lyme arthritis generally resolves spontaneously within several years; permanent joint damage is uncommon. Because of molecular mimicry with synovial tissue proteins, a minority of patients have persistent chronic arthritis (≥1 y of continuous joint inflammation) despite an adequate course of antibiotic therapy and clearance of the organism.
  - Untreated disease may progress to **chronic neuroborreliosis**, causing an axonal polyneuropathy, with spinal radicular pain or distal paresthesias. Lyme encephalopathy manifests as subtle cognitive defects and problems in mood, memory, or sleep. CSF inflammation is typically absent. Unlike Lyme arthritis, chronic neurologic Lyme can persist for >10 years if not treated.
- A small subset of patients continues to have subjective symptoms—mainly musculoskeletal pain, fatigue, and cognitive difficulties—which is referred to as "**post–Lyme disease syndrome**." These symptoms do not respond to additional or prolonged antibiotic therapy.

Diagnostic Testing

- Diagnosis of Lyme disease is difficult and relies on a combination of clinical presentation, epidemiology, and serologic studies. **Although Lyme should never be diagnosed based on subjective symptoms alone, the physical finding of EM in the appropriate geographic setting is pathognomonic for early Lyme disease.** *Borrelia* can be detected by PCR from a tissue biopsy of EM. Blood, joint, and CSF cultures are very insensitive and should not be used.
- **Suspected cases of late disease must be supported with serology** because clinical findings are often nonspecific. Enzyme-linked immunosorbent assay (ELISA) is used to detect IgG and IgM antibodies, followed by confirmation by Western blot. Pretest probability based on clinical syndrome, epidemiologic considerations, and physical findings is an important consideration.
  - IgM begins to rise at 2 weeks after infection and declines after 2 months. However, IgM should not be used to diagnose disease beyond 1 month of symptoms because of an unacceptably high false positive rate.

○ IgG rises at 6 to 8 weeks after infection and persists for life. A negative IgG titer rules out late disease. Early antibiotic treatment blocks the rise of antibody titers.

- Neuroborreliosis can be specifically confirmed by reference laboratories by demonstrating a CSF-to-serum Lyme antibody ratio of >1. In Lyme arthritis, PCR of the synovial fluid is often positive. Repeat PCR for test of cure is not recommended, as *Borrelia* DNA can often be detected after successful treatment.

TREATMENT

- Tick avoidance and removal of an embedded tick within 36 hours are the most important steps in prevention.
- Postexposure prophylaxis with a single dose of doxycycline 200 mg PO is 87% effective in preventing Lyme disease if given within 72 hours after a tick bite in hyperendemic areas.[9]
- The preferred oral regimen for treatment of most stages in nonpregnant adults is **doxycycline** 100 mg PO twice daily, in part because it can also treat other potentially cotransmitted infections (e.g., ehrlichiosis, anaplasmosis, Rocky Mountain spotted fever [RMSF]). Alternatives include azithromycin 500 mg PO daily, amoxicillin 500 mg PO three times daily, or cefuroxime 500 mg PO twice daily.
- Preferred parenteral regimens include ceftriaxone 2 g IV daily or penicillin G 3 to 4 million units IV every 4 hours.
- Treatment route and duration vary by clinical syndrome.
  ○ **Early disease** with EM: oral regimen for 14 days.
  ○ **Isolated cranial nerve palsy** without CSF abnormality: oral regimen for 14 days.
  ○ **Neuroborreliosis or high-degree atrioventricular block:** parenteral regimen for 14 to 28 days.
  ○ **Late arthritis:** oral regimen for 28 days. An oral or parenteral regimen may be repeated once in the case of recurrent arthritis after treatment is completed. Chronic arthritis after treatment may require anti-inflammatory medications or surgical synovectomy.
- After appropriate antibiotic therapy, chronic subjective symptoms of post-Lyme disease syndrome **do not respond to further antibiotic therapy** as compared with placebo. These patients should be treated symptomatically rather than with prolonged courses of antibiotics.

SPECIAL CONSIDERATIONS

- Southern Tick-Associated Rash Illness is a syndrome resembling early Lyme disease that has been associated with lone star tick (*Amblyomma americanum*) bites. No causative agent has been identified.
- The rash resembles EM, except the central clearing is more prominent and the major symptom is fatigue.
- Lone star ticks are distributed across the Southern and Eastern United States. Patients with a compatible syndrome and epidemiologic exposure can be treated with the same antibiotic regimens as early Lyme disease although efficacy is uncertain.

Rocky Mountain Spotted Fever

GENERAL PRINCIPLES

- RMSF is the most common rickettsial disease in the United States, caused by the obligate intracellular gram-negative bacterium *Rickettsia rickettsii*.
- The disease manifests as a diffuse vasculitis and if untreated can be fulminant and fatal.

- The endemic areas are east of the Rocky Mountains, most commonly in the Carolinas, Maryland, Oklahoma, and Virginia. The principal vectors are the dog tick (*Dermacentor variabilis*) in the East and wood tick (*Dermacentor andersoni*) in the West. Approximately 600 to 1200 cases occur throughout the United States each year, with peak incidence in April through September, although winter cases can be seen in southern states.

DIAGNOSIS

Clinical Presentation

- The presentation can be nonspecific and is easily mistaken for a viral syndrome, drug allergy, or meningococcemia. Around 60% of cases recall a history of tick bite.[14]
- After incubation (2-14 d), initial symptoms include fever, malaise, myalgia, headache, nausea, diarrhea, and abdominal pain.
- Approximately 2 to 7 days after symptom onset, the classic rash begins as red macules that initially have a centripetal distribution on the extremities, including the palms of the hands and soles of the feet. The rash then spreads centrally, and macules can transform into petechiae or purpura. Around 10% of cases can occur without the classic rash, particularly among African Americans and the elderly.[15,16]
- As the disease progresses, conjunctivitis, lymphadenopathy, and hepatosplenomegaly are common physical examination findings. Severe disease can include aseptic meningitis, renal failure, myocarditis, acute respiratory distress syndrome, and digital ischemia. Those at higher risk for these complications include men, the elderly, alcoholics, and patients with glucose-6-phosphate dehydrogenase deficiency.

Diagnostic Testing

- The diagnosis can be made pathologically by immunofluorescence staining or PCR of skin biopsies.
- Retrospective serologic diagnosis of RMSF requires demonstration of a fourfold convalescent rise in antibodies against the rickettsial organisms by latex agglutination or immunofluorescence.
- Routine laboratory findings are varied and nonspecific, including hyponatremia, elevated creatinine, elevated transaminases and bilirubin, anemia, thrombocytopenia, and coagulopathy. The peripheral WBC count can vary widely.

TREATMENT

- In heavily endemic areas, there should be a low threshold for empiric treatment because of the potential for rapid lethality and a lack of accurate rapid tests. Mortality is 22% without treatment and 6% with appropriate treatment.[17]
- **The drug of choice for all ages is doxycycline**, 100 mg PO twice daily for 7 days or until 3 days after fever resolution. IV doxycycline should be used for severe disease.[17] Doxycycline has the advantage of covering unrecognized tick-borne coinfections such as ehrlichiosis, anaplasmosis, and Lyme disease. Chloramphenicol is a second-line agent.
- Pediatric cases should be treated with doxycycline because of the potential for rapid lethality and the low likelihood of tooth staining with a 7-day course of doxycycline.
- Tetracyclines are generally contraindicated in pregnancy; however, they may be considered for severe RMSF. IV chloramphenicol (50-100 mg/kg per day in four divided doses) is an alternative option for severe disease, although chloramphenicol may be associated with gray baby syndrome if given during the third trimester. Oral chloramphenicol (500 mg every 6 hours) is not available in the United States.
- No vaccine is available, and there is no consensus on postexposure prophylaxis for RMSF after a tick bite.

Human Ehrlichiosis and Anaplasmosis

GENERAL PRINCIPLES

- Human ehrlichiosis is a severe multisystem disease caused by small intracellular gram-negative rods. **Human monocytic ehrlichiosis (HME)** is caused by monocyte infection with *Ehrlichia chaffeensis*, whereas **human granulocytic anaplasmosis (HGA)** is due to granulocyte infection with *Anaplasma phagocytophilum*. *Ehrlichia ewingii* is an unusual cause of ehrlichiosis seen primarily in immunocompromised patients.
- Small mammals are the natural reservoir for these organisms. Geographic distribution of disease follows that of the tick vectors. *E. chaffeensis* is transmitted by *A. americanum* (lone star tick) and may also be occasionally transmitted by other tick vectors such as *D. variabilis* (dog tick). *A. phagocytophilum* is transmitted by the same vectors as Lyme disease: on the East Coast the deer tick (*I. scapularis*) and on the West Coast the western black-legged tick (*I. pacificus*).

DIAGNOSIS

Clinical Presentation

- Definitive diagnosis can be difficult and may involve significant delay. The recognition of a compatible clinical syndrome in a patient from an endemic region during the spring or summer should provide the basis for initiating empiric therapy while awaiting laboratory confirmation.
- **HME and HGA are nearly identical in their clinical presentation.** Initial symptoms typically include fever, severe headache, and myalgias. Nausea and vomiting are frequent; abdominal pain is rare. Cough and arthralgias are also common.
- Severe disease is seen most often in immunocompromised patients. It can manifest with mental status changes, renal failure, respiratory failure, heart failure, and/or disseminated intravascular coagulation (DIC).
- A faint maculopapular rash occurs in approximately 30% of HME cases but is very unusual in HGA. Petechiae are uncommon unless they are a result of thrombocytopenia or DIC. Rash is much more common in children, occurring in approximately two-thirds of infections.[17]
- Hepatomegaly and lymphadenopathy are rare physical findings.

Diagnostic Testing

- Diagnosis is typically made by PCR of the blood or serology (a single indirect fluorescent antibody titer of >1:256 or fourfold convalescent rise 13 d after the onset of symptoms).
- Examination of the buffy coat can allow direct observation of morulae in the cytoplasm of monocytes in HME or granulocytes in HGA, which is diagnostic. **Direct observation of morulae is common in HGA but unusual in HME.** Culture is extremely low yield.
- Routine laboratory findings are nonspecific and similar to those of other tick-borne illnesses. However, characteristic laboratory findings including leukopenia and thrombocytopenia, notably without anemia, and mildly elevated transaminases are frequently present and suggestive of infection when patients present with a compatible illness in endemic areas during the summer.
- If clinically compatible findings are present and epidemiologically appropriate, coinfection with other tick-borne illnesses should be considered and the appropriate testing performed.

TREATMENT

- **Doxycycline** 100 mg PO or IV every 12 hours is the drug of choice for HGA and HME, even in children.[8,17,18] This also provides treatment for RMSF, which presents similarly and could potentially be cotransmitted by dog ticks. Treatment should be continued for 10 days or at least 3 days once afebrile, whichever is longer.
- Rifampin and chloramphenicol are second-line agents in patients who cannot receive doxycycline. In pregnancy, rifampin can be used for mild cases of ehrlichiosis; however, as for RMSF, doxycycline should still be strongly considered to treat life-threatening infections.

Babesiosis

GENERAL PRINCIPLES

- Infection by protozoa of the genus *Babesia* (primarily *B. microti* in the United States and *B. divergens* in Europe) occurs during the summer and fall months. This intraerythrocytic infection causes a febrile malaria-like syndrome with hemolysis.
- The primary tick vectors are ixodid ticks; therefore, coinfection with Lyme disease or HGA is possible and should be considered when evaluating a patient with an atypical presentation in the appropriate epidemiologic setting.

DIAGNOSIS

Clinical Presentation

- Clinical presentation of *B. microti* ranges from an asymptomatic infection to severe and life-threatening disease with high parasitemia. Incubation typically ranges from 1 to 6 weeks after inoculation by a feeding tick. *B. divergens* tends to present as fulminant life-threatening illness.
- **Mild illness** is characterized by gradual onset of high fever, fatigue, and malaise. Other associated symptoms can include headache, myalgia, arthralgia, cough, neck stiffness, nausea, vomiting, or diarrhea.
- **Severe illness** is usually seen in older patients, those with splenectomy or are immunocompromised, and patients who are coinfected with *B. burgdorferi*. Potential complications of severe disease include DIC, acute respiratory distress syndrome, renal failure, and splenic infarction.
- Physical examination will reveal high fever in most patients, which can be intermittent or constant. Hepatosplenomegaly may be noted. Other findings such as jaundice and splinter hemorrhages are unusual except in severe cases. Rash is unusual and should prompt evaluation for Lyme coinfection.

Diagnostic Testing

- Diagnostic testing should include routine blood chemistries, blood counts, and examination of peripheral smears. Routine urinalysis may reveal hemoglobinuria. Liver enzymes are typically elevated.
- Common hematologic findings include a variable WBC count, thrombocytopenia, and evidence of hemolytic anemia, with low hematocrit, low haptoglobin, high total bilirubin, and reticulocytosis. Peripheral smear may reveal parasitemia as high as 80% in asplenic patients. Severe disease manifestations correlate with severe anemia (<10 mg/dL) and high parasitemia (>10%), although the level of parasitemia does not predict the severity of anemia.

- Laboratory confirmation is made by PCR-based detection of parasitemia or by microscopic examination of Wright- or Giemsa-stained thin blood smears by experienced personnel. Some *Babesia* forms, especially the ring forms of *B. microti*, can appear similar in appearance to those of *Plasmodium falciparum*; attention to distinguishing features, such as the absence of schizonts and gametocytes, and the characteristic appearance of merozoite "Maltese Cross" tetrads help to confirm *Babesia*. Serology using indirect immunofluorescence with a titer ≥1:64 can be useful to confirm the diagnosis after clearance of parasitemia. Concurrent testing for Lyme disease or HGA should also be considered if the epidemiologic setting is appropriate.

TREATMENT

- Treatment is indicated for patients who have parasitemia detected by PCR or direct microscopy and should not be administered for seropositivity alone.
- Treatment of *B. microti* requires combination therapy with **atovaquone** 750 mg PO twice daily plus **azithromycin** 250 mg PO daily after 500 mg to 1 g oral loading dose on day 1 (mild disease) or quinine 650 mg PO every 6 to 8 hours plus clindamycin 300 to 600 mg IV every 6 hours or 600 mg PO three times daily (mild or severe disease). Immunocompromised patients with mild disease should receive atovaquone and high-dose azithromycin 500 mg to 1 g IV or PO daily.
- *B. divergens* should be treated as for severe disease.[8]
- Mild disease should be treated for 7 to 10 days. Severe disease should be treated for 2 weeks beyond clearance of parasitemia. Refractory or relapsing disease and immunocompromised patients should be treated for at least 6 weeks, including 2 weeks beyond clearance of parasitemia.
- While treating severe disease, daily examination of hematocrit and peripheral smear should be performed to follow response to therapy.
- Partial or complete exchange transfusion should be considered for severe disease with high-grade parasitemia (>10%), severe anemia (<10 mg/dL), or evidence of organ failure.
- Symptoms that persist 3 months after completion of treatment should be evaluated by repeat PCR and thin smear examination to rule out relapsing or persistent infection. This typically occurs in asplenic or immunocompromised patients.

Other Tick-Borne Illnesses

- **Tick-borne relapsing fever** is caused by many species of the spirochete *Borrelia* transmitted in remote areas of the western United States.
  - A 2- to 3-mm eschar develops at the site of the tick bite, and high fever begins after an incubation period of approximately 1 week. The febrile period lasts 3 to 6 days and is followed by a rapid defervescence.
  - Rash develops as the fever resolves in up to half of the patients.
  - If untreated, patients will relapse after an afebrile period of approximately 8 days, with an average of three to five relapses.
  - Diagnosis is by blood culture or by Giemsa- or Wright-stained thick and thin blood smears.
  - Treatment of mild cases is 10 days of tetracycline or erythromycin. Neurologic symptoms should be treated with parenteral penicillin or ceftriaxone for 14 to 28 days.
- **Tick paralysis** is a noninfectious, rapidly ascending paralysis caused by a neurotoxin that affects acetylcholine transmission at the neuromuscular junction. It is secreted into the bloodstream by an actively feeding, engorged *Dermacentor* tick.
  - The illness is rapid in onset, within hours of the first tick exposure.
  - Additional symptoms include ataxia, loss of tendon reflexes, and late-stage cranial nerve and diaphragmatic muscle weakness.

○ Mortality is approximately 10%, and children are more often and more severely affected.

○ Tick paralysis is often confused with Guillain–Barré syndrome; however, the rapid course of the paralysis and the concomitant ataxia differentiate it from Guillain–Barré and other acute paralytic illnesses.

○ The potentially fatal illness can be completely cured within hours by removal of the offending tick.

○ A variant caused by *Ixodes holocyclus* in Australia should be treated with antitoxin before removal to avoid transient worsening of symptoms after removal.

Other Zoonotic Infections

Bartonellosis

GENERAL PRINCIPLES

- Bartonellosis is caused by six species of *Bartonella*, a small, fastidious intracellular gram-negative bacillus. *Bartonella henselae* and *Bartonella quintana* cause most human diseases in the United States.
- Children are the primary risk group for **cat-scratch disease** (CSD). Special populations include the homeless, who can develop louse-borne **urban trench fever**, and patients with advanced HIV, who can develop complications such as **bacillary angiomatosis and peliosis hepatis**.
- Cats are the major reservoir for *B. henselae*.
- *B. quintana* is transmitted by the body louse. Humans are the primary reservoir of this pathogen, which disproportionally affects socially vulnerable populations such as the urban homeless.
- Transmission occurs by scratches (especially by kittens) and bites, as well as bites from lice, fleas, and ticks.

DIAGNOSIS

Clinical Presentation

- *B. henselae* primarily causes CSD. This usually begins as a single or few vesicular, papular, or pustular lesions, appearing 3 to 10 days after a cat bite or scratch. This is followed by painful regional lymphadenitis (usually a single fluctuant cervical or axillary node) and mild constitutional symptoms, including fever. In patients with systemic disease or prolonged fever, lymphadenopathy is less common. Hepatosplenomegaly is sometimes seen.
- CSD is a common cause of prolonged **fever of unknown origin** (FUO) in children.
- *B. quintana* is the cause of urban trench fever, an undifferentiated febrile illness with headache, body pain, and conjunctival injection. This can be a single self-limited episode or, more classically, a chronic debilitating relapsing illness with episodes that last around 5 days each.
- Unusual manifestations of *Bartonella* infection may occur in 5% to 10% of cases, which can include culture-negative endocarditis, oculoglandular infections (especially uveitis), arthritis, and neurologic syndromes.
- Endocarditis and bacteremia may be associated with conjunctival injection, maculopapular rash, lymphadenopathy, or hepatosplenomegaly. Leukocytosis and thrombocytopenia may be present. Native valves are most commonly affected in endocarditis.
- Neurologic deficits are uncommon but can carry significant morbidity. Encephalopathy can manifest with headache, mental status changes, seizure, and focal or generalized neurologic deficits including hemiplegia and ataxia. Other unusual sequelae are retinal neuritis and transverse myelitis.

- Patients with advanced HIV can develop unusual forms of disseminated bartonellosis. **Bacillary angiomatosis** is characterized by dark violaceous subcutaneous vascular nodules, which may be numerous. These **can be easily mistaken for the lesions of Kaposi sarcoma**. Visceral, neurologic, and bone involvement of bacillary angiomatosis can be seen. **Peliosis hepatis** is a visceral manifestation of disseminated bartonellosis that presents as vomiting, diarrhea, hepatosplenomegaly, and fever.

Diagnostic Testing

- **PCR** of tissue is very sensitive and specific. It is of particular use on heart valve tissue to diagnose culture-negative endocarditis due to *Bartonella* species, as it is not affected by prior use of antibiotics.
- **Serology** can be very useful for diagnosis of CSD. Positive IgM (≥1:16) or high IgG titer (>1:256) suggests current *Bartonella* infection. Decreases in antibody titer should follow 10 to 14 days after antibiotic treatment. An IgG titer of >1:800 suggests chronic infection.
- Cross-reactivity occurs among *Bartonella*, *Chlamydia*, and *Coxiella* species. This can lead to confusion between similar disease presentations of the various organisms, such as inguinal CSD and lymphogranuloma venereum.
- False negatives may occur in patients who are immunocompromised.
- Culture is difficult and low yield, requiring special media and growth conditions, and taking from 2 to 6 weeks to incubate. It is therefore not useful in the diagnosis of routine CSD; however, it may play a role in the diagnosis of other clinical manifestations, such as FUO, encephalitis, endocarditis, peliosis, or bacillary angiomatosis. Lysis-centrifugation (isolator) tubes can increase the yield of blood cultures. In vitro antibiotic susceptibility does not correlate well to clinical response.
- Tissue biopsy can be helpful. Lymph node biopsy can reveal granulomata with stellate necrosis, and the organism can be seen with silver stains. Bacillary angiomatosis and peliosis hepatis have characteristic patterns of blood vessel proliferation on pathologic examination.

TREATMENT

- CSD is almost always self-limited; however, symptoms can last several weeks. Treatment with antibiotics is reserved for patients with extensive or painful lymphadenopathy. The drug of choice for limited CSD is **azithromycin** 500 mg PO daily on day 1 followed by 4 days of 250 mg PO daily. Alternative medications include erythromycin, doxycycline, trimethoprim–sulfamethoxazole, or a fluoroquinolone.[19]
- Disseminated CSD or trench fever requires at least 4 weeks of therapy. Peliosis hepatis and bacillary angiomatosis require 3 to 4 months of therapy. Retinitis is treated for 4 to 6 weeks with a combination of rifampin and doxycycline or azithromycin.[19]
- Endocarditis is treated with ceftriaxone and gentamicin and/or doxycycline for 6 weeks. Valve replacement is often required.[19]

Brucellosis

GENERAL PRINCIPLES

- Human brucellosis is caused by a group of small, aerobic, nonmotile, non–spore-forming, intracellular gram-negative coccobacilli belonging to the genus *Brucella*. The most important animal reservoirs are ruminant animals such as cattle and goats.
- Transmission occurs by exposure to infected animals (especially placental tissue and vaginal secretions) or consumption of contaminated dairy products.

- Human disease in the United States is typically diagnosed in Latin American migrant workers or travelers who consume **unpasteurized cheese and milk products. Abattoir workers, farmers, and veterinarians** are also at increased risk.
- Endemic disease is found in the Mediterranean, Middle East, and Latin American regions.

DIAGNOSIS

Clinical Presentation

- The clinical manifestations can vary significantly, from an undulant undifferentiated febrile illness to focal complications of large joints, genitourinary, neurologic, cardiac, and hepatosplenic systems.
- Untreated subacute and chronic infection can present months to more than 1 year after inoculation.
- Manifestations can be seen in any organ system. However, most patients with acute disease report sudden or gradual onset of malaise, high fever, chills, sweats, fatigue, weakness, arthralgias, and myalgias. Symptoms of extreme fatigue, malodorous sweat, and depression are classically associated with this disease, can be severe, and can persist after successful treatment.
- Physical examination may include splenomegaly and lymphadenopathy (usually axillary, cervical, and supraclavicular). Osteoarticular complaints are common, and sacroiliitis or arthritis of large weight-bearing joints is characteristic. Orchitis may also occur in infected men.

Diagnostic Testing

- Laboratory findings are nonspecific but can include anemia, thrombocytopenia, and elevated liver enzymes. WBC counts can vary significantly.
- **Culture is considered the gold standard but is difficult** and yields decrease with duration of infection. Cultures may be observed for ≥4 weeks, although most cultures will turn positive within 16 days by modern techniques.[20] Culture of bone marrow aspirate and use of lysis-centrifugation tubes can improve yield. When brucellosis is suspected, the laboratory should be alerted so special precautions can be implemented to prevent aerosol infection of laboratory workers.
- **Serology** is an insensitive method of detection; agglutination titer of >1:160 or fourfold change in titer indicates infection. ELISA is more sensitive but must be confirmed by agglutination assay. Relapse can be detected by demonstrating a rise in agglutination titer.

TREATMENT

- Treatment requires combination antibiotic therapy that can achieve good intracellular penetration. The best clinical outcomes are seen with **doxycycline** 100 mg PO twice daily **plus rifampin** 600 to 900 mg PO daily for 6 weeks, **plus gentamicin** 5 mg/kg daily for 7 days.[21,22]
- Trimethoprim-sulfamethoxazole plus an aminoglycoside is the preferred treatment for children aged <8 years. Pregnant women have been successfully treated with rifampin 900 mg PO daily as monotherapy.

Tularemia

GENERAL PRINCIPLES

- The small gram-negative coccobacillus *Francisella tularensis* is enzootic in rabbits and other small rodent reservoirs in the United States.

- It can be transmitted to humans in a variety of ways: contact with infected animal tissues (e.g., skinning rabbits), inhalation of aerosolized particles, contact with contaminated food or water, and bites of infected ticks, mammals, mosquitoes, or deer flies.
- Approximately 50% of cases are attributed to bites from *A. americanum*, *D. andersoni*, and *D. variabilis* ticks.
- Incidence is declining in the United States. Most cases are reported in the Midwest, particularly Oklahoma, Missouri, and Arkansas.
- Inadvertent spread can occur in the microbiology laboratory setting. Person-to-person transmission does not occur.

DIAGNOSIS

Clinical Presentation

- The clinical manifestations of tularemia depend on the route of inoculation.
  - **Ulceroglandular:** Regional lymphadenopathy and necrotic, painful, erythematous ulcers occur at the site of inoculation.
  - **Glandular:** Tender, localized lymphadenopathy without skin or mucosal involvement.
  - **Oculoglandular:** Painful conjunctivitis with preauricular, submandibular, or cervical lymphadenopathy secondary to conjunctival inoculation by contaminated fingers, splashes, or aerosols. Vision loss is rare.
  - **Typhoidal/Systemic:** A more severe febrile illness that manifests with chills, headache, myalgias, sore throat, anorexia, nausea, vomiting, diarrhea, abdominal pain, and cough. Pulmonary involvement is common. Severe cases can progress to hyponatremia, rhabdomyolysis, renal failure, and sepsis. Lymphadenopathy and skin involvement are absent.
  - **Pharyngeal:** Sore throat, cervical and retropharyngeal lymphadenopathy, and, rarely, a mild pseudomembranous pharyngitis result from direct pharyngeal contact with contaminated food, water, or droplets.
  - **GI:** Persistent, fulminant diarrhea secondary to consumption of contaminated food or water; can be fatal.
  - **Pneumonic:** Lobar or diffuse pneumonia secondary to inhalation of the organism (rare) or hematologic spread of any of the above forms, especially ulceroglandular or typhoidal.
- In general, initial systemic manifestations include fever, chills, and low back pain. Temperature–pulse dissociation is a classic finding. Multiple symptom complexes may occur simultaneously.

Diagnostic Testing

- Diagnosis is usually made serologically with any one titer of >1:160 or a fourfold increase in convalescent titers.
- *F. tularensis* can be grown from a number of different specimens but is difficult to culture and is rarely seen on Gram stain. Moreover, the laboratory should be forewarned when tularemia is suspected, as the organism can be transmitted to laboratory workers by aerosol from actively growing cultures.

TREATMENT

- **The treatment of choice is streptomycin,** 15 mg/kg IM every 12 hours for 10 days. Gentamicin 5 mg/kg IV daily is nearly as effective. Other aminoglycosides are also excellent therapeutic choices.[23]
- **Fluoroquinolones** are rapidly being accepted as good alternative therapies.
- Relapses are more common after treatment with tetracyclines and chloramphenicol monotherapies. Cephalosporins are ineffective.
- Tularemia meningitis should be treated with an aminoglycoside plus IV chloramphenicol.

Leptospirosis

GENERAL PRINCIPLES

- Leptospirosis is **presumed to be the most ubiquitous zoonosis worldwide**. Most disease is observed in the tropical developing world, especially in the Americas and in Asia.
- Infected animal reservoirs, particularly rats, livestock, and dogs, become infected with spirochetes of the genus *Leptospira* and shed the organism in urine, where it is highly concentrated. Direct contact with infected animals or contaminated water or soil leads to human infection.
- This disease is endemic in rural subsistence farmers, and seasonal epidemics can be seen in urban slum environments as a result of flooding and poor sanitation. In the developed world, risk groups include farmers, abattoir workers, and veterinarians. Additionally, recreational exposure to contaminated water can cause sporadic or clustered disease. Sporadic cases are also reported in the urban poor in the United States.
- Most US cases are found in Hawaii.

DIAGNOSIS

Clinical Presentation

- Clinical presentation after a 5- to 14-day incubation period ranges from subclinical or undifferentiated febrile illness to life-threatening disease with multiorgan failure. This disease is characteristically biphasic, with an early nonspecific febrile phase, followed by progression to severe late manifestations in a minority of patients.
- **Early-phase** symptoms typically begin with abrupt onset of high fever, severe myalgias, and frontal headache. Other associated symptoms may include abdominal pain, nausea, vomiting, diarrhea, or cough.
- **Late-phase** disease occurs in 5% to 15% of patients and can include life-threatening complications such as shock, severe hemorrhage, respiratory failure, myocarditis, and severe nonoliguric renal failure associated with electrolyte wasting.
  - **Weil disease** is a severe form of late-phase disease that is characterized by a triad of jaundice, acute renal failure, and hemorrhage.
  - Acute respiratory distress syndrome and leptospirosis pulmonary hemorrhage syndrome, characterized by massive pulmonary hemorrhage and respiratory failure, are increasingly recognized complications.
  - Anicteric late-phase disease is milder and self-limited, typically characterized by abrupt fever, myalgias, and intense headache with or without aseptic meningitis.
- Physical examination may reveal hepatosplenomegaly or lymphadenopathy in a minority of patients. The finding of **conjunctival suffusion** (i.e., hyperemia of the conjunctival vessels and chemosis) is a pathognomonic finding that is seen in 30% of cases.[24] Jaundice is a poor prognostic sign and should prompt observation for development of acute renal failure and hemorrhage.

Diagnostic Testing

- Routine diagnostic testing in early-phase illness is nonspecific.
- In late-phase disease, laboratory studies may reveal severe thrombocytopenia and anemia, but minimally abnormal coagulation studies, even in the case of severe hemorrhage. WBC count is variable. Chemistry studies may reveal severe renal failure, as well as hypokalemia and other electrolyte derangements. Total bilirubin is typically elevated out of proportion to serum transaminases and alkaline phosphatase.
- Laboratory confirmation is challenging, in most settings requiring a fourfold rise in **antibody titers by microagglutination testing** (MAT) **or culture of the organism** from blood, urine, or CSF. Both of these methods provide only retrospective confirmation, as culture is difficult and can take several weeks.

- A single acute-phase MAT titer of >1:100 is indicative of infection; however, it may reflect prior infection in endemic settings.
- Detection of IgM by ELISA or immunofluorescence testing can also provide supportive evidence of acute infection.
- PCR is highly sensitive, especially during early infection, but is not widely available.

TREATMENT

- Management should include aggressive supportive care and vigilance for severe complications. Severe disease requires hospitalization, and icteric leptospirosis requires intensive care unit management with cardiac monitoring. Daily or continuous dialysis is an important component of management when renal failure occurs.
- Mild leptospirosis can be treated orally with **doxycycline** 100 mg twice daily or amoxicillin 500 mg three times daily.[25]
- Severe leptospirosis should be treated with IV **penicillin** 1.5 million units every 6 hours or **ceftriaxone** 1 g daily.[26] A Jarisch–Herxheimer reaction can occur but is typically mild.
- Chemoprophylaxis with doxycycline offers an alternative prevention strategy for persons with exposure in high-risk areas of endemic disease.[27]

Plague

GENERAL PRINCIPLES

- Plague is caused by the gram-negative bacillus *Yersinia pestis*.
- Naturally acquired plague occurs rarely in the southwestern and western United States after exposure to infected animals.

DIAGNOSIS

- Plague takes one of three forms:
  - **Bubonic.** Local painful lymphadenitis (bubo) and fever (15% case fatality ratio)
  - **Septicemic** disease. Can cause peripheral necrosis and DIC (i.e., "black death"). Usually from progression of bubonic disease (30%-50% case fatality ratio)
  - **Pneumonic.** Severe pneumonia with hemoptysis preceded by initial influenza-like illness (50% case fatality ratio, nearing 100% when treatment is delayed). Pneumonic disease can be transmitted from person to person and would be expected after inhalation of aerosolized *Y. pestis*
- Diagnosis is confirmed by isolation of *Y. pestis* from blood, sputum, or CSF. Local infection control and public health departments should be notified immediately when plague is suspected.

TREATMENT

- Treatment should start at first suspicion of plague as rapid initiation of antibiotics improves survival.
- Agents of choice are **gentamicin** 5 mg/kg IV/IM daily or a 2 mg/kg loading dose then 1.7 mg/kg IV/IM every 8 hours with appropriate drug level monitoring; **ciprofloxacin** 400 mg IV every 8 to 12 hours; **levofloxacin** 500 mg IV once daily; or **moxifloxacin** 400 mg IV once daily.[28]
- Alternatives include streptomycin, doxycycline, and chloramphenicol.
- Oral therapy can be started after clinical improvement, for a total course of 10 to 14 days or until 2 days after the fever subsides, whichever is longer.

- **Postexposure prophylaxis** is recommended for close contacts of pneumonic plague patients or persons with direct contact with infected body fluids or tissues. Recommended regimens are doxycycline 100 mg PO twice daily or ciprofloxacin 500 mg PO twice daily for 7 days after exposure.[28]

Anthrax

GENERAL PRINCIPLES

- Spores from the gram-positive *Bacillus anthracis* germinate at the site of entry into the body, causing inhalational, cutaneous, or GI anthrax.
- Natural transmission can occur through butchering and eating infected animals, usually leading to cutaneous ("Woolsorter's disease") and GI disease.

DIAGNOSIS

- Inhalational anthrax (45% case fatality rate) presents initially with influenza-like illness, GI symptoms, or both, followed by fulminant respiratory distress and multiorgan failure.
- Cutaneous anthrax is characterized by a painless black eschar with surrounding edema.
- Diagnosis of inhalational disease is suggested by a widened mediastinum without infiltrates on chest radiography and confirmed by blood culture. Cutaneous and GI disease are also diagnosed by culture of blood or tissue. Local infection control and public health officials should be immediately notified for confirmed cases.

TREATMENT

- Immediate antibiotic initiation on first suspicion of inhalational anthrax reduces mortality.
- Empiric therapy should be either **ciprofloxacin** 400 mg IV every 12 hours or **doxycycline** 100 mg IV every 12 hours **plus two other antibiotics that are active against *B. anthracis*** (e.g., penicillin, clindamycin, and/or vancomycin).[29]
- Oral therapy with ciprofloxacin 500 mg PO twice daily or doxycycline 100 mg PO twice daily and one other active agent should be started after improvement and continued for 60 days to reduce the risk of delayed spore germination.
- Uncomplicated cutaneous anthrax can be treated with oral ciprofloxacin 500 mg twice daily or doxycycline 100 mg twice daily for the same duration.
- **Postexposure prophylaxis** is recommended for anyone exposed to anthrax. Dual therapy with ciprofloxacin 500 mg twice daily and doxycycline 100 mg twice daily is recommended for 60 days after exposure. Clindamycin, penicillin VK, or amoxicillin are alternatives if the organism is susceptible.[30]

Q Fever

GENERAL PRINCIPLES

- Q fever is caused by *Coxiella burnetii*, an obligate intracellular gram-negative bacillus found in the feces and body fluids of infected animals, most commonly ruminant animals. Placental tissue has especially high concentrations of the organism.
- Infection is uncommon in the United States but widespread throughout the world.
- Infection typically occurs via inhalation of infected material, such as dust contaminated by infected fluids or tissue. Risk groups include farmers, veterinarians, and abattoir workers.

DIAGNOSIS

Clinical Presentation

- **Acute Q fever** is characterized by the abrupt onset of high fever, severe headache, and influenza-like symptoms. Chest pain and GI distress are also seen. Liver function abnormalities and pneumonia are common sequelae of acute Q fever. **Most acute infections will resolve spontaneously.**
- **Chronic Q fever** can occur long after the initial infection, often years later. *C. burnetii* endocarditis is a cause of **culture-negative endocarditis** and most commonly affects patients with prosthetic or otherwise abnormal heart valves or patients with compromised immunity. Other forms of chronic Q fever include pneumonia, hepatitis, and chronic fatigue. **Chronic Q fever carries high morbidity and mortality.**

Diagnostic Testing

- Diagnosis is made by **serology** to detect one of two antigenic phases. Antibodies directed against phase II antigens appear rapidly and high antibody levels indicate acute Q fever. Phase I antibodies indicate continuous exposure to *C. burnetii* antigens and are highest in chronic Q fever. Both phase I and phase II antibodies persist long after the initial infection.
- Local infection control and the public health department should be immediately notified for confirmed cases.

TREATMENT

- Treat acute Q fever with **doxycycline** 100 mg PO twice daily for 2 to 3 weeks. Treatment is most effective if initiated within the first days of illness. Ciprofloxacin and a macrolide with or without rifampin are alternatives. Treatment should be restarted if symptoms relapse.[31]
- Chronic Q fever requires prolonged therapy with **doxycycline 100 mg PO twice daily and hydroxychloroquine** 200 mg PO three times daily for at least 18 months, until phase I IgG titer falls to below 1:200. This may require 3 years of therapy or more.[32]

Ectoparasites

Scabies

GENERAL PRINCIPLES

- Scabies is caused by the human mite *Sarcoptes scabiei*.
- Symptoms are caused by host hypersensitivity to the eggs and excreta of gravid females, who create linear burrows into the skin.
- Transmission of scabies results from close person-to-person contact. The mite does not survive >24 hours without a host, therefore, transmission by sharing contaminated clothing or bedding does occur but is not efficient.
- Although scabies is more common in persons living in crowded conditions and poverty, it is not limited to this population; outbreaks occur in households, hospitals, nursing homes, and day care centers.

DIAGNOSIS

- The clinical presentation is characterized by an **intensely pruritic rash**. Small excoriated papular lesions are typically found in the finger webs, wrists, elbows, and along skin folds. **Burrows may be noted, particularly in the finger webs.** Pruritus is typically worse at night or after a hot shower or bath. In the immunocompromised, a severe form called "Norwegian scabies" can occur.

- Diagnosis requires identification of the organisms or their eggs and fecal pellets. This is best accomplished by placing a drop of mineral oil on a lesion, scraping it with a scalpel, and examining the specimen under a microscope. Burrows may be identified by applying dark ink from a felt-tip or fountain pen. After cleansing with an alcohol pad, the ink may be partially retained in the burrows.

TREATMENT

- The treatment of choice for all patients older than 2 months is **5% permethrin cream**, which should be applied from the chin to the toes and washed off after 8 hours. This should be repeated 1 to 2 weeks after the first treatment.[33]
- Washing all bedding and potentially infected clothes in hot water can prevent reinfection.
- A single dose of **ivermectin** 200 μg/kg PO is also effective and may be helpful in refractory infestations or for immunocompromised patients with severe manifestations. A second dose can be repeated in 10 days.[33]

Pediculosis (LICE)

GENERAL PRINCIPLES

- Pediculosis is the term given to infestation by lice of the genus *Pediculus* or *Phthirus*. There are three species in these two genera that are most often implicated in human disease: *Pediculus humanus corporis* (the body louse), *P. humanus capitis* (the head louse), and *Phthirus pubis* (the crab louse).
- Lice are wingless insects with three pairs of legs, each terminating with a curved claw. Lice grasp the clothes or hairs of their hosts and obtain a blood meal. The bite is painless; symptoms are caused by hypersensitivity to the insects' saliva. Sensitization and development of symptoms occur approximately 1 month after the initial infestation.
- Transmission of lice also results from close person-to-person contact; certain populations are more affected by each of these organisms (e.g., body lice in those with poor hygiene, head lice in school children, and pubic lice in sexually active individuals).

DIAGNOSIS

- The clinical presentation depends on the site of infection; on the head, it is characterized by localized pruritus and crusted lesions. Body lice and pubic lice result in discrete areas of erythematous or bluish maculopapular rash.
- Diagnosis of pediculosis is made by identifying the eggs, or "nits," at the sites of the lesions. The use of a magnifying glass may be helpful in differentiating the nits from other artifacts, such as dandruff, dried hair spray, or casts of sebum from the hair follicle.

TREATMENT

- The treatment of choice for pediculosis is **1% permethrin cream** to affected areas. Alternative therapies include 0.5% malathion and 1% lindane. However, these agents are less effective and more toxic.[33]
- Oral **ivermectin** can also be used for severe or refractory cases as for scabies (see above).[33]
- Combs and brushes should be sterilized with hot water (65°C [149°F]) for 5 to 15 minutes. Clothing and bedding should also be sterilized with hot water and dried (54°C [129.2°F]) for 30 to 45 minutes.

REFERENCES

1. Goldstein EJC. Bite wounds and infection. *Clin Infect Dis.* 1992;14:633-638.
2. Abrahamian FM, Goldstein EJ. Microbiology of animal bite wound infections. *Clin Microbiol Rev.* 2011;24:231-246.
3. Manning SE, Rupprecht CE, Fishbein D, et al. Human rabies prevention—United States, 2008: recommendations of the Advisory Committee on Immunization Practices. *MMWR Recomm Rep.* 2008;57(RR-3):1-28.
4. Noah DL, Drenzek CL, Smith JS, et al. Epidemiology of human rabies in the United States, 1980 to 1996. *Ann Intern Med.* 1998;128:922-930.
5. Rupprecht CE, Briggs D, Brown CM, et al. Use of a reduced (4-dose) vaccine schedule for post-exposure prophylaxis to prevent human rabies: recommendations of the Advisory Committee on Immunization Practices. *MMWR Recomm Rep.* 2010;59(RR-2):1-9.
6. Willoughby RE, Tieves KS, Hoffman GM, et al. Survival after treatment of rabies with induction of coma. *N Engl J Med.* 2005;352:2508-2514.
7. Jackson AC. Treatment of rabies. In: Hirsch MS, Morven SE, Mitty J, eds. *UpToDate.* Waltham, MA: UpToDate Inc; 2017. http://www.uptodate.com. Accessed October 17, 2017.
8. Wormser GP, Dattwyler RJ, Shapiro ED, et al. The clinical assessment, treatment, and prevention of Lyme disease, human granulocytic anaplasmosis, and babesiosis: clinical practice guidelines by the Infectious Diseases Society of America. *Clin Infect Dis.* 2006;43:1089-1134.
9. Nadelman RB, Nowakowski J, Fish D, et al. Prophylaxis with single-dose doxycycline for the prevention of Lyme disease after an *Ixodes scapularis* tick bite. *N Engl J Med.* 2001;345:79-84.
10. Steere AC, Sikand VK. The presenting manifestations of Lyme disease and outcomes of treatment. *N Engl J Med.* 2003;348:2472-2474.
11. Halperin JJ. Nervous system Lyme disease. *Infect Dis Clin North Am.* 2008;22:261-274.
12. Fish AE, Pride YB, Pinto DS. Lyme carditis. *Infect Dis Clin North Am.* 2008;22:275-288.
13. Steere AC, Schoen RT, Taylor E. The clinical evolution of Lyme arthritis. *Ann Intern Med.* 1987;107:725-731.
14. Dalton MJ, Clarke MJ, Holman RC, et al. National surveillance for Rocky Mountain spotted fever, 1981–1992: epidemiologic summary and evaluation of risk factors for fatal outcome. *Am J Trop Med Hyg.* 1995;52:405-413.
15. Helmick CG, Bernard KW, D'Angelo LJ. Rocky Mountain spotted fever: clinical, laboratory, and epidemiological features of 262 cases. *J Infect Dis.* 1984;150:480-488.
16. Sexton DJ, Corey GR. Rocky Mountain "spotless" and "almost spotless" fever: a wolf in sheep's clothing. *Clin Infect Dis.* 1992;15:439-448.
17. Biggs HM, Behravesh CB, Bradley KK, et al. Diagnosis and management of tickborne rickettsial diseases: Rocky mountain spotted fever, ehrlichiosis, and anaplasmosis—United States: a practical guide for physicians and other health-care and public health professionals. *MMWR Recomm Rep.* 2016;65(2):1-44.
18. Thomas RJ, Dumler JS, Carlyon JA. Current management of human granulocytic anaplasmosis, human monocytic ehrlichiosis and *Ehrlichia ewingii* ehrlichiosis. *Expert Rev Anti Infect Ther.* 2009;7:709-722.
19. Rolain JM, Brouqui P, Koehler JE, et al. Recommendations for treatment of human infections caused by *Bartonella* species. *Antimicrob Agents Chemother.* 2004;48:1921-1933.
20. Mangalgi S, Sajjan A. Comparison of three blood culture techniques in the diagnosis of human brucellosis. *J Lab Physicians.* 2014;6(1):14-17
21. Franco MP, Mulder M, Gilman RH, Smits HL. Human brucellosis. *Lancet Infect Dis.* 2007;7:775-786.
22. Skalsky K, Yahav D, Bishara J, et al. Treatment of human brucellosis: systematic review and meta-analysis of randomised controlled trials. *BMJ.* 2008;336:701-704.
23. Nigrovic LE, Wingerter SL. Tularemia. *Infect Dis Clin North Am.* 2008;22:489-504.
24. Katz AR, Ansdell VE, Effler PV, et al. Assessment of the clinical presentation and treatment of 353 cases of laboratory-confirmed leptospirosis in Hawaii, 1974–1998. *Clin Infect Dis.* 2001;33:1834-1841.
25. McClain JB, Ballou WR, Harrison SM, Steinweg DL. Doxycycline therapy for leptospirosis. *Ann Intern Med.* 1984;100:696-698.
26. Suputtamongkol Y, Niwattayakul K, Suttinont C, et al. An open, randomized, controlled trial of penicillin, doxycycline, and cefotaxime for patients with severe leptospirosis. *Clin Infect Dis.* 2004;39:1417-1424.

27. Sehgal SC, Sugunan AP, Murhekar MV, et al. Randomized controlled trial of doxycycline prophylaxis against leptospirosis in an endemic area. *Int J Antimicrob Agents*. 2000;13:249-255.

28. Centers for Disease Control and Prevention. *Plague: Resources for Clinicians*. Atlanta: Centers for Disease Control and Prevention; 2015. https://www.cdc.gov/plague/healthcare/clinicians.html. Accessed January 18, 2018.

29. Inglesby TV, Henderson DA, Bartlett JG, et al. Anthrax as a biological weapon: medical and public health management. *JAMA*. 1999;281:1735-1745.

30. Hendricks KA, Wright ME, Shadomy SV, et al. Centers for Disease Control and Prevention expert panel meetings on prevention and treatment of anthrax in adults. *Emerg Infect Dis*. February 2014. http://dx.doi.org/10.3201/eid2002.130687. Accessed January 18, 2018.

31. Gikas A, Kokkini S, Tsioutis C. Q fever: clinical manifestations and treatment. *Expert Rev Anti Infect Ther*. 2010;8:529-539.

32. Karakousis PC, Trucksis M, Dumler JS. Chronic Q fever in the United States. *J Clin Microbiol*. 2006;44:2283-2287.

33. Diaz JH. The epidemiology, diagnosis, management, and prevention of ectoparasitic diseases in travelers. *J Travel Med*. 2006;13:100-111.

Protozoal Infections

17

Derek Yee and F. Matthew Kuhlmann

INTRODUCTION

- Protozoa are unicellular organisms infecting billions of people globally. Most cases occur in developing countries; however, travel and migration can lead to cases anywhere in the world.
- Table 17-1 provides a brief description of the most common protozoal infections.

TABLE 17-1	SUMMARY OF PROTOZOA INFECTIONS		
Protozoa (Disease)	Clinical Manifestations	Diagnosis	Treatment
Vector-borne protozoa			
Plasmodium spp. (malaria)	Fever, prostration, anemia	Blood smear, rapid antigen testing	Multiple options depending on species and local resistance
Toxoplasma gondii (toxoplasmosis)	Fever, lymphade-nopathy, severe manifestations in immunocompro-mised or pregnant patients	Direct parasite detection, serol-ogy, or PCR	Pyrimethamine, sulfadiazine with folinic acid
Babesia spp. (babesiosis)	Fever, anemia, malaise	Direct detection of parasite on blood smear or PCR	Atovaquone plus azith-romycin OR quinine plus clindamycin
Leishmania spp. (cutaneous or mucocutaneous leishmaniasis)	Ulcer with heaped border	Direct parasite detection on skin biopsy	Variable, depen-dent on species and geography
Leishmania spp. (visceral leishmaniasis)	Fever, hepatosplenomegaly	Direct parasite detection or serology	Variable, depen-dent on species and geography
Trypanosoma cruzi (Chagas disease)	Acute cellulitis followed by cardio-megaly, megacolon, or megaesophagus years later	Direct detection of parasites in acute phases, serology in chronic phases	Benznidazole or nifurtimox

(Continued)

TABLE 17-1	SUMMARY OF PROTOZOA INFECTIONS (CONTINUED)		
Protozoa (Disease)	Clinical Manifestations	Diagnosis	Treatment
Trypanosoma brucei rhodesiense (East African sleeping sickness)	Acute onset of fever, lymphadenopathy, and mental status changes	Direct detection of parasites in blood or CSF	Suramin for acute disease. Melarsoprol for CNS disease
Trypanosoma brucei gambiense (West African sleeping sickness)	Fevers, lymphadenopathy, and pruritus in the acute stage	Direct detection of parasites in blood or CSF	Pentamidine for acute disease
	Progressive mental status changes over months to years (chronic)		Late stage treated with eflornithine and nifurtimox
Free-living ameba			
Acanthamoeba spp.	Granulomatous amebic encephalitis, keratitis	Biopsy and/or culture	Propamidine and surgical debridement (keratitis)
Balamuthia mandrillaris	Meningoencephalitis	Biopsy or postmortem	Amphotericin
Naegleria fowleri	Meningoencephalitis	CSF analysis for trophozoites	Amphotericin, rifampin, and azoles
Intestinal protozoa			
Entamoeba spp. (amebiasis)	Bloody diarrhea, abdominal pain, liver abscess	Microscopic stool examination. Antibody detection by EIA	Metronidazole followed by paromomycin (United States) for cyst eradication
Endolimax nana	Nonpathogenic	Stool microscopy	None
Iodamoeba bütschlii	Nonpathogenic swine protozoa	Stool microscopy	None
Blastocystis hominis	Controversial pathogen. May cause bloating, diarrhea, abdominal pain	Microscopic stool examination	Controversial, metronidazole or TMP-SMX may be tried
Giardia lamblia (synonymous with *Giardia intestinalis*) (giardiasis)	Bloating, diarrhea, abdominal pain, malabsorption, nausea	Microscopic stool examination. Fecal immunoassays	Metronidazole

TABLE 17-1	SUMMARY OF PROTOZOA INFECTIONS (CONTINUED)		
Protozoa (Disease)	Clinical Manifestations	Diagnosis	Treatment
Dientamoeba fragilis	Diarrhea, abdominal pain	Stool microscopy	Metronidazole or paromomycin
Cryptosporidium spp. (cryptosporidiosis)	Watery diarrhea and abdominal pain, especially immuno-compromised (e.g., AIDS)	Microscopic stool examination using acid-fast staining, smaller; DFA; enzyme immunoassays to detect antigens in stools	Self-limiting; nitazoxanide in AIDS
Cyclospora cayetanensis	Chronic diarrhea, abdominal pain, bloating	Stool microscopy with acid-fast staining, larger	TMP-SMX
Isospora belli	Watery diarrhea and abdominal pain (life-threatening in AIDS)	Microscopic stool examination using acid-fast staining, ovoid	TMP-SMX
Enterocytozoon bieneusi	Chronic, watery diarrhea and abdominal pain, especially in HIV	Microscopic stool examination, electron micros-copy of small bowel biopsy	Albendazole
Encephalitozoon spp.	Rare cause of per-sistent diarrhea	Stool microscopy	Albendazole

CNS, central nervous system; CSF, cerebrospinal fluid; DFA, direct fluorescent anti-body; EIA, enzyme immunoassay; PCR, polymerase chain reaction; TMP-SMX, trimethoprim–sulfamethoxazole.

Malaria

GENERAL PRINCIPLES

Epidemiology

- An estimated 148 to 304 million infections occurred worldwide, resulting in 235,000 to 639,000 deaths in 2015.[1] Most deaths occur in children living in sub-Saharan Africa.
- Each species inhabits distinct geographical regions with unique clinical characteristics and treatments.
- A detailed map of malarious regions can be found on the CDC web site (www.cdc.gov/travel) or in their travel reference, the CDC Yellow Book.

Etiology

Five species of malaria cause disease in humans:

- *Plasmodium falciparum*: Worldwide distribution, high mortality
- *Plasmodium vivax*: Most common in Asia, Central and South America, and Oceania
- *Plasmodium ovale*: Mainly in West Africa
- *Plasmodium malariae*: Rare cause of disease, found in Africa and Southeast Asia
- *Plasmodium knowlesi*: Simian malaria rarely causing infections in Southeast Asia

Pathophysiology

- Transmission is via bites from female *Anopheles* mosquitoes. Less common means of transmission include blood transfusion, transplantation, shared needle use, or congenital transmission.
- Life cycles:
  - Sexual stages (sporogony) occur in the mosquito.
  - Asexual stages (schizogony) occur in the mammalian host as briefly described in the following:
    - Sporozoites are injected by the mosquito and infect hepatocytes. After 1 to 3 weeks, hepatocytes rupture, releasing merozoites into the bloodstream, which invade red blood cells (RBCs). Dormant liver stages (hypnozoites) occur with *P. ovale* and *P. vivax* infections.
    - Intraerythrocytic ring forms replicate, releasing additional merozoites and causing RBC lysis.
    - Merozoites infect additional RBCs or differentiate into gametocytes, which are taken up by biting mosquitoes to complete the life cycle.
- Host consequences:
  - RBC lysis generates many symptoms.
  - Glycolipid release induces cytokine production, leading to systemic symptoms including fever.
  - RBC lysis is cyclical, leading to classical descriptions of quotidian fever (occurring daily as with *P. falciparum*) or tertian fever (every other day for *P. vivax* and *P. ovale*).
  - Decreased production of RBCs contributes to profound anemia as well as RBC lysis.
  - Infected RBCs are sequestered in the microvasculature, causing renal failure, tissue hypoxia, and central nervous system (CNS) pathology.
  - Severity of symptoms depends in part on the type of RBC infected.
    - *P. falciparum*: Infects any RBC, causes severe infection
    - *P. vivax*: Reticulocytes only, less severe infection
    - *P. malariae*: Mature RBCs, mild chronic infection

Risk Factors

- Indigenous patients at risk for severe malaria include pregnant women and nonimmune children; sickle cell disease or thalassemia may be protective.
- Travelers at high risk for severe malaria are pregnant, older than 50, or indigenous persons returning home.

Prevention

- Prevention of malaria depends upon types of exposures and risk of acquiring disease.
- For patients living in endemic regions:
  - Insecticide-impregnated bed nets prevent malaria and other vector-borne diseases.
  - Intermittent treatment during pregnancy reduces the risk of placental disease.

- For travelers to endemic regions:
  - Chemoprophylaxis is indicated based on level of risk.
  - Protective clothing (long-sleeved shirts and pants) should be worn.
  - Sleeping under a bed net is advised when accommodations place one at risk.
  - Insect repellents can provide added protection against biting mosquitoes.

DIAGNOSIS

Clinical Presentation

History
- Malaria presents with nonspecific symptoms including fever and prostration.
- Any patient returning from or residing in endemic regions should be evaluated for malaria.
- The type of prophylaxis and adherence to the prophylactic regimen help determine risk of malaria.
- Usual presentation is 1 to 2 weeks after exposure; longer incubation times or recrudescence (especially with *P. vivax* or *P. ovale*) can occur.
- Factors indicative of severe malaria include mental status changes, changes in urine color, or palpitations.

Physical Examination
- Pallor, jaundice, tachycardia, systolic murmurs, or shortness of breath may indicate hemolytic anemia.
- Signs of severe malaria include dark urine, pulmonary rales, disorientation, altered mental status, focal neurologic deficits, or papilledema.

Diagnostic Criteria

Severe or complicated malaria includes any of the following:

- Cerebral malaria with coma, encephalopathy, seizures, focal neurologic deficits, or altered consciousness
- Acute renal failure with acute tubular necrosis or macroscopic hemoglobinuria (blackwater fever)
- Acute pulmonary edema with acute respiratory distress syndrome (ARDS), which may occur up to 2 to 3 days after starting therapy
- Hypoglycemia
- Severe anemia (hemoglobin <5 g/dL)
- Spontaneous bleeding, thrombocytopenia (<100,000/µL)
- Metabolic acidosis
- Shock
- Hyperparasitemia (>5%)

Differential Diagnosis

The differential is quite broad; other common illnesses include dengue fever, leptospirosis, meningococcal sepsis, or typhoid fever.

Diagnostic Testing

- Complete blood counts and comprehensive metabolic panels should be obtained.
- **Thick and thin blood smears are the gold standard**; obtain multiple samples, especially during fever. **Intraerythrocytic ring forms or schizonts** on microscopy confirm the diagnosis and can identify the plasmodial species.
- Rapid diagnostic tests identify plasmodial antigens in the blood and are a good alternative when skilled microscopy is not available.

- A positive test is highly specific and can identify *P. falciparum*.
- A false negative may occur with low parasitemia and repeat testing may be necessary.
- Polymerase chain reaction (PCR) is not yet routinely used in clinical diagnostics.
- Lumbar puncture may be needed to rule out meningoencephalitis; the cerebrospinal fluid profile in cerebral malaria is benign, usually with elevated protein.

TREATMENT

- Therapy must be initiated as soon as possible.
- Infectious disease consultation should be considered in severe malaria.
- Treatment of **uncomplicated malaria due to *P. falciparum***[2,3]
  - For chloroquine-sensitive areas: Chloroquine 600 mg base orally followed by 300 mg base at 6, 24, and 48 hours
  - For chloroquine-resistant areas (oral treatment):
    - Artemether–lumefantrine (20 mg artemether, 120 mg lumefantrine), for weight ≥35 kg, four tablets at 0 and 8 hours followed by four tablets twice daily for 2 days
    - Outside the United States, artemisinin-based combination therapy is considered first-line treatment.
    - Atovaquone–proguanil (250 mg atovaquone/100 mg proguanil) four tablets daily for 3 days
    - Quinine (542 mg base) three times daily for 3 to 7 days PLUS one of the following:
      - Tetracycline 250 mg four times daily for 7 days
      - Doxycycline 100 mg twice daily for 7 days
      - Clindamycin 20 mg base/kg/d divided into three doses daily × 7 days, sulfadoxine–pyrimethamine (25/1.25 mg base/kg) one dose
      - Side effects of quinine include tinnitus, hearing loss, confusion, other CNS effects, thrombocytopenia, hypotension, and cardiotoxicity.
  - As a third-line agent, mefloquine can be used in combination with artesunate or doxycycline.
- **Malaria due to *P. vivax* or *P. ovale*:**
  - Chloroquine or atovaquone–proguanil PLUS primaquine 30 mg base daily for 14 days in patients with normal glucose-6-phosphate dehydrogenase (screen before treatment).
  - If acquired in Papua New Guinea or Indonesia, treat with atovaquone–proguanil, quinine sulfate plus doxycycline, or mefloquine.
- **Complicated malaria:**
  - Quinidine gluconate 6.25 mg base/kg loading dose IV over 1 to 2 hours, then 0.0125 mg base/kg/min continuous infusion for at least 24 hours, PLUS doxycycline, tetracycline, or clindamycin as above. A baseline ECG should be obtained prior to initiating therapy.
  - Artesunate (2.4 mg/kg IV at 0, 12, and 24 h followed by daily treatment) can be acquired as an investigational drug through the CDC (Centers for Disease Control and Prevention) because of unavailability or intolerance of quinidine.

Prophylaxis

Prophylaxis in travelers: Chemoprophylaxis for malaria depends on the presence of chloroquine resistance (more details can be found in the CDC web site). In general, the drugs used for prophylaxis are as follows:

- Atovaquone/proguanil to start 1 to 2 days before traveling and 7 days after returning. Side effects are uncommon, usually mild gastrointestinal (GI) discomfort. Contraindicated in women who are pregnant or breast-feeding a child weighing less than 5 kg.
- Chloroquine 300 mg once weekly, to start 1 week before traveling and to continue 4 weeks after returning. Used in pregnancy but only in chloroquine-sensitive malaria.

- Doxycycline 100 mg PO daily, started 1 day before travel and continued for 4 weeks after returning. Photosensitivity and gastrointestinal distress may limit use. Cannot be used in pregnant women and children less than age 8 years.
- Mefloquine 250 mg PO weekly, started 2 weeks prior and continued 4 weeks after traveling. Use with caution in people with psychiatric and seizure disorders because of neuropsychiatric side effects.

REFERRAL

The CDC Malaria Hotline can be reached at (770) 488 to 7788 and at http://www.cdc.gov/MALARIA/.

Babesiosis

GENERAL PRINCIPLES

Epidemiology

- Babesiosis is a zoonotic tick-borne infection caused by *Babesia* spp., which infect RBCs.
- Infections occur both in Europe and in North America; European infections tend to be more severe.
- North American infections:
  - Caused by *Babesia microti* and are frequently asymptomatic
  - Share *Ixodes* tick vector with *Borrelia burgdorferi*, making co-infections common
- *Babesia divergens* is commonly found in Europe.

Pathophysiology

- Transmission occurs after *Ixodes* tick bites but can also rarely occur through blood transfusions or congenital transmission.
- Massive RBC lysis leads to hemolytic anemia, resulting in hyperbilirubinemia, hemoglobinuria, and acute tubular necrosis.
- Thrombocytopenia, pulmonary edema, and ARDS can also be seen.
- Severe disease occurs in the elderly, immunocompromised, or asplenic patient.
- The only effective means of prevention is tick avoidance by using insect repellants and covering exposed areas of the skin.

DIAGNOSIS

Clinical Presentation

History

- Fever, chills, sweats, headache, body aches, loss of appetite, nausea, or fatigue occur 1 to 3 weeks after exposure.
- A history of tick bite in an endemic region is helpful but not necessary.
- A history of splenectomy or immunodeficiency increases the risk for severe infection.

Physical Examination

- Fever, hepatomegaly, splenomegaly, and evidence of anemia are potential findings.
- In severe disease, findings of acute respiratory distress or congestive heart failure may be present.

Differential Diagnosis

- Malaria, leptospirosis, viral hepatitis, and other tick-borne diseases should be considered.
- Intraerythrocytic *Babesia* organisms are frequently confused with *P. falciparum*.

Diagnostic Testing

- Complete blood cell count may reveal mild to severe anemia, thrombocytopenia, atypical lymphocytes, leukopenia, or leukocytosis.
- Haptoglobin and reticulocyte count may be decreased.
- Transaminitis and indirect hyperbilirubinemia may be present.
- Hemoglobinuria or proteinuria may be present.
- Microscopic detection on blood smear is routinely used for diagnosis:
  - The percent parasitemia can be as high as 80% in splenectomized patients but may not correlate directly with disease severity.
  - Classically, "Maltese cross" forms are identified on microscopy but are not always present.
- Several PCR-based diagnostic tests are becoming more readily accepted as an alternative to microscopy.

TREATMENT

- *B. microti* infections tend to be subclinical and treatment may not be indicated.
- In cases of prolonged symptoms, **atovaquone** (750 mg orally twice daily for 7–10 d) **PLUS azithromycin** (500 mg orally on day 1 followed by 250 mg daily for 6 d) OR **quinine** (650 mg orally three times daily for 7 d) **PLUS clindamycin** (600 mg orally three times daily for 7 d) for more severe disease.[4]
- In severe cases, exchange transfusion may be indicated.

Toxoplasmosis

GENERAL PRINCIPLES

- *Toxoplasma gondii* causes toxoplasmosis.
- Toxoplasmosis is usually a self-limiting disease but reactivates or disseminates in HIV-positive patients or other immunosuppressed patients such as organ transplant recipients.
- Primary infection in nonimmune mothers can cause severe congenital abnormalities.
- Ocular toxoplasmosis is another common presentation, caused by disease reactivation.

Epidemiology

- Toxoplasmosis occurs worldwide, especially where raw or undercooked meats are consumed.
- In the United States, approximately 1% of domestic cats shed *Toxoplasma* cysts and 11% to 31% of humans are seropositive.

Pathophysiology

- Transmission occurs by ingesting cysts in undercooked meat, ingesting food contaminated with sporocysts, congenitally, or through transplantation.
- Life cycle:
  - Sporocysts are shed in cat feces.
  - Tachyzoites are actively replicating parasites that form cysts in host tissues.
  - Dormant stages are referred to as bradyzoites.

Prevention

- Cook food to appropriate temperatures.
- Wash fruits and vegetables before eating.
- Freeze meat for several days before cooking.

- Do not feed cats raw or undercooked meat.
- Wear gloves when gardening or during contact with soil.
- Pregnant women should avoid changing litter boxes or contact with kittens.

DIAGNOSIS

Clinical Presentation

History
- Primary infection in immunocompetent hosts is usually asymptomatic. Some patients may note fever, fatigue, or lymphadenopathy. Symptoms of primary infection are similar to infectious mononucleosis.[5]
- Reactivation in AIDS patients presents as fever, headache, worsening mental status, and focal neurologic deficits in patients with CD4 cell counts <100 cells/mL. As disease progresses, other organ systems may be involved.
- Ocular toxoplasmosis presents as a sudden blurring of vision.
- The risk of congenital infection increases with gestational age. Severe manifestations occur in <10% of maternal infections and include hydrocephalus, mental retardation, and even death. Infected infants may develop ocular disease later in life.

Physical Examination
- Immunocompetent patients most commonly present with bilateral, symmetrical, non-tender cervical lymphadenopathy.
- Ophthalmologic examination of acute ocular toxoplasmosis typically includes findings of iritis, vitritis, and chorioretinitis.

Differential Diagnosis

CNS (central nervous system) reactivation can be confused with brain abscess, metastasis, lymphoma, and tuberculosis.

Diagnostic Testing

In acute infection, detection of IgM antibodies or isolation of *T. gondii* from body fluids confirms the diagnosis.

- Chronically infected individuals may have cysts present in tissue.
- Reactivation in HIV is diagnosed by the following:
  ○ A compatible clinical syndrome with consistent lesions on radiography and response to empirical therapy, or
  ○ Demonstration of the parasite by biopsy or cerebrospinal fluid PCR
- Risk of congenital infection is determined by positive maternal IgM testing or positive PCR of amniotic fluid.

TREATMENT

- The standard treatment consists of 2 to 4 weeks of **pyrimethamine (200 mg PO first dose then 100 mg PO daily), sulfadiazine (1 g every 6 h), or clindamycin, and supplementation with folinic acid** (10–25 mg PO) to avoid pyrimethamine-induced bone marrow toxicity. In immunocompetent hosts, treatment of acute infection does not alter outcomes.
- Pregnant women should be treated with spiramycin (3 g/d) throughout pregnancy. If fetal infection has been detected, further therapy with sulfadiazine and pyrimethamine is indicated.
- In AIDS patients, therapy is similar to standard therapy in immunocompetent hosts but should be continued for 6 weeks followed by chronic maintenance therapy.
- Ocular disease requires consultation with an ophthalmologist.

Leishmaniasis

GENERAL PRINCIPLES

- The three main types of disease are as follows:
  - Cutaneous leishmaniasis (the most common form) resulting in ulcerative skin lesions
  - Visceral leishmaniasis causing severe disease of the reticuloendothelial system
  - Mucocutaneous leishmaniasis in which severe ulcerative lesions of the mucosa develop
- Living in or traveling to an endemic region is the essential risk factor.
- Protective clothing and insect repellants are the only means of prevention.

Epidemiology

- Cutaneous leishmaniasis:
  - Occurs in the Middle East, Africa, and Central and South America; caused by several *Leishmania* species
  - Occurs in travelers to endemic countries and military personnel
- Visceral leishmaniasis:
  - Frequently caused by *Leishmania donovani* or *Leishmania infantum/tropica*
  - Untreated symptomatic disease is frequently fatal and is a major cause of death, especially in children.
  - Occurs in India, Bangladesh, Sudan, Brazil, and the Mediterranean coast
- Mucocutaneous leishmaniasis: Occurs primarily in South America; usually caused by *Leishmania brasiliensis*
- Various mammals provide an animal reservoir for most *Leishmania* spp. (e.g., dogs or rodents).

Pathophysiology

- Transmission occurs primarily through the bites of female sandflies, rarely by blood transfusion or needle sharing.
- Life cycle: Sandflies inject infectious metacyclic promastigotes that differentiate into intracellular amastigotes residing within host macrophages.
- Host consequences:
  - The immune response is central to the development of pathology within the mammalian host.
    - Th2 responses generally lead to symptomatic disease or nonhealing lesions.
    - Th1 responses result in spontaneous cure.
  - Disease resolution leads to lifelong immunity, but reactivation can occur in the setting of immunosuppression.
  - Secondary bacterial infections are a frequent cause of death in visceral leishmaniasis.

DIAGNOSIS

Clinical Presentation

History

- Cutaneous disease: Patients notice a papule that appears weeks to months after the bite, which eventually ulcerates. Dissemination can occur in immunocompromised patients.
- Mucocutaneous disease:
  - Patients present with a cutaneous lesion that heals spontaneously.
  - Mucosal lesions develop weeks to years after exposure.

- Visceral disease:
  - Patients present with fever, weight loss, massive hepatosplenomegaly, and pancytopenia.
  - Hyperpigmentation of the skin may occur, leading to the term *kala-azar*, or "black fever."

Physical Examination
- Cutaneous disease:
  - Shallow painless ulcers with a heaped-up border occur on exposed extremities or face.
  - Mucosal evaluation is important in patients from Central and South America.
  - Satellite lesions and lymphadenopathy can also occur.
- Visceral disease: Hepatosplenomegaly is a hallmark of the disease.

Differential Diagnosis

- Cutaneous disease: Various fungal, bacterial, or malignant conditions should be considered.
- Visceral disease: Typhoid fever, miliary tuberculosis, brucellosis, malaria, and acute schistosomiasis are all possibilities.

Diagnostic Testing

- Visceral disease may be associated with hypergammaglobulinemia, leukopenia, anemia, thrombocytopenia, and/or hypoalbuminemia.
- The gold standard for diagnosis is **culture of parasites** from ulcers (cutaneous or mucocutaneous) or bone marrow/splenic aspirates (visceral).
- PCR testing or demonstration of parasites on histopathology provides adjunctive diagnostic confirmation.
- Immunodiagnostics:
  - Cutaneous disease: Not recommended.
  - Visceral disease: Antibody detection using enzyme-linked immunosorbent assay (ELISA), immunofluorescence antibody test (IFAT), or recombinant kinesin antigen (rK39) dipstick is used if other approaches are negative.[6]

TREATMENT

- Cutaneous disease:
  - Because spontaneous resolution of cutaneous ulcers frequently occurs, treatment may not be necessary.
  - In all cases, lesions affecting function or cosmetics (such as the face) should be treated to prevent further disfiguration.
- Visceral and mucocutaneous disease: Treatment is indicated in all symptomatic patients.
- Treatment options[7]:
  - Antimonials: Pentavalent antimonials have been the mainstay of therapy for many years. Their use is limited by multiple toxicities and widespread resistance. In the United States, **sodium stibogluconate** (Pentostam) is available from the CDC.
  - Miltefosine: Is the only oral agent for treatment of visceral disease. It is particularly effective in India and adjacent regions of South Asia where resistance to pentavalent antimonials is present.
  - Amphotericin B: **Liposomal amphotericin B** is the treatment of choice for visceral leishmaniasis.
- There is no universally applicable treatment of choice for cutaneous or mucocutaneous disease. Treatment can be complex and consultation with a specialist in Leishmaniasis is indicated.
- Treatment failures occur in patients with HIV or other immunosuppression.
- Mucocutaneous leishmaniasis is difficult to treat, with relapses being common.

American Trypanosomiasis

GENERAL PRINCIPLES

- American trypanosomiasis (Chagas disease) is a protozoan infection caused by *Trypanosoma cruzi.*
- Disease is divided into two main phases:
  - Acute disease—in which cutaneous manifestations of disease predominate with minimal mortality
  - Chronic disease—in which symptoms of end-stage organ failure develop with high mortality rates

Epidemiology

- Chagas disease affects around 6 million people, primarily in Central and South America.[8]
- Globally, *T. cruzi* is frequently detected in migrant populations.
- In the United States, more than 2000 cases have been confirmed through screening the blood supply.

Pathophysiology

- Transmission:
  - Primarily vector-borne through the bite of the reduviid bug, also known as the **kissing bug (*Triatoma* spp.).**
  - Transmission also occurs through blood transfusion, transplantation, and congenitally.
  - Oral transmission from food contaminated by triatome feces is increasingly recognized.
  - Various mammals including dogs and rodents serve as reservoirs of infection.
- Life cycle:
  - Triatomines deposit feces containing infectious trypomastigotes near the site of a blood meal.
  - Scratching or other behaviors help trypomastigotes infect the host through breaches in skin or mucosal membranes.
  - Trypomastigotes differentiate into intracellular amastigotes in various host tissues, primarily cardiac myocytes and GI smooth muscle cells.
- Host consequences:
  - Acute infection occurs days or weeks after exposure; local swelling, similar to cellulitis, is followed by malaise, fever, and anorexia.
  - Chronic infection appears years after the indeterminate stage.
  - **The immune response to chronically infected tissues likely causes end-organ disease** such as cardiomegaly, megaesophagus, and megacolon. This occurs in 20% to 30% of infected patients.

Prevention

- Campaigns utilizing insecticide in homes and outbuildings have been highly effective.
- Bed nets prevent insects from biting, which mostly occurs at night.

DIAGNOSIS

Clinical Presentation

History
- A high level of suspicion based on epidemiologic risk factors is necessary.
- In endemic regions, acute infection commonly occurs in children.
- In chronic stages, adults may describe symptoms of heart failure, palpitations, severe constipation, vomiting after meals, dysphagia, or odynophagia.

Physical Examination

- Acute phase: Cutaneous swellings known as chagomas form at the initial site of parasite entry. **Facial swelling with periorbital edema and conjunctivitis is a specific manifestation of acute Chagas disease**, also known as Romaña sign. Local lymphadenopathy or hepatosplenomegaly may also be present.
- Chronic infection: Physical examination findings depend on the specific organs affected.
  - Cardiac disease may manifest as heart failure or an arrhythmia.
  - GI disease may result in abdominal tenderness or distension.
  - Reactivation of chronic disease occurs in immunocompromised patients and can result in meningoencephalitis with altered mental status.

Differential Diagnosis

- Acute infection: Infectious mononucleosis, acute HIV, periorbital cellulitis, allergic reaction to triatomine bites
- Chronic infection: dilated cardiomyopathy by other causes, achalasia, congenital aganglionosis (Hirschsprung disease), hypothyroidism, or severe esophagitis

Diagnostic Testing

- Acute infection: Parasites may be directly visualized on thick blood smears; PCR on blood remains investigational.
- Chronic infection:
  - Serology: At least two distinct serologic tests are required to diagnose Chagas disease in the appropriate clinical setting.
  - PCR on infected tissues is experimental.
  - Direct visualization on biopsy of infected tissues is extremely insensitive but highly specific.
- ECG and echocardiogram may be indicated to evaluate for cardiac involvement.
- Barium swallow/enema may be performed to identify abnormalities of the alimentary tract.

Treatment

- Treatment with **benznidazole** is highly effective in acute stages and can prevent complications of chronic Chagas disease.[9]
- All serologically confirmed cases of chronic Chagas disease should be offered treatment unless there are contraindications or end-stage disease.
- Benznidazole is the first-line treatment (5–7 mg/kg/d in two divided doses for 60 d); rash and dermatitis are frequent side effects.
- Nifurtimox (8–10 mg/kg/d in three or four divided doses for 90–120 d) has many toxicities including psychological disturbances and GI upset.
- Both benznidazole and nifurtimox are contraindicated during pregnancy.
- Sequela of chronic Chagas disease should be treated with medical or surgical approaches.
  - Cardiac disease: Antiarrhythmics should be administered in consultation with cardiology.
  - GI disease: Conservative approaches and laxatives may provide symptomatic relief; surgical approaches may be indicated.

COMPLICATIONS

Complications of chronic disease include the following:

- Cardiac: ventricular arrhythmias, heart block, severe heart failure, and death from cardiac disease
- GI: constipation, aspiration, and inability to eat

MONITORING/FOLLOW-UP

Serologic reversion occurring within 1 year for acute disease or several years for chronic disease suggests cure.

Amebiasis

GENERAL PRINCIPLES

Epidemiology

- *Entamoeba histolytica* causes intestinal amebiasis manifested by amebic dysentery or liver abscess.
- *E. histolytica* occurs in tropical countries or areas with poor sanitation worldwide.
- It affects around 500 million people worldwide, with an annual mortality of 40,000 to 100,000 persons.[10] Estimates vary because of colonization with the morphologically indistinct but nonpathogenic *Entamoeba dispar.*
- The prevalence in the United States is 1% to 2%.
- The main risk groups are travelers, immigrants, men who have sex with men, and institutionalized persons.
- Proper water treatment and sanitation dramatically reduces the incidence of disease.

Pathophysiology

- Transmission: *E. histolytica* is spread by the fecal–oral route when cysts are ingested.
- Life cycle:
  ○ Cysts are ingested and resist the acidic environment of the stomach.
  ○ In the small intestine, trophozoites are released that mature and eventually form new cysts.
- Host consequences:
  ○ When trophozoites invade the bowel mucosa, they release enzymes that cause tissue lysis. Symptoms develop 2 to 6 weeks after cyst ingestion.
  ○ Submucosal lesions enlarge and form "teardrop" ulcers.
  ○ Dissemination occurs upon entry into the portal circulation.
  ○ The most frequent site of systemic disease is the liver, where abscesses form.

DIAGNOSIS

Clinical Presentation

History
- Most disease is asymptomatic, patients can become carriers but most clear carriage within a year.
- Acute infection: crampy lower abdominal discomfort, flatulence, tenesmus, with bloody or mucoid diarrhea
- Extraintestinal manifestations:
  ○ Liver abscess:
    ▪ Most common extraintestinal site of infection; occurs more frequently in adults
    ▪ Amebic abscess of the liver is characterized by the abrupt onset of right upper quadrant pain, weight loss, and high fever.
  ○ Rarely, *E. histolytica* may infect other tissues such as the lungs, brain, peritoneum, or pericardial space.

Physical Examination
- A tender, enlarged liver may be appreciated in amebic abscess of the liver.
- Some patients may develop an ameboma, a tender and palpable submucosal mass of granulation tissue, often mistaken for malignancy.

Differential Diagnosis

- Causes of dysentery include *Shigella*, *Escherichia coli*, *Salmonella*, *Campylobacter*, and some *Vibrio* species.
- Amebic liver abscess must be differentiated from pyogenic liver abscess, carcinoma, or echinococcal disease.

Diagnostic Testing

- Microscopic identification of cysts and trophozoites in the stool remains a common method of diagnosis. Importantly, *E. histolytica* is indistinguishable from *E. dispar* in stool, and additional confirmatory tests are needed.
- Antigen detection and PCR are available and can aid in the diagnosis and differentiation from *E. dispar*.
- Serology may be negative in patients with acute disease and should be repeated in 5 to 7 days.
- Hepatic abscesses can be detected with either ultrasound or CT; aspiration may reveal material resembling anchovy paste.

TREATMENT

Medical Management

- **Iodoquinol or paromomycin** (in the United States) will eradicate **cysts** in asymptomatic carriers.
- **Metronidazole** 500 to 750 mg by mouth three times a day for 10 to 14 days should be followed by iodoquinol or paromomycin to eradicate cysts in patients with **colitis** or **liver abscess**.

Surgical Management

- Abscesses can be drained either surgically or by percutaneous intervention.
- Ruptured abscess or bacterial superinfection should be treated surgically.

Giardiasis

GENERAL PRINCIPLES

Epidemiology

- *Giardia duodenalis* is the cause of giardiasis (historical names include *Giardia lamblia* and *Giardia intestinalis*).
- It occurs worldwide, infecting mostly humans but also other mammals.
- Outbreaks in day care centers are common.
- Hikers in the Rocky Mountains (United States) are also at risk.

Pathophysiology

- Transmission occurs through fecal–oral routes.
- Life cycle:
  - Cysts are ingested from contaminated food or water and release trophozoites in the duodenum.
  - The trophozoite then attaches to the GI tract wall, causing disease manifestations.
- Host consequences:
  - Inflammation of the duodenal mucosa leads to malabsorption of protein and fat.
  - Humoral immunity is thought to be important. Patients with hypogammaglobulinemia develop prolonged infections that respond poorly to therapy.

Prevention

- The cysts persist for months in the environment.
- Chlorination does not kill the cysts, but they can be removed by filtration.

DIAGNOSIS

Clinical Presentation

- The majority of patients are asymptomatic carriers.
- Symptoms occur after an incubation period of 1 to 3 weeks. Commonly, patients complain of bloating, abdominal pain, nausea, flatulence, emesis, and diarrhea. Symptoms usually resolve spontaneously.
- Chronically infected children may have retarded growth and development.

Differential Diagnosis

The differential diagnosis includes other parasitological causes of chronic diarrhea such as strongyloidiasis, cryptosporidiosis, cyclosporiasis, or microsporidiosis.

Diagnostic Testing

- The gold standard for diagnosis is **direct detection of parasites in the stool** by an experienced microscopist.
- ELISA-based antigen detection has largely replaced microscopy in most laboratories because of equivalent performance and ease of use.

TREATMENT

Metronidazole is the treatment of choice. Multiple alternative agents are available but can be difficult to find in the United States.

REFERENCES

1. WHO Global Malaria Programme. *World Malaria Report: 2016.* Geneva: World Health Organization; 2016. http://apps.who.int/iris/bitstream/10665/252038/1/9789241511711-eng.pdf?ua=1. Accessed 01 November 2017.
2. WHO. *Guidelines for the Treatment of Malaria.* 3rd ed. Geneva: World Health Organization; 2015. http://www.who.int/malaria/publications/atoz/9789241549127/en/. Accessed 12 December 2017.
3. Centers for Disease Control and Prevention. *CDC Yellow Book 2018: Health Information for International Travel.* New York: Oxford University Press; 2017.
4. Vannier E, Krause PJ. Human babesiosis. *N Engl J Med.* 2012;366:2397-2407.
5. Dubey JP, Jones JL. *Toxoplasma gondii* infection in humans and animals in the United States. *Int J Parasitol.* 2008;38:1257-1278.
6. Mandal J, Khurana S, Dubey ML, et al. Evaluation of direct agglutination test, rk39 Test, and ELISA for the diagnosis of visceral leishmaniasis. *Am J Trop Med Hyg.* 2008;79:76-78.
7. Aronson N, Herwaldt BL, Libman M, et al. Diagnosis and treatment of leishmaniasis: clinical practice guidelines by the Infectious Diseases Society of America (IDSA) and the American Society of Tropical Medicine and Hygiene (ASTMH). *Clin Infect Dis.* 2016;63:1539.
8. Chagas disease in Latin America: an epidemiological update based on 2010 estimates. *Wkly Epidemiol Rec.* 2015, 90(6);33-44.
9. Bern C, Montgomery SP, Herwaldt BL, et al. Evaluation and treatment of Chagas disease in the United States: a systematic review. *JAMA.* 2007;298:2171-2181.
10. Stanley SL. Amoebiasis. *Lancet.* 2003;361:1025-1034.

Helminthic Infections

18

Carlos Mejia-Chew and Philip Budge

INTRODUCTION

- Helminths (Greek for "worms") are common in poorer regions of tropical and subtropical developing countries, with soil-transmitted helminths (ascaris, whipworm, and hookworm) contributing the greatest disease burden.[1]
- Travel and immigration lead to cases in nonendemic countries such as North America and Europe.[2] Additionally, some helminths remain endemic in temperate countries.
- In general, disease severity depends on extent of exposure as most worms, with the major exception of Strongyloides, do not replicate within a host. The presence of eosinophilia generally relates to increased worm burden and tissue invasion (may not be observed with helminthes that reside only in the gastrointestinal lumen or contained in cystic structures).
- Helminths are classified as follows:
  ○ **Nematodes** (roundworms):
    ▪ Intestinal worms: *Ascaris lumbricoides*, *Trichuris trichiura* (whipworm), *Ancylostoma duodenale* (hookworm), *Necator americanus* (hookworm), *Strongyloides stercoralis*, and *Enterobius vermicularis* (pinworm) are a few examples.
    ▪ Blood and tissue worms: *Trichinella spiralis*, filarial roundworms (e.g., *Onchocerca volvulus* and *Wuchereria bancrofti)*, and *Toxocara* spp., among others.
  ○ **Trematodes** (flukes):
    ▪ Intestinal: *Fasciolopsis buski*, *Echinostoma ilocanum*.
    ▪ Blood and tissue: *Schistosoma* spp., *Clonorchis sinensis*, *Opisthorchis viverrini Paragonimus* spp., *Fasciola* spp.
  ○ **Cestodes** (tapeworms):
    ▪ Intestinal: *Taenia* spp. and *Diphyllobothrium latum.*
    ▪ Tissue (larval): *Taenia solium* (pork tapeworm) and *Echinococcus* spp.
- Helminth infections most likely to present in adults in the United States will be discussed. Additional helminths are briefly described in Table 18-1.

Cysticercosis

GENERAL PRINCIPLES

- The cestode *T. solium* is the only helminth infection in which the human can be host for both adult tapeworms and larval cysts[3] (see "Transmission" below).
- Adult worm infections (taeniasis) are limited to the intestines.
- **Larval infections (cysticercosis)** can lead to severe disease in the central nervous system (**neurocysticercosis**) or calcifications in muscle tissue.

Epidemiology

- High-prevalence areas of *T. solium* include Central and South America and Southeast Asia. Meat inspections and improved sanitation have eliminated the disease in many developed countries.
- In the United States, cases occur **primarily in immigrants from Central and South America.**

TABLE 18-1	OVERVIEW OF CLINICALLY IMPORTANT INFECTIONS CAUSED BY HELMINTHS		
Classification	Helminth disease	Clinical manifestations	Diagnosis	Treatment
Intestinal nematodes (roundworms)	*Ascaris lumbricoides*	Asymptomatic infections are common. Other symptoms include abdominal pain and intestinal obstruction (largest intestinal nematode). Pulmonary symptoms occur during larval migration, inducing asthma-like symptoms (Löffler syndrome). Eosinophilia is present during larval migration through host tissues.	Identify eggs in stools by microscopy. Patients may see adult worms in their feces.	Albendazole 400 mg single dose
	Trichuris trichiura (whipworm)	Range from asymptomatic to abdominal pain, dysentery, and rectal prolapse (in children). Eosinophilia suggests coinfections.	Identify eggs in stools by microscopy	Mebendazole 100 mg q12h for 3 d
	Ancylostoma duodenale and *Necator americanus* (hookworm)	Range from asymptomatic to severe. Pulmonary symptoms and eosinophilia may occur (Löffler syndrome). Heavy infections cause iron deficiency anemia.	Identify eggs or larvae in stool by microscopy	Albendazole 400 mg single dose
	Strongyloides stercoralis	Symptoms include abdominal pain, pulmonary complaints, or other life-threatening disease in hyperinfection syndrome (see text).	Identify worms in feces or sputum. Serology may be helpful.	Ivermectin 200 µg/kg/d for 2 d
	Enterobius vermicularis (pinworm)	Perianal itching in children upon external egg deposition	Identify eggs on the perianal area using the "tape test"	Treat entire household with albendazole. Repeat treatment in 2–3 wk may be necessary.

Filarial nematodes	*Wuchereria bancrofti* *Brugia malayi* Lymphatic filariasis	Extreme lymphatic swelling including elephantiasis of the lower extremities and hydrocele	Nocturnal thick blood smear to identify the microfilariae Serology	Albendazole plus ivermectin or DEC[a]; rule out concurrent *Loa loa* infection before treatment. or Doxycycline 100mg q12h for 6 wk (to kill endosymbiont *Wolbachia*)
	Loa loa	Calabar swellings (transient cutaneous swellings typically near joints or in the arms) are the hallmark of infection. Worms may migrate across conjunctiva.	Daytime blood smear	Surgical extraction if the worm is in the eye. Treatment depends on burden of infection.
	Onchocerca volvulus (onchocerciasis or river blindness)	Subcutaenous nodules, pruritis, occasionally with leopard skin. River blindness (keratitis, anterior uveitis and/or chorioretinitis).	Identify worms in skin snips	Ivermectin (if no coinfection with *Loa loa*) or Doxycycline
Other nematodes	*Toxocara canis* (visceral larva migrans)	Abdominal pain and hepatomegaly; see text for additional detail	Compatible history and serology	Albendazole 400 mg q12h for 5 d
	Ancylostoma braziliense (cutaneous larva migrans)	Pruritic serpiginous rash, usually of the lower extremities	Based on clinical suspicion	Albendazole 400 mg daily x 3–7 d, or ivermectin 200 µg/kg once
	Trichinella spiralis (trichinosis)	Classically described as myalgias, periorbital edema, and eosinophilia. CK elevated due to myositis. Heavier disease burden associated with cachexia and CNS disease.	Demonstration of larvae in muscle tissue or serology	Albendazole 400 mg q12h x14 d, plus steroids

(Continued)

TABLE 18-1   OVERVIEW OF CLINICALLY IMPORTANT INFECTIONS CAUSED BY HELMINTHS (CONTINUED)

Classification	Helminth disease	Clinical manifestations	Diagnosis	Treatment
	Dracunculus medinensis (guinea worm)	Blisters form upon exposure to water followed by emergence of the worm in the wound	Identify worms in blisters or ulcers	Slow extraction of the worm (can take days to weeks)
	Anisakis and *Pseudoterranova* spp. (anisakiasis)	Intense abdominal pain after eating undercooked fish. Eosinophilia is rare.	Identify worms on endoscopy; serology helpful in chronic cases	Worm removal by endoscopy or albendazole
Trematodes (flukes)	*Schistosoma* spp. (schistosomiasis)	*Schistosoma hematobium*: hematuria, bladder cancer Other *Schistosoma* spp.: hepatomegaly, fibrosis, liver failure	Identify eggs in stool or urine Serology	See text
	Opisthorchis viverrini and *Clonorchis sinensis* (liver flukes)	Generally asymptomatic; increased risk of hepatomegaly and cholangiocarcinoma	Identify eggs on stool microscopy	Praziquantel 25 mg/kg q8h for 2 d
	Paragnonimus spp. (lung flukes) *P. kellicotti* is endemic in North America	Subacute pneumonia mimicking tuberculosis; transient cutaneous migrations	Direct detection of eggs in sputum, feces, or pleural fluid Serology	Praziquantel 25 mg/kg q8h for 2 d
	Fasciola hepatica and *Fasciola gigantica* Fascioliasis (liver flukes)	Symptoms range from asymptomatic infections to diarrhea, coughing, hepatomegaly, and right upper quadrant pain with eosinophilia	Serology is quite helpful as egg detection in feces can be difficult	Two doses of triclabendazole 10 mg/kg/dose, separated by 12–24 hours

Cestodes (tape worms)	T. solium (pork) or T. saginatum (beef) Taeniasis	Abdominal pain, passing worm segments	Identify eggs or proglottids in feces	Praziquantel 5–10 mg/kg once
	T. solium Cysticercosis	CNS and other tissue lesions, seizures	Clinical suspicion	See text
	Echinococcus granulosus (cystic echinococcosis)	Large cysts form leading to symptoms in the affected organ. The liver is the primary organ infected. Can disseminate when cysts rupture.	Positive serology with associated cysts on imaging	Individualized approach based on WHO stage-specific classification for both liver and lung disease.
	Echinococcus multilocularis (alveolar echinococcosis, exclusive to North America)	Parasitic tumors involving the liver, lungs, spleen, heart, or other organs	Serology CT may be helpful	Surgical removal of cyst and long-term albendazole
	Diphyllobothrium latum (fish tapeworm)	Frequently asymptomatic; abdominal pain; classically (but rarely) vitamin B12 deficiency	Identify eggs or proglotids in feces (largest tapeworm that infects humans)	Praziquantel Niclosamide
	Hymenolepis nana or Hymenolepis diminuta	Mild abdominal pain, anorexia, diarrhea, and eosinophilia	Identify eggs in stool examination	Single-dose praziquantel 25 mg/kg, repeated in 10 d

[a]DEC is only available in the United States through the CDC, and its use can increase the risk of precipitating blindness if the individual is coinfected with *Onchocerca volvulus*.

CNS, central nervous system; CK, creatine kinase; CT, computed tomography; DEC, diethylcarbamazine.

Pathophysiology

- Transmission of *T. solium* occurs through two separate routes
  - **Ingestion of infected meats** containing cysts **leads to taeniasis** (intestinal tapeworm infection), which is usually asymptomatic.
  - **Ingestion of eggs (or proglottids)** through fecal–oral transmission **leads to cysticercosis**, which can be life-threatening.
- Life cycle
  - When humans ingest infected meat, larvae are released from their cysts and attach to the gut mucosa. There, the worms mature and develop characteristic proglottids, the hermaphroditic reproductive segments of tapeworms, which release eggs in feces.
  - Eggs shed by humans are ingested by foraging pigs. Ingested eggs of *T. solium* differentiate into larvae (oncospheres), which cross the gut mucosa and disseminate to other tissues forming cysts, termed cysticerci.
  - Human ingestion of undercooked meat containing cysticerci completes the life cycle.
  - When humans unwittingly assume the pig's role and ingest eggs (via fecal–oral contamination), cysticerci develop in human tissue.
- Effects on the host
  - Like most cestode infections, **taeniasis** results in long-term chronic asymptomatic infections, allowing for prolonged shedding of eggs.
  - In contrast, **cysticercosis** causes significant pathology, which can include ocular disease, meningitis, and brain and spinal cord lesions.
  - **Neurocysticercosis** is the most frequently diagnosed form of *T. solium* infections, often presenting as new-onset seizures caused by inflammation surrounding a CNS cyst. Focal neurologic deficits can also develop, depending on cyst location.

Risk Factors

- Pork consumption is a risk factor for taeniasis.
- Risk factors for cysticercosis include poor hygiene, living in endemic regions, taeniasis, or household contacts with taeniasis.

Prevention

- Prevention strategies include the following:
  - Improved sanitation and meat inspections.
  - Avoiding consumption of undercooked pork prevents taeniasis.
  - Treatment of taeniasis reduces the risk of cysticercosis.
- No vaccines are available.

DIAGNOSIS

Clinical Presentation

History
- Taeniasis is generally asymptomatic; patients may pass proglottids in their stool for years.
- Cysticercosis may have protean manifestations ranging from vague neurologic symptoms to seizures and rarely symptoms from other infected organs.
- The peak incidence of neurocysticercosis occurs between ages 30 and 40 years.

Physical Examination
- Various neurologic manifestations may be found depending on the location of the CNS lesion.
- Rapid paralysis may occur with spinal lesions.
- Subcutaneous lesions may be identified.

Diagnostic Criteria

- Stool O&P detects taeniasis.
- Brain imaging detects neurocysticercosis.
- Serology can confirm exposure but does not differentiate active from prior infection.

Differential Diagnosis

The differential includes any space-occupying brain lesion, subarachnoid hemorrhage, bacterial abscess, toxoplasmosis, nocardiosis, malignancy, and septic emboli.

Diagnostic Testing

Laboratories

- Peripheral eosinophilia is usually not present in cysticercosis or taeniasis.
- Cerebrospinal fluid analysis may reveal lymphocytic pleocytosis or eosinophils and elevated protein.
- Serologic testing is frequently indicated.
  - **The enzyme-linked immunoelectrotransfer blot (EITB)** assay in serum is highly sensitive (98%), more so than in CSF (90%), but only in patients with ≥2 live parasites in the CNS.
  - Sensitivity drops from 50 to 60% in cases with a single intracranial cysticercus.
  - Enzyme-linked immunosorbent assay (ELISA) has cross-reactivity with both *Taenia saginata* (beef tapeworm) and *Echinococcus.*
  - For taeniasis, at least three stool examinations are recommended to increase detection rate of eggs.

Imaging

- CT scan of the brain can show the typical lesions that are generally small or calcified with a bright central spot of the protoscolex.
- MRI provides more detail and may assist in identifying the etiology of CNS lesions.

TREATMENT

- Treatment is not always indicated, and infectious disease consultation is strongly recommended.
- When indicated, **dual therapy with albendazole plus praziquantel** is the most effective regimen.[4]
- Corticosteroids, started 24 hours before antiparasitic therapy and maintained for 1 to 2 weeks, with subsequent taper are recommended to reduce brain edema caused by the death of the parasite.
- Antiepileptics should usually be continued for at least 6 to 12 months after the last seizure episode.[5]

Strongyloidiasis

GENERAL PRINCIPLES

- *S. stercoralis* and *Strongyloides fuelleborni* are intestinal nematodes causing human strongyloidiasis.
- Unlike other nematodes, *Strongyloides* **replicates within the human host allowing for persistence of infection indefinitely without re-exposure.**
- Overwhelming **hyperinfection syndrome** occurs in immunocompromised patients.

Epidemiology

- Strongyloidiasis affects 30 to 100 million people globally, mostly in tropical and subtropical regions.[6]
- It is uncommon in developed countries with adequate sanitation.
- It is frequently found in rural areas, institutional settings, and lower socioeconomic groups.
- Most cases in the United States are imported by travelers and immigrants, but endemic cases have been reported in Kentucky and Tennessee.

Pathophysiology

- Transmission: Filariform larvae penetrate skin from contaminated soil.
- Life cycle:
  - After skin penetration, larvae migrate to the lung where they mature and then travel up to the trachea where they are swallowed to finally reach the small bowel mucosa.
  - In the small bowel, female adult worms produce eggs that are either excreted in the feces or develop into filariform larvae within the intestines. **The internally developed filariform larvae can penetrate the intestinal mucosa and perpetuate infection inside the host (autoinfection).**
- Effects on the host:
  - Immune response to *Strongyloides* is broad, inducing both cell-mediated and humoral responses coinciding with eosinophilia.
  - Immunosuppression by steroids, malignancies, or drugs leads to **hyperinfection syndrome** where worms invade many other organ systems.
  - Gram-negative sepsis or meningitis are associated with gut epithelial disruption or dissemination of bacteria by the worms as they migrate through host tissues.
  - Pneumonia or other pulmonary manifestations may occur when worms migrate through the lungs.

Risk Factors

- For strongyloidiasis: walking barefoot in endemic areas, contact with human waste or sewage
- For hyperinfection syndrome: various forms of immunodeficiency, as well as coinfection with human T-lymphotropic virus (HTLV)-1. Advanced HIV disease itself is not a strong risk factor for disseminated disease.

Prevention

- Improved sanitation to prevent open defecation.
- Avoid walking barefoot or swimming in areas potentially infested with *Strongyloides* larvae (i.e., contaminated by human stool).

DIAGNOSIS

Clinical Presentation

History
- Manifestations of strongyloidiasis can range from abdominal pain to pulmonary complaints.
- A pruritic lesion can develop at the sight of entry.
- Pulmonary symptoms occur shortly thereafter and resolve spontaneously.
- Chronic infections in immunocompetent hosts are often asymptomatic.
- Mental status changes and gram-negative meningitis are associated with disseminated strongyloidiasis (hyperinfection syndrome).

Physical Examination
- Signs of pneumonia may be observed.
- Recurrent rashes known as "larva currens" may occur. They present as a linear eruption that is intensely pruritic, lasting several hours before spontaneous resolution.[7]

Differential Diagnosis

The differential includes chronic causes of diarrhea, duodenitis, and colitis.

Diagnostic Testing

Laboratories
- Peripheral eosinophilia varies throughout the course of the infection.
- In immunocompromised hosts, eosinophilia may not be present and loss of eosinophilia portends a worse prognosis.
- Direct parasitological confirmation of larvae in the stool or lungs confirms the diagnosis. A minimum of three stool examinations are frequently required to make a diagnosis.
- Serologic tests detect antibodies in suspected cases but cannot distinguish active from prior infection.
- Screening for disease may be indicated in high-risk patients who will become immunosuppressed.

Imaging
Various abnormalities may be seen depending on the disease manifestation.

- Pulmonary infiltrates on chest radiograph
- Duodenitis on CT scan or esophagogastroduodenoscopy
- CNS infarcts in hyperinfection syndromes with dissemination

TREATMENT

- All disease should be treated.
- The drug of choice for uncomplicated disease is **ivermectin** (200 µg/kg/d for 2–3 d); hyperinfections require prolonged treatment courses and the advice of specialists.[7]
- Follow-up examinations for cure are recommended.
- Empiric treatment for high-risk patients who will undergo immunosuppression is frequently advised.

Toxocariasis

GENERAL PRINCIPLES

Epidemiology
- *Toxocara canis* and *Toxocara catis* are intestinal nematodes of dogs and cats that cause toxocariasis or visceral larva migrans (VLM) in humans.
- In the United States, the overall seroprevalence rate is about 14%.[8]
- Young children are especially vulnerable due to dirt pica (geophagia), poor hygiene, or frequent contact with dogs.
- Treating infected dogs and cats reduces the number of eggs and the potential burden for humans.

Pathophysiology
- Transmission: Ingestion of parasite eggs from contaminated soil
- Life cycle: Eggs excyst and larvae migrate through the circulation to the pulmonary system where they migrate up the trachea and are swallowed. In dogs and cats, adult worms develop in the intestine and shed eggs in the stool, which contaminate the environment.
- In humans larvae migrate to different tissues (liver, lung, heart, muscle, brain, and eyes) and are unable to develop into adult worms.
- Effects on the host: Larvae migrate but become trapped in host tissues, primarily the liver, where they are killed by granulomatous reactions from the host.

DIAGNOSIS

Clinical Presentation

- Most infected people are asymptomatic or have transient symptoms.
- Severity of symptoms depends on extent of exposure and resultant worm burden.
- Two clinical syndromes occur in children, VLM and ocular toxocariasis (OT).
  - VLM presents with episodes of fever, coughing and wheezing, anemia, eosinophilia, urticaria, and/or hepatomegaly.
  - OT presents as an inflamed tissue mass resembling a tumor. Patients present with loss of vision, strabismus, and/or retinal lesions.

Differential Diagnosis

- For VLM: infection with other helminths that migrate through tissues (ascariasis, hookworm, strongyloidiasis), asthma, and rheumatologic diseases (e.g., eosinophilic granulomatosis with polyangiitis).
- For OT: retinoblastoma and other causes of chorioretinitis.

Diagnostic Testing

- Leukocytosis with eosinophilia and hypergammaglobulinemia may be present in VLM.
- **The detection of larvae in tissue or body fluid samples is diagnostic but uncommon.**
- **Serology (ELISA) is commonly used but cannot distinguish between current and prior infection** and may cross-react with other helminths. Sensitivity is poor in OT and neurotoxocariasis; testing vitreous/aqueous humor or CSF may improve sensitivity.[9]
- Chest radiography may show nonspecific pulmonary infiltrates.
- Abdominal ultrasound may identify granulomas in the liver.

TREATMENT

- Although most patients recover with supportive care and anti-inflammatory medications, treatment of acute infection is recommended to prevent larvae from migrating to neural tissue.
- **Albendazole 400 mg PO twice daily × 5 days is recommended for VLM.**
- For OT, treatment of acute disease may help prevent vision loss but damage is irreversible.[9]

Schistosomiasis

GENERAL PRINCIPLES

- Schistosomiasis, also known as bilharzia, is caused by trematodes (flukes) of the genus *Schistosoma*.
- There are two main clinical forms of Schistosomiasis: urogenital (*S. haematobium*) and intestinal (*S. mansoni* and *S. haematobium*).
- Heavy infections can lead to liver fibrosis and portal hypertension.
- Praziquantel is the treatment of choice for schistosomiasis.

Epidemiology

- Approximately 230 million people globally are affected.[10]
- Persons swimming in contaminated freshwater are at highest risk for disease.
- Distribution of their intermediate snail vector determines the *Schistosoma* spp. present.
  - *S. mansoni*: Africa, South America, and parts of the Caribbean

- *Schistosoma haematobium*: Africa and the Middle East
- *Schistosoma japonicum* and *Schistosoma mekongi*: Southeast Asia
- Appropriate snail hosts are not present in the United States, but cases are frequently diagnosed in travelers and immigrants.

Pathophysiology

- Transmission: Occurs when cercariae in fresh water penetrate human skin.
- Life cycle
  - Cercariae penetrate skin, migrate through host tissues, and develop into adult worms within the mesenteric (*S. mansoni and others*) or perivesicular (*S. haematobium*) venules.
  - Female adult worms are wrapped by male worms *in copula*, allowing the female eggs to be fertilized and later released through the urine (*S. haematobium*) or feces (all other species).
  - In fresh water, eggs develop into miracidia, which enter the snail intermediate host, eventually developing into cercariae, which are released into the aqueous environment to perpetuate the cycle.
- Effects on the host: host pathology develops due to a granulomatous inflammatory response to adult worms and eggs within host tissues.
  - *S. mansoni*, *S. japonicum*, and *S. mekongi* **reside within mesenteric veins,** where their eggs can be swept into the portal vein, leading to periportal fibrosis and portal hypertension.
  - *S. haematobium* resides within the **bladder wall**, leading to hematuria and increased risk of bladder cancer. Urogenital infection in women also increases the risk of HIV infection.

DIAGNOSIS

Clinical Presentation

- Manifestations of chronic disease depend on the infecting species.
- Severity of symptoms depends on extent of exposure and worm burden.

History

- Swimmer's itch is a local dermatitis usually seen within a day of swimming in infected water. This pruritic rash may last for over a week and can also occur after exposure to avian schistosomes in the United States (Great Lakes).
- Acute schistosomiasis (**Katayama fever**) is a self-limited febrile illness that develops 4 to 8 weeks after exposure in response to the release of eggs from young adult worms. Symptoms can include myalgias, arthralgias, headache, abdominal pain, and diarrhea.
- *S. haematobium* infection may be asymptomatic or cause hematuria, frequency, dysuria, and incontinence.
- Intestinal schistosomiasis may result in chronic abdominal pain and diarrhea.
- Hepatic schistosomiasis may present with symptoms of portal hypertension.

Physical Examination

- Rashes may occur with acute disease.
- Women with *S. haematobium* may have polyps on external genitalia.
- In intestinal schistosomiasis, hepatomegaly, splenomegaly, and stigmata of portal hypertension can be seen.
- For *S. japonicum*, CNS disease or pulmonary findings occur in a minority of patients.

Differential Diagnosis

Geography and exposure history provide useful clues, as other helminthic infections can present similarity.

Diagnostic Testing

- Eosinophilia is frequent; anemia may occur with chronic blood loss.
- With *S. haematobium*, urinalysis may reveal hematuria.
- Definitive diagnosis is made by identifying schistosome eggs in the stool or urine.
- Serologic tests are available but are unable to differentiate between acute and chronic infections. They may be useful in acute disease before maturation of adult worms.
- Abdominal imaging may detect hepatomegaly, fibrosis, or portal hypertension.
- Other imaging modalities for pulmonary or CNS disease.

TREATMENT

- All patients with schistosomiasis should be offered therapy.
- **Praziquantel** is the drug of choice. A dose of 40 mg/kg/d administered in 1 to 2 doses for ×1 day is effective against both *S. mansoni* and *S. haematobium*. Other species may require a higher dose (60 mg/kg/d).[10]
- For travelers, treatment should be at least 6 to 8 weeks after the most recent exposure as immature larvae are not as sensitive to praziquantel as adults.
- Repeat screening examinations followed by repeat therapy within 3 to 6 weeks may be indicated to kill late-maturing worms.
- Management of hepatic, pulmonary, or urinary complications should be treated accordingly.
- Infectious disease consultation is advised for management of cases in the United States.

REFERENCES

1. Hotez PJ, Alvarado M, Basáñez M-G, et al. The global burden of disease study 2010: interpretation and implications for the neglected tropical diseases. *PLoS Negl Trop Dis.* 2014;8(7):e2865. doi:10.1371/journal.pntd.0002865.
2. Starr MC, Montgomery SP. Soil-transmitted helminthiasis in the United States: a systematic review – 1940–2010. *Am J Trop Med Hyg.* 2011;85(4):680-684. doi:10.4269/ajtmh.2011.11-0214.
3. Garcia HH, Gonzalez AE, Evans CAW, Gilman RH. Taenia solium cysticercosis. *Lancet.* 2003;362:547-556. doi:10.1016/S0140-6736(03)14117-7.
4. Garcia HH, Nash TE, Del Brutto OH. Clinical symptoms, diagnosis, and treatment of neurocysticercosis. *Lancet Neurol.* 2014;13(12):1202-1215. doi:10.1016/S1474-4422(14)70094-8.
5. Sharma M, Singh T, Mathew A. Antiepileptic drugs for seizure control in people with neurocysticercosis. *Cochrane Database Syst Rev.* 2015;(3). doi:10.1002/14651858.CD009027.pub2.
6. Olsen A, van Lieshout L, Marti H, et al. Strongyloidiasis–the most neglected of the neglected tropical diseases? *Trans R Soc Trop Med Hyg.* 2009;103(10):967-972. doi:10.1016/j.trstmh.2009.02.013.
7. Toledo R, Muñoz-Antoli C, Esteban JG. Strongyloidiasis with emphasis on human infections and its different clinical forms. *Adv Parasitol.* 2015;88:165-241. doi:10.1016/bs.apar.2015.02.005.
8. Hotez PJ, Wilkins PP. Toxocariasis: America's most common neglected infection of poverty and a helminthiasis of global importance? *PLoS Negl Trop Dis.* 3(3):e400. doi:10.1371/journal.pntd.0000400.
9. Ma G, Holland C V, Wang T, et al. Human toxocariasis. *Lancet Infect Dis.* 2017. doi:10.1016/S1473-3099(17)30331-6.
10. Colley DG, Bustinduy AL, Secor WE, King CH. Human schistosomiasis. *Lancet.* 2014;383:2253-2264. doi:10.1016/S0140-6736(13)61949-2.

Infection Prevention

19

Caline S. Mattar and Michael J. Durkin

GENERAL PRINCIPLES

Decades of improvements in infection prevention have resulted in significant decreases in health care–associated infections (HAIs); however, they remain a constant threat to hospitalized patients, resulting in significant morbidity and mortality and increases in health care costs. The Centers for Disease Control and Prevention (CDC) estimates that 5% to 10% of hospitalized patients develop an HAI, corresponding to approximately 2 million HAIs associated with nearly 100,000 deaths annually in US hospitals.[1,2] The emergence of pathogens such as severe acute respiratory syndrome coronavirus, avian influenza, epidemic influenza, Middle East Respiratory Syndrome and changes in existing pathogens (e.g., multidrug-resistant gram-negative organisms, methicillin-resistant *Staphylococcus aureus* [MRSA], *Clostridium difficile*) create an ongoing need for more efficient and effective infection prevention practices in both community and hospital settings.[3]

INFECTION PREVENTION STRATEGIES

- Current infection prevention strategies consist of two main sets of precautions: **standard precautions and transmission-based precautions.**[3]
  - ○ Standard precautions should be used with all patients who are admitted to the hospital. Frequent hand-washing with good technique is the most important factor in effective control of horizontal transmission of most pathogens.[4-6]
    - ▪ The current hand hygiene recommendations by the World Health Organization define the following as key moments to perform hand hygiene: 1-before touching a patient, 2-before clean/aseptic procedures, 3-after body fluid exposure/risk, 4-after touching a patient, and 5-after touching patient surroundings.
    - ▪ Gloves are not a substitute for hand hygiene. Wearing gloves is required when health care workers (HCWs) anticipate contact with body substances, mucous membranes, and nonintact skin of patients.
    - ▪ Additional precautions such as gowns and eye/face protection (i.e., masks and goggles) are indicated when splashes of body substances or blood are possible.
    - ▪ Standard precautions were developed not only for the prevention of transmission of blood-borne pathogens (e.g., HIV, hepatitis B, and hepatitis C) through percutaneous and mucous membrane contacts but also to protect against exposure to other pathogens.[3]
  - ○ Transmission-based precautions include contact precautions, droplet precautions, and airborne precautions.[3] These are designed to control the spread of infectious organisms not adequately controlled by standard precautions alone.
    - ▪ **Contact precautions** are recommended for patients infected or colonized with epidemiologically significant organisms that are transmitted by direct patient contact or by contact with items in the patient environment. The elements of contact precautions include wearing gowns and gloves when in a patient's room, using dedicated equipment that stays in the patient's room, and private room assignment or cohorting patients if private rooms are unavailable. Contact precautions should be used for patients with MRSA and other multidrug-resistant pathogens.

- **Droplet precautions** are indicated for infections that are spread by large respiratory droplets, such as *Neisseria meningitidis*, *Haemophilus influenza*, and influenza virus. HCWs should wear surgical/isolation masks when entering the room of a patient on droplet precautions.
- **Airborne precautions** are indicated for infections spread by small airborne particles. As these infectious particles can remain in the air for prolonged periods of time, negative-pressure ventilation rooms are required and HCWs must wear an N95 mask that can filter the small particles. Tuberculosis, measles, and chicken pox (varicella zoster virus) are common pathogens requiring airborne precautions.
- The CDC-Healthcare Infection Control Practices Advisory Committee (HICPAC) provides guidelines on isolation precautions for hospitals, including an appendix listing the type and duration of precautions needed for selected infections and conditions.[3]
- The type of precautions indicated for select clinically important pathogens is shown in Table 19-1.[3,7]

COMMON HAIs AND PREVENTION STRATEGIES

- An important aspect of hospital infection control is the development of preventive strategies to curtail the acquisition and transmission of HAIs.
- **HAIs are generally defined as infections occurring more than 48 hours after hospital admission** (the definition might be changed by the type of HAI and the incubation period of causative pathogens).
- The most common types of HAIs are **central line–associated bloodstream infections,**[8,9] **catheter-associated urinary tract infections,**[10,11] **surgical site infections,**[12,13] **ventilator-associated pneumonia,**[14,15] and ***C. difficile* infection.**[16] These infections result in increased health care costs, morbidity, and mortality.
- Prevention of HAIs is extremely important as these are frequently caused by multi-drug-resistant pathogens such as MRSA, vancomycin-resistant enterococci, multi-drug-resistant gram-negative organisms, and *C. difficile*.[17]
- Besides meticulous hand hygiene and implementation of proper isolation precautions, there are detailed guidelines which outline preventive strategies for each HAI.

OCCUPATIONAL HEALTH AND INFECTION PREVENTION

- Occupational health is closely linked to infection prevention. HCWs are at risk for being exposed to various types of infections during patient care. Prompt action may be necessary for assessment of a HCW exposed to infectious pathogens.
- **The most important strategy to protect HCWs from potentially infectious pathogens is prevention of the exposure.** This is achieved through adherence to all advised standard and transmission-based precautions as outlined above.[3]
- In addition, **vaccination against certain pathogens is a crucial component** of an occupational health program. Vaccinations recommended for HCWs include measles/mumps/rubella, varicella, hepatitis B, pertussis, and influenza.
  - Influenza vaccination of HCWs is an important method to prevent transmission of influenza to patients.
  - HCWs should receive annual influenza vaccination unless they have a medical contraindication.[18-20]
- Among pathogens commonly seen in the setting of occupational exposure, blood-borne pathogens including hepatitis B virus (HBV), hepatitis C virus (HCV), and HIV are particularly important.[21,22]

| TABLE 19-1 | ISOLATION PRECAUTIONS FOR SELECTED INFECTIONS AND CONDITIONS | |

Infection/Condition	Type	Precautions Duration
Multidrug-resistant pathogens (MRSA, MDR-GNR)	Contact	CN
Clostridium difficile infection	Contact	DI
Conjunctivitis, acute viral (acute hemorrhagic)	Contact	DI
Epiglottitis due to *Haemophilus influenza*	Droplet	U (24 h)
Hepatitis A virus, diapered or incontinent patients	Contact	F[a]
Herpes simplex virus		
Encephalitis	Standard	
Mucocutaneous, disseminated or primary, severe	Contact	DI
Influenza		
Seasonal influenza	Droplet	DI
Avian (H5N1) influenza	Airborne	F[b]
Pandemic influenza (2009 H1N1)	Droplet	DI
Measles (rubeola), all presentations	Airborne	DI
Meningitis		
Haemophilus influenzae, known or suspected	Droplet	U (24 h)
Neisseria meningitidis, known or suspected	Droplet	U (24 h)
Other diagnosed bacterial	Standard	
Meningococcal pneumonia	Droplet	U (24 h)
Meningococcemia (meningococcal sepsis)	Droplet	U (24 h)
Pneumococcal diseases	Standard	
Parvovirus B19	Droplet	F[c]
Pertussis (whooping cough)	Droplet	U (5 d)
Rabies	Standard	
Respiratory syncytial virus infection, infants, young children, or immunocompromised adults	Contact	DI
Streptococcal disease (group A streptococcus), skin, wound, or burn		
Major (no dressing or uncontained drainage)	Contact	U (24 h)
Minor or limited (contained drainage)	Standard	
Tuberculosis		
Extrapulmonary, draining lesion (including scrofula)	Standard	

(Continued)

TABLE 19-1	ISOLATION PRECAUTIONS FOR SELECTED INFECTIONS AND CONDITIONS (CONTINUED)		
Extrapulmonary, meningitis	Standard	
Pulmonary or laryngeal disease, confirmed or suspected	Airborne	F[d]
Skin test positive, without evidence of pulmonary disease	Standard	
Varicella zoster virus[e]		
Varicella (chickenpox)	Airborne and contact	F[f]
Zoster		
Localized in immunocompromised patient, disseminated	Airborne and contact	F[e]
Localized in normal patient	Standard	
Wound infections		
Major (no dressing or uncontained drainage)	Contact	DI
Minor or limited (contained drainage)	Standard	

Adapted from Siegel JD, Rhinehart E, Jackson J, Chiarello L. *2007 Guideline for Isolation Precautions: Preventing Transmission of Infectious Agents in Healthcare Settings.* Atlanta, GA: Centers for Disease Control and Prevention; 2007.

[a]Maintain precautions in infants and children younger than three years of age for the duration of hospitalization; in children aged 3 to 14, for 2 weeks after onset of symptoms; for children over age 14 years, for 1 week after onset of symptoms.

[b]See http://www.cdc.gov/flu/avianflu/ for current avian influenza guidance. Accessed May 22, 2012.

[c]Maintain precautions for the duration of hospitalization when chronic disease occurs in an immunocompromised patient. For patients with transient aplastic crisis or red cell crisis, maintain precautions for 7 days. Duration of precautions for immunosuppressed patients with persistently positive polymerase chain reaction test not defined, but transmission has occurred.

[d]Discontinue precautions ONLY when the patient is on effective therapy, is improving clinically, AND has three consecutive negative sputum smears collected on different days; or tuberculosis is ruled out.

[e]Maintain precautions until all lesions are crusted.

[f]Persons susceptible to varicella are at risk for varicella when exposed to patients with herpes zoster lesions or varicella and should not enter the room.

MDR-GNR, multidrug-resistant gram negative rod; MRSA, methicillin-resistant *Staphylococcus aureus.* Duration of precautions: CN, until off antibiotics and culture negative; DI, duration of illness; F, see footnote; U, until time specified after initiation of effective therapy.

○ The risks for a HCW acquiring infection after a contaminated percutaneous exposure to HBV, HCV, or HIV are approximately 30% (for an unvaccinated HCW), 3%, and 0.3%, respectively.

○ High-risk exposures include those from an infected source with high viremia or exposures involving a large-bore hollow needle, deep puncture, or large amount of visible blood.

- **Postexposure prophylaxis** is available for certain high-risk infections. Postexposure prophylaxis can include vaccination (e.g., HBV), use of infused immunoglobulin (IVIG) (e.g., HBV, varicella), and/or chemoprophylaxis with antimicrobials and anti-viral agents (e.g., pertussis and influenza).
- The pathogens that require postexposure prophylaxis and the type of postexposure prophylaxis are shown in Table 19-2.[22]

TABLE 19-2	POSTEXPOSURE PROPHYLAXIS FOR SELECTED ORGANISMS OR INFECTION	
Infection or Condition	Postexposure Prophylaxis	Comments
Hepatitis B (known HBsAg-positive source)		
Percutaneous injury:		
Unvaccinated health care worker (HCW)	HBIG × 1 and HBV vaccine series	If HBIG is indicated, it should be administered as soon as possible (prefera-bly within 24 h)
Previously vaccinated:		
Known responder	No treatment	
Known nonresponder	HBIG × 2 (previously revac-cinated) OR HBIG × 1 and initiate revaccination (not previously revaccinated)	
Antibody response unknown	Test exposed person for anti-HBsAb. If adequate HBsAb response (≥10 mIU/mL), no treatment; if inad-equate HBsAb response (<10 mIU/mL), HBIG × 1 and vaccine booster	
HIV body substance exposure		
HIV positive	Three drug postexposure prophylaxis[a]	For details of regimens for postexposure prophylaxis, see the guidelines from the USPHS[22]
Delayed exposure report(beyond 72 h from exposure)	Benefits of PEP undefined, case-by-case basis	

(Continued)

TABLE 19-2	POSTEXPOSURE PROPHYLAXIS FOR SELECTED ORGANISMS OR INFECTION (CONTINUED)	
Infection or Condition	**Postexposure Prophylaxis**	**Comments**
Unknown source	Use of PEP should be decided on a case-by-case (considering severity of exposure and epidemiologic likelihood of HIV exposure)	
Known or suspected resistance of the source virus to antiretrovirals	Provision of PEP should be delayed while awaiting resistance testing	Selection of antiretrovirals to which the source virus is unlikely to be resistant
Hepatitis C body substance exposure	No evidence of benefit of therapy (e.g., immunoglobulin or antiviral therapy) for postexposure prophylaxis; consider early treatment if seroconversion	
Influenza virus	Consider giving influenza vaccination and antiviral agents (e.g., oseltamivir and zanamivir)	Vaccination should be considered for exposed nonimmune HCW Chemoprophylaxis may vary by location, season, and drug susceptibility
Bordetella pertussis	Azithromycin 500 mg PO daily × 5 d or erythromycin 40 mg/kg PO daily (maximum 2 g/d) in four divided doses for 14 d For nonimmune HCW, Tdap should also be given	Does not require work restriction for exposed, asymptomatic HCW For infected HCW, they may return to work after receiving effective therapy for at least 5 d
Varicella zoster virus	Consider varicella virus vaccine within 3 d after exposure For nonimmune immunocompromised HCW, consider giving VZIG within 96 h after exposure	Day 8–21 after exposure, nonimmune HCW must not work or must not have direct patient contact and must work only with immune persons away from patient care areas For HCWs who received IVIG, restrict work until day 28 Giving the vaccine does not change the work restriction

TABLE 19-2	POSTEXPOSURE PROPHYLAXIS FOR SELECTED ORGANISMS OR INFECTION (CONTINUED)	
Infection or Condition	Postexposure Prophylaxis	Comments
Measles virus	For HCWs who have not received two doses of measles vaccine, consider giving MMR vaccine within 3 d after exposure	Day 5–21 after the exposure, nonimmune HCW must be excluded from work setting Giving vaccine after exposure does not change work restriction
Rubella virus	No prophylaxis is recommended	Rubella vaccine or immunoglobulin is not proven to prevent infection after exposure Day 7–21 after exposure, nonimmune HCW must not work or must not have direct patient contact and must work only with immune persons away from patient care areas
Mumps virus	No prophylaxis is recommended	Vaccine or immunoglobulin is not proven to prevent infection after exposure Day 12–26 after exposure, HCW must not work or must not have direct patient contact and must work only with immune persons away from patient care areas
Meningococcal disease	Ciprofloxacin 20 mg/kg (maximum 500 mg) PO single dose or rifampin 10 mg/kg (maximum 600 mg) PO q12h for 2 d or ceftriaxone 250 mg IM in a single dose	For pregnant HCW, IM ceftriaxone should be used Local antimicrobial susceptibility for *N. meningitides* should be checked as ciprofloxacin-resistant strains have been reported in the United States.

Adapted from Kuhar DT, Henderson DK, Struble KA, et al. Updated U.S. Public Health Service guidelines for the management of occupational exposures to HIV and recommendations for postexposure prophylaxis. *Infect Control Hosp Epidemiol.* 2013;34:875-892.

[a]Two nucleoside reverse transcriptase inhibitors (NRTIs) and one integrase inhibitor (INSTI) is the preferred regimen.

HBIG, hepatitis B immunoglobulin; HBsAb, hepatitis B surface antibody; HBsAg, hepatitis B surface antigen; HBV, hepatitis B virus; IVIG, intravenous immunoglobulin; MMR, measles/mumps/rubella vaccination; Tdap, tetanus, diphtheria, and acellular pertussis vaccination; VZIG, varicella zoster immunoglobulin.

REFERENCES

1. Klevens RM, Edwards JR, Richard CL, et al. Estimating health care-associated infections and deaths in U.S. hospitals, 2002. *Public Health Rep.* 2007;122:160–166.
2. Centers for Disease Control and Prevention. Healthcare-Associated Infections. http://www.cdc.gov/hai/. Accessed January 2, 2018.
3. Siegel JD, Rhinehart E, Jackson J, Chiarello L. *2007 Guideline for Isolation Precautions: Preventing Transmission of Infectious Agents in Healthcare Settings.* Atlanta, GA: Centers for Disease Control and Prevention; 2007. http://www.cdc.gov/hicpac/2007IP/2007isolation Precautions.html. Accessed January 2, 2018.
4. Centers for Disease Control and Prevention. Guideline for hand hygiene in health-care settings. Recommendations of the Healthcare Infection Control Practices Advisory Committee and the HICPAC/SHEA/APIC/IDSA Hand Hygiene Task Force. *MMWR Recomm Rep.* 2002;51(RR-16):1-45.
5. *WHO Guidelines on Hand Hygiene for Health Care.* Geneva: World Health Organization; 2009. http://whqlibdoc.who.int/publications/2009/9789241597906_eng.pdf. Accessed April 25, 2018.
6. Centers for Disease Control and Prevention. Hand Hygiene Training Tools. http://www.cdc.gov/handhygiene/training.html. Accessed January 4, 2018.
7. Centers for Disease Control and Prevention. Information on Avian Influenza. http://www.cdc.gov/flu/avianflu/. Accessed April 25, 2018.
8. Marschall J, Mermel LA, Classen D, et al. Strategies to prevent central line-associated bloodstream infection in acute care hospitals. *Infect Control Hosp Epidemiol.* 2008;29:S22-S30.
9. O'Grady NP, Alexander M, Burns LA, et al. *Guidelines for Prevention of Intravascular Catheter-Related Infections, 2011.* Atlanta, GA: Centers for Disease Control and Prevention; 2011. https://www.cdc.gov/infectioncontrol/guidelines/BSI/index.html. Accessed April 25, 2018.
10. Lo E, Nicolle L, Classen D, et al. Strategies to prevent catheter-associated urinary tract infections in acute care hospitals. *Infect Control Hosp Epidemiol.* 2008;29:S41-S50.
11. Gould CV, Umscheid CA, Agarwal RK, et al. *Guideline for Prevention of Catheter-Associated Urinary Tract Infections 2009.* Atlanta, GA: Centers for Disease Control and Prevention; 2009. https://www.cdc.gov/infectioncontrol/guidelines/CAUTI/index.html. Accessed April 25, 2018.
12. Anderson DJ, Podgorny K, Berrios-Torres SI, et al. Strategies to prevent surgical site infections in acute care hospitals. *Infect Control Hosp Epidemiol.* 2014; 35(6):605-627.
13. Berrios-Torres SI, Umscheid CA, Bratzler DW, et al. Centers for Disease Control and Prevention guideline for the prevention of surgical site infection, 2017. *JAMA Surg.* 2017;152(8):784-791.
14. Klompas M, Branson R, Eichenwald EC, et al. Strategies to prevent ventilator-associated pneumonia in acute care hospitals: 2014 update. *Infect Control Hosp Epidemiol.* 2014;35(8):915-936.
15. Tablan OC, Anderson LJ, Besser R, et al. Guidelines for preventing health-care–associated pneumonia, 2003: recommendations of CDC and the Healthcare Infection Control Practices Advisory Committee. *MMWR Recomm Rep.* 2004;53(RR-3):1-36.
16. Dubberke ER, Gerding DN, Classen D, et al. Strategies to prevent *Clostridium difficile* infections in acute care hospitals. *Infect Control Hosp Epidemiol.* 2008;29:S81-S92.
17. Siegel JD, Rhinehart E, Jackson J, Chiarello L. *Management of Multidrug-Resistant Organisms in Healthcare Settings, 2006.* Atlanta, GA: Centers for Disease Control and Prevention; 2006. http://www.cdc.gov/infectioncontrolguidelines/MDRO/index.html. Accessed January 4, 2018.
18. Centers for Disease Control and Prevention. Prevention Strategies for Seasonal Influenza in Healthcare Settings. http://www.cdc.gov/flu/professionals/infectioncontrol/healthcaresettings.htm. Accessed January 5, 2018.
19. Grohskopf LA, Sokolow LZ, Broder KR, et al. Prevention and control of influenza: recommendations of the Advisory Committee on Immunization Practices (ACIP). *MMWR Recomm Rep.* 2017;66(RR-5):1-20.
20. Talbot TR, Babcock H, Caplan AL, et al. Revised SHEA position paper: influenza vaccination of healthcare personnel. *Infect Control Hosp Epidemiol.* 2010;31:987-995.
21. U.S. Public Health Service. Updated U.S. Public Health Service guidelines for the management of occupational exposures to HBV, HCV, and HIV and recommendations for postexposure prophylaxis. *MMWR Recomm Rep.* 2001;50(RR-11):1-52.
22. Kuhar DT, Henderson DK, Struble KA, et al. Updated U.S. Public Health Service guidelines for the management of occupational exposures to HIV and recommendations for postexposure prophylaxis. *Infect Control Hosp Epidemiol.* 2013;34:875-892.

Antimicrobial Agents

David J. Ritchie, Maren Cowley, and
Nigar Kirmani

20

INTRODUCTION

- This chapter highlights key information for antibacterials, antimycobacterials, antifungals, and antivirals and is intended to serve as a quick reference to assist prescribers in the clinical use and monitoring of the agents discussed.
- The content of this chapter is derived from numerous primary, secondary, and tertiary sources. Additional information on products mentioned in this chapter may be obtained from the American Hospital Formulary Service, the Physicians' Desk Reference, Lexicomp, The Pharmacologic Basis of Therapeutics, relevant product package inserts, Drug Prescribing in Renal Failure: Dosing Guidelines for Adults and Children, and a variety of other print-based sources.
- Definitions used consistently throughout the chapter include CrCl, creatinine clearance; CVVHD, continuous venovenous hemodialysis; HD, hemodialysis; PD, peritoneal dialysis; TB, tuberculosis; MDR, multidrug-resistant; MSSA, methicillin-susceptible *Staphylococcus aureus*; MRSA, methicillin-resistant *S. aureus*; ESBL, extended-spectrum β-lactamase; FDA, Food and Drug Administration

Antibacterial Agents

β-LACTAMS

- The main adverse effects are gastrointestinal (GI) disturbances, hypersensitivity reactions, and phlebitis.
- Hematologic disturbances, seizures, electrolyte abnormalities, liver function test (LFT) abnormalities, and interstitial nephritis may also rarely occur.
- Patients receiving high doses of β-lactams should have their neurologic status monitored continuously for the presence of seizure activity.
- Serum creatinine (Cr) should be periodically monitored to assess dosing appropriateness and for interstitial nephritis.
- Complete blood counts (CBCs) should also be monitored for evidence of bone marrow suppression, as should the appearance of the skin for rash.
- Serum electrolytes should also be periodically monitored, as electrolyte disturbances may occur.

PENICILLINS

Amoxicillin

Amoxicillin is similar in spectrum to ampicillin but is more active than ampicillin against *Salmonella* and less active against *Shigella*.

Dosing and Administration
- The usual dosage range is 250 to 500 mg PO q8h or 500 to 875 mg PO q12h.
- *Renal dosing:*

- ◦ CrCl 10 to 50 mL/min: 250 to 500 mg q8-12h
- ◦ CrCl <10 mL/min: 250 to 500 mg q24h
- ◦ HD: 250 to 500 mg q24h, with the daily dose administered after dialysis on dialysis days
- ◦ PD: 250 mg q12h
- ◦ CVVHD: 250 to 500 mg q24h

Amoxicillin/Clavulanic Acid

The addition of clavulanic acid to amoxicillin extends the spectrum of amoxicillin to include β-lactamase-producing strains of methicillin-sensitive *S. aureus* (MSSA), enterococci, anaerobes, *Haemophilus influenzae*, *Moraxella catarrhalis*, and some gram-negative bacilli. Amoxicillin/clavulanic acid is an oral agent of choice for bite wound infections and for step-down therapy of polymicrobial infections not involving *Pseudomonas aeruginosa*, as it does not cover *Pseudomonas*.

Dosing and Administration
- The usual dosage range is (1) 250 to 500 mg q8h or 500 to 875 mg PO q12h of the oral tablets; (2) 90 mg/kg per day divided q12h of the suspension; or (3) 2000 mg PO q12h of the Augmentin XR tablet formulation.
- *Renal dosing:*
  - ◦ CrCl 15 to 30 mL/min: usual dose q12h
  - ◦ CrCl 5 to 15 mL/min: usual dose q24h
  - ◦ CrCl <5 mL/min: usual dose q48h
  - ◦ HD: 250 to 500 mg q24-48h, with the daily dose on dialysis days administered after dialysis
  - ◦ PD: 250 mg q12h
  - ◦ CVVHD: 250 to 500 mg q24h

Key Monitoring and Safety Information
The chewable tablets and oral suspension formulations contain aspartame and should thus be used cautiously in patients with phenylketonuria.

Ampicillin

Ampicillin is considered the drug of choice for treatment of infections caused by susceptible strains of enterococci and *Listeria monocytogenes*.

Dosing and Administration
- The usual dosage range for IV ampicillin is 8 to 12 g/d administered in divided doses q4-6h or as a continuous infusion. The usual dose of oral ampicillin is 250 to 500 mg PO q6h.
- *Renal dosing:*
  - ◦ CrCl of 10 to 50 mL/min: usual dose q6-8h
  - ◦ CrCl <10 mL/min: usual dose q12-24h
  - ◦ HD: 1 to 2 g IV q12-24h, with one of the daily doses on dialysis days administered after dialysis
  - ◦ PD: 250 mg to 2 g q12h
  - ◦ CVVHD: 1 to 2 g q6-12h

Ampicillin/Sulbactam

The addition of sulbactam to ampicillin extends or restores the spectrum of ampicillin to include β-lactamase-producing strains of MSSA, enterococci, anaerobes, *H. influenzae*, *M. catarrhalis*, and some gram-negative bacilli. The sulbactam component is also active against some strains of multidrug-resistant *Acinetobacter*.

Dosing and Administration
- The usual dosage is 1.5 to 3 g IV q6h.
- *Renal dosing:*
  - CrCl 15 to 29 mL/min: 1.5 to 3 g q12h
  - CrCl 5 to 14 mL/min: 1.5 to 3 g IV q24h
  - HD: 1.5 to 3 g IV q24h, with the daily dose on dialysis days administered after dialysis
  - PD: 1.5 to 3 g IV q24h
  - CVVHD: 1.5 to 3 g q8h

Dicloxacillin

Dicloxacillin is a drug of choice for treating minor MSSA infections, but the agent has minimal activity against enterococci and gram-negative bacteria.

Dosing and Administration
The usual dosage range is 125 to 500 mg PO q6h. No dosage adjustments are required in renal insufficiency or dialysis.

Nafcillin

Nafcillin is a drug of choice for treating MSSA infections, but the agent has minimal activity against enterococci and gram-negative bacteria.

Dosing and Administration
The usual dosage range for IV nafcillin is 8 to 12 g/d. Dose reduction should be considered in patients with significant hepatic impairment. No dosage adjustments are required in renal failure or dialysis.

Key Monitoring and Safety Information
Nafcillin may be more prone to causing neutropenia than other penicillins.

Oxacillin

Oxacillin is a drug of choice for treating MSSA infections, but the agent has minimal activity against enterococci and gram-negative bacteria.

Dosing and Administration
The usual dosage range for IV oxacillin is 8 to 12 g/d. Dose reduction should be considered in patients with significant hepatic impairment. No dosage adjustments are required in renal failure or dialysis.

Key Monitoring and Safety Information
Oxacillin may be more prone to causing drug-induced hepatitis than other penicillins. LFTs should be obtained periodically to monitor for hepatic effects, especially in patients receiving ≥12 g/d.

Penicillin G

Penicillin G remains among the drugs of choice for syphilis, *Pasteurella multocida*, *Actinomyces*, and some other anaerobic infections. Penicillin is the drug of choice for group A streptococcal pharyngitis and for prophylaxis of rheumatic fever and poststreptococcal glomerular nephritis.

Dosing and Administration
- The usual dosage range for IV penicillin G is 12 to 30 million U/d administered in divided doses q2-4h or as a continuous infusion. The dose of oral penicillin VK is 250 to 500 mg q6h. The usual dose of procaine penicillin is 0.6 to 1.2 million U/d. The usual dose of benzathine penicillin is 1.2 to 2.4 million U administered intermittently.

- *Renal dosing:*
  - CrCl 10 to 50 mL/min: 75% of the normal daily dose
  - CrCl <10 mL/min: 25% to 50% of the normal daily dose
  - HD: 2 to 3 million U/d, with one of the daily doses administered after dialysis on dialysis days
  - PD: 20% to 50% of the normal daily dose
  - CVVHD: 75% of the normal daily dose

Key Monitoring and Safety Information

Hyperkalemia (particularly with penicillin G potassium) and hypokalemia (with penicillin G sodium) may occur. Although the potassium salt is the more commonly used penicillin G preparation, the sodium salt should be given in the setting of hyperkalemia or azotemia.

Piperacillin/Tazobactam

Piperacillin, an extended-spectrum penicillin, has improved gram-negative activity over other penicillin derivatives, including *P. aeruginosa*. The addition of tazobactam to piperacillin enhances the spectrum to include β-lactamase-producing strains of anaerobes, gram-negative bacilli, staphylococci, and enterococci.

Dosing and Administration

- The usual dosage is 3.375 to 4.5 g IV q6h.
- *Renal dosing:*
  - CrCl 10 to 50 mL/min: 2.25 g q6-8h
  - CrCl <10 mL/min: 2.25 g IV q8h
  - HD: 2.25 g q8h, with one of the daily doses on dialysis days administered after dialysis
  - PD: 4.5 g q12h
  - CVVHD: 4.5 g q8h

CARBAPENEMS

Carbapenems have an extremely broad spectrum of activity against most strains of anaerobes, gram-negative bacilli, and gram-positive cocci, including strains of these organisms that produce a variety of β-lactamases.

Key Monitoring and Safety Information for All Carbapenems

Seizures may occur, particularly in patients with renal failure and prior central nervous system (CNS) disorders. Patients receiving carbapenems should have their neurologic status monitored continuously for the presence of seizure activity. Serum Cr should be closely monitored to assess dosing appropriateness in an effort to decrease seizure risk. Patients allergic to penicillin may exhibit cross-hypersensitivity reactions with carbapenems. Coadministration of carbapenems with valproic acid may cause valproic acid serum levels to decline, which may increase risk of breakthrough seizures in patients receiving valproic acid for seizures.

Doripenem

Doripenem is slightly more potent than meropenem for *P. aeruginosa*, and doripenem susceptibility testing of *P. aeruginosa* strains resistant to other carbapenems is warranted. However, doripenem does not provide reliable coverage against methicillin-resistant *S. aureus* (MRSA), *Enterococcus faecium*, and *Stenotrophomonas maltophilia*.

Dosing and Administration:

- The usual dose is 500 mg every 8 hours.
- *Renal dosing:*
  - CrCl 30 to 49 mL/min: 250 mg over 1 hour q8h
  - CrCl 11 to 29 mL/min: 250 mg over 1 hour q12h

- ○ CrCl ≤10 mL/min: No specific recommendations are available
- ○ HD/PD/CVVHD: No specific recommendations are available

Ertapenem

Ertapenem does not provide reliable coverage against *P. aeruginosa*, *Acinetobacter*, *enterococci*, MRSA, and *S. maltophilia* and is not suitable for empiric therapy of nosocomial infections.

Dosing and Administration:
- The usual dosage is 1 g IV q24h.
- *Renal dosing:*
  - ○ CrCl ≤30 mL/min: 500 mg q24h
  - ○ HD: 500 mg q24h, with the daily dose on dialysis days administered after each dialysis
  - ○ PD: 500 mg q24h
  - ○ CVVHD: 1 g q24h

Imipenem/Cilastatin

Imipenem does not provide reliable coverage against MRSA, *E. faecium*, and *S. maltophilia*, and is only weakly active against *Proteus*, *Providencia*, and *Morganella*. Cilastatin is microbiologically inactive but is added to prevent renal metabolism by dehydropeptidase I, thus increasing urinary levels of imipenem.

Dosing and Administration
- The usual dosage is 500 mg IV q6h or 1000 mg q6-8h
- *Renal dosing:*
  - ○ HD: 200 mg q6h or 500 mg q12h
  - ○ PD: 250 mg q12h
  - ○ CVVHD: 250 mg q6h or 500 mg q6-8h

Meropenem

Compared with imipenem, meropenem has slightly more activity against gram-negative organisms and slightly less activity against gram-positive organisms. However, meropenem does not provide reliable coverage against MRSA, *E. faecium*, and *S. maltophilia*.

Dosing and Administration
- Meropenem may be administered as an IV bolus or infusion over 30 to 180 minutes. The usual dose is 1 g q8h or 500 mg q6h for systemic infections and 2 g q8h for meningitis.
- *Renal dosing:*
  - ○ CrCl 10 to 50 mL/min: 1 to 2 g q12h
  - ○ CrCl <10 mL/min: 1 to 2 g q24h
  - ○ HD: 1 to 2 g q24h, with the daily dose given after dialysis on dialysis days
  - ○ PD: 1 to 2 g q24h
  - ○ CVVHD: 1 to 2 g q12h

Meropenem/Vaborbactam

Meropenem/vaborbactam contains a carbapenem and a cyclic boric acid β-lactamase inhibitor. The addition of vaborbactam increases the spectrum of meropenem to include *Klebsiella pneumoniae* carbapenemase (KPC)-producing Enterobacteriaceae. This product is FDA-approved for complicated urinary tract infections (UTIs), including pyelonephritis, but should be reserved for treatment of infections caused by multidrug-resistant organisms that are susceptible to meropenem/vaborbactam.

Dosing and Administration
- The recommended dose is 4 g (meropenem 2 g and vaborbactam 2 g) every 8 hours as an IV infusion over 3 hours.
- *Renal dosing:*

- ○ CrCl 30 to 49 mL/min: 2 g q8h
- ○ CrCl 15-29 mL/min: 2 g q12h
- ○ CrCl <15 mL/min: 1 g q12h
- ○ HD: 1 g q12h, with one of the daily doses given after dialysis on dialysis days
- ○ CVVHD/PD: No specific recommendations are available

MONOBACTAMS

Aztreonam

Aztreonam possesses a clinically relevant spectrum of activity that encompasses only gram-negative bacteria, including many strains of *P. aeruginosa*. Aztreonam does not provide reliable coverage against gram-positive or anaerobic bacteria and is also not stable to (1) AmpC chromosomal cephalosporinases produced by *Enterobacter*, *Citrobacter freundii*, or *Serratia* or (2) extended-spectrum plasmid-mediated β-lactamases (ESBLs) produced by *Klebsiella*, *Escherichia coli*, and many other gram-negative bacilli. An inhalational formulation of aztreonam is available to improve respiratory symptoms in cystic fibrosis patients with *P. aeruginosa* airway infection.

Dosing and Administration
- The usual dosage is 1 to 2 g IV q8h. The dose of the inhalational formulation is 75 mg three times daily (at least 4 h apart) for 28 days.
- *Renal dosing:*
  - ○ CrCl 10 to 50 mL/min: 50% of the usual daily dose IV
  - ○ CrCl <10 mL/min: 25% of the usual daily dose IV
  - ○ HD: 1 g IV q24h, with the daily dose on dialysis days administered after dialysis
  - ○ PD: 25% of the usual daily dose IV
  - ○ CVVHD: 1 g IV q12h

Key Monitoring and Safety Information
In contrast to cephalosporins and carbapenems, aztreonam is considered safe to use in patients with a history of serious β-lactam allergy. The inhalational formulation is only minimally absorbed systemically, but necessitates bronchodilator pretreatment to minimize the likelihood of bronchospasm.

CEPHALOSPORINS

- First-generation cephalosporins have activity against streptococci, MSSA, and many community-acquired *E. coli*, *Klebsiella* spp., and *Proteus* spp. These agents have limited activity against other enteric gram-negative bacilli and anaerobes.
- Second-generation cephalosporins have expanded coverage against enteric gram-negative bacilli and anaerobes (cefotetan and cefoxitin only).
- Third-generation cephalosporins have even broader coverage against enteric aerobic gram-negative bacilli, and most retain adequate activity against streptococci. However, these agents are not reliable for treatment of organisms producing AmpC β-lactamases regardless of the results of susceptibility testing.
- The fourth-generation cephalosporin, cefepime, provides broad-spectrum activity against aerobic gram-negative bacilli, including *P. aeruginosa* and many gram-negative bacilli resistant to third-generation cephalosporins, including those producing AmpC β-lactamases.
- **Ceftaroline** is the first β-lactam available for clinical use in the United States with activity against MRSA and is classified as a cephalosporin with anti-MRSA activity.
- There are two cephalosporin-β-lactamase inhibitor combination products (ceftolozane-tazobactam, ceftazidime-avibactam) that possess activity against many multidrug-resistant gram-negative bacteria, including *P. aeruginosa*.

- All cephalosporins have been associated with anaphylaxis, interstitial nephritis, anemia, and leukopenia. All patients should be asked about penicillin or cephalosporin allergies. Patients allergic to penicillins may have a cross-hypersensitivity reaction to cephalosporins. Prolonged therapy (>2 wk) is typically monitored with weekly serum Cr and CBCs.
- Patients receiving cephalosporins, particularly at high doses and in the presence of renal failure, should have their neurologic status monitored continuously for the presence of seizure activity. Serum Cr should be periodically monitored to assess dosing appropriateness. CBCs should also be monitored for evidence of bone marrow suppression, as should the appearance of the skin for evidence of rash.

FIRST-GENERATION CEPHALOSPORINS

Cefazolin

Cefazolin possesses activity against streptococci, MSSA, and many *E. coli*, *Klebsiella* spp., and *Proteus* spp. Cefazolin does not have activity against MRSA, enterococci, *P. aeruginosa*, and many other gram-negative organisms that produce a variety of β-lactamases.

Dosing and Administration
- The usual dosage is 1 to 2 g IV q8h.
- *Renal dosing:*
  - CrCl 10 to 50 mL/min: 1 g q12h
  - CrCl <10 mL/min: 1 g q24h
  - HD: 1 g q24h, with the daily dose on dialysis days administered after dialysis or 2 to 3 g thrice weekly after each regular thrice-weekly HD session.
  - PD: 500 mg IV q12h
  - CVVHD: 1 g q12h

Cephalexin
Dosing and Administration
- The usual dosage is 250 to 500 mg PO q6h.
- *Renal dosing:*
  - CrCl 10 to 50 mL/min: 250 to 500 mg q8 to 12h
  - CrCl <10 mL/min: 250 to 500 mg q12-24h
  - HD: 250 to 500 mg q12-24h, with one of the daily doses on dialysis days administered after dialysis
  - PD: 250 to 500 mg q12-24h
  - CVVHD: No specific recommendations are available

SECOND-GENERATION CEPHALOSPORINS

Cefaclor
Dosing and Administration
- The usual dosage is 250 to 500 mg PO q8h for the standard-release preparation or 375 mg q12h for the extended-release preparation.
- *Renal dosing:*
  - CrCl 10 to 50 mL/min: 50% to 100% of the usual daily dose
  - CrCl <10 mL/min: 50% to 100% of the usual daily dose
  - HD: 250 mg q8h, with one of the daily doses on dialysis days administered after dialysis
  - PD: 250 to 500 mg PO q8h
  - CVVHD: 250 mg PO q8h

Key Monitoring and Safety Information
Cefaclor has been associated with serum sickness–like reactions (0.5%), most commonly in children of age <6 years. Symptoms of this reaction include rash, arthritis, arthralgia, and fever usually occurring 2 to 11 days into therapy. Symptoms typically resolve within a few days after discontinuation.

Cefotetan

Cefotetan is classified chemically as a cephamycin. A unique aspect of cefotetan is its coverage against anaerobes, including many *Bacteroides fragilis*. Cefotetan is active against many ESBL-producing gram-negative bacteria, but clinical data supporting use of cefotetan for their treatment are limited.

Dosing and Administration
• The usual dosage is 1 to 2 g IV q12h.
• *Renal dosing:*
  ○ CrCl 10 to 50 mL/min: 1 to 2 g q24h
  ○ CrCl <10 mL/min: 1 to 2 g IV q48h
  ○ HD: 1 g q24h, with the daily dose on dialysis days administered after dialysis
  ○ PD: 1 g IV q24h
  ○ CVVHD: 1 to 2 g q24h

Key Monitoring and Safety Information
Cefotetan may cause bleeding and the disulfiram reaction (when administered concomitantly with alcohol) due to an *N*-methylthiotetrazole side chain contained on the molecule.

Cefoxitin

Cefoxitin is classified chemically as a cephamycin. A unique aspect of cefoxitin is its coverage against anaerobes, including many *B. fragilis*. Cefoxitin is also active against most ESBL-producing gram-negative bacteria, but clinical data supporting treatment of these organisms are limited.

Dosing and Administration
• The usual dosage is 1 to 2 g IV q6 to 8h.
• *Renal dosing:*
  ○ CrCl 10 to 50 mL/min: 1 to 2 g q8 to 12h
  ○ CrCl <10 mL/min: 1 to 2 g q24-48h
  ○ HD: 1 g q24-48h, with the daily dose on dialysis days administered after dialysis
  ○ PD: 1 g IV q24h
  ○ CVVHD: 1 to 2 g q8 to 12h

Cefuroxime IV

Dosing and Administration
• The usual dosage is 750 mg to 1.5 g IV q8h.
• *Renal dosing:*
  ○ CrCl 10 to 50 mL/min: 750 mg to 1.5 g q8 to 12h
  ○ CrCl ≤10 mL/min: 750 mg to 1.5 g q24h
  ○ HD: 750 mg to 1.5 g q24h, with the daily dose on dialysis days administered after dialysis
  ○ PD: 750 mg to 1.5 g q24h
  ○ CVVHD: 1 g IV q12h

Cefuroxime Axetil PO

Dosing and Administration
• The usual dosage is 250 to 500 mg PO q12h.
• *Renal dosing:*

- ○ CrCl 10 to 50 mL/min: 250 to 500 mg PO q12h
- ○ CrCl ≤10 mL/min: 250 to 500 mg PO q12h
- ○ HD: 250 to 500 mg PO q12h, with one of the daily doses on dialysis days administered after dialysis
- ○ PD: 250 to 500 mg PO q12h
- ○ CVVHD: No specific recommendations are available

THIRD-GENERATION CEPHALOSPORINS

Cefdinir

Dosing and Administration
- The usual dosage is 600 mg PO q24h or 300 mg PO q12h.
- *Renal dosing:*
  - ○ CrCl 10 to 50 mL/min: 300 mg q24h
  - ○ CrCl <10 mL/min: 300 mg q48h
  - ○ HD: 300 mg q48h, with the daily dose on dialysis days administered after dialysis
  - ○ PD: 300 mg q48h
  - ○ CVVHD: No specific recommendations are available

Cefditoren Pivoxil

Dosing and Administration
- The usual dosage is 200 to 400 mg PO q12h with food.
- *Renal dosing:*
  - ○ CrCl 10 to 50 mL/min: 200 mg q12-24h
  - ○ CrCl <10 mL/min: 200 mg q24h
  - ○ HD: 200 mg q24h
  - ○ PD; CVVHD: No specific recommendations are available

Key Monitoring and Safety Information
Cefditoren decreases serum levels of carnitine, the clinical significance of which is unknown. However, carnitine levels normalize after 7 to 10 days. The tablets are formulated with sodium caseinate (milk protein) and should be avoided in patients with a history of milk protein sensitivity.

Cefixime

Cefixime was used as an alternative therapy for uncomplicated gonorrhea in combination with single-dose oral azithromycin. This regimen is less effective than preferred CDC-endorsed gonorrhea treatments.

Dosing and Administration
- The usual dosage is 400 mg PO q24h or 200 mg PO q12h.
- *Renal dosing:*
  - ○ CrCl 21 to 60 mL/min: 300 mg q24h
  - ○ CrCl <20 mL/min: 200 mg q24h
  - ○ HD: 300 mg q24h, with the daily dose on dialysis days administered after dialysis
  - ○ PD: 200 mg PO q24h
  - ○ CVVHD: No specific recommendations are available

Key Monitoring and Safety Information
Cefixime is 30% to 50% absorbed orally and causes diarrhea in up to 27% of patients.

Cefotaxime

Cefotaxime is an alternative to ceftriaxone for empiric treatment of community-acquired pneumonia and bacterial meningitis.

Dosing and Administration
- The usual dosage is 1 g IV q6-8h for most infections and 2 g q4h for treatment of meningitis.
- *Renal dosing:*
  ○ CrCl 10 to 50 mL/min: 1 to 2 g q6 to 12h
  ○ CrCl <10 mL/min: 1 to 2 g q24h
  ○ HD: 1 g q24h, with the daily dose on dialysis days administered after dialysis
  ○ PD: 1 g q24h
  ○ CVVHD: 1 g q12h

Cefpodoxime Proxetil

Dosing and Administration
- The usual dosage is 100 to 400 mg PO q12h.
- *Renal dosing:*
  ○ CrCl 10 to 50 mL/min: 100 to 400 mg q24h
  ○ CrCl <10 mL/min: 100 to 400 mg q24h
  ○ HD: 100 to 400 mg q24-48h, with the daily dose on dialysis days administered after dialysis
  ○ PD: 100 to 400 mg PO q24h
  ○ CVVHD: No specific recommendations are available

Ceftazidime

Ceftazidime possesses clinically important activity against *P. aeruginosa* and is effective for treatment of infections caused by this organism. It is only weakly active against most gram-positive bacteria, including MSSA.

Dosing and Administration
- The usual dosage is 1 to 2 g q8h for most infections and 2 g q8h for treatment of gram-negative meningitis.
- *Renal dosing:*
  ○ CrCl 10 to 50 mL/min: 1 to 2 g q12-24h
  ○ CrCl <10 mL/min: 1 to 2 g q24h
  ○ HD: 1 g q24-48h is recommended, with the daily dose on dialysis days administered after dialysis
  ○ PD: 500 mg q24h
  ○ CVVHD: 1 to 2 g q12h

Ceftriaxone

Ceftriaxone is a drug of choice for community-acquired pneumonia and empiric treatment of bacterial meningitis. The combination of ceftriaxone and ampicillin IV may be used for treatment of ampicillin-susceptible *Enterococcus faecalis* endocarditis. Ceftriaxone IM is the treatment of choice for gonorrhea (along with azithromycin).

Dosing and Administration
The usual dosage is 1 to 2 g IV q24h for most infections and 2 g q12h for treatment of meningitis and ampicillin-susceptible *E. faecalis* endocarditis. No dosage adjustments are recommended in renal failure or dialysis.

Key Monitoring and Safety Information
Ceftriaxone may cause biliary sludging and stones because of its high extent of biliary excretion and resultant precipitation with bile salts. Owing to its biliary excretion,

ceftriaxone frequently causes diarrhea. Intravenous ceftriaxone and intravenous calcium-containing products should not be coadministered in neonates because of risk of lung and/or kidney precipitation of ceftriaxone-calcium salts.

FOURTH-GENERATION CEPHALOSPORIN

Cefepime

Cefepime possesses clinically important activity against streptococci, MSSA, and gram-negative bacilli, including *P. aeruginosa* and other AmpC β-lactamase-producing strains.

Dosing and Administration
- The usual dosage is 1 to 2 g q8 to 12h for most infections and 2 g q8h for use in febrile neutropenia.
- *Renal dosing:*
  - CrCl 10 to 50 mL/min: 1 to 2 g q24h
  - CrCl <10 mL/min: 500 mg to 1 g q24h
  - HD: 500 mg to 1 g q24h, with the daily dose on dialysis days administered after dialysis or 2 g after each thrice-weekly regular dialysis session
  - PD: 500 mg to 1 g q24h
  - CVVHD: 1 to 2 g q12h

CEPHALOSPORIN WITH ANTI-MRSA ACTIVITY

Ceftaroline

Ceftaroline is the first β-lactam antibiotic approved by the FDA to have clinically useful activity against MRSA. Ceftaroline is also active against many drug-resistant pneumococci and is FDA-approved for treatment of community-acquired pneumonia. However, ceftaroline is not active against gram-negative bacteria producing ESBLs, AmpC β-lactamase (including *P. aeruginosa*), or class A or B carbapenemases (including *K. pneumoniae* carbapenemases), enterococci, or anaerobes.

Dosing and Administration
- The usual dosage is 600 mg IV q12h.
- *Renal dosing:*
  - CrCl 30 to 49 mL/min: 400 mg q12h
  - CrCl 15 to 29 mL/min: 300 mg q12h
  - CrCl ≤14 mL/min: 200 mg q12h
  - HD: 200 mg q12h, with one of the daily doses given after dialysis on dialysis days
  - PD: No specific recommendations are available
  - CVVHD: No specific recommendations are available

Key Monitoring and Safety Information
Ceftaroline has a safety profile similar to other cephalosporins.

CEPHALOSPORINS WITH BETA-LACTAMASE INHIBITORS

Ceftazidime-avibactam

The addition of avibactam, a β-lactamase inhibitor, enhances the gram-negative spectrum of ceftazidime to include AmpC β-lactamase-, ESBL-, and KPC-producing strains, in addition to many strains of multidrug-resistant *P. aeruginosa*. Ceftazidime-avibactam has minimal activity against anaerobes and gram-positive bacteria. It is useful for treatment of infections caused by multidrug-resistant gram-negative pathogens testing or expected to be sensitive to ceftazidime-avibactam when safety and/or effectiveness concerns exist with other agents.

Dosing and Administration
- The usual dosage is 2.5 g IV 8h.
- *Renal dosing:*
  - CrCl 31 to 50 mL/min: 1.25 g q8h
  - CrCl 16 to 30 mL/min: 0.94 g q12h
  - CrCl 6 to 15 mL/min: 0.94 g q24h
  - CrCl <5 mL/min: 0.94 g q48h
  - HD: 0.94 g q48h, administered after dialysis on dialysis days

Ceftolozane-tazobactam

Ceftolozane-tazobactam is active against many strains of *P. aeruginosa* that are resistant to other agents, as well as some ESBL-producing Enterobacteriaceae. This agent is not reliably active against anaerobes and Gram-positive bacteria. Ceftolozane-tazobactam is FDA-approved for complicated UTIs and complicated intra-abdominal infections in combination with metronidazole but is best used for treatment of infections caused by multidrug-resistant *P. aeruginosa* when safety and/or effectiveness concerns exist with other agents.

Dosing and Administration
- The usual dosage is 1.5 g IV q8h.
- *Renal dosing:*
  - CrCl 30 to 50 mL/min: 750 mg IV q8h
  - CrCl 15 to 29 mL/min: 375 mg IV q8h
  - CrCl <10 mL/min: no data
  - HD: The usual dose is a one-time loading dose of 750 mg followed by 150 mg IV q8h, with one of the daily doses given shortly after dialysis on dialysis days

MACROLIDES AND AZALIDES

Macrolides and azalides possess activity against many typical and atypical community respiratory tract pathogens, including *Streptococcus pneumoniae*, *Mycoplasma pneumoniae*, *Chlamydia pneumoniae*, and *Legionella pneumophila*. In addition, clarithromycin and azithromycin provide coverage against *H. influenzae* as well as *Mycobacterium avium* complex (MAC) infections. Adverse effects include GI disturbances, elevations in LFT and hepatic dysfunction, IV site reactions, rash, and, rarely, ototoxicity at high sustained doses.

Azithromycin

In addition to its activity against typical and atypical community respiratory tract pathogens, azithromycin is useful for treatment of MAC infection and some sexually transmitted infections including chlamydia, pelvic inflammatory disease, and chancroid.

Dosing and Administration
The usual dosage is 250 to 500 mg PO q24h or 500 mg IV q24h. Dosage adjustments are not required for renal failure or dialysis.

Key Monitoring and Safety Information
Unlike erythromycin and clarithromycin, azithromycin does not inhibit cytochrome P450 hepatic enzymes and is not associated with drug interactions involving this mechanism. Azithromycin has been safely used in pregnant women.

Clarithromycin

In addition to its activity against typical and atypical community respiratory tract pathogens, clarithromycin is useful for treatment of MAC infection and *Helicobacter pylori*–associated peptic ulcer disease.

Dosing and Administration

- The usual dosage is 250 to 500 mg PO q12h or 1000 mg PO q24h for the extended-release formulation.
- *Renal dosing:*
  ○ CrCl 10 to 50 mL/min: 250 to 500 mg q12-24h
  ○ CrCl <10 mL/min: 250 to 500 mg q24h
  ○ HD: 250 to 500 mg q24h, with the daily dose on dialysis days administered after dialysis
  ○ PD: 250 to 500 mg q12-24h
  ○ CVVHD: 250 to 500 mg q12-24h

Key Monitoring and Safety Information

Clarithromycin is a significant inhibitor of hepatic cytochrome P450 enzymes and can increase serum levels of carbamazepine, HMG-CoA reductase inhibitors, cyclosporine, tacrolimus, theophylline, warfarin, ergotamine, dihydroergotamine, triazolam, and many other drugs. Clarithromycin should be avoided in pregnancy.

Erythromycin

Erythromycin does not provide reliable coverage against *H. influenzae*, but it does possess clinically useful activity against *Chlamydia trachomatis* and *Campylobacter*.

Dosing and Administration

The usual dosage of erythromycin is 250 to 500 mg PO q6h (base, estolate, stearate), 333 mg PO q8h (base), or 400 mg PO q6h (ethylsuccinate). The usual IV dose of erythromycin lactobionate is 500 mg to 1 g IV q6h. Dosage reduction in patients with hepatic failure may be advisable. Dosage reduction is not required in renal failure or dialysis.

Key Monitoring and Safety Information

Erythromycin causes increased gastric motility and is poorly tolerated. It is a significant inhibitor of hepatic cytochrome P450 enzymes and can increase serum levels of many drugs (similar to clarithromycin above).

AMINOGLYCOSIDES

- Aminoglycosides are used as adjunctive agents in severe infections caused by gram-negative aerobes and may also be used to provide synergistic activity with β-lactams or vancomycin in the treatment of severe gram-positive infections. These agents have diminished activity in the low-pH/low-oxygen environment of abscesses and do not have activity against anaerobes. Their use is limited by significant nephrotoxicity and ototoxicity. Resistance to one aminoglycoside is not routinely associated with resistance to all members of this class.
- Traditional dosing of aminoglycosides is q8h, with the upper end of the dose range reserved for life-threatening infections. Peak and trough levels should be obtained with the third or fourth dose and then every 3 to 4 days along with a serum Cr. Increasing serum Cr or peaks/troughs out of the acceptable range require immediate attention.
- Extended-interval dosing of aminoglycosides is an alternative method of administration. A drug concentration is obtained 6 to 14 hours after the first dose, and a nomogram (Figure 20-1)[1] is consulted to determine the subsequent dosing interval. Monitoring includes obtaining another drug concentration 6 to 14 hours after a dose every week and a serum Cr thrice weekly. In patients who are not responding to therapy, a 12-hour level should be checked. If that 12-hour level is undetectable, extended-interval dosing should be abandoned in favor of traditional dosing. For obese patients (actual weight >20% above ideal body weight [IBW]), an obese dosing weight (ODW) should be used for determining doses in either traditional or extended-interval dosing as follows: ODW = IBW + 0.4 (actual weight−IBW).

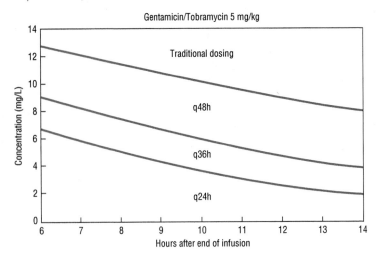

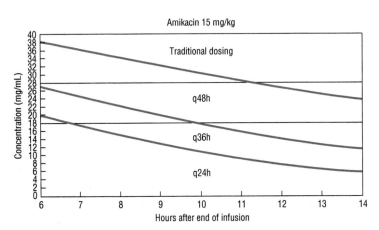

FIGURE 20-1 Nomograms for extended-interval aminoglycoside dosing. Adapted from Bailey TC, Little JR, Littenberg B, et al. A meta-analysis of extended-interval dosing versus multiple daily dosing of aminoglycosides. *Clin Infect Dis.* 1997;24(5):786-795.

Key Monitoring and Safety Information for Aminoglycosides

- Nephrotoxicity occurs more commonly after ≥5 days of therapy and is characterized by a reduction in glomerular filtration rate (GFR). Risk factors include hypotension, duration of therapy, associated liver disease, increased serum concentrations, advanced age, and coadministration of other nephrotoxic agents. The renal dysfunction noted is generally nonoliguric and is usually reversible with discontinuation of the agent. Serum Cr should be monitored closely as well as serum drug levels, with the dose and frequency adjusted accordingly.
- Ototoxicity associated with aminoglycosides is usually irreversible and may be vestibular or auditory. The hearing loss typically affects high-tone frequencies. Vestibular

damage may manifest as nystagmus, vertigo, nausea, or vomiting. Aminoglycosides may also rarely cause neuromuscular blockade. Underlying conditions or the use of other medications that affect the neuromuscular junction enhances this effect. Hypokalemia and hypomagnesemia may also occur. Patients receiving aminoglycosides for extended periods (usually >14 d) should have baseline and regularly scheduled audiometric studies to assess for ototoxicity. Patients receiving other nephrotoxic or ototoxic agents should receive aminoglycosides with caution and be monitored closely.

- Aminoglycosides can cause fetal harm when given to pregnant women. These agents are able to cross the placenta and may cause otologic damage. These agents should only be used during pregnancy if the potential benefits outweigh the possible risks to the fetus.

Amikacin

Amikacin has in vitro activity against a wide range of aerobic gram-negative bacilli, including some organisms resistant to other aminoglycosides. Amikacin is also useful in the treatment of infections caused by *Nocardia asteroides*, MAC, and certain species of rapid-growing mycobacteria (*Mycobacterium chelonae* and *Mycobacterium fortuitum*). As with other aminoglycosides, amikacin lacks activity against anaerobes and *S. maltophilia*.

Dosing and Administration

- The usual multiple daily dose regimen is 5 to 7.5 mg/kg q8-12h. Serum peaks and troughs should be measured once the patient is at steady state. Serum peaks should be 20 to 30 μg/mL, with troughs of 5 to 10 μg/mL. Amikacin may also be given as 15 mg/kg doses administered infrequently. A random serum concentration should be checked 6 to 14 hours after the initial dose. The subsequent dosing interval should then be adjusted based on this random concentration using a nomogram (see Figure 20-1).[1]
- *Renal dosing:*
  - CrCl 10 to 50 mL/min: 5 to 7.5 mg/kg q12-78h per levels
  - CrCl <10 mL/min: 5 to 7.5 mg/kg q48-72h per levels
  - HD: 2.5 to 7.5 mg/kg after dialysis on dialysis days only as per levels
  - PD: 5 to 7.5 mg/kg × 1, with serial level monitoring
  - CVVHD: 5 to 7.5 mg/kg q24-48h, with serial level monitoring

Gentamicin

Gentamicin is the most established and commonly used aminoglycoside for **synergistic therapy with cell wall–active antibiotics** in the treatment of serious gram-positive infections.

Dosing and Administration

- The usual multiple daily dose regimen is 1 to 1.7 mg/kg q8h. Serum peaks and troughs should be measured once the patient is at steady state. Serum **peaks** should be 3 to 4 μg/mL for gram-positive synergy and 6 to 10 μg/mL for gram-negative infections. **Troughs** should be <1 μg/mL. Gentamicin may also be given as 5 mg/kg doses administered infrequently. A random serum concentration should be checked 6 to 14 hours after the initial dose. The subsequent dosing interval should then be adjusted based on this random concentration using a nomogram (see Figure 20-1).[1]
- *Renal dosing:*
  - CrCl 10 to 50 mL/min: 1 to 1.7 mg/kg q12-48h per levels
  - CrCl <10 mL/min: 1 to 1.7 mg/kg q48-72h per levels
  - HD: 0.5 to 1.7 mg/kg after dialysis on dialysis days only as per levels
  - PD: 1 to 1.7 mg/kg, with serial level monitoring
  - CVVHD: 1 to 1.7 mg/kg q12-48h, with serial level monitoring

Streptomycin

Streptomycin can be used clinically as an alternative agent for tuberculosis, for synergistic therapy of enterococcal endocarditis in the setting of high-level gentamicin resistance, and for tularemia.

Dosing and Administration
- Tuberculosis:
  - Daily therapy: 15 mg/kg per day (maximum, 1 g)
  - Twice-weekly therapy: 25 to 30 mg/kg (maximum, 1.5 g)
  - Thrice-weekly therapy: 25 to 30 mg/kg (maximum, 1.5 g)
- Synergy for Endocarditis: 15 mg/kg per day divided q12h in combination with cell wall–active agent (e.g., penicillin, ampicillin, and vancomycin)
- Tularemia
  - 15 mg/kg q12h
  - *Renal dosing:*
    - CrCl 10 to 50 mL/min: dose q24-72h per levels
    - CrCl <10 mL/min: dose q72-96h per levels
    - HD: 50% of the usual dose should be administered after dialysis on dialysis days only as per levels
    - PD: Usual dose × 1, with serial level monitoring
    - CVVHD: Usual dose q24-72h, with serial level monitoring

Key Monitoring and Safety Information
Peaks should be 20 to 35 µg/mL, and troughs should be <5 to 10 µg/mL. Intramuscular injections of streptomycin are often painful, and hot, tender masses may develop at sites of injection. The drug may also be administered IV.

Tobramycin

The activity of tobramycin against some strains of *Acinetobacter* spp. and *P. aeruginosa* may be greater than that of gentamicin.

Dosing and Administration
- The usual multiple daily dose regimen is 1 to 1.7 mg/kg q8h. Serum peaks and troughs should be measured once the patient is at steady state. Serum peaks should be 6 to 10 µg/mL for gram-negative infections. Troughs should be <1 µg/mL. Tobramycin may also be given as 5 mg/kg doses administered infrequently. A random serum concentration should be checked 6 to 14 hours after the initial dose. The subsequent dosing interval should then be adjusted based on this random concentration using a nomogram (Figure 20-1).[1]
- *Renal dosing:*
  - CrCl 10 to 50 mL/min: 1 to 1.7 mg/kg q24-48h per levels
  - CrCl <10 mL/min: 1 to 1.7 mg/kg q48-72h per levels
  - HD: 0.5 to 1.7 mg/kg after dialysis on dialysis days only as per levels
  - PD: 1 to 1.7 mg/kg, with serial level monitoring
  - CVVHD: 1 to 1.7 mg/kg q24-48h, with serial level monitoring

FLUOROQUINOLONES

Fluoroquinolones are well absorbed orally, with serum levels that approach parenteral therapy for several of these agents. Fluoroquinolones are active against Enterobacteriaceae, but only ciprofloxacin, levofloxacin, and delafloxacin are active against *P. aeruginosa*. Fluoroquinolones have activity against atypical community respiratory tract pathogens, but only moxifloxacin, gemifloxacin, levofloxacin, and delafloxacin are considered reliable for pneumococcus. Delafloxacin is the only fluoroquinolone with clinically reliable activity against MRSA.

Key Monitoring and Safety Information

- The main adverse effects with fluoroquinolones include nausea, CNS disturbances (e.g., drowsiness, headache, restlessness, and dizziness, especially in the elderly), rashes, and phototoxicity. Patients should be counseled to use caution when performing tasks requiring alertness or coordination. Excess sunlight should also be avoided.
- These agents can cause prolongation of the QTc interval and should not be used in patients with known conduction abnormalities on ECG, patients with bradycardia, those with uncorrected hypokalemia, and those receiving class IA or III antiarrhythmic agents. They should also be used with caution in patients receiving agents that may have an additive effect in prolonging the QT interval (e.g., erythromycin, antipsychotics, and tricyclic antidepressants [TCAs]) and in patients with ongoing proarrhythmic conditions (e.g., significant bradycardia and acute myocardial ischemia). Patients at risk should be monitored closely with the use of ECGs. In patients with hepatic dysfunction or receiving other hepatotoxic drugs, LFTs should be monitored. Fluoroquinolones should not be used routinely in patients aged <18 years or in pregnant or lactating women. They can cause an age-related arthropathy and should be discontinued in patients who develop joint pain or tendinitis (most commonly the Achilles tendon), which may include the possibility of tendon rupture. Myasthenia gravis exacerbations, peripheral neuropathy, aortic ruptures or tears, and hypoglycemia may also occur with fluoroquinolones.
- Aluminum- and magnesium-containing antacids, sucralfate, bismuth, oral iron, oral calcium, oral zinc, and enteral nutritional formulas can markedly impair absorption of oral quinolones when administered simultaneously. Staggering oral fluoroquinolone doses by at least 2 to 6 hours from these preparations is recommended.

Ciprofloxacin

Ciprofloxacin has in vitro activity against a wide range of gram-negative aerobes, including Enterobacteriaceae, *P. aeruginosa*, and other non-Enterobacteriaceae, although resistance may occur. Ciprofloxacin is considered to be the most clinically established **oral antibiotic for treatment of *P. aeruginosa* infections**. However, it is relatively inactive against streptococci and anaerobes and therefore should not be used as monotherapy of community respiratory tract, skin, or abdominal infections.

Dosing and Administration

- For most infections, an oral dose of 500 mg q12h may be used. For more severe or complicated infections, up to 750 mg q12h may be used. For uncomplicated acute cystitis, doses of 100 to 250 mg q12h or 500 mg qd of the extended-release formulation for 3 days have been used successfully. The usual IV dose is 400 mg IV q12h. For more severe infections, doses of 400 mg q8h have been used.
- *Renal dosing:*
  - CrCl <30 mL/min: 50% of the usual dose
  - HD: 200 to 250 mg q12h, with one of the daily doses administered after dialysis on dialysis days
  - PD: 200 to 250 mg q8h
  - CVVHD: 400 mg q24h

Gemifloxacin

Gemifloxacin activity against *S. pneumoniae* is significantly greater than that of ciprofloxacin and levofloxacin and slightly better than that of moxifloxacin. It is not reliably active against *P. aeruginosa* and is only available orally.

Dosing and Administration

- The usual dosage is 320 mg PO q24h.
- *Renal dosing:*

- CrCl 10 to 50 mL/min: 160 to 320 mg q24h
- CrCl <10 mL/min: 160 mg q24h
- HD: 160 mg q24h, with the daily dose given after dialysis on dialysis days
- PD: 160 mg q24h
- CVVHD: 160 to 320 mg q24h

Key Monitoring and Safety Information

Skin rash occurs in 2.8% of patients, and approximately 10% of these cases are severe. The incidence of skin rash may be >15% in women under age 40 who receive 10 days of therapy. Women, patients under age 40 years, and postmenopausal women receiving hormone replacement therapy are at increased risk of rash.

Levofloxacin

Levofloxacin activity against *S. pneumoniae* is greater than that of ciprofloxacin but less than that of gatifloxacin and moxifloxacin. Levofloxacin activity against *P. aeruginosa* is inferior to that of ciprofloxacin. Levofloxacin is active against *C. trachomatis* and is an alternative treatment for this infection.

Dosing and Administration
- The usual recommended dose is 500 mg IV or PO q24h. Doses of 750 mg q24h have been used for complicated skin and skin structure infections and pneumonia.
- *Renal dosing:*
  - CrCl 20 to 49 mL/min: 500 to 750 mg × 1, then 250 to 500 mg q24h
  - CrCl 10 to 19 mL/min: 500 to 750 mg × 1, then 250 to 500 mg q48h
  - HD: 250 to 500 mg q48h
  - PD: 250 to 500 mg q48h
  - CVVHD: 500 mg q48h

Moxifloxacin

Moxifloxacin has greater activity against *S. pneumoniae* than ciprofloxacin and levofloxacin. Moxifloxacin is not reliably active against *P. aeruginosa*. Moxifloxacin has activity against anaerobes, including *B. fragilis*, but resistance is frequent. Moxifloxacin should not be used for UTIs due to its minimal urinary excretion.

Dosing and Administration:
- The usual dose is 400 mg q24h. No dosage adjustments are required in renal failure or dialysis.

Delafloxacin

Delafloxacin possesses activity against both MRSA and *P. aeruginosa*. While clinical evidence is limited, in vitro data reveal that delafloxacin has a broad range of activity against gram-positive, gram-negative, and anaerobic organisms. The FDA has approved delafloxacin to treat acute bacterial skin and skin structure infections.

Dosing and Administration
- The usual dosage is 450 mg PO q12h, or 300 mg IV q12h.
- *Renal dosing:*
  - CrCl 15 to 30 mL/min: 200 mg IV q12h, no dosage adjustments for oral administration
  - CrCl <15 mL/min: use not recommended
  - HD/PD/CVVDH: use not recommended

Key Monitoring and Safety Information

Delafloxacin did not shown potential for prolongation of the QT interval or phototoxicity in early clinical trials.

TETRACYCLINES AND GLYCYLCYCLINE

Doxycycline

Doxycycline is the treatment of choice for most rickettsial infections, including Rocky Mountain spotted fever and ehrlichiosis and can also be used to treat *Chlamydia*, *Mycoplasma*, syphilis, and outpatient community-acquired pneumonia. The drug may also be active against some multidrug-resistant gram-negative bacteria, including some *Acinetobacter* and *Klebsiella*, warranting susceptibility testing with this agent against such strains.

Dosing and Administration

The usual dose is 100 mg PO/IV q12h. No dosage adjustments are required in renal failure or dialysis.

Key Monitoring and Safety Information

GI disturbances and photosensitivity are common side effects. Esophageal ulceration, hepatic impairment, and pseudotumor cerebri may also occur. Doxycycline should not be given routinely to children because of its ability to discolor tooth enamel. Aluminum- and magnesium-containing antacids, sucralfate, bismuth, oral iron, oral calcium, oral zinc, and enteral nutritional formulas can markedly impair absorption of oral doxycycline when administered simultaneously. Staggering oral doxycycline doses by at least 2 to 6 hours from these preparations is recommended.

Oral doxycycline should be administered with a full glass of water to decrease the possibility of esophageal ulceration. The drug should be avoided in pregnancy. It is distributed in breast milk and should be avoided in nursing mothers.

Minocycline

Minocycline is used clinically for acne, nocardiosis, leprosy, and *Mycobacterium marinum* infections. The drug may also be active against some multidrug-resistant gram-negative bacteria, including some *Acinetobacter*, *Klebsiella*, and *Stenotrophomonas*, warranting susceptibility testing with this agent against these strains.

Dosing and Administration

The usual dose is 200 mg PO/IV × 1, then 100 mg PO/IV q12h. No dosage adjustment is required in renal failure or dialysis.

Key Monitoring and Safety Information

- Vestibular disturbances occur more frequently with minocycline as compared with other tetracyclines.
- GI disturbances and photosensitivity are common side effects.
- Esophageal ulceration, hepatic impairment, and pseudotumor cerebri may also occur.
- Minocycline should not be given to children because of its ability to discolor tooth enamel.
- Aluminum- and magnesium-containing antacids, sucralfate, bismuth, oral iron, oral calcium, oral zinc, and enteral nutritional formulas can markedly impair absorption of oral minocycline when administered simultaneously. Staggering oral minocycline doses by at least 2 to 6 hours from these preparations is recommended.
- Oral minocycline should be administered with a full glass of water to decrease the possibility of esophageal ulceration.
- The drug should be avoided in pregnancy. It is distributed in breast milk and should be avoided in nursing mothers.

Tigecycline

Tigecycline is a glycylcycline antibiotic that is US FDA-approved for treatment of abdominal and skin/skin structure infections, as well as community-acquired pneumonia. The drug does not have activity against *P. aeruginosa* and has been shown to be ineffective for ventilator-associated pneumonia (VAP). The drug has also been associated with break-through bacteremias, which may be due to its very low blood concentrations. Tigecycline was also linked with increased all-cause mortality across phase 3 and 4 clinical trials. In vitro susceptibility to this agent should be documented as resistance may occur.

Dosing and Administration

The usual dose is 100 mg × 1, then 50 mg q12h. The dose should be reduced to 100 mg × 1, then 25 mg q12h for severe hepatic failure. There are no dosage adjustments in renal failure or dialysis.

Key Monitoring and Safety Information

The most common adverse effects are nausea and vomiting, diarrhea, and headache. Hepatic dysfunction and pancreatitis may also occur. Patients allergic to tetracyclines may be cross-allergic to tigecycline. Tigecycline should not be given routinely to children because of its ability to discolor tooth enamel. The drug should be avoided in pregnancy. It is likely distributed in breast milk and should be avoided in nursing mothers.

OTHER ANTIBACTERIALS

Nitrofurantoin

Nitrofurantoin is an oral antibiotic useful for uncomplicated UTIs. This drug is frequently active against enterococci and *E. coli* that are resistant to other agents. It has minimal activity against *P. aeruginosa*, *Serratia*, or *Proteus*. Nitrofurantoin should not be used for pyelonephritis or any other systemic infections due to its poor systemic availability.

Dosing and Administration

The usual dose is 50 to 100 mg four times a day for the macrocrystals and 100 mg q12h as the dual-release formulation. The drug should be avoided in patients with CrCl <60 mL/min, as these patients do not achieve adequate urinary concentrations and are at increased risk for toxicity.

Key Monitoring and Safety Information

Peripheral neuropathy, pulmonary reactions, hepatotoxicity, hemolytic anemia, brown urine, and rash may also occur. Probenecid and sulfinpyrazone may decrease the efficacy of nitrofurantoin by decreasing its renal elimination. Magnesium trisilicate antacids may decrease the absorption of nitrofurantoin. Although nitrofurantoin has been used for UTI suppressive therapy, this practice should be avoided because prolonged therapy is associated with chronic pulmonary syndromes that can be fatal. The drug should be avoided in pregnant women at term or when labor is imminent due to risk of hemolysis. It is also contraindicated in children aged <1 month due to hemolysis risk. The drug is distributed in breast milk.

Trimethoprim–Sulfamethoxazole

Trimethoprim–sulfamethoxazole (TMP-SMX) is a combination antibiotic (IV or PO) with a 1:5 ratio of TMP to SMX. This combination agent is commonly used for uncomplicated UTIs and is the treatment of choice for *Pneumocystis jiroveci* pneumonia (PCP), *Nocardia*, and *Stenotrophomonas maltophilia* infections. Many strains of MRSA are susceptible to TMP-SMX, but the drug is not reliably active against *Streptococcus pyogenes* and should be avoided for uncomplicated cellulitis treatment.

Dosing and Administration

- The usual dose is 160 mg TMP/800 mg SMX q12h. For PCP and other serious systemic infections, the dose is 15 mg/kg per day based on the TMP component.
- *Renal dosing:*

- CrCl 10 to 50 mL/min: Usual dose q12h
- CrCl <10 mL/min: Usual dose q24h
- HD: Dose q24h, with one of the usual daily doses on dialysis days administered after dialysis
- PD: usual dose q24h
- CVVHD: 2.5 to 10 mg/kg q12h

Key Monitoring and Safety Information

- GI disturbances, hypersensitivity reactions, and hematologic abnormalities are common side effects. Headache, hepatitis, interstitial nephritis, hyperkalemia, hyponatremia, and obstructive uropathy may also occur.
- TMP/SMX may cause a "pseudo" renal failure through competition with serum Cr for tubular secretion. Isolated serum Cr elevations in the absence of alteration in other renal function parameters should raise suspicion of this effect.
- TMP-SMX can increase the hypoprothrombinemic effect of warfarin.
- TMP-SMX can also potentiate the activity of phenytoin and oral hypoglycemic agents.
- Oral TMP-SMX should be administered with a full glass of water to decrease the possibility of crystalluria.
- The drug should be avoided when possible in pregnancy, particularly during the third trimester, to minimize the possibility of kernicterus. It is distributed in breast milk and should be avoided in nursing mothers, particularly with infants <2 months.
- If there is uncertainty with TMP/SMX dosing, serum concentrations of TMP/SMX can be monitored. Suggested serum peak concentrations of TMP and SMX are 5 to 15 and 100 to 150 µg/mL, respectively. Suggested serum trough concentrations of TMP and SMX are 2 to 8 and 75 to 120 µg/mL, respectively.

Clindamycin

Clindamycin has a predominantly gram-positive spectrum similar to that of erythromycin, with inclusion of activity against some anaerobes. Clindamycin also provides activity against some MRSA isolates and is useful for treatment of minor infections caused by this organism. Clindamycin is also used for toxoplasmosis in combination with pyrimethamine and for *Pneumocystis* in combination with primaquine, typically in sulfa-allergic patients. Metronidazole is preferred for intraabdominal infections due to its superior activity against *B. fragilis* relative to clindamycin.

Dosing and Administration

The usual dosage is 300 to 450 mg PO q6-8h or 600 to 900 mg IV q8h. No dosage adjustments are required in renal failure or dialysis.

Key Monitoring and Safety Information

GI disturbances (including *Clostridium difficile* colitis), elevations in LFTs, IV site reactions, and rash may occur. Clindamycin may enhance the activity of neuromuscular blockers and should be used cautiously in this setting.

Metronidazole

Metronidazole is more active against gram-negative versus gram-positive anaerobes but does possess activity against *C. difficile* and *Clostridium perfringens*. It can be used to treat bacterial vaginosis and as an alternative for treatment of *C. difficile* infection. It is also commonly used in combination with other antibiotics to treat intra-abdominal infections and brain abscesses, as well as *Giardia*, *Entamoeba histolytica*, and *Trichomonas vaginalis* infections.

Dosing and Administration

The usual dose is 250 to 500 mg PO/IV q6-12h. A single 2000 mg dose may be used to treat trichomoniasis. Dosage reduction is suggested in severe hepatic failure. No dosage adjustments are required in renal failure or dialysis.

Key Monitoring and Safety Information

GI disturbances (e.g., nausea, vomiting, diarrhea, and dysgeusia), disulfiram-like reactions to alcohol, and mild CNS disturbances (headache, restlessness) may occur. Rarely, seizures and peripheral neuropathy may occur. Metronidazole can increase the procoagulant effects of warfarin. Concomitant administration of metronidazole with disulfiram may result in psychosis and confusion and should be avoided.

Vancomycin

Vancomycin provides clinically useful activity against most important gram-positive pathogens, including streptococci, enterococci, MRSA, and drug-resistant pneumococci. This agent is a drug of choice for empiric therapy of suspected MRSA infection and remains a mainstay of therapy for treatment of gram-positive infections in β-lactam-allergic patients. In vitro susceptibility to this agent should be documented as nonsusceptible strains have been reported.

Dosing and Administration

- The usual dose of vancomycin is 15 mg/kg of actual body weight IV q12h. Attempts should be made to limit daily doses of vancomycin to under 4 g/d, as nephrotoxicity risk increases beyond this limit.
- *Renal failure:*
  - CrCl 10 to 50 mL/min: 15 mg/kg intermittently per serum concentrations
  - CrCl <10 mL/min: 15 mg/kg intermittently per serum concentrations
  - HD: 15 mg/kg after dialysis, with redosing when the concentration drops below 15 to 20 μg/mL
  - PD: 15 mg/kg with redosing when the concentration drops below 15 to 20 μg/mL
  - CVVHD: 15 mg/kg q24h with close serum concentration monitoring and dose titration

Key Monitoring and Safety Information

- The main side effects of vancomycin are phlebitis and rash.
- Nephrotoxicity can occur, and concurrent administration of vancomycin with other potentially nephrotoxic drugs may potentiate these side effects.
- Leukopenia, very rare ototoxicity, and red man syndrome (flushing of the upper body with rapid administration of the drug) are other adverse effects.
- Serum trough concentrations should be obtained one to two times weekly. Patients with rapidly changing renal function may need more frequent serum-level monitoring. Serum Cr should also be regularly monitored to assess dosing appropriateness. Doses should be adjusted to maintain the trough concentration between 15 and 20 μg/mL for treatment of serious infections. Trough concentrations <10 μg/mL are considered subtherapeutic, whereas trough concentrations >20 μg/mL and daily doses >4 g appear to be associated with increased nephrotoxicity.

Linezolid

Linezolid is broadly active against gram-positive bacteria, including streptococci, MSSA, MRSA, coagulase-negative staphylococci, and enterococci (including vancomycin-resistant enterococci [VRE]). Linezolid or vancomycin is recommended for the treatment of hospital-acquired pneumonia (HAP) and VAP caused by MRSA. Linezolid also has unique activity against some mycobacteria and *Nocardia*. Linezolid has been associated with increased mortality in the treatment of IV line–related bacteremia and should be avoided in that setting. In vitro susceptibility to this agent should be documented as non-susceptible strains have been reported.

Dosing and Administration

The recommended dose is 600 mg IV or PO q12h. No dosage adjustments are required in renal failure or dialysis.

Key Monitoring and Safety Information

Thrombocytopenia occurs commonly in patients receiving courses of >2 weeks. Anemia and leukopenia may also occur. These may return to pretreatment values following discontinuation of the drug. Lactic acidosis may occur, as can peripheral and optic neuropathy (especially with long-term use). Linezolid is a reversible, nonselective monoamine oxidase inhibitor. The consumption of large amounts of tyramine in the diet should be avoided to prevent possible elevations in blood pressure. Linezolid also has the potential for interaction with adrenergic and serotonergic agents, causing a risk of serotonin syndrome in patients receiving concomitant serotonergic agents, such as selective serotonin reuptake inhibitors and other antidepressants. CBCs should be monitored regularly in patients receiving linezolid, especially in patients receiving this medication for durations >2 weeks, those with preexisting myelosuppression, and those receiving concomitant drugs that cause bone marrow suppression.

Tedizolid

Tedizolid is an oxazolidinone similar to linezolid which is active against some linezolid-resistant strains. It has activity against MSSA, MRSA, MRSE, streptococcal species (Group A, B and *S. anginosus* group), enterococci (VSE [vancomycin-susceptible] and VRE). It was noninferior to linezolid for treatment of ABSSSI (acute bacterial skin and skin structure infection) and was licensed for this indication in 2014.

Dosing and Administration

The usual dose is 200 mg once daily for 6 days, given intravenously or orally. No dosage adjustment is necessary for renal failure.

Key Monitoring and Safety Information

The most common effects are headache, nausea, and diarrhea. Thrombocytopenia and anemia can occur, but at a lesser frequency than linezolid. It is a weak MAO inhibitor, and appears to have less potential for serotonergic interactions than linezolid.

Daptomycin

Daptomycin, a lipopeptide antibiotic, is broadly active against gram-positive bacteria, including streptococci, MSSA, MRSA, and enterococci, including VRE. Daptomycin is a viable option for *S. aureus* bacteremia and endocarditis and has also emerged as a preferred agent for **treatment of serious VRE infections**. In vitro susceptibility to this agent should be documented as nonsusceptible strains have been reported. Daptomycin is bound by pulmonary surfactant and should **not** be used for the treatment of pneumonia.

Dosing and Administration

- The usual dosage is 4 to 10 mg/kg IV q24h, as dictated by infection type.
- *Renal dosing:*
  - CrCl <30 mL/min: usual dose q48h
  - HD: usual dose after each regular thrice weekly dialysis session
  - PD: usual dose q48h
  - CVVHD: 8 mg/kg q48h

Key Monitoring and Safety Information

Elevations in creatine phosphokinase (CPK) as well as muscle pain and weakness may occur, necessitating baseline and serial (weekly) monitoring of CPK. The drug should be discontinued in patients with unexplained myopathy and a CPK >1000 U/L and in patients without muscle symptoms who have CPK >2000 U/L. Daptomycin has also been associated with the development of eosinophilic pneumonia, and occurrence of new pulmonary symptoms during therapy should raise suspicion for the possibility of this adverse effect. Receipt of HMG-CoA reductase inhibitors in combination with daptomycin may increase the risk of myopathy and should be avoided if possible. Combined use of daptomycin and HMG-CoA reductase inhibitors necessitates more frequent CPK monitoring.

Telavancin

Telavancin is a lipoglycopeptide antibiotic that is broadly active against gram-positive bacteria, including streptococci, MSSA, MRSA, and heteroresistant vancomycin-intermediate *S. aureus* (VISA). The drug is not reliably active against VRE. Telavancin is effective for complicated skin and skin structure infections, as well as HAP and VAP. The drug has also been anecdotally effective for bacteremia, bone and joint infections, and endocarditis.

Dosing and Administration
- The usual dose is 10 mg/kg q24h.
- *Renal dosing:*
  - CrCl 30 to 50 mL/min: 7.5 mg/kg q24h
  - CrCl 10 to 29 mL/min: 10 mg/kg q24h
  - CrCl <10 mL/min: No specific recommendations are available
  - HD: No specific recommendations are available, but a dose of 10 mg/kg after each thrice-weekly regular dialysis session has been used
  - PD/CVVHD: No specific recommendations are available

Key Monitoring and Safety Information
- The most common adverse effects are nausea and vomiting, taste disturbances, and foamy urine.
- Nephrotoxicity may also occur and warrants regular serum Cr monitoring.
- Each dose should be administered over 1 hour to prevent red man syndrome.
- The drug is also associated with a minor QTc interval prolongation; use caution with other drugs that can prolong the QTc interval, and avoid in patients with conditions associated with risk of ventricular arrhythmias.
- Telavancin can also falsely prolong the prothrombin time, international normalized ratio, activated partial thromboplastin time, activated clotting time, or coagulation-based factor Xa tests. These tests should be obtained immediately before or within 6 hour before the next dose of telavancin.
- Patients allergic to vancomycin may be cross-allergic to telavancin.

Dalbavancin

Dalbavancin is a new lipoglycopeptide similar to vancomycin. It is active against gram-positive bacteria including MRSA, MRSE, VISA, many streptococci, enterococci but **not** VRE. It does not have any activity against gram-negative bacteria. It is approved for treatment of ABSSI, where it has been shown to be noninferior to vancomycin and linezolid.

Dosing and Administration
- It has an extended half-life allowing for once a week dosing. A 2 dose regimen of 1000 mg initially, followed by 500 mg 1 week later has been used. A single dose regimen of 1500 mg is also effective.
- Renal failure: Cr Clearance < 30 mL/min: 750 mg initially followed by 375 mg on day 8.

Key Monitoring and Safety Information
The most common adverse effects include nausea, headache, diarrhea and rash, and red man syndrome. Occasional ALT elevations occur, and LFTs should be monitored on therapy. The drug should be avoided in patients with a history of glycopeptide allergy and discontinued if an allergic reaction occurs.

Oritavancin

Oritavancin is a new lipoglycopeptide with a very prolonged half-life. It is active against MRSA, MRSE, VRSA, VISA, and both VSE and **VRE**. Clinical trials have shown non-inferiority to vancomycin in the treatment of skin and soft tissue infection, and it was approved for this indication in 2014.

Dosing and Administration
1200 mg intravenously as a single dose. It has not been studied in patients with Cr clearance < 30 mL/min.

Key Monitoring and Safety Information
The most common adverse effects are headache, nausea, diarrhea, and red man syndrome. It can increase levels of warfarin and omeprazole and decrease levels of midazolam and dextromethorphan. Caution should be exercised in reviewing laboratory coagulation tests as it binds to the phospholipid reagent. Heparin is contraindicated during the first 48 hours of oritavancin administration.

Quinupristin/Dalfopristin

Quinupristin/dalfopristin may have activity against some antibiotic-resistant gram-positive organisms, including MRSA, *E. faecium*, and multidrug-resistant *S. pneumoniae*. The drug has minimal activity against *E. faecalis*. In vitro susceptibility to this agent should be documented as nonsusceptible strains have been reported.

Dosing and Administration
The recommended dose is 7.5 mg/kg IV q8-12h. Dosage reduction is suggested in severe hepatic failure. No dosage adjustments are required in renal failure or dialysis.

Key Monitoring and Safety Information
The main adverse effects are arthralgias and myalgias (which are frequent and often force discontinuation of therapy), IV site pain and thrombophlebitis (common when the drug is administered through the peripheral vein), and elevated LFTs. Quinupristin/dalfopristin is an inhibitor of CYP3A4 and can increase serum levels of drugs metabolized by that enzyme, including but not limited to carbamazepine, HMG-CoA reductase inhibitors, cyclosporine, tacrolimus, midazolam, triazolam, calcium channel blockers, and many other drugs.

Colistin

Colistin is a bactericidal polypeptide antibiotic that acts by disrupting the cell membrane of gram-negative bacteria. This drug has a role in the **treatment of multiple drug-resistant gram-negative bacilli** (except *Proteus, Serratia, Providencia*, and *Burkholderia*). However, colistin **should only be given under guidance of an experienced clinician**, as parenteral therapy has significant CNS side effects and potential nephrotoxicity. Inhaled colistin is better tolerated with only mild upper airway irritation and has some efficacy as adjunctive therapy for *P. aeruginosa*. The drug is **not active** against gram-positive bacteria.

Dosing and Administration
- The usual dose of colistin IV is 2.5 to 5 mg/kg per day divided into two to four doses, with a maximum dose of 5 mg/kg per day. The usual dose of inhaled colistin is 75 to 150 mg inhaled two to three times daily.
- *Renal dosing:*
  - CrCl 50 to 80 mL/min: 2.5 to 3.8 mg/kg per day divided q12h
  - CrCl 10 to 49 mL/min: 2.5 mg/kg per day divided q12h
  - CrCl <10 mL/min: 1.5 mg/kg q36h
  - HD: 2 mg/kg after each dialysis session

○ PD: 0.75 to 1.5 mg/kg per day
○ CVVHD: 2.5 mg/kg q48h

Key Monitoring and Safety Information

Nephrotoxicity, neurotoxicity (paresthesias, neuromuscular blockade), and hypersensitivity reactions are the most significant adverse effects, necessitating careful monitoring during therapy. Serum Cr should be monitored daily early in therapy and at regular intervals for the duration of therapy. Ideally, colistin should not be coadministered with aminoglycosides, other known nephrotoxins, or neuromuscular blockers due to possible potentiation of toxicity.

Chloramphenicol

Chloramphenicol is a bacteriostatic antibiotic that binds to the 50S ribosomal subunit, blocking protein synthesis in susceptible bacteria. It has broad activity against aerobic and anaerobic gram-positive and gram-negative bacteria, including *S. aureus*, enterococci, and enteric gram-negatives. It is also active against spirochetes, *Rickettsia*, *Mycoplasma*, and *Chlamydia*. Chloramphenicol is used almost exclusively as alternate therapy for serious VRE infections caused by strains susceptible to chloramphenicol. Because of its excellent CNS penetration, it may also play a role for meningitis caused by *Francisella tularensis* or *Yersinia pestis*.

Dosing and Administration

The usual adult dose of chloramphenicol is 25 mg/kg IV q6h, up to a maximum dose of 1 g IV q6h. No dosage adjustments are required in renal failure or dialysis.

Key Monitoring and Safety Information

Potential adverse effects include idiosyncratic aplastic anemia (~1/30,000) and dose-related bone marrow suppression. Peak drug levels (1 h post-infusion) should be checked every 3 to 4 days (goal peak <25 mcg/mL) and doses adjusted accordingly. Dosage adjustment is necessary in the presence of significant liver disease. This antibiotic has major drug interactions.

Fosfomycin

Fosfomycin is a bactericidal oral antibiotic that kills bacteria by inhibiting an early step in cell wall synthesis. It has a spectrum of activity that includes most urinary tract pathogens, including *P. aeruginosa*, *Enterobacter* species, and enterococci (including VRE), and some multidrug-resistant gram-negative bacteria. It is most useful for treating uncomplicated UTIs in women with susceptible strains of *E. coli* or *E. faecalis*. The single-dose sachet formulation should not be routinely used to treat pyelonephritis or systemic infections.

Dosing and Administration

The usual dose is a 3-g sachet dissolved in cold water PO once.

Key Monitoring and Safety Information

Adverse events include diarrhea. It should not be taken with metoclopramide, which interferes with fosfomycin absorption.

Antimycobacterial Agents

PREFERRED AGENTS

Ethambutol

Ethambutol (ETH) is used primarily for the treatment of TB and MAC infection.

Dosing and Administration

- Please see Table 20-1
- *Renal dosing:*

TABLE 20-1	ETHAMBUTOL DOSING		
Dosing Interval	**Ideal Body Weight Range (kg)**		
	40–55	56–75	76–90
Daily	800	1200	1600[a]
3×/wk	1200	2000	2400[a]
2×/wk	2000	2800	4000[a]

[a]Maximum dose irrespective of body weight.

- CrCl <30 mL/min: usual dose 3 times weekly
- HD: 15 to 20 mg/kg after each dialysis
- PD: 15 to 20 mg/kg q48h
- CVVHD: 15 to 20 mg/kg q24-36h

Key Monitoring and Safety Information

The primary adverse effect of ETH is a dose-dependent **optic neuritis**, which may manifest unilaterally or bilaterally as decreased red/green perception, decreased visual acuity, and visual field defects. At baseline, patients receiving ETH should have visual acuity and color perception tested. Vision should be tested monthly, with each eye tested separately. ETH is not recommended in children in whom visual acuity cannot be monitored.

Isoniazid

Isoniazid (INH) is the mainstay of treatment and prevention of TB. Both MAC and *M. marinum* are resistant to INH.

Dosing and Administration

For treatment of *Mycobacterium tuberculosis*, the recommended daily dose is 5 mg/kg up to a maximum dose of 300 mg/d. For twice-weekly regimens, the recommended dose is 15 mg/kg per dose up to a maximum of 900 mg/dose. No dosage adjustments are required in renal failure or dialysis. The drug should be avoided in severe liver disease. Dosage reduction in milder forms of liver impairment may be warranted.

Key Monitoring and Safety Information

- The incidence of **hepatitis with INH increases with age and alcohol consumption**. Increases in transaminase levels may be seen, but these effects generally **do not necessitate holding the medication unless the transaminase levels are three to five times the upper limit** of normal. Baseline and monthly LFTs should be performed in patients receiving INH. Patients should be monitored for signs and symptoms of liver toxicity, such as weakness, jaundice, dark urine, decreased appetite, nausea, and vomiting. The hepatotoxicity of INH may be increased by the concurrent administration of rifampin.
- **Peripheral and optic neuritis** may also occur with INH; patients should be monitored for numbness, tingling, burning, pain in hands or feet, and blurred or loss of vision. These effects occur more frequently in slow acetylators, diabetes mellitus, and poor nutrition. The concurrent administration of pyridoxine (vitamin B6) at doses of 25 to 50 mg PO daily may help avoid these adverse effects. Other potential side effects of INH include hypersensitivity reactions (e.g., fever and rash), hematologic reactions (e.g., agranulocytosis, eosinophilia, thrombocytopenia, and anemia), arthritic symptoms,

encephalopathy, and convulsions. INH has a direct inhibitory effect on peripheral and central dopa decarboxylase and can increase parkinsonian symptoms in patients taking levodopa. INH is distributed in breast milk. Breast-fed infants of INH-treated mothers should be monitored for adverse effects.

Pyrazinamide

Pyrazinamide (PZA) is used clinically for the treatment of TB and is relied on for its ability to shorten treatment regimens down to 6 months.

Dosing and Administration
- Please see Table 20-2
- *Renal dosing:*
  - CrCl < 30 mL/min: Usual dose three times weekly
  - HD: Usual dose three times weekly after dialysis
  - PD: Usual dose q24h
  - CVVHD: Usual dose q24h

Key Monitoring and Safety Information
A possible serious adverse effect of this agent is **hepatotoxicity** manifested as increases in serum aminotransferases, jaundice, hepatitis, fever, anorexia, malaise, liver tenderness, hepatomegaly, discolored urine and/or stools, or pruritis. Hepatotoxicity appears to be dose-related and may occur at any time during therapy. Patients with hepatic dysfunction or risk factors for chronic liver disease may be at higher risk. PZA causes hyperuricemia by inhibiting the renal excretion of uric acid and should be avoided in patients with acute gout. Nongout polyarthralgia has been reported to occur in up to 40% of patients receiving pyrazinamide. Baseline LFTs as well as uric acid concentration should be obtained before initiation of therapy and repeated at periodic intervals.

Rifampin

Rifampin (RIF) is active in vitro against a number of mycobacterial species, including *M. tuberculosis*, *Mycobacterium bovis*, *M. marinum*, *Mycobacterium kansasii*, and some strains of *M. fortuitum*, *MAC*, and *Mycobacterium leprae*. The drug also has in vitro activity against many gram-positive bacteria, including *S. aureus* and *Bacillus anthracis*. In vitro activity is also seen against some gram-negative bacteria, including *Neisseria meningitidis*, *H. influenzae*, *Brucella melitensis*, and *L. pneumophila*.

Dosing and Administration
The usual dose of RIF for the treatment of TB is 600 mg once daily IV or PO or 600 mg twice weekly as part of multidrug therapy. A dose of 300 mg PO/IV q8h is recommended for synergistic treatment of staphylococcal prosthetic valve endocarditis. No dosage

TABLE 20-2	PYRAZINAMIDE DOSING		
Dosing Interval	**Ideal Body Weight Range (kg)**		
	40–55	56–75	76–90
Daily	1000	1500	2000[a]
3×/wk	1500	2500	3000[a]
2×/wk	2000	3000	4000[a]

[a]Maximum dose irrespective of body weight.

adjustments are required in renal failure or dialysis. Dosage adjustment in severe hepatic failure should be considered.

Key Monitoring and Safety Information
- The most common adverse effects of RIF are GI disturbances. RIF may also cause increases in LFTs. **Hepatitis** and jaundice have been reported in patients with pre-existing liver disease or in those who have received concomitant hepatotoxic agents. Baseline LFTs should be performed and repeated periodically during therapy with RIF to assess for hepatotoxicity.
- Thrombocytopenia, leukopenia, hemolytic anemia, hemolysis, hemoglobinuria, and decreased hemoglobin concentrations have occurred with RIF therapy. Hypersensitivity reactions characterized by a flu-like syndrome have also occurred, as has renal failure. A reddish-orange discoloration of body fluids, including urine, sputum, sweat, and tears, occurs with RIF. This effect may lead to permanent staining of soft contact lenses.
- RIF is a **potent inducer of cytochrome P4503A4** as well as 1A2, 2C9, 2C18, 2C19, and 2D6 and has many drug interactions. Decreases in plasma concentrations are seen with numerous agents. Medications profiles should be screened for potential drug interactions before RIF is initiated.

Rifabutin

Rifabutin is a RIF antimycobacterial agent similar to RIF that is used to treat TB and MAC infections in HIV-positive patients who are receiving antiretroviral therapy, as it has fewer drug–drug interactions than RIF (see Chapter 12, Human Immunodeficiency Virus and Acquired Immunodeficiency Syndrome).

Dosing and Administration
The usual dose is 300 mg PO q24h. The dose should be reduced to 150 mg PO q24h for CrCl < 30 mL/min.

Key Monitoring and Safety Information
Patients should be warned about the reddish-orange discoloration of body fluids, and contact lenses should not be worn during treatment. Rash, GI disturbances, hematologic disturbances, hepatitis, and interstitial nephritis can occur. Uveitis has also been associated with rifabutin. This agent also has major drug interactions but is considered less prone to drug interactions than RIF.

Antifungal Agents

AMPHOTERICIN B PREPARATIONS

- Amphotericin B is active against a wide range of fungi, including yeasts and molds. In vitro activity is seen against *Aspergillus* spp., *Blastomyces dermatitidis, Coccidioides immitis, Cryptococcus neoformans, Histoplasma capsulatum, Paracoccidioides brasiliensis,* and most species of *Candida*. High minimal inhibitory concentration values and clinical resistance have been seen with *Pseudallescheria boydii, Fusarium* spp., *Candida lusitaniae,* and *Trichosporon* spp. The drug is available as a conventional deoxycholate formulation and as different lipid formulations, which have been designed to minimize toxicity while preserving the therapeutic efficacy of amphotericin B.
- **Infusion-related adverse effects** may occur and include fever, chills, rigors, malaise, generalized aches, nausea, vomiting, and headache. Premedication with aspirin, ibuprofen, and acetaminophen may blunt these effects. Antihistamines may also be useful, likely due to the sedating effect. Other infusion-related adverse effects include hypotension, hypothermia, and bradycardia. Thrombophlebitis may also be seen at the site of infusion.

- **Decreases in GFR** occur early during therapy and may occur in up to 80% of patients. Renal function may return to normal but may take months in some patients. This may be prevented with sodium loading. Pre- and postdose normal saline (500–1000 mL) has been employed for this use. Tubular toxicity may also occur and is manifest as **hypokalemia, hypomagnesemia, and renal tubular acidosis**. Nephrotoxic agents (e.g., aminoglycosides, cyclosporine, tacrolimus, and pentamidine) may result in acute deterioration of renal function when given with amphotericin B preparations. Agents causing electrolyte disturbances, such as hypokalemia seen with loop diuretics, should be used cautiously in patients being treated with amphotericin B. Electrolytes (especially potassium and magnesium) should be closely monitored during therapy.
- A normocytic, normochromic anemia may be seen well after initiation of therapy. Ventricular arrhythmias have been seen in patients with hypokalemia, those receiving rapid infusions, and patients with renal failure. Neurotoxic effects include confusion, incoherence, delirium, depression, psychotic behavior, convulsions, tremors, blurred vision, and loss of hearing. Administration during pregnancy has resulted in increased serum Cr levels in infants. Renal function should be closely monitored in neonates born to mothers who have received amphotericin B.

Amphotericin B Deoxycholate

Owing to its increased toxicities relative to the lipid-based formulations of amphotericin B, intravenous conventional amphotericin B use has been largely supplanted by lipid formulations of the drug. However, conventional amphotericin B is still reasonably used for local administration, including continuous bladder irrigation or intravitreal injection.

Dosing and Administration

Usual daily doses are 0.5 to 1 mg/kg, with escalation from lower doses to higher doses at the start of therapy. An absolute maximum dose of 1.5 mg/kg per day should never be exceeded. Infusions should be over a period of ≥4 to 6 hours. No dosage adjustments are required in renal failure or dialysis.

Key Monitoring and Safety Information

Conventional amphotericin B is the most toxic formulation of amphotericin B.

Amphotericin B Lipid Complex

Amphotericin B lipid complex (ABLC) consists of amphotericin B complexed to lipid bilayers that results in a ribbon structure.

Dosing and Administration

The recommended dose is 5 mg/kg per day IV at a rate of 2.5 mg/kg per hour. No dosage adjustments are required in renal failure or dialysis.

Key Monitoring and Safety Information

Other adverse effects that have been reported with ABLC include abnormalities in hepatic function, as manifested by elevations in alkaline phosphatase, conjugated bilirubin, and transaminases.

Liposomal Amphotericin B

Liposomal amphotericin B (LAmB) is the **only true "liposomal" preparation** of the three lipid preparations available.

Dosing and Administration

The recommended dose of LAmB is 3 to 5 mg/kg per day for the treatment of systemic fungal infections. Infusions may be given over 1 hour. Doses of 3 mg/kg per day have been used for empiric therapy of suspected fungal infections in febrile neutropenia. No dosage adjustments are required in renal failure or dialysis.

Key Monitoring and Safety Information

LAmB may be associated with less frequent nephrotoxicity and infusion-related reactions versus other amphotericin B formulations. Other adverse effects that have been reported with LAmB include chest pain, abnormalities in hepatic function, as manifested by elevations in alkaline phosphatase, conjugated bilirubin, and transaminases.

AZOLES

Fluconazole

Fluconazole is a triazole antifungal generally considered to be fungistatic, with its principal activity against *Candida* spp. and *Cryptococcus* spp. However, *C. krusei* is intrinsically resistant to fluconazole, and *C. glabrata* has dose-dependent sensitivity. Fluconazole has activity against *Coccidioides immitis*, but it has limited activity against *H. capsulatum*, *B. dermatitidis*, and *Sporothrix schenckii* and no activity against *Aspergillus* spp. or other molds.

Dosing and Administration
- The usual dosage is 100 to 400 mg/d. A single 150-mg oral dose is effective for vaginal candidiasis.
- *Renal dosing:*
  - CrCl ≤50 mL/min: 50% of the usual daily dose q24h
  - HD: 100% of the usual daily dose after each dialysis session or 50% of the usual daily dose administered daily (after dialysis session on dialysis days)
  - PD: 50% of the usual daily dose q24h
  - CVVHD: 100% of the usual daily dose q24h

Key Monitoring and Safety Information
- **Hepatitis, cholestasis, and fulminant hepatic failure** have been reported to occur rarely in patients receiving fluconazole. Mild increases in LFTs have been reported to occur and are generally reversible. LFTs should be performed at baseline and monitored during prolonged courses of fluconazole. Prolongation of the QTc interval may also occur.
- Fluconazole is a substrate of the CYP3A4 isoenzyme and may also **inhibit metabolism of other medications** metabolized by this isoenzyme. RIF has been shown to decrease the area under the curve (AUC) and half-life of fluconazole (25% and 20%, respectively). Fluconazole may also decrease the metabolism of TCAs, carbamazepine, certain benzodiazepines, warfarin, cyclosporine, tacrolimus, phenytoin, and oral sulfonylurea agents.
- Fluconazole at multiple daily dosing should be avoided in pregnancy. Pregnant patients should be informed of the potential hazards of fluconazole. Fluconazole is distributed into breast milk, with concentrations approaching those achieved in plasma. Because of this, it is recommended that fluconazole not be used in nursing women.

Itraconazole

Itraconazole is a triazole antifungal agent active against clinically important *Aspergillus* spp. Itraconazole also has in vitro activity against *B. dermatitidis*, *H. capsulatum*, *C. immitis*, *S. schenckii*, and *C. neoformans*.

Dosing and Administration

The usual dose is 200 to 400 mg/d. For severe infection, loading doses of 200 mg 3 times daily for the first 3 days is recommended. The liquid formulation is not significantly affected by lack of gastric acidity or food and is more reliably absorbed as compared with the capsules. No dosage adjustments are required in renal failure or dialysis.

Key Monitoring and Safety Information
- Serious **hepatotoxicity**, including liver failure, has been reported rarely in patients receiving itraconazole with or without preexisting liver disease.

- Congestive heart failure, peripheral edema, and pulmonary edema have been reported secondary to a dose-related negative inotropic effect.
- Hypokalemia ranging from mild to severe has also been reported in patients receiving itraconazole for systemic fungal infections.
- Itraconazole **inhibits the metabolism of other drugs metabolized by the CYP3A4** isoenzyme. Concomitant use of itraconazole with quinidine or dofetilide is contraindicated because of potential for arrhythmias. Itraconazole is also contraindicated in patients receiving atorvastatin, lovastatin, and simvastatin because of the potential for rhabdomyolysis and in patients receiving certain benzodiazepines because of the potential for prolonged sedative and hypnotic effects. Itraconazole should be used with caution with other agents that are metabolized by CYP3A4 or with medications that may induce or inhibit the metabolism of itraconazole. The medication profiles of patients receiving itraconazole should be carefully reviewed for potential drug interactions.
- Itraconazole should be used for the treatment of systemic fungal infections in pregnancy only when the benefits outweigh the risks to the fetus. Itraconazole is distributed into breast milk. Patients receiving oral itraconazole should have LFTs performed at baseline and at regular intervals throughout the course of therapy. Potassium levels should also be monitored due to the risk of hypokalemia. Monitoring of signs and symptoms of congestive heart failure should also occur in patients receiving prolonged courses of therapy. Prolongation of the QTc interval may also occur.
- Serum itraconazole **trough concentration monitoring** is advised to verify absorption and therapeutic levels. Desired trough concentrations are at least 1 μg/mL.

Posaconazole

Posaconazole is a triazole antifungal active against *Aspergillus* spp and zygomycetes. Posaconazole is also active against many *Candida* spp., *C. neoformans*, *B. dermatitidis*, *C. immitis*, and *H. capsulatum*. Posaconazole is also effective for prophylaxis of invasive fungal infections in hematopoietic stem cell transplant recipients with graft versus host disease and in patients with hematologic malignancies experiencing prolonged neutropenia following chemotherapy.

Dosing and Administration

Posaconazole is available as an oral delayed-release tablet, oral suspension, and intravenous formulation. The usual dose for the delayed-release tablet and IV formulation is 300 mg q12h on day 1, followed by 300 mg q24h thereafter. The usual oral suspension dose for fungal prophylaxis is 200 mg three times daily. No dosage adjustments are required in renal failure, dialysis, or hepatic failure.

Key Monitoring and Safety Information

- Each oral suspension dose must be taken within 20 minutes of either a full meal or dose of a liquid nutritional supplement or an acidic carbonated beverage (e.g., ginger ale). Patients receiving posaconazole should have LFTs performed at baseline and at regular intervals, especially if a long course of therapy is undertaken, as **hepatotoxicity** may occur. Prolongation of the QTc interval may also occur.
- Despite the fact that posaconazole is not metabolized by CYP450 enzymes, numerous **drug interactions** still exist because of its effects on UDP-glucuronidation and p-glycoprotein efflux. Rifabutin, phenytoin, cimetidine, and efavirenz significantly reduce posaconazole exposure and should not be coadministered unless benefit clearly outweighs risk. **Sirolimus is contraindicated** with posaconazole due to dramatically increased sirolimus exposure. Cyclosporine and tacrolimus dose reduction to 75% and 33% of normal, respectively, is recommended if these drugs are used with posaconazole. Posaconazole is also likely to interact with many other drugs, including ergot alkaloids, vinca alkaloids, certain HMG-CoA reductase inhibitors, certain calcium channel

blockers, and digoxin. Monitoring for adverse effects of midazolam and protease inhibitors is required with concomitant posaconazole.

- Posaconazole should only be used during pregnancy if the potential benefits outweigh the possible risks.
- Serum posaconazole trough concentration monitoring is advised to verify absorption and therapeutic levels. Desired trough concentrations are at least 0.7 to 1.25 μg/mL.

Voriconazole

Voriconazole is a triazole antifungal active against *Aspergillus* spp., *Candida* spp., including *C. krusei. C. neoformans, B. dermatitidis, C. immitis,* and *H. capsulatum.*

Dosing and Administration

- For invasive aspergillosis and infections caused by *Fusarium* spp. and *Scedosporium apiospermum*, a loading dose of 6 mg/kg IV every 12 hours for two doses followed by 4 mg/kg IV every 12 hours is recommended by the manufacturer.
- Oral doses of 200 to 300 mg every 12 hours may be given once the patient is able to tolerate oral medications.
- Moderate renal impairment (CrCl of 30–50 mL/min) does not affect the pharmacokinetics of voriconazole. Accumulation of the IV excipient sulfobutyl ether β-cyclodextrin sodium may occur in patients with moderate to severe renal failure. As a result, the IV formulation should not be used in patients with CrCl <50 mL/min unless the benefits outweigh the risks. In these circumstances, the oral formulation may be used instead. No pharmacokinetic-based dosage adjustments are required in renal failure or dialysis.

Key Monitoring and Safety Information

- **Transient visual disturbances**, including blurred vision, changes in light perception, photophobia, and visual hallucinations, have been reported to occur in clinical trials. These may be dose-related and occur with the first few doses. Patients should be warned of the possible visual disturbances associated with the use of this agent. Other potential adverse events include **elevations in LFTs**, skin rash, periostitis, GI disturbances, and prolongation of the QTc interval. Patients receiving voriconazole should have LFTs performed at baseline and at regular intervals, especially if a long course of therapy is undertaken, as hepatotoxicity may occur.
- Voriconazole is both a **substrate and inhibitor** of CYP2C9, 2C19, and 3A4 isoenzymes. Caution should be used when administering voriconazole with agents that are metabolized or inhibited/induced by the same pathways. RIF, rifabutin, and phenytoin have been shown to induce the metabolism of voriconazole. The metabolisms of cyclosporine, sirolimus, tacrolimus, warfarin, and omeprazole are inhibited by voriconazole. Monitoring for potential drug interactions should also be performed prospectively.
- Voriconazole can cause fetal harm if administered during pregnancy. Women becoming pregnant while receiving voriconazole should be informed of potential fetal risk.
- Serum voriconazole concentration monitoring is advised to verify absorption and therapeutic levels. Desired trough concentrations are ≥ 1 to 5.5 μg/mL.

Isavuconazole

Isavuconazonium sulfate-prodrug of isavuconazole is an azole with broad-spectrum antifungal activity that is US FDA-approved for treatment of invasive aspergillosis and invasive mucormycosis.

Dosing and Administration

The usual dose is 372 mg isavuconazonium sulfate (equivalent to 200 mg isavuconazole) PO/IV q8h for 48 hours, then 372 mg isavuconazonium sulfate (equivalent to 200 mg isavuconazole) PO/IV q24h. No dose adjustments are required in renal insufficiency.

Key Monitoring and Safety Information
- The oral formulation has a 98% oral bioavailability with absorption unaffected by food. The IV formulation does not contain a solubilizing cyclodextrin vehicle and can therefore be freely administered in patients with CrCl < 50 mL/min.
- Other adverse events, as with other azoles, include **elevations in LFTs**, skin rash, and GI disturbances.
- Patients should have LFTs performed at baseline and at regular intervals, as hepatotoxicity may occur.
- Unlike other azole antifungals, isavuconazole does not prolong the QTc interval and actually can cause a minor QTC interval shortening.
- The agent is a **substrate and inhibitor** of CYP3A4 and has the potential for drug interaction mediated by this route of metabolism.

Echinocandins

Echinocandins are active against *Aspergillus* spp. as well as most *Candida* spp. These agents do not have clinically meaningful activity against *C. neoformans*, *Histoplasma*, *Blastomyces*, *Coccidioides*, and *Mucor* species.

Anidulafungin
Dosing and Administration
The usual dose is 200 mg once, followed by 100 mg q24h. No dosage adjustments are recommended in renal failure or dialysis or in the setting of even severe hepatic failure.

Key Monitoring and Safety Information
To minimize risk of infusion-related reactions (e.g., rash, urticaria, flushing, dyspnea, and hypotension), the drug should be administered no quicker than 1.1 mg/min. Patients should be monitored for clinical evidence of hepatic dysfunction, including with periodic LFTs. Anidulafungin is not a significant substrate, inhibitor, or inducer of cytochrome P450 enzymes and is not expected to be associated with clinically relevant drug interactions occurring via this mechanism.

Caspofungin
Dosing and Administration
- Caspofungin is administered as a loading dose of 70 mg IV on day 1, followed by 50 mg IV daily thereafter.
- Infusions should be given over approximately 1 hour.
- No dosage adjustments are required in renal failure or dialysis.
- Patients with moderate hepatic insufficiency (Child–Pugh score 7–9) should receive the initial loading dose of 70 mg and then 35 mg IV daily thereafter.

Key Monitoring and Safety Information
Infusion-related reactions (i.e., pruritus, erythema, induration, and pain) and headache may occur. **Increases in LFTs** are the most commonly reported laboratory adverse effects. When administered concurrently with cyclosporine, the AUC of caspofungin has been reported to increase 35%. Owing to elevations in LFTs observed with concurrent administration of cyclosporine, the manufacturer does not recommend coadministration. Reduced caspofungin concentrations have been observed with concomitant administration of enzyme inducers or mixed enzyme inducers/inhibitors. Reduced concentrations have been observed with efavirenz, nelfinavir, nevirapine, phenytoin, rifampin, dexamethasone, or carbamazepine. Caspofungin

should be avoided in the first trimester of pregnancy. Patients should be monitored for allergic reactions, infusion-related toxicities and evidence of hepatic dysfunction, including with periodic LFTs.

Micafungin

Dosing and Administration

The usual dose is 100 mg q24h. No dosage adjustments are recommended in renal failure or dialysis or in the setting of even severe hepatic failure.

Key Monitoring and Safety Information

To minimize risk of infusion-related reactions (e.g., rash, pruritis, and facial swelling), the drug should be administered over 1 hour. Patients should be monitored for clinical evidence of **hepatic dysfunction**, including with periodic LFTs. Micafungin is not a clinically significant substrate, inhibitor, or inducer of most cytochrome P450 enzymes.

OTHER ANTIFUNGALS

Flucytosine

Flucytosine is a fluorinated pyrimidine antifungal that is primarily used as **adjunctive therapy for cryptococcal meningitis**. The drug is also active in vitro against some strains of *C. albicans, C. glabrata, C. parapsilosis, C. tropicalis,* and *C. neoformans,* whereas *C. krusei* may be resistant. This agent is an alternative treatment for candiduria.

Dosing and Administration

- The recommended dose is 100 mg/kg per day divided q6h.
- *Renal dosing:*
  ○ CrCl 10 to 50 mL/min: 25 mg/kg q12-24h
  ○ CrCl <10 mL/min: 25 mg/kg q24-48h
  ○ HD: 25 mg/kg after each dialysis session
  ○ PD: 0.5 to 1 g q24h
  ○ CVVHD: 25 mg/kg q12-24h

Key Monitoring and Safety Information

- **Bone marrow suppression**, including leukopenia and thrombocytopenia, is the main serious complication of flucytosine. This may occur more frequently in patients with peak concentrations >100 µg/mL. It may also occur more commonly in patients with underlying hematologic disorders, those with concurrent myelosuppression, or those receiving nephrotoxic agents that may decrease the clearance of flucytosine.
- Flucytosine may also cause **GI adverse effects**. Severe nausea, vomiting, diarrhea, and anorexia may occur. Elevations in LFTs may occur but appear to be dose-related and are generally reversible.
- Hematologic tests, renal function tests, and LFTs should be performed before and at frequent intervals during therapy.
- Nephrotoxic agents may decrease the renal clearance of flucytosine, leading to accumulation and toxicity. When given in combination with such agents, flucytosine **peak serum levels** should be monitored along with renal function, and dosage adjustments should be made accordingly. Peak serum levels should be obtained after the fifth dose. Concentrations of 25 to 100 µg/mL should be maintained. Peak serum levels should be monitored throughout therapy, especially in patients with signs of toxicity or a change in renal function or those with myelosuppression.
- Flucytosine should only be used in pregnancy when the potential benefits outweigh the possible risks. It is not known whether flucytosine is distributed into breast milk.

Antiviral Agents

Antiretroviral agents used in the treatment of HIV disease are discussed in detail in Chapter 12.

GENERAL ANTIVIRALS

Acyclovir

Acyclovir antiviral activity is limited to herpesviruses. Its greatest activity is against herpes simplex virus (HSV)-1, HSV-2, and varicella zoster virus (VZV).

Dosing and Administration
- The usual dose is 200 to 800 mg three to five times daily or 5 to 10 mg/kg IV q8h.
- *Renal dosing:*
  - CrCl 10 to 50 mL/min: Usual dose q12-24h
  - CrCl <10 mL/min: 50% dose q24h
  - HD: 50% dose q24h, with the daily dose administered after dialysis on dialysis days
  - PD: 50% dose q24h
  - CVVHD: 5 to 10 mg/kg q24h

Key Monitoring and Safety Information
- Reversible **nephropathy** due to crystallization of the drug in the renal tubules is an uncommon adverse effect seen after IV administration. Pre-existing renal insufficiency, dehydration, and bolus dosing may increase the risk of nephrotoxicity. This effect may be avoided by appropriately adjusting doses for renal dysfunction.
- **CNS toxicity** has been reported in the form of tremors, delirium, and seizures. This may be seen with high doses, in patients with impaired renal function, and in the elderly.
- Phlebitis has been associated with IV infusions.
- Acyclovir is distributed into breast milk, and concentrations may be higher than concurrent maternal plasma levels. Acyclovir should be used with caution in nursing mothers and only when clearly indicated.
- Renal function should be monitored at baseline and during therapy. Patients should also be monitored for seizure activity, especially those undergoing high-dose therapy, those with renal dysfunction, or those with a history of seizures.

Cidofovir

Cidofovir has in vitro and in vivo inhibitory activity against a broad spectrum of herpesviruses, including HSV-1, HSV-2, VZV, cytomegalovirus (CMV), Epstein–Barr virus (EBV), papillomaviruses, polyomaviruses, and adenoviruses. Its use is limited by toxicity.

Dosing and Administration
- The induction dose of cidofovir is 5 mg/kg infused over 1 hour once weekly for 2 consecutive weeks. This is followed by a maintenance dose of 5 mg/kg infused over 1 hour once every other week.
- To reduce the risk of **nephrotoxicity, probenecid must be used concomitantly**. The recommended dose is 2 g 3 hours before the cidofovir dose, followed by 1-g doses administered at 2 and 8 hours after the completion of the infusion for a total dose of 4 g.
- Patients should also receive 1 L 0.9% sodium chloride over 1 to 2 hours immediately before each cidofovir infusion. For patients who can tolerate it, a second infusion of 1 L 0.9% sodium chloride should be initiated concomitantly with or immediately after the cidofovir dose and should be infused over 1 to 3 hours.

- Cidofovir is **contraindicated** in patients with a serum Cr of >1.5 mg/dL, a CrCl of ≤55 mL/min or a urine protein concentration ≥100 mg/dL. If renal function changes during therapy, the dose should be reduced to 3 mg/kg for an increase in serum Cr of 0.3 to 0.4 mg/dL above baseline.

Key Monitoring and Safety Information
- Dose-related **nephrotoxicity** is the principal side effect of IV cidofovir and is characterized by proteinuria, azotemia, glycosuria, and metabolic acidosis.
- Fanconi syndrome may also occur.
- Proteinuria may occur in up to 50% of patients receiving maintenance doses of 5 mg/kg every other week; elevated serum Cr may occur in 15%.
- **Neutropenia** may occur in 20% of patients. Other adverse effects when combined with probenecid include fever, nausea, emesis, diarrhea, headache, rash, asthenia, anterior uveitis, and ocular hypotony.
- Topical application is associated with burning, pain, pruritus, and occasionally ulceration. Concurrent use of nephrotoxic agents increases the risk of nephrotoxicity.
- Cidofovir has mutagenic, gonadotoxic, embryotoxic, and teratogenic effects and is considered a potential human carcinogen. It may cause infertility in humans. It is unknown whether cidofovir is excreted in breast milk.
- Serum Cr concentration and urine protein should be determined within 48 hours before each dose. Proteinuria may be an early sign of nephrotoxicity. Owing to neutropenia associated with cidofovir, it is recommended that leukocyte counts with differentials be monitored during therapy. It is also recommended that signs and symptoms of uveitis be monitored along with intraocular pressure and visual acuity.

Famciclovir

Famciclovir is converted to the active triphosphate form of penciclovir, which has activity against HSV-1, HSV-2, and VZV.

Dosing and Administration
- The usual dose for treatment of HSV or VZV infection is 500 mg q8-12h. Chronic suppressive therapy doses are 125 to 250 mg q12h.
- *Renal dosing:*
  - CrCl 10 to 50 mL/min: Usual dose q12-24h
  - CrCl <10 mL/min: 50% dose q24h
  - HD: 50% dose q24h, with the daily dose administered after dialysis on dialysis days
  - PD: No specific recommendations are available
  - CVVHD: No specific recommendations are available

Key Monitoring and Safety Information
Famciclovir appears to be well tolerated in both immunocompetent and immunocompromised patients. The most common adverse effects reported include headache, nausea, and diarrhea, which are generally mild to moderate in severity.

Foscarnet

Foscarnet is active against HSV-1, HSV-2, VZV, and CMV. Because it does not require phosphorylation by thymidine kinase, foscarnet remains active against many resistant strains of HSV and CMV and is used primarily for resistant herpesviruses.

Dosing and Administration
- CMV Retinitis: The recommended dose is 60 mg/kg infused over 1 hour q8h or 90 mg/kg infused over 1.5 to 2 hours q12h for 14 to 21 days. This induction regimen is followed by a maintenance regimen of 90 to 120 mg/kg per day infused over 2 hours.

- Acyclovir-Resistant Mucocutaneous Herpes Simplex Virus: The recommended dose is 40 mg/kg q8-12h for 14 to 21 days.
- Herpes Zoster in Immunocompromised Patients: The recommended dose is 40 mg/kg q8h for 10 to 21 days or until complete healing occurs. Higher doses of 60 mg/kg q8h have also been used.
- *Renal dosing:* Please see Tables 20-3 and 20-4
  ○ HD: 45 to 65 mg/kg per dose postdialysis (three times/wk)
  ○ PD: suggest 6 mg/kg q8 hours
  ○ CVVHD: 60 mg/kg q24-48h

Key Monitoring and Safety Information
- The major dose-limiting side effect of foscarnet is **nephrotoxicity** with azotemia, mild proteinuria, and sometimes acute tubular necrosis. Renal function should be meticulously monitored during therapy and converted to Cr clearance in mL/min per kilogram body weight to allow dosage adjustments to be made according to specific manufacturer guidelines. Renal impairment usually begins during the second week of therapy and is reversible within 2 to 4 weeks after cessation of the medication in most patients. Concurrent administration with other nephrotoxic drugs (e.g., amphotericin B, cidofovir, aminoglycosides, and IV pentamidine) may result in additive nephrotoxicity.
- Metabolic abnormalities may include hypocalcemia or hypercalcemia, hypophosphatemia or hyperphosphatemia, hypomagnesemia, and hypokalemia. Concurrent use with IV pentamidine also may increase the risk of hypocalcemia. Potential CNS side effects include headache, tremor, irritability, seizures, and hallucinations. Other side effects may include fever, rash, diarrhea, nausea, vomiting, abnormal LFTs, anxiety, fatigue, and genital ulcerations.
- Foscarnet should be administered by an infusion pump at a rate not exceeding 1 mg/kg per minute. Patients should be **adequately hydrated** before and during administration

TABLE 20-3	INDUCTION DOSING OF FOSCARNET IN PATIENTS WITH VARYING RENAL FUNCTION			
CrCl in mL/min per kilogram	Herpes Simplex Virus		Cytomegalovirus	
	Equivalent mg/kg to 40 mg/kg q12h	Equivalent mg/kg to 40 mg/kg q8h	Equivalent mg/kg to 60 mg/kg q8h	Equivalent mg/kg to 90 mg/kg q12h
>1.4	40 q12h	40 q8h	60 q8h	90 q12h
>1–1.4	30 q12h	30 q8h	45 q8h	70 q12h
>0.8–1	20 q12h	35 q12h	50 q12h	50 q12h
>0.6–0.8	35 q24h	25 q12h	40 q12h	80 q24h
>0.5–0.6	25 q24h	40 q24h	60 q24h	60 q24h
>0.4–0.5	20 q24h	35 q24h	50 q24h	50 q24h
<0.4	NR	NR	NR	NR

NR, not recommended.

TABLE 20-4	MAINTENANCE DOSING OF FOSCARNET IN PATIENTS WITH VARYING RENAL FUNCTION	
CrCl in mL/min per kilogram	Equivalent mg/kg to 90 mg/kg once Daily	Equivalent mg/kg to 120 mg/kg once Daily
>1.4	90 q24h	120 q24h
>1–1.4	70 q24h	90 q24h
>0.8–1	50 q24h	65 q24h
>0.6–0.8	80 q48h	105 q48h
>0.5–0.6	60 q48h	80 q48h
≥0.4–0.5	50 q48h	65 q48h
<0.4	NR	NR

NR, not recommended.

to minimize the risk of nephrotoxicity. A total of 750 to 1000 mL normal saline or 5% dextrose should be administered before the first dose. With additional doses of 90 to 120 mg/kg, 750 to 1000 mL of fluid should be administered concurrently with each dose; 500 mL of fluid should be administered with each dose of 40 to 60 mg/kg. Renal function, electrolytes, and CBCs should be monitored at least two to three times a week during induction therapy and at least once every 1 to 2 weeks during maintenance therapy.
• The drug should only be used in pregnant women when the potential benefits outweigh the potential risks. It is not known whether foscarnet is distributed in breast milk.

Ganciclovir

Ganciclovir is a potent inhibitor of CMV replication, with inhibitory concentrations 10- to >50-fold lower than acyclovir for CMV strains. Ganciclovir also has inhibitory activity against HSV-1, HSV-2, EBV, and VZV.

Dosing and Administration
• For the treatment of CMV disease, the induction dose is 5 mg/kg q12h for 2 to 3 weeks, followed by a maintenance dose of 5 mg/kg per day IV; or 6 mg/kg IV 5 d/ wk. Intravitreal injection of ganciclovir may also be used for the treatment of CMV retinitis.
• *Renal dosing*:
  ○ CrCl 10 to 50 mL/min: 25% to 50% dose q24h
  ○ CrCl <10 mL/min: 25% dose three times weekly
  ○ HD: 25% dose after each regular dialysis session (three times weekly)
  ○ PD: 25% dose three times weekly
  ○ CVVHD: 1.25 to 2.5 mg/kg q12-24h

Key Monitoring and Safety Information
• **Myelosuppression** is the principal dose-limiting toxicity, with neutropenia occurring in 15% to 40% of patients and thrombocytopenia in 5% to 20%. These effects are usually reversible with drug cessation. Neutrophil counts and platelet counts should be monitored every 2 days during twice-daily dosing of ganciclovir and at least weekly thereafter.

Neutrophil counts should be monitored daily in patients who have previously experienced leukopenia. Ganciclovir should not be administered if the absolute neutrophil count falls below 500 cells/μL or if the platelet count falls below 25,000/μL.

- Potential **CNS side effects** (e.g., headache, behavioral changes, convulsions, and coma) may occur in 5% to 15% of patients. Other side effects include infusion-related phlebitis, azotemia, anemia, rash, fever, LFT abnormalities, nausea, vomiting, and eosinophilia.
- Ganciclovir should be used in pregnancy only when potential benefit outweighs risk. It is not known whether ganciclovir is distributed in breast milk. Because of the potential for serious adverse reactions in breast-fed infants, it is recommended that nursing mothers discontinue nursing while they are receiving the drug and that they do not resume nursing until ≥72 hours after the last dose.

Valacyclovir

Valacyclovir is an acyclovir prodrug with antiviral activity limited to herpesviruses. Its greatest activity is against HSV-1, HSV-2, and VSV.

Dosing and Administration
- The dose for treatment of herpes zoster infection is 1000 mg PO q8h for 7 days. The dose for treatment of genital HSV infection is 1000 mg PO q12h for 10 days for initial episodes and 500 mg PO daily for 5 days for recurrent episodes.
- *Renal dosing:*
  ○ CrCl 10 to 50 mL/min: Usual dose q12-24h
  ○ CrCl <10 mL/min: 500 mg q24h
  ○ HD: 500 mg q24h, with the daily dose after dialysis on dialysis days
  ○ PD: 500 mg q24h
  ○ CVVHD: 500 mg q24h

Key Monitoring and Safety Information
Adverse effects are similar to those noted with acyclovir. **Thrombotic thrombocytopenic purpura** with hemolytic uremic syndrome has occurred in immunocompromised patients receiving high doses of valacyclovir. Renal function should be monitored at baseline and during therapy. Patients should also be monitored for seizure activity, especially those undergoing high-dose therapy, those with renal dysfunction, and those with a history of seizures.

Valganciclovir

Valganciclovir is a ganciclovir prodrug that is a potent inhibitor of CMV replication. Ganciclovir also has inhibitory activity against HSV-1, HSV-2, and VZV. It is very bioavailable and achieves high serum concentrations.

Dosing and Administration
- For the treatment of active CMV retinitis in patients with normal renal function, the induction dose is 900 mg (two 450-mg tablets) twice daily for 21 days with food. After the induction dose, or in patients with inactive CMV retinitis, the recommended maintenance dosage is 900 mg once daily with food.
- *Renal dosing:*
  ○ Please See Table 20-5
  ○ HD/PD/CVVHD: It is recommended to avoid valganciclovir in these situations

Key Monitoring and Safety Information
Adverse effects are similar to those noted with ganciclovir. Other adverse effects associated with valganciclovir include diarrhea, nausea, vomiting, abdominal pain, headache, and pyrexia. Because valganciclovir is considered a potential teratogen and carcinogen in humans, caution should be observed in handling broken tablets. Tablets should not be broken or crushed, and direct contact of broken or crushed tablets should be avoided.

TABLE 20-5	VALGANCICLOVIR RENAL DOSING	
CrCl (mL/min)	Induction Dose	Maintenance Dose
≥60	900 mg twice daily	900 mg daily
40–59	450 mg twice daily	450 mg daily
25–39	450 mg daily	450 mg q2d
10–24	450 mg q2d	450 mg twice weekly

ANTI-INFLUENZA AGENTS

Oseltamivir

Oseltamivir is a neuraminidase inhibitor that is **active against both influenza A and B virus.**

Dosing and Administration
- The recommended treatment dose of oseltamivir is 75 mg PO q12h for a total of 5 days. It should be initiated **within 48 hours of symptom onset.**
- *Renal dosing:*
  - CrCl <30 mL/min: 75 mg q48h
  - HD: 30 mg three to four times weekly
  - PD: 30 mg one to two times weekly
  - CVVHD: 75 mg q12h

Key Monitoring and Safety Information
The main side effects are nausea and vomiting. These GI side effects usually occur after the first dose and resolve after 1 to 2 days with continued dosing. They may be reduced by taking oseltamivir with food. Oseltamivir should only be used in pregnancy when the potential benefits outweigh the possible risks. In animal studies, both the prodrug and active drug have been found distributed in breast milk. Caution is recommended if used in nursing mothers.

Peramivir

Peramivir is an intravenous neuraminidase inhibitor that is active against influenza A and B. The agent is US FDA-approved for single-dose treatment of **acute, uncomplicated influenza** in adults who have been symptomatic for up to 2 days. The agent has not been proven to be effective for serious influenza requiring hospitalization.

Dosing and Administration
The recommended dose is 600 mg IV as a single-dose treatment.

Key Monitoring and Safety Information
Potential adverse effects include diarrhea, **skin reactions**, behavioral disturbances, neutrophils < 1000/µL, hyperglycemia, CPK elevation, and elevation of hepatic transaminases.

Zanamivir

Zanamivir is an **inhalational** neuraminidase inhibitor active against both influenza A and B virus.

Dosing and Administration
Zanamivir is given via two inhalations of dry powder (5 mg/inhalation for a total of 10 mg) q12h for the treatment of influenza A and B infection. A Rotadisk is loaded into the supplied plastic breath-activated Diskhaler inhalation device. One blister is pierced,

and zanamivir is dispersed into the airstream created by inhalation of the patient. Each Rotadisk contains four blister packets of 5 mg and supplies enough medication for 1 day. Optimal response to therapy is seen when zanamivir is initiated within 2 days of symptom onset. No dosage adjustments are required in renal failure or dialysis.

Key Monitoring and Safety Information

In patients with underlying airway disease, **bronchospasm and allergic-like reactions** have been reported. As a result, caution should be used when zanamivir is used in patients with underlying airway diseases, such as asthma and chronic obstructive pulmonary disease. Patients with airway diseases should be instructed to have a fast-acting bronchodilator available when inhaling zanamivir and to discontinue use and contact their physician if they experience worsening respiratory symptoms.

REFERENCE

1. Bailey TC, Little JR, Littenberg B, et al. A meta-analysis of extended-interval dosing versus multiple daily dosing of aminoglycosides. *Clin Infect Dis.* 1997;24(5):786-795.

Antimicrobial Stewardship

21

Kevin Hsueh and Michael J. Durkin

INTRODUCTION

Antimicrobials have radically changed the landscape of human disease. Previously lethal bacterial infections are now often curable. However, antibiotics have also become some of the most frequently misused drugs in modern medicine. Studies suggest that up to 50% of antimicrobial use is inappropriate.[1,2] This misuse is not without consequence.[3] Carbapenem-resistant enterobacteriaceae, antibiotic-resistant gonorrhea, and the spread of epidemic *Clostridium difficile* infection are all in part manifestations of antibiotic overuse.[4] A major strategic response to these threats has been the development of antimicrobial stewardship: the organized effort to reduce the adverse impact of antimicrobial use by optimizing appropriate antibiotic use. This chapter outlines core principles and activities of antimicrobial stewardship.

GENERAL PRINCIPLES

- **Appropriate antimicrobial therapy**: The "5 D's" of appropriate antibiotic utilization is a common strategy for measuring appropriateness of therapy[5]:
  - **Appropriate diagnosis**: Antimicrobials are frequently inappropriately utilized for noninfectious or viral conditions. It is essential for clinicians to identify the **correct diagnosis** and determine if antibiotics will provide a benefit to the patient.
  - **Appropriate drug**: All antimicrobials have a limited number of organisms they are effective against, known as their spectrum of activity. They also often have limitations to their activity, absorption, distribution, clearance, adverse reactions, and pharmacologic parameters, making them more or less suitable for certain infections and patients. Appropriate drug selection attempts to maintain vigorous **clinical efficacy** against the indicated infection, while minimizing the risk of collateral damage. This often means selecting antimicrobials with the **narrowest spectrum** of activity needed to target the organism(s) of concern.
  - **Appropriate dose**: Antimicrobials typically have recommended doses that correspond with the minimum tissue drug concentrations needed to address each infective indication. Appropriate selection of dose and frequency maximize clinical utility while minimizing adverse drug events.
  - **Appropriate duration**: The appropriate duration of antimicrobial therapy for each indication is the minimum effective duration needed for consistent cure or control of an infection. Modern studies have shown that **shorter durations** are often as effective as traditional longer courses. For example, research has consistently demonstrated that courses as short as 5 days are noninferior to longer regimens in the treatment of pneumonia.[6]
  - **Appropriate de-escalation**: Initial antimicrobial regimens are generally empiric and include broad-spectrum antibiotics. However, as the patient clinically improves and/or confirmatory diagnostic data are obtained, **antibiotic regimens can often be de-escalated** to a more targeted, narrow-spectrum antibiotic.[7]

- **Antimicrobial Stewardship Program** (ASP): An ASP is a formal body charged with improving antimicrobial use. Currently, most US hospitals have an ASP due to regulatory requirements. Most established ASPs share joint leadership between a physician and a pharmacist. ASP programs in acute care hospitals should be integrated into hospital operations.[9] The Centers for Disease Control and Prevention (CDC) has defined seven core elements that stewardship programs need to have in order to be effective[8]:
- **CDC core elements of hospital ASPs**
  - ○ **Leadership commitment**: Dedicated human, financial, and information technology resources are necessary for the success of an ASP.
  - ○ **Accountability**: A single appointed leader should be responsible for program outcomes.
  - ○ **Drug expertise**: Formal training in either infectious diseases and/or antimicrobial stewardship is necessary.
  - ○ **Action**: Implementing interventions to improve antimicrobial use should be a priority of the ASP.
  - ○ **Tracking**: Antimicrobial use and outcomes should be monitored by the ASP.
  - ○ **Reporting**: Antibiotic use metrics should be shared with appropriate staff and providers.
  - ○ **Education**: Clinical staff education about appropriate antimicrobial use and antimicrobial resistance is paramount.

COMMON STEWARDSHIP STRATEGIES

- Efforts to improve antimicrobial use can generally be broken into two broad categories. **Decision support**, or efforts to transparently guide care providers toward ordering antibiotics in an appropriate fashion, and **direct intervention**, where the stewardship program clearly intervenes on specific cases of antimicrobial use. Frequent fields involved in stewardship interventions include infectious diseases, medical informatics, hospital epidemiology, pharmacy, microbiology, nursing, and medical education.[10]
- **Decision support** are interventions that aim to encourage appropriate antimicrobial use by providers without clear case-by-case intervention by a stewardship program. Commonly used decision support tools include:
  - ○ **Institutional guidelines**: Guidelines on antimicrobial use can take the form of infection-specific guidelines, such as guidance on antimicrobial selection, dosing, and duration for common conditions (e.g., community-acquired pneumonia, neutropenic fever).
  - ○ **Antibiograms**: Stewardship programs play a critical role in publicizing, developing, and interpreting antibiograms, which display historical local bacterial resistance patterns for common pathogens.
  - ○ **Selective reporting of resistance profiles**: The manner in which bacterial sensitivity results are reported can significantly influence provider ordering decisions. An overly broad array of options can cause decision paralysis, whereas inclusion of suboptimal options can increase the likelihood of their selection. Selective reporting (sometimes called cascade reporting) minimizes reported agents to a subset of narrow-spectrum agents).[11]
  - ○ **Computerized decision support**: It is a large subset of decision support, generally including a range of interventions meant to guide providers into writing appropriate antimicrobial orders while dissuading them from inappropriate usage.
    - ▪ **Order sets**: Predefined bundles of orders, often for a specific indication (e.g., pneumonia), act as in situ guidelines for the provider, defining appropriate antimicrobial regimens. They often incorporate default values for dosing and duration, improving adherence to clinical practice guidelines.

- **Condition-specific alerts**: Computer interventions that use contextual information about the patient trigger alerts or recommended actions. The most basic type of these alerts is the drug-interaction warning that is a feature of almost all modern computerized order entry systems.
  - **Rapid diagnostic tests**: Timely and/or point-of-care diagnostics allow clinicians to tailor antimicrobial therapy sooner. For example, procalcitonin results can help providers narrow antibiotics by differentiating between bacterial and viral conditions.
- **Direct intervention**: Most classic stewardship interventions directly target specific antibiotic orders and may include:
  - **Up-front restriction/preauthorization**: This intervention requires providers to consult (or obtain approval from) a separate service in order for the patient to receive a specific antimicrobial. Usually, the consulted service is either an infectious diseases physician or pharmacist. The authorizing service is charged with quickly assessing whether the requested agent is appropriate for the intended therapy and recommending alternatives when available.
  - **Prospective audit and feedback** (PAF): PAF involves the stewardship team reviewing antibiotic orders within a set period of time after the order is placed, often between 24 to 72 hours afterward. PAF is considered one of the core stewardship interventions along with up-front restriction, and can either complement it or be used alone.[12]
  - **Antimicrobial time-out**: This intervention is a forced, periodic re-evaluation for the ordering provider of the need for antimicrobial therapy. Electronic means for enforcing this type of re-evaluation include pop-up alerts that occur after a standard period of time and preset limits to antimicrobial durations.
  - **Inappropriate use alerts**: Inappropriate use alerts are computerized flags that trigger when a specific combination of elements occur in a patient's electronic medical record. Common alerts include those for duplicative anaerobic or beta-lactam coverage, and screening for anti–methicillin-resistant *Staphylococcus aureus* agents in patients with only methicillin-sensitive *S. aureus* culture isolates.

STEWARDSHIP TRACKING METRICS

- One of the main duties of a stewardship program is the tracking of antimicrobial usage patterns and associated outcomes. Antimicrobial-associated metrics commonly tracked by an ASP fall into three broad categories[13]:
- **Antimicrobial utilization**: Antimicrobial utilization is a measurement of the quantity of antimicrobial use within a specified context. There are multiple different ways to measure antimicrobial use:
  - **Days of therapy** (DOT): This metric estimates cumulative antibiotic exposure by calculating the number of days a patient has received any specific antibiotic. It is often paired with the denominator of patient days (number of days a patient is in a particular location).
  - **Defined daily dose** (DDD): This metric estimates antibiotic use based on cumulative physical quantity of drug being used divided by a standardized estimate of "normal" daily individual antibiotic use as defined by the World Health Organization to create an estimate of the number of ideal patients treated per day.
- **Stewardship process metrics**: In evaluating the efficacy of a stewardship intervention, an ASP should rely on antimicrobial utilization metrics alone.
  - **Intervention rate**: The most basic process metric to track for any intervention is the intervention rate. This is mostly applicable to direct interventions by the ASP.
  - **Intervention characteristics**: For many interventions, additional granular information about the individual instances are needed to fully make use of the data. Additional useful characteristics include antibiotic and infection targeted, the recommended course of action, and the success/acceptance rate.

- **Outcomes metrics:** Outcomes metrics are data points that attempt to measure the secondary impacts of stewardship interventions on the medical system. Common outcomes metrics used by ASPs include:
  - **Antimicrobial appropriateness:** Usually measured as a percentage of antimicrobial starts which are appropriate (or conversely, inappropriate) and can be global or specific to indications or drugs.
  - **Costs:** Impact of antimicrobial stewardship efforts on medical expenditure is one of the most common outcomes monitored by stewardship programs.
  - **Microbiology:** *C. difficile* infection (CDI) rates are tightly linked to antimicrobial utilization, and an effective ASP may see a reduction in CDI rates in the hospital.
  - **Patient-level outcomes:** Length of stay, readmission rate, and mortality rate are routinely monitored by most hospitals and thus often available for use by ASPs.

STEWARDSHIP REPORTING AND EDUCATION

- Stewardship reporting to stakeholders is a crucial responsibility of an ASP.
- **Government reporting:** The CDC has recently implemented a voluntary national reporting and tracking system for hospitals nationwide called the Antimicrobial Use and Resistance Module (AUR Module). It allows for broad reporting on antimicrobial usage patterns within acute care hospitals, as well as antimicrobial resistance reporting from hospital microbiology laboratories. The AUR Module includes a benchmarking tool called the **standardized antimicrobial administration ratio** (SAAR), which is one of the first efforts to compare antimicrobial usage patterns.
- **Leadership reporting:** ASPs are required to report their progress to hospital leadership. This generally involves periodic updates within hospital committees.
- **Individual reporting:** ASP will often provide feedback to hospital-specific providers, provider groups, or wards. One of the most common methods of reporting is called benchmarking where providers or units are compared to peers. Benchmarking has also been successfully used in outpatient settings to improve antibiotic prescribing.[14]

REFERENCES

1. Scheckler WE, Bennett JV. Antibiotic usage in seven community hospitals. *JAMA.* 1970;213:264-267.
2. Braykov NP, Morgan DJ, Schweizer ML, et al. Assessment of empirical antibiotic therapy optimisation in six hospitals: an observational cohort study. *Lancet Infect Dis.* 2014;14:1220-1227.
3. Penicillin's finder assays its future: Sir Alexander Fleming says improved dosage method is needed to extend use other scientists praised self-medication decried. *The New York Times* [Internet]. June 26, 1945 [cited 2018 May 30]. Available at https://www.nytimes.com/1945/06/26/archives/penicillins-finder-assays-its-future-sir-alexander-fleming-says.html (last accessed 7/5/18).
4. Centers for Disease Control and Prevention (CDC). *Antibiotic Resistance Threats in the United States, 2013* [Internet]. Atlanta: CDC; 2013. Available at http://www.cdc.gov/drugresistance/threat-report-2013/pdf/ar-threats-2013-508.pdf (last accessed 7/5/18).
5. Doron S, Davidson LE. Antimicrobial Stewardship. *Mayo Clin Proc* 2011;86:1113-1123.
6. Uranga A, España PP, Bilbao A, et al. Duration of antibiotic treatment in community-acquired pneumonia: a multicenter randomized clinical trial. *JAMA Intern Med.* 2016;176:1257-1265.
7. Stevens DL, Bisno AL, Chambers HF, et al. Practice guidelines for the diagnosis and management of skin and soft tissue infections: 2014 update by the Infectious Diseases Society of America. *Clin Infect Dis.* 2014;59:e10-e52.
8. Pollack LA, Srinivasan A. Core elements of hospital antibiotic stewardship programs from the Centers for Disease Control and Prevention. *Clin Infect Dis.* 2014;59:S97-S100.
9. Dellit TH, Owens RC, McGowan JE, et al. Infectious Diseases Society of America and the Society for Healthcare Epidemiology of America guidelines for developing an institutional program to enhance antimicrobial stewardship. *Clin Infect Dis.* 2007;44:159-177.
10. Barlam TF, Cosgrove SE, Abbo LM, et al. Implementing an antibiotic stewardship program: guidelines by the Infectious Diseases Society of America and the Society for Healthcare Epidemiology of America. *Clin Infect Dis.* 2016;62:e51-e77.

11. McNulty CAM, Lasseter GM, Charlett A, et al. Does laboratory antibiotic susceptibility reporting influence primary care prescribing in urinary tract infection and other infections? *J Antimicrob Chemother*. 2011;66:1396-1404.

12. Doernberg SB, Abbo LM, Burdette SD, et al. Essential resources and strategies for antibiotic stewardship programs in the acute care setting. *Clin Infect Dis*. 2018;67(8):1168-1174. [Epub ahead of print].

13. Spivak ES, Cosgrove SE, Srinivasan A. Measuring appropriate antimicrobial use: attempts at opening the black box. *Clin Infect Dis*. 2016;63:1639-1644.

14. Linder JA, Meeker D, Fox CR, et al. Effects of behavioral interventions on inappropriate antibiotic prescribing in primary care 12 months after stopping interventions. *JAMA*. 2017;318:1391-1392.

What was Old is New Again: Arboviruses and Hemorrhagic Fevers

22

Michael Tang and Steven J. Lawrence

Arboviruses

GENERAL PRINCIPLES

- Arboviruses are arthropod-borne viruses.
- Major vectors are mosquitoes and ticks.
  - *Aedes aegypti* and *A. albopictus* are the most important mosquito vectors.
    - They are aggressive daytime biters
    - They prefer urban settings
    - They are rare in the United States except for Florida, the Gulf Coast, and the Southwest
  - Vector control is important for disease control.
- Endemicity is defined by geographic range of vectors.
- Explosive epidemics occur when first introduced into a region.
- Centers for Disease Control and Prevention (CDC) is an excellent source for updated transmission risk areas.

DIAGNOSIS

Clinical Presentation

- Fever, rash, and joint/muscle pains are common.
- Arbovirus infections should be considered in recently returned travelers from endemic areas.

Diagnostic Testing

- Confirmation of specific diagnosis is difficult.
- Local public health departments may help with testing.
- Polymerase chain reaction (PCR) is available for some arboviral infections to confirm current infection.
- Most rely on convalescent serology to confirm recent infection. Cross-reactivity between flaviviruses is common, making serologic diagnosis more challenging.

TREATMENT

Treatment is primarily supportive as there are no licensed antiviral drugs available for arbovirus infections.

PREVENTION

Mosquito avoidance while in endemic areas is key to prevention.

- Apply at least 20% DEET on exposed skin
- Apply permethrin to clothing
- Use mosquito bed nets at nighttime
- Decrease breeding by draining standing water sources

Dengue Virus

GENERAL PRINCIPLES

Epidemiology

- An estimated 390 million infections per year occur worldwide, although the true burden of disease is unknown.
- It is endemic in more than 100 countries in Asia, the Pacific, the Americas, Africa, and the Caribbean.
- An estimated 500,000 cases of Dengue hemorrhagic fever (DHF) occur per year, with 22,000 deaths primarily in children.[1]

Pathophysiology

- RNA virus, in the Flaviviridae family. There are four serotypes; infection with one serotype does not protect against others.
- *Aedes* mosquitoes are primary vectors.
- Rare cases of transmission occur through organ transplant, blood transfusion, and maternal–fetal vertical transmission.
- DHF or dengue shock syndrome (DSS) are seen in secondary infections by a different serotype. Mechanism is related to antibody-dependent enhancement of virus infection in Fc receptor-bearing cells and subsequent increased capillary permeability.[2]

Risk Factors

- Travel to areas endemic for dengue.
- Young age, female, high BMI, MHC Class 1 genetic variant and secondary infection by different serotypes are risk factors for severe dengue.

DIAGNOSIS

Clinical Presentation

- Nonspecific symptoms (fever, headache, myalgias, maculopapular or petechial rash) occur after a 3 to 7 day incubation period and last 3 to 7 days. Prominent arthralgias ("breakbone fever") are common.
- DHF/DSS occurs after defervescence in ~0.4% of cases. Presents with volume overload, liver failure, mucosal hemorrhage, myocarditis, ARDS, and encephalopathy.
- Case fatality rate is >20% if untreated, but ~2.5% when treated with supportive measures.[2]
- Laboratory findings
  - ○ Mild to moderate thrombocytopenia and leukopenia with moderate elevation of aminotransferases (AST/ALT) may be seen in the initial febrile phase.
  - ○ Common findings of severe disease include increasing hematocrit, hypoalbuminemia, severe thrombocytopenia, elevated aPTT, and low fibrinogen.

Differential Diagnosis

Other arbovirus infections, measles, rubella, enterovirus, adenovirus, influenza, typhoid, malaria, leptospirosis, viral hepatitis, rickettsial disease.

Diagnostic Criteria

World Health Organization 2009 Classification[3]:

- Travel/exposure to endemic areas with fever and ≥2 of the following:
  - ○ Nausea and vomiting
  - ○ Rash

- ○ Leukopenia
- ○ Headache, eye pain, muscle ache, or joint pain
- ○ Positive tourniquet sign
- Dengue with warning signs – The above criteria plus any of the following:
  - ○ Severe abdominal pain
  - ○ Persistent vomiting
  - ○ Clinical fluid accumulation (ascites/pleural effusion)
  - ○ Mucosal bleeding
  - ○ Liver enlargement (>2 cm)
  - ○ Lethargy
  - ○ Increase in hematocrit with decrease in platelet count
- Severe Dengue – dengue with at least one of the following:
  - ○ Plasma leakage leading to shock or fluid accumulation with respiratory distress
  - ○ Severe bleeding
  - ○ Severe organ involvement including AST/ALT>1000, impaired consciousness, or organ failure

Diagnostic Testing
- PCR for active infection.
- Acute and convalescent serology for recent infection.
- May require consultation with state or local health department.

TREATMENT[2]

- Supportive treatment is key, with appropriate triaging of patients based on severity of disease.
  - ○ Avoid nonsteroidal anti-inflammatory drugs (NSAIDs) or aspirin. Use acetaminophen to control fevers.
  - ○ Ensure adequate hydration.
  - ○ No indication for steroids or platelet transfusion.
- Patients at high risk of complications (pregnancy, infancy, diabetes, poor social situation, advanced age, renal failure) may require inpatient management.
- Severe dengue requires ICU management.
  - ○ Close monitoring of vital signs, oxygen saturation, and renal and hepatic function.
  - ○ Aggressive IV crystalloid replacement even in absence of hypotension.
  - ○ Hematocrit-driven colloid infusions or packed red blood cell transfusions may be necessary.

PREVENTION

- Mosquito avoidance measures (See Arboviruses – General Principles).
- A dengue vaccine is available in some countries but not licensed in the United States.

Zika Virus

GENERAL PRINCIPLES
Epidemiology
- It was a rare cause of sporadic disease before 2007.
- It is endemic to many African and Southeast Asian countries.
- Since 2007, there have been several large outbreaks on the Pacific Islands and Central/South America with a large proportion of the population impacted (>1 million people affected in Brazil).[4]

Pathophysiology
- RNA virus, in the Flaviviridae family.
- *Aedes* mosquitoes are the primary vector.
- Nonmosquito transmission
  - Vertical transmission from a pregnant woman to her fetus
  - Sexual transmission – viral RNA can be found in sperm of some men for many months after convalescence[5]
  - Blood transfusions, particularly in endemic or epidemic areas
- Congenital Zika Syndrome results from transplacental infection of fetal progenitor neuronal stem cells.

Risk Factors for Congenital Zika Syndrome
- Infection during first trimester of pregnancy imparts highest risk but can occur from infections later in pregnancy.[5]

DIAGNOSIS

Clinical Presentation
- Most infections are asymptomatic.
- Incubation period is 3 to 14 days. Common symptoms are fever, maculopapular rash, conjunctivitis, arthralgias (particularly of small joints) and headache. Symptoms may last from days to weeks.
- Guillain–Barre syndrome is a rare complication.[6]
- Congenital Zika infection[5]:
  - Results from fetal infection in utero.
  - Spectrum of disease ranges from severe microcephaly with partially collapsed skull and severe developmental delays to vision/hearing deficiencies and limb deformities

Diagnostic Testing
- Testing is recommended for patients with compatible symptoms who may have been exposed to Zika recently by travel or sexual contact.
- Testing recommendations, particularly for pregnant women, may change with improved understanding of congenital Zika syndrome, changing incidence of Zika, and new diagnostic testing options. Refer to the CDC website for the most up-to-date recommendations.
- PCR for active infection.
- Acute and convalescent serology for recent infection.
- May require consultation with state or local health department.

TREATMENT

- No specific antiviral treatment is available for Zika virus disease.
- Rest, fluids, analgesics, and antipyretics as needed.
- Avoid NSAIDS or aspirin until dengue has been ruled out.
- Protect from mosquito exposure during first week of illness to prevent local transmission.

PREVENTION

Mosquito avoidance measures (See Arboviruses – General Principles).

West Nile Virus

GENERAL PRINCIPLES

Epidemiology

- It is widely spread throughout the Americas, the Middle East, Africa, South Asia, and Australia.[7]
- It has been seen throughout the continental United States.
- Incidence varies from year to year.

Pathophysiology

- RNA virus of the Flaviviridae family
- Culex mosquitoes are primary vectors. They are most active at dusk and more common in wooded areas.
- Rare transmission occurs through organ transplantation.
- Transmission by blood transfusions has been largely eliminated by universal screening.
- Neuroinvasive disease occurs in an estimated 1/150 cases.[8] Unclear mechanism of entry for neuroinvasive disease.

Risk Factors

Risk factors for neuroinvasive disease: Age over 60 years, malignancy, diabetes, hypertension, chronic kidney disease, and posttransplant are risk factors for serious neurologic illness.

DIAGNOSIS

Clinical Presentation

- Most infections are asymptomatic.
- Incubation is 2 to 14 days, can be longer in immunocompromised patients.
- 20% develop fever, headache, body aches, joint pains with or without rash. May have prolonged course of fatigue and weakness.
- Severe illness occurs in less than 1% of patients.
  - Meningitis – headache, nuchal rigidity
  - Encephalitis – confusion, tremors, seizures, obtundation
  - Paralysis – asymmetric flaccid weakness similar to poliomyelitis
  - Cerebrospinal fluid (CSF) findings – lymphocytic pleocytosis
  - Brain MRI findings – normal or variable abnormalities in basal ganglia, thalamus, brain stem, or anterior spinal cord
  - Case fatality rate ~10% (higher for encephalitis)
  - Long-term sequelae are common in survivors.

Diagnostic Testing

- West Nile virus–specific IgM antibody in serum or CSF
  - Typically detectable 3 to 8 days after illness onset and persist up to 90 days.[8]
  - False positives with recent St Louis encephalitis or dengue infection, or recent receipt of yellow fever vaccine.
- PCR tests on CSF, blood, and tissue can be used in early disease through state public health laboratories or the CDC but have limited sensitivity.[7]

TREATMENT

- There are no specific antivirals. No clear benefit of interferon, IVIG, or corticosteroids.
- Supportive care
  - Hydration and pain control
  - In patients with encephalitis, monitoring for increased intracranial pressure and seizures.
  - Patients with encephalitis and poliomyelitis should be monitored for airway protection and neuromuscular respiratory failure.

PREVENTION

Mosquito avoidance measures (See Arboviruses – General Principles).

Chikungunya

GENERAL PRINCIPLES

Epidemiology

- It is endemic with frequent epidemics in South and Southeast Asia, Africa, and certain southern European countries.
- It was introduced into the Americas in 2014 with explosive epidemics in many Central and South American countries.

Pathophysiology

- RNA Alphavirus belonging to the Togaviridae family.
- *Aedes* mosquitoes are primary vectors
- Nonmosquito transmission is rare. Rare vertical transmission largely limited to women who are viremic at the time of delivery, but no evidence of transmission from breast milk.

Risk Factors

- Those at increased risk for severe disease include neonates exposed intrapartum, older adults, and persons with hypertension, diabetes, and cardiovascular disease.
- Deaths are rare and are generally only seen with older adults.

DIAGNOSIS

Clinical Presentation[9]

- Incubation is 3 to 7 days. A minority of infections are asymptomatic.
- Fever, maculopapular rash, severe symmetric polyarthralgias of distal joints, headache, fatigue, and lymphadenopathy are common and last ~1 week.
- Laboratory findings – Leukopenia, thrombocytopenia, hypocalcemia, mild transaminitis.
- Prolonged RA-like polyarticular distal small joint arthritis.[10]
  - Occurs in ~25% of cases
  - Steroid nonresponsive
  - May have association with HLA B27
- Rare complications include myocarditis, meningoencephalitis, hemorrhage, Guillain–Barre syndrome, acute flaccid paralysis, uveitis, and retinitis.
- Neonatal infection: Neurologic disease, hemorrhage, myocardial disease.

Diagnostic Testing

- PCR can be used in the first week of disease to confirm acute infection.
- Acute and convalescent serology for recent infection.
- May require consultation with state or local health department.

TREATMENT

- Supportive treatment with rest, fluids, and NSAIDs.
- Protect from mosquito exposure during first week of illness to prevent local transmission.

PREVENTION

Mosquito avoidance measures (See Arboviruses – General Principles).

Yellow Fever

GENERAL PRINCIPLES

Epidemiology[11]

Endemic with occasional large epidemics in several countries in Africa and South America, with 20 to 30x greater risk in African countries.

Pathophysiology

- RNA virus of the Flaviviridae family.
- *Aedes* and Haemagogus mosquitoes are primary vectors.

Risk Factors

- Suspected increased susceptibility in Caucasian patients.[11]
- Immunocompromised patients at higher risk of severe disease.

DIAGNOSIS

Clinical Presentation

- Incubation period is 3 to 6 days.
- Majority of yellow fever virus infections are asymptomatic or only a mild illness.
- Sudden onset of high fever, headache, chills, back pain, body aches, nausea, vomiting fatigue, and weakness for ~3 days occurs.
- Bradycardia in relation to elevated body temperature (Faget sign) is a characteristic finding.
- Elevated PT and PTT, thrombocytopenia, and hyperbilirubinemia may also occur. Elevated transaminases may last for months.
- 15% of patients develop severe disease.
  - Nausea, vomiting, epigastric pain, jaundice, encephalopathy, and shock.
  - Hemorrhagic manifestations are possible (e.g., hematemesis, melena, hematuria, ecchymoses, epistaxis).
  - 20% to 50% case fatality rate for patients with severe disease.

Diagnostic Testing[12]

- PCR can be used in the first few days of illness to confirm acute infection.
- Acute and convalescent serology for recent infection. False positives from prior vaccination or other flavivirus infections.
- May require consultation with state or local health department.

TREATMENT

- No specific antiviral treatment.
- Supportive treatment with fluids, rest, and antipyretics. Avoid NSAIDS which may increase the risk of bleeding.
- Protect from mosquito exposure during first 5 days of illness to prevent local transmission.

PREVENTION[12]

- Live-attenuated virus vaccine
  - Recommended for people age >9 months who are traveling or living in areas at risk for transmission in South America and Africa.
  - Vaccine may be required for entry into certain countries.
  - Protection is lifelong in most patients though some may require boosters.
  - Contraindicated in immunocompromised patients.
  - Rare adverse events include yellow fever vaccine–associated viscerotropic disease (1/250,000) and yellow fever vaccine–associated neurologic disease (1/125,000).
- Mosquito avoidance measures (See Arboviruses – General Principles).

Hemorrhagic Fever Viruses

Ebola Virus

GENERAL PRINCIPLES

Epidemiology

- Discovered in 1976 in the Democratic Republic of Congo.
- Sporadic outbreaks occurred in Central Africa involving <500 cases.
- From 2014 to 2016 West Africa epidemic had >28,000 cases and >11,000 deaths.[13]
- Rare cases in the United States have been isolated to recent travelers and health care workers from epidemic areas and health care workers who were involved in the care of infected patients.

Pathophysiology

- RNA virus in the Filovirus family.
- Marburg virus is a closely related filovirus causing a disease similar to Ebola virus disease (EVD).
- Transmission
  - Direct contact with blood or body fluids from infected animal or human.
  - Epidemic index cases often associated with bush meat.
  - Patients are not infectious before symptom onset.
  - Sexual transmission possible – virus particles can persist in semen >12 months after symptom onset.[14]
- Virus can persist in other immune-privileged sites, including the eye and CNS. Associated with rare relapse of symptomatic illness in these sites months after convalescence.

Risk Factors

Any exposure to blood or body fluids of patients or animals infected with Ebola virus.

- Health care providers
- Close family contacts
- Persons involved with traditional burial rituals[15]

DIAGNOSIS

Clinical Presentation[16]

- Incubation period is 2 to 21 days
- EVD
  - Initial – nonspecific fever, headache, rash, abdominal pain, myalgias
  - GI phase is common – severe vomiting, large volume diarrhea, dehydration
  - Hemorrhagic fever – 18% with bleeding or bruising
  - Occasional neurologic disease – encephalopathy, seizures
  - Laboratory findings – leukopenia, thrombocytopenia, transaminitis, anemia, DIC, renal failure, and electrolyte abnormalities
  - Case fatality rate varies from 20% in advanced health care settings to >70% in minimal care settings.

Diagnostic Testing

- PCR has high sensitivity for active infection and is predictive of infectiousness.
- Consultation with local or state public health department is necessary if EVD is suspected.

TREATMENT

- Supportive care with attention to aggressive hydration, electrolyte repletion, and symptomatic treatment has been shown to significantly improve survival.
- Several investigational antiviral agents have been tested, but none are licensed.

PREVENTION

- Community engagement is key to successfully controlling outbreaks, including case management, infection prevention and control practices, surveillance and contact tracing. Appropriate use of high-level personal protective equipment is critical for the safe provision of care to EVD patients.
- Male survivors should use condoms until they have two separate semen tests negative by PCR at least 1 week apart.
- A vaccine, rVSV-ZBOV, was shown to be effective in preventing infection via ring vaccination trial during an outbreak in Guinea and Sierra Leone.[17]

REFERENCES

1. Dengue. https://www.cdc.gov/dengue/index.html. Accessed 10/12/2017.
2. Simmons CP, Farrar JJ, Nguyen vV, Wills B. Dengue. *N Engl J Med.* 2012;366(15):1423-1432. doi:10.1056/NEJMra1110265.
3. World Health Organization. *Dengue: Guidelines for Diagnosis, Treatment, Prevention and Control*; 2009. Available athttp://www.who.int/tdr/publications/documents/dengue-diagnosis.pdf (last accessed 6/15/18).
4. Zika virus spreads to new areas – region of the Americas, May 2015–January 2016. *MMWR Morb Mortal Wkly Rep.* 2016;65:55-58.
5. Petersen LR, Jamieson DJ, Powers AM, Honein MA. Zika virus. *N Engl J Med.* 2016;374(16):1552-1563. doi:10.1056/NEJMra1602113.
6. Cao-Lormeau VM, Blake A, Mons S, et al. Guillain-Barré syndrome outbreak associated with Zika virus infection in French Polynesia: a case-control study. *Lancet.* 2016;387(10027):1531. [Epub 2016 March 2].
7. West Nile Virus: Information for Health Care Providers. https://www.cdc.gov/westnile/healthcare-providers/index.html. Accessed 10/12/2017.
8. Peterson LR, Brault AC, Nasci RS. West Nile virus: review of the literature. *JAMA.* 2013;310(3):308-315. doi:10.1001/jama.2013.8042.

9. Staples J, Breiman RF, Powers AM. Chikungunya fever: an epidemiological review of an re-emerging infectious disease. *Clin Infect Dis.* 2009;49(6):942-948.

10. Rodríguez-Morales AJ, Cardona-Ospina JA, Fernanda Urbano-Garzón S, Sebastian Hurtado-Zapata J. Prevalence of post-chikungunya infection chronic inflammatory arthritis: a systematic review and meta-analysis. *Arthritis Care Res (Hoboken).* 2016;68(12):1849.

11. Monath TP, Vasconcelos PF. Yellow fever. *J Clin Virol.* 2015;64.

12. Yellow Fever. https://www.cdc.gov/yellowfever/index.html. Accessed 10/12/2017.

13. CDC: Ebola. https://www.cdc.gov/vhf/ebola/index.html. Accessed 10/12/2017.

14. Diallo B, Sissoko D, Loman NJ, et al. Resurgence of Ebola virus disease in Guinea linked to a survivor with virus persistence in seminal fluid for more than 500 days. *Clin Infect Dis.* 2016;63(10):1353. [Epub 2016 September 1].

15. Ebola transmission linked to a single traditional funeral ceremony – Kissidougou, Guinea, December, 2014–January 2015. *Morb Mortal Wkly Rep.* 2014;64:386-388.

16. CDC – Ebola Virus Disease (EVD) Information for Clinicians in U.S. Healthcare Settings. https://www.cdc.gov/vhf/ebola/healthcare-us/preparing/clinicians.html. Accessed 12/1/2017.

17. Henao-Restrepo AM, Longini IM, Egger M et al. Efficacy and effectiveness of an rVSV-vectored vaccine in preventing Ebola virus disease: final results from the Guinea ring vaccination, open-label, cluster-randomised trial. *Lancet.* 2017;389(10068):505-518.

Index

Note: Page numbers followed by "f" indicate figures and "t" indicate tables.